Praise for this book

"This excellent text really is a must for anyone involved in health research. It is truly multidisciplinary in its scope, drawing on a breadth of relevant research from health economics, to epidemiology to psychology which is beyond the scope of most books on research methods. Yet in spite of the wealth of material included it is written and presented in an accessible way so that it will be an invaluable source for those with a background in either qualitative or quantitative research and from students to experienced researchers."

Robert J. Edelmann, Professor of Forensic and Clinical psychology, Roehampton University, UK

"Health service researchers - new and old - will be delighted by this new edition of a popular and useful text. There is new content but also updated material making this practically useful as a resource at any stage of the research trajectory. While health is the focus the book is hugely valuable to researchers in cognate areas, such as social care, education and housing. The book meets its own high standards in being easy to follow, well indexed and containing interesting examples of approaches. The limitations of different methods are also honestly reported. A 'must have' for the book shelf."

Jill Manthorpe, Professor of Social Work, King's College London, UK

"When first published in 1997, this volume was the first systematic overview of research methods used in the health field. In its updated 4th Edition it remains vital and, if anything, more important given the growing number of researchers and students investigating health issues and health services. It provides an impressively comprehensive overview of health research methods in which the wealth and variety of experience of the author shines through at every point. Qualitative, quantitative and mixed methods are appraised and explained with unpartisan authority and rigour, and the volume covers everything from multidisciplinary collaboration in health service evaluation through the Delphi technique of consensus development to the health economics needed to evaluate costing."

Paul Stenner, Professor of Social Psychology, The Open University, UK

Research Methods in Health:
Investigating Health and Health Services

FOURTH EDITION

Ann Bowling

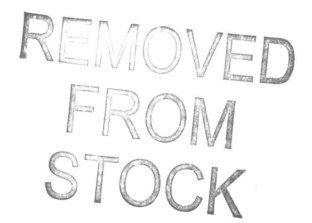

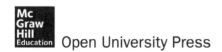
Open University Press

Open University Press
McGraw-Hill Education
McGraw-Hill House
Shoppenhangers Road
Maidenhead
Berkshire
England
SL6 2QL

email: enquiries@openup.co.uk
world wide web: www.openup.co.uk

and Two Penn Plaza, New York, NY 10121-2289, USA

First published 1997
Second edition published 2002
Third edition published 2009
First published in this fourth edition 2014

A catalogue record of this book is available from the British Library

ISBN-13: 978-0-335-26274-8
ISBN-10: 0-335-26274-0
eISBN: 978-0-335-26275-5

Library of Congress Cataloging-in-Publication Data
CIP data applied for

Typeset by Aptara, Inc.

Contents

SECTION II The philosophy, theory and practice of research 129

SECTION III Quantitative research: sampling and research methods 189

SECTION IV The tools of quantitative research   273

Preface to the fourth edition

This book is more than a text on research methods. It is an introduction to the theoretical concepts, as well as the descriptive and analytic research methods, that are used by the main disciplines engaged in research on health and health services. In order to understand why the various research methods are used, it is important to be aware of the conceptual backgrounds and scientific philosophies of those involved in research and evaluation, in particular in demography, epidemiology, health economics, psychology and sociology.

The fourth edition, while essentially similar to the earlier editions, includes updated classic and more recent references, and additional reference to key methodological developments, including realistic evaluation, stepped wedge trials, Zelen's design in trials, critical appraisal and evidence-based health care. The book is aimed at students and researchers of health and health services, health professionals and the policy-makers who have the responsibility for applying research findings, and who need to know how to judge the soundness of that research. The idea for the book, and its structure, are grounded in my career as a researcher on health and health service issues, and the valuable experience this has provided in meeting the challenges of research on people and organisations in real-life settings.

The varying terminology used by members of different disciplines in relation to the same research methods is often confusing. This variation simply reflects the multidisciplinary nature of this whole area, and the specialised languages of each discipline. While no descriptor can be labelled as incorrect, the multitude of them, especially when not clearly defined, can easily lead to confusion. Therefore, I have tried to justify the terminology used where it differs from that in other disciplines. Towards the end of the book I have included a glossary which I hope will prove useful for readers coming across unfamiliar terms. Readers wishing to explore methodological topics in more depth are referred to Bowling and Ebrahim (2005).

Acknowledgements

I would like to thank Professor Ian Rees Jones for his earlier collaboration and advice on the chapters on economics and needs assessment. I am, as ever, grateful to the editorial staff at Open University Press for their positive and enthusiastic support for this undertaking, and to Susan Dunsmore for her helpful and thorough copy editing.

Investigating health services and health: the scope of research

'Would you tell me, please, which way I ought to go from here?', asked Alice.

'That depends a good deal on where you want to get to', said the cat.

Lewis Carroll (1865) *Alice's Adventures in Wonderland*

Introduction

Research is the systematic and rigorous process of enquiry which aims to describe phenomena and to develop and test explanatory concepts and theories. Ultimately it aims to contribute to a scientific body of knowledge. More specifically, in relation to the focus of this book, it aims to improve health, health outcomes and health services.

The book aims to provide an overview of the range of research methods that are used in investigations of health and health services. Ultimately the purpose is to guide the reader in choosing an appropriate research method and design in order to address a particular research question. However, it is not possible to place research methods in a hierarchy of excellence, as different research methods are appropriate for addressing different research questions.

If the research question is descriptive, for example, 'What is the health status of population X?', then a cross-sectional survey of a sample of that population is required to provide population estimates. The survey method will also enable the answers to secondary questions to be estimated for that population (e.g. 'Are men more likely than women to report poor health status?') and certain (non-causal) types of hypotheses to be tested (e.g. 'Men will be X times more likely than women to report good health status'). If the research question is 'Do women have worse health outcomes than men following acute myocardial infarction (AMI)?', then a prospective, longitudinal survey of identified men and women who had suffered an AMI would be undertaken in order to be able to compare their health outcomes over time in the future.

If the research aims to find out information on a topic about which little is known, or is too complex or sensitive for the development of standardised instruments, then qualitative methods (e.g. observational methods, in-depth interviews and/or focus groups) may be more appropriate (e.g. 'Is there quality of life on long-stay psycho-geriatric wards?'; 'Are there dehumanising care practices in long-stay institutions?'; 'How do doctors prioritise their patient caseload?').

And if the research aims to investigate cause-and-effect issues, then an experimental design is, in theory, required (e.g. 'Do women aged 75+ have worse health outcomes than men aged 75+ following thrombolysis therapy for acute myocardial infarction?'; 'Do patients with osteoarthritis of the knee benefit from physiotherapy?'; 'Are specialists' outreach clinics held in general practitioners' surgeries as cost-effective as specialists' out-patient clinics in hospitals?'). While the double-blind, randomised controlled trial (RCT) is the true experimental design, and most appropriate for addressing these types of questions, there are also situations in which this method is unrealistic, impractical or inappropriate and other well-designed analytic (as opposed to descriptive) methods have to be employed instead (see Chapter 10). For some cause-and-effect questions, the RCT may be the most appropriate research design but it would be unethical to randomise people to interventions that are unacceptable, and the issue must therefore be addressed using other methods, such as a prospective, longitudinal survey of a population (e.g. 'Does drinking spirits increase the risk of heart disease?').

Finally, research methods should not be seen in isolation from each other. A triangulated or combined methodological approach to addressing different facets of a research issue, using different methods which complement each other, is increasingly recommended as a means of establishing the external validity of the research. In the same way in which prospective, longitudinal surveys can inform the results from RCTs, so qualitative research findings can enhance quantitative survey data by placing the latter into real social contexts and enhancing understanding of relevant social processes.

The importance of using triangulated research methods is enhanced by the multifaceted nature of health, and the multidisciplinary character of research on health and health services. This includes investigations by anthropologists, demographers, epidemiologists, health economists, health geographers, health policy analysts, health psychologists, historians, medical sociologists, statisticians and health professionals (clinicians, nurses, physiotherapists, and so on). Specialists in public health medicine play a key role in health services research, as they are equipped with a range of research skills, including epidemiology. In Britain and in some other countries, they also have responsibility for assessing needs for health services in specific geographical areas, and advising purchasers on effective health care. There is a close working relationship between researchers investigating health and health services and health professionals, particularly in relation to the development of measures of clinical outcomes and the appropriateness of health care interventions.

One consequence of this multidisciplinary activity is that a wide range of qualitative and quantitative, descriptive and analytical research methods is available. This diversity should enrich the approach to research design, although there has been a tendency in research on health services to focus mainly on the experimental method. All methods have their problems and limitations, and the over-reliance on any one method, at the expense of using multiple research methods, to investigate the phenomenon of interest can lead to 'a very limited tool box' (Pope and Mays 1993), sometimes with questionable validity (Webb *et al.* 1966), and consequently to a limited understanding of the phenomena of interest.

It is necessary at this point to distinguish between the terms *health research* and *health services research*.

Health research

Health research has been defined in relation to health generally. As well as having an emphasis on health services, it has an important role in informing the planning and operation of services aiming to achieve health (Hunter and Long 1993). As Davies (1991) observes:

> ❝the process [of] obtaining systematic knowledge and technology . . . can be used for the improvement of the health of individual groups. It provides the basic information on the state of health and disease of the population; it aims to develop tools to prevent and cure illness and mitigate its effects, and it attempts to devise better approaches to health care for the individual and the community. ❞

The broader aspects of health research are described in Chapters 2, 3 and 4 (e.g. in relation to health needs and sociological and psychological aspects of health).

Health systems and health services research

There is no accepted definition of a health system, and it has been variously defined in terms of the structures used to deliver health care, the geographical boundaries of the latter, or the strategies used to attain population health (Nolte *et al.* 2005). Health systems research has thus been defined fairly broadly as: 'ultimately concerned with improving the health of a community, by enhancing the efficiency and effectiveness of the health system as an integrated part of the overall process of socio-economic development' (Varkevisser *et al.* 1991).

In Britain and the USA the general focus is on health services research, rather than on health systems research. Health services research is defined more narrowly in relation to the relationship between health service delivery and the health needs of the population: for example, as 'the identification of the health care needs of communities and the study of the provision, effectiveness and use of health services' (Medical Research Council, see Clarke and Kurinczuk 1992). While there is an overlap with health research, health services research needs to be translated into action to be of value and should 'transcend the R (acquiring knowledge) and the D (translating that knowledge into action) divide' (Hunter and Long 1993).

Each of these definitions emphasises the multidisciplinary nature of health research, health systems research and health services research. Health services research, for example, has been described as 'a space within which disciplines can meet' (Pope 1992), and as an area of applied research, rather than a discipline (Hunter and Long 1993).

Within these definitions, the topics covered in Chapters 1, 4 and 5, on evaluating health services, health needs and their assessment (the latter also comes within the definition of broader health research) and the costing of health services, are encompassed by health services research. Chapter 2, on social research on health, and Chapter 3, on quality of life, also fall within both health research and health services research. Not everyone would agree with these definitions and distinctions. For example, some might categorise the assessment of needs as health research rather than health services research. What is important is not the distinctions and overlaps between these branches of research, but a respect for each discipline in relation to its contribution to a multidisciplinary body of knowledge about health and disease, health systems as a whole and health services.

Finally, it should be pointed out that research on health services is not insulated from the society within which it is placed. It is often responsive to current policy and political issues (see Cartwright 1992), and is thus dependent upon decisions taken by others in relation to research topics and research funding. While it is common for researchers to initiate new research ideas, much of the funding for this research comes from government bodies, who tend to prioritise research and development on a local or national basis. The research topics are rarely value-free. The research findings are also disseminated to members of a wide range of professional, voluntary and management groups. In relation to this multidisciplinary nature, the agenda for research and the consumers of the research findings, it contrasts starkly with the traditional biomedical model of research.

Section contents

CHAPTER 1

Evaluating health services: multidisciplinary collaboration

Chapter contents

Introduction

Research on health and health services ranges from descriptive investigations of the experience of illness and people's perceptions of health and ill health (known as research on health, or health research) to evaluations of health services in relation to their appropriateness, effectiveness and costs (health services research). However, these two areas overlap and should not be rigidly divided, as it is essential to include the perspective of the lay person in health service evaluation and decision-making. Other related fields of investigation include audit, quality assurance and the assessment of needs for health services (usually defined in terms of the need for effective services), which come under the umbrella of health research but also have a crucial link with health services research. Audit and quality assurance are not strictly research in the sense of contributing to a body of scientific knowledge and adherence to rigorous methods of conducting research (quantitative or qualitative). Instead they are concerned with monitoring in order to ensure that predefined standards of care are met. They are increasingly important activities with the emphasis on clinical governance in health care (Lugon and Secker-Walker 1999). They are described briefly below with the other main areas of research activity.

Health services research

It was explained in the introduction to Section I that health services research is concerned with the relationship between the provision, effectiveness and efficient use of health services and the health needs of the population. It is narrower than health research. More specifically, health services research aims to produce reliable and valid research data on which to base appropriate, effective, cost-effective, efficient and acceptable health services at the primary and secondary care levels. The phrase health technology assessment has been coined to describe the wider evaluation of health care interventions in terms of both their costs and their effectiveness.

The research knowledge acquired needs to be developed into action if the discipline is to be of value; hence the emphasis throughout industry and service organisations on 'research *and* development'. The focus is generally on:

- the relationships between the population's need and demand for health services, and the supply, use and acceptability of health services;
- the processes and structures, including the quality and efficiency, of health services;
- the appropriateness and effectiveness of health service interventions, in relation to effectiveness and cost-effectiveness, including patients' perceptions of outcome in relation to the effects on their health, health-related quality of life and their satisfaction with the outcome.

These areas of research are addressed in more detail in this chapter and in the other chapters included in Section I.

Health services research is distinct from audit and quality assurance, though they share the same concepts in relation to the evaluation of structure, process and outcome. Audit and quality assessment aim to monitor whether predefined and agreed standards have been met. Health services research has evaluation – rather than monitoring – as its aim. Health services research is also broader than traditional clinical research, which directly focuses on patients in relation to their treatment and care. Clinical research has traditionally focused on biochemical indicators, and more recently, and in selected specialties only, on the measurement of the broader quality of life of the patients. Health services research investigates the outcome of medical interventions from social, psychological, physical and economic perspectives. It has also been cogently argued that health services research should be concerned with the evaluation of the health sector in the broadest sense, and not limited to health services alone (Hunter and Long 1993).

Quality assessment and audit will be described next, followed by the concepts central to the latter and to health services research: the evaluation of the structure, process and outcome, including appropriateness, of health services.

The assessment of quality

The quality of care for the purposes of health care evaluation can be defined in relation to its effectiveness with regard to improving the patient's health status, and how well it meets professionals' and the public's standards about how the care should be provided (Donabedian 1980).

Approaches include performance indicators and assessment, and patient surveys. Systematic evaluations of quality follow Donabedian's (1980) or Maxwell's (1984) broader approaches. Donabedian focused on the measurement of *structure* (inputs and resources, such as staffing, buildings, funding); *process* (service delivery, organisation and use, including resources – e.g. rates of consultations and referrals, waiting times, admission and discharge procedures, prescribing practices); *output* (productivity and throughput, including discharge rates, access, effectiveness, equity); and *outcome* (death, disease, disability, discomfort, dissatisfaction). Maxwell described six dimensions of quality: *appropriateness*; *social acceptability* (patients' views, met expectations); *effectiveness* (consistent with desired effect); *relevance to need*; *equity*; and *accessibility* (siting, language, disability-friendly). Broader definitions are shown in Box 1.1.

Box 1.1 Modern definitions of quality of care

Higginson (1994) stated that quality of care needs to include humanity, as well as effectiveness, acceptability, equity, accessibility and efficiency. Building on work by Shaw (1989) and Black (1990), she defined quality of health care in broad terms:

- effectiveness (achieving the intended benefits in the population, under usual conditions of care);
- acceptability and humanity (to the consumer and provider);
- equity and accessibility (the provision and availability of services to everyone likely to benefit (in 'need'));
- efficiency (greatest benefit for least cost).

Higginson adds that patient empowerment might also be included, in order that they may increase their control over the services received, and each patient should be offered care that is appropriate.

Quality is clearly relevant to health services research. Quality assurance and medical and clinical audit are all initiatives to establish and maintain quality in health care, and also involve the evaluation of structure, process and outcome in relation to quality.

Audit

Audit is directed at the maintenance and achievement of quality in health care. Audit aims to improve patient outcome, to develop a more cost-effective use of resources and to have an educational function for health professionals. In theory, it should lead to change in clinical practice by encouraging a reflective culture of reviewing current practice, and by inducing changes which lead to better patient outcomes and satisfaction.

Suggested criteria for undertaking an audit include: the issue addressed should be a common, significant or serious problem; any changes following audit should be likely to benefit patients and to lead to greater effectiveness; the issue is relevant to professional practice or development; there is realistic potential for improvement; and the end result is likely to justify the investment of the time and effort involved (Clinical Resource and Audit Group 1994). Investigators of audit have reported that most audit has focused on process, rather than structure or outcomes (e.g. Packwood 1995).

Medical audit, clinical audit, quality assurance and clinical governance

Audit consists of reviewing and monitoring current practice, and evaluation (comparison of performance) against agreed predefined standards (Standing Committee on Postgraduate Medical Education 1989). It is divided into medical and clinical audit, and is related to quality assurance. These have become commonplace in the British National Health Service (NHS) and are now built into the structure of provider units (e.g. hospitals and, increasingly, general practice). These three concepts have been clarified by Higginson (1994) (see Box 1.2.):

Box 1.2 Study of three concepts in audit

- Medical audit is the systematic critical analysis of the quality of *medical* care, including a review of diagnosis, and the procedures used for diagnosis, clinical decisions about the treatment, use of resources and patient outcome (Secretaries of State for Health, Wales, Northern Ireland and Scotland 1989a). Examples of medical audit include analyses of avoidable deaths, and the assessment of medical decision-making, resources and procedures used in relation to patient outcome.
- Clinical audit is conducted by doctors (medical audit) *and* other health care professionals (e.g. nurses, physiotherapists, occupational and speech therapists), and is the systematic critical analysis of the quality of clinical care. It includes collecting information to review diagnosis and the procedures used for diagnosis, clinical decisions about the treatment, use of resources and patient outcome (Secretaries of State for Health, Wales, Northern Ireland and Scotland 1989a).
- Quality assurance is a clinical and management approach which involves the systematic monitoring and evaluation of predefined and agreed levels of service provision. Quality assurance is the definition of standards, the measurement of their achievement and the mechanisms employed to improve performance (Shaw 1989). Medical and clinical audit is usually one part of a quality assurance programme. Quality assurance usually implies a planned programme involving the whole of a particular health service.

Audit can be carried out internally by organisations, members of a discipline (peer review), individuals who systematically review their work or that of their teams, or external bodies (e.g. purchasers for contract monitoring, or professional bodies). Certain criteria need to be met for conducting successful audit, including: effective clinical leadership;

strategic direction (vision, strategy, objectives and planning); audit staff and support (e.g. high calibre, right skill mix, reward, staff development); basic structures and systems (e.g. business planning); training and education; understanding and involvement (e.g. communication, leadership and so on); and organisational environment (e.g. structure, relationships) (Walshe 1995).

The process of audit

The process of audit involves multiple methods, such as document searching and analysis (e.g. analysis of complaints files, random or systematic selection of nursing and medical records for routine reviews), analysis of routine data, clinical case reviews and presentations in team meetings (see Hopkins 1990, for a review). It can also include the collection of information by focus groups of patients or by questionnaire, for example, patient satisfaction, patient-assessed outcome (see Riordan and Mockler 1996, for an example of this in an audit of a psycho-geriatric assessment unit). While quantitative research methodology is most appropriate for audit, much can also be gained by supplementing this with qualitative methods such as observation (e.g. visits to wards and clinics to assess quality by observation). The design of audits should also aim to be scientifically and methodologically rigorous (Russell and Wilson 1992; Department of Health 1993b).

Clinical governance

Clinical governance is a framework through which health care organisations are accountable for the quality and standard of the health care they provide. This is implemented by having systems in place to ensure best practice based on evidence-based medicine; clinical audit (measuring practice against predefined standards); monitoring and minimising risk; having systems for protecting patient confidentiality; education and training to enable staff competencies; providing good working conditions; being responsive to patients' needs; encouraging, and listening to, their feedback; being open about information and having formalised complaints procedures; and by patient and public involvement in service planning.

Evaluation

Evaluation is the use of the scientific method, and the rigorous and systematic collection of research data, to assess the effectiveness of organisations, services and programmes (e.g. health service interventions) in achieving predefined objectives (Shaw 1980). Evaluation is central to health services research and audit. It is *more* than audit because it aims to record not only what changes occur, but also what led to those changes. Evaluation can be divided into two types: formative and summative. Formative evaluation involves the collection of data while the organisation or programme is active, with the aim of developing or improving it. Summative evaluation involves collecting data about the active (or terminated) organisation or programme with the aim of deciding whether it should be continued or repeated (a health promotion activity or screening programme) (Kemm and Booth 1992).

As the starting point in all research, including evaluation, the investigator needs to first of all match the appropriate research methods to the questions or issues under investigation. When an intervention has high levels of homogeneity across contexts, or different settings, then the experimental method may be the appropriate research method (e.g. as in many drug trials). However, as heterogeneity increases, experimental methods are less helpful for establishing effectiveness. Many health and social care interventions, for example, experience high levels of contextual variation, are complex interventions, and attempts to standardise them, in attempts to force them to fit into experimental design paradigms, are likely to lead to lack of external validity, or generalisability. A different approach to evaluating the effectiveness of complex interventions is needed, in order to understand the situations within and mechanisms by which interventions work. (See sections on complex interventions in Chapter 10 and realistic evaluation in Chapter 19.)

Structure, process and outcome

The evaluation of health services has traditionally been based on the collection of data about the structure, processes, outputs and outcomes of services (Donabedian 1980). Structure refers to the organisational framework for the activities; process refers to the activities themselves; outputs relate to productivity, and outcome refers to the impact (effectiveness) of the activities of interest (e.g. health services and interventions) in relation to individuals (e.g. patients) and communities. Health outcome relates to the impact of the service on the patient (effectiveness). The structure and process of services can influence their effectiveness. These concepts have been clearly described in relation to the evaluation of health services by St Leger *et al.* (1992).

Thus, it is often necessary to measure structure and process in order to interpret the outcome of the care. For example, the collection of qualitative and quantitative descriptive data about process and structure is essential if the investigator wishes to address the question of whether – and how – the outcome was caused by the activity itself, and/or by variations in the structure, or the way it was organised or delivered (process). These data can enhance the influence of the research results. These concepts, and their operationalisation, are described below.

Structure and inputs

The structure of an organisation refers to the buildings, inputs such as equipment, staff, beds and the resources needed to meet defined standards. The assessment of quality will be in relation to their numbers, type and suitability. It is represented in economic terms by its fixed costs (see Chapter 5). The operationalisation of this concept requires measurement of the raw materials forming the inputs. These can be operationalised in relation to the distribution of staff, their mix in relation to level of training, grade and skill, availability, siting and type of buildings (e.g. hospitals, clinics and type), facilities and equipment, numbers and types of services, consumables (e.g. medication) used and other types of capital and financial resources.

Data on structure and inputs can be obtained by questionnaire and document analysis. The study design might be a descriptive survey or the data might be collected within an experimental design comparing organisations in relation to outcome.

Process and outputs

The process refers to how the service is organised, delivered and used. It is assessed in medical audit in relation to deviation from predefined and agreed standards. It includes accessibility (e.g. proximity to public transport, waiting lists), the way in which personnel and activities interact, and interaction between personnel and patients. In other words, it is the documentation and analysis of dynamic events and interactions. Data on processes are essential for the evaluation of whether scarce health service resources are used efficiently.

The types of data to be collected include outputs (e.g. the activities that occur through the use of the resources in the system). These can be operationalised in relation to rates of productivity for hospital discharge, number and type of supplies given (e.g. medication, equipment), the number of patient–professional contacts and their type, the number of home visits, average lengths of hospital stay, length of consultation, medical and surgical intervention rates, waiting lists and waiting times. Donabedian (1980) included accessibility as a process indicator (e.g. levels of use by different population groups, adequacy and appropriateness of services provided). The analysis of process also involves the collection of data about the quality of the relationship, and communications, between professional and professional, and professional and patient (e.g. timely provision of information to general practitioners (GPs) about their patients' treatment/discharge, provision of information to patients), the plans or procedures followed and documentation.

Some of the information can be extracted from records and, increasingly, computer databases, combined with checks with patients and professionals in relation to its accuracy and completeness. Alternatively, it can be collected by asking patients to provide the information. Appropriate methods include questionnaire surveys and document analyses.

Appropriateness and inappropriateness

Appropriateness is relevant to outcome. Appropriateness of health care interventions has been variously defined. Investigators at Rand in the USA defined it in terms of whether the expected health benefit of the procedure exceeds its expected negative health consequences by a sufficiently wide margin to justify performing the procedure, excluding considerations of financial cost (Chassin 1989). The view of the British NHS Executive is that appropriateness of care refers to the selection, on the basis of the evidence, of interventions of demonstrable effectiveness that are most likely to lead to the outcome desired by the individual patient (Hopkins 1993). The definition used in Britain often includes consideration of resources (Chantler *et al.* 1989; Maxwell 1989), and of the individuality of the patient. There is no consensus internationally on a definition of appropriateness.

The emphasis in health services research is on the measurement of the appropriateness of, as well as the effectiveness of, interventions in the broadest sense. Policy-makers, purchasers and providers of health services aim, in theory, to identify the most appropriate treatments and services to deliver and purchase (outcome assessment) and the level of need in the population for the interventions, and to monitor their provision and mode of delivery (measurement of processes and structure). Patients themselves also want to know whether the treatment will work and whether they will recover – as well as where to go for their treatment. The difficulties at policy level stem from the relative dearth of research data on appropriateness and effectiveness. Appropriateness is not limited to interventions, but also applies to organisational factors. For example, there is an increasing literature on the appropriateness of length of hospital inpatient stays (Houghton *et al.* 1997).

All medical treatments aim to save or prolong life, to relieve symptoms, to provide care and/or to improve health-related quality of life. However, the assessment of health outcomes and appropriateness of treatments has been given impetus by the increasing evidence about high rates of inappropriate treatments. For example, in the USA, relatively high levels of inappropriateness rates have been found in relation to surgical interventions for coronary heart disease (Chassin *et al.* 1987; Winslow *et al.* 1988; Smith 1990). High levels of inappropriate care and wide variations in practice (e.g. intervention rates) have been documented in the UK in relation to various procedures (Brook *et al.* 1988; Anderson and Mooney 1990; Coulter *et al.* 1993). While Brook (1994) argued that there is too much literature on medical *practice* for doctors to assimilate routinely, it is also the case that there is insufficient research evidence on the *appropriateness* of many medical interventions. Methods for developing *consensus* on appropriateness criteria are described in Chapter 19.

Outcome

Health service outcomes are the effects of health services on patients' health (e.g. their health gain) as well as patients' evaluations of their health care. Reliable and valid information on outcomes of health services is essential for audit, as well as for purchasing policies. Donabedian (1980) defined health outcome as a *change* as a result of antecedent health care. This is a narrow definition, though widely used, and excludes the maintenance of patients in a stable condition, which can also be a valid aim of treatment. It also excludes many health promotion and prevention activities. Outcome refers to the effectiveness of the activities in relation to the achievement of the intended goal. Purchasing debates in health care have focused on health care costs in relation to broader 'health gains' or 'benefits' from the treatments and interventions that are being contracted for.

There is similar debate about the definition and measurement of outcome in relation to social care and input from social services. Outcome is more complex in the context of social care, and also in the case of long-term health care, than it is with specific, time-limited treatments and interventions. In relation to social care, and long-term health care, the objective is to measure what difference this made to the recipient's life in the broadest sense (Qureshi *et al.* 1994).

Health outcome measurement has traditionally focused on survival periods, toxicity, bio-chemical indicators and symptom rates, relapses, various indicators of physical and psychological morbidity, and easily measured social variables (e.g. days off work or school, number of bed days, hospital readmission rates, other indicators of health service use). Lohr (1988) defined outcome in relation to death, disease, disability, discomfort and dissatisfaction ('the five Ds'), and argued that measurement instruments should focus on each of these concepts. However, the trend now is to incorporate positive indicators (e.g. degrees of well-being, ability, comfort, satisfaction), rather than to focus entirely on negative aspects of outcome.

Broader measures of outcome

In health and social services research, more positive criteria of quality of life are increasingly being incorporated into the broader assessment of outcome. Treatment and care need to be evaluated in terms of whether they are more likely to lead to an outcome of a life worth living in social, psychological and physical terms. Health and ill health are a consequence of the interaction of social, psychological and biological events (sometimes called the bio-psychosocial model of ill health). Thus each of these elements requires measurement in relation to: patients' perceived health status and health-related quality of life (physical, psychological and social); reduced symptoms and toxicity; and patients' (and carers' where appropriate) satisfaction with the treatment and outcome (see Chapter 3). Thus, the assessment of outcome needs to incorporate both the medical model and the patient's perspective.

Health and health-related quality of life

Health status and health-related quality of life are two distinct conceptual terms which are often used interchangeably. Health status is one domain of health-related quality of life. The definition of health status traditionally focused on physical morbidity and mental health, and was negative in its operationalisation. Because the current usage of health status implies a multifaceted concept, it overlaps with the broader concept of health-related quality of life. Both can encompass physical health (e.g. fitness, symptoms, signs of disease and wellness), physical functioning (ability to perform daily activities and physical roles), social functioning and social health (relationships, social support and activities), psychological well-being (depression, anxiety), emotional well-being (life satisfaction, morale, control, coping and adjustment) and perceptions. It is increasingly accepted that an instrument which encompasses the above domains is measuring health-related quality of life, rather than a narrower aspect of physical or mental health status (see WHOQOL Group 1993; Bowling 2001, 2005a). In addition, the concepts of perceived health status, quality of life and health-related quality of life can be complex to analyse as they might be mediated by several interrelated variables, including self-related constructs (e.g. self-efficacy, self-esteem, perceived control over life) and subjective evaluations could be influenced, in theory, by cognitive mechanisms (e.g. expectations of life, level of optimism or pessimism, social and cultural values, aspirations, standards for social comparisons of one's circumstances in life). Few investigators have taken these variables, and their interplay, into account, though associations between expectations of treatment and patient outcome, and between level of optimism and patients' coping strategies, have been reported (Higginson 2000; Koller *et al.* 2000).

Health-related quality of life as an outcome measure broadens outcome towards considering the impact of the condition and its treatment on the person's emotional, physical and social functioning and lifestyle. It addresses the question of whether the treatment leads to a life worth living, and it provides a more subjective, patient-led baseline against which the effects of interventions can be evaluated. It can only do this, however, if the measurement scale reflecting its components is valid, reliable, precise, specific, responsive to change and sensitive. A universal questionnaire to elicit the relevant information for a number of conditions would need to be of enormous length. Disease-specific quality of life scales are needed, not simply for greater brevity, but to ensure sensitivity to sometimes small, but clinically significant, changes in health status and levels of disease severity. A quality of life measure used in research on health and health care should be able to inform the investigator of the effects of the condition or treatment on the patient's daily, as well as long-term, life. It should also be capable of providing information on whether, and to what extent, any gains in survival time among patients with life-threatening conditions are at the expense of reductions in quality of life during the period of the treatment and in the long term.

A disease-specific, or condition-specific instrument will have a narrower focus generally, but contain more details of relevance to the area of interest. If the investigator is interested in a single disease or condition, then a disease-specific indicator is appropriate, though if the respondent has multiple health problems it may be worth combining it with a generic measure. If the research topic covers more than one condition, or general health, then generic measures might be more appropriate. It is not possible in this short space to recommend specific measures; generic and disease-specific measures have been reviewed by the author elsewhere (Bowling 2001, 2005a). The theoretical influences which shaped the development of health status and health-related quality of life scales are described briefly in Chapter 3.

Patient-reported outcomes

Due to the conceptual confusion resulting from overlapping concepts in health status, generic quality of life and health-related quality of life scales, investigators tend to refer to any end-points derived from patient reports as 'patient-reported outcome' measures (Patrick 2003; Acquadro and Jambon 2005; Fitzpatrick *et al.* 2006), or more specifically as self-reported health instruments (Fitzpatrick *et al.* 2006). These more generic terms include generic and disease-specific health status, all specific measures of physical and mental functioning, quality of life and health-related quality of life, as well as experiences of health care and treatment (e.g. patient expectations, satisfaction, preferences, adherence). The MAPI Trust in Lyon, France (www.mapi-trust.org), produces a patient-reported outcomes newsletter, in place of its previous quality of life newsletter (Acquadro and Jambon 2005; www.pro-newsletter.com), and maintains a patient-reported outcomes validated instruments database (PROVIDE).

Summary of main points

- Research: a systematic and rigorous process of enquiry. It aims to describe processes and develop explanatory concepts and theories, in order to contribute to a scientific body of knowledge.
- Health services research: aims to produce reliable and valid research data on which to base appropriate, effective, cost-effective, efficient and acceptable health services.
- Quality of care: effectiveness at improving patients' health status and how well it meets predefined and agreed standards about how the care should be provided.
- Audit: directed at the maintenance and achievement of quality in health care. It consists of review and monitoring of current practice, and evaluation against standards.

- Medical audit: the systematic critical analysis of the quality of medical care. Clinical audit is the systematic critical analysis of the quality of clinical care by all health care professionals.
- Quality assurance: a clinical and management approach which is the systematic monitoring and evaluation of predefined and agreed levels of service provision.
- Evaluation: the use of scientific method, and the rigorous and systematic collection of research data to assess the effectiveness of organisations, services and programmes in achieving predefined objectives.
- Evaluation is *more* than audit because it aims to record not only what changes occur, but also what led to those changes.
- The evaluation of health services is usually based on collecting data about the structure, process and outcomes of services, as well as the appropriateness of the services.
- Outcome should usually include measurement of the impact of the condition and the intervention on the broader health-related quality of life of the patient.

Key questions

1 Define research.
2 Distinguish between health research, health systems research and health services research.
3 What are the key components of health services research?
4 Distinguish between evaluation and audit.
5 What is the difference between audit and quality assurance?
6 Distinguish between the structure, process and outcome of health services.
7 What are health service inputs and outputs?
8 What are the main domains of health-related quality of life which should be included in the measurement of health outcomes?

Key terms

appropriateness
audit
clinical audit
disease-specific quality of life
equity
evaluation
health research
health services research
health status
health systems
health technology assessment

health-related quality of life
inputs
medical audit
outcome
outputs
patient-based outcomes
process
quality assurance
quality of life
structure

Recommended reading

Black, N. (2009) Health services research: the gradual encroachment of ideas, *Journal of Health Services Research and Policy,* 14: 120–3.

Black, N., Brazier, J., Fitzpatrick, R. and Reeve, B. (eds) (1998) *Health Services Research Methods: A Guide to Best Practice.* London: BMJ Publishing.

Bowling, A. (2001) *Measuring Disease: A Review of Disease-specific Quality of Life Measurement Scales,* 2nd edn. Buckingham: Open University Press.

Donabedian, A. (1980) *Explorations in Quality Assessment and Monitoring,* Vol. 1: *The Definition of Quality and Approaches to its Assessment.* Ann Arbor, MI: Health Administration Press.

Green, J. and Brown, J. (2005) *Principles of Social Research.* Maidenhead: Open University Press.

Higginson, I. (1994) Quality of care and evaluating services, *International Review of Psychiatry,* 6: 5–14.

Hunter, D.J. and Long, A.F. (1993) Health research, in W. Sykes, M. Bulmer and M. Schwerzel (eds) *Directory of Social Research Organizations in the UK.* London: Mansell.

Jenkinson, C. (ed.) (1997) *Assessment and Evaluation of Health and Medical Care.* Buckingham: Open University Press.

Long, A. (1994) Assessing health and social outcomes, in J. Popay and G. Williams (eds) *Researching the People's Health.* London: Routledge.

Maxwell, R.J. (1984) Quality assessment in health, *British Medical Journal,* 288: 1471.

Nolte, E., McKee, M. and Wait, S. (2005) Describing and evaluating health systems, in A. Bowling and S. Ebrahim (eds) *Handbook of Health Research Methods: Investigation, Measurement and Analysis.* Maidenhead: Open University Press.

Smith, S., Sinclair, D., Raine, R. and Reeves, B. (2005) *Health Care Evaluation.* Maidenhead: Open University Press.

St Leger, A.S., Schnieden, H. and Wadsworth-Bell, J.P. (1992) *Evaluating Health Services' Effectiveness.* Buckingham: Open University Press.

CHAPTER 2

Social research on health: sociological and psychological concepts and approaches

Chapter contents

Introduction

The focus of this chapter is on society and the individual in relation to some of the main social and psychological theories and concepts of health and illness. It is important to understand lay definitions and theories of health and illness, and the factors that influence behaviour, when measuring the effectiveness of health services, as well as when developing health services which aim to be acceptable to people. There is little point in developing services, or measuring the patient's outcome of health care, without an understanding of how people's beliefs and expectations about health, illness and therapeutic regimens might conflict with those of health professionals (thereby influencing the take-up of services and adherence to therapies).

The aim of describing the contribution of sociology and psychology is to increase awareness of the richness of approaches to research on health and disease, and to enhance understanding of why different quantitative and qualitative research methods are used. Readers are referred to Jones (1994), Cockerham (1995), Stroebe (2000) and Cockerham and Scambler (2010) for more comprehensive and critical overviews of relevant sociological and psychological perspectives.

Sociological and psychological research on health

Psychology is the scientific study of behaviour and mental processes. *Sociology* is the study of social life and behaviour. Unlike psychologists, sociologists are divided into those who focus on developing a theoretical, academic discipline (known as the 'sociology *of* medicine' or, more recently, as the 'sociology *of* health'), and those who focus on applied research and analysis, and aim to contribute to contemporary issues on health and health care, alongside health care practitioners ('sociology *in* medicine') (see Strauss 1957; Cockerham 1995; Jefferys 1996). The latter are involved in applying their knowledge to issues in health research and health services research.

Social scientists who investigate health and health services aim to understand people's perceptions, behaviours and experiences in the face of health and illness, their experiences of health care, their coping and management strategies in relation to stressful events (e.g. illness), their societal reactions to illness and the functioning of health services in relation to their effects on people. Social research on health is highly relevant to health services research, and should not be divorced from it. As Popay and Williams (1993) have argued in relation to health research generally:

> [It] is of central relevance to our understanding of both the process and the outcomes of health and social care, including initiatives in health promotion and prevention. This research has a major contribution to make, particularly in the assessment of health and social need, the measurement of patient assessed outcomes, and the assessment of the public's views of priorities in health care.

A wide range of qualitative and quantitative, descriptive and analytic methods are used. The choice of method is dependent on the perspective of the investigator, as well as on what is appropriate to the research situation. The measurement of health and disease has traditionally been based on quantitative methodology. Social sciences have generally developed alongside the natural and physical sciences, and favour the use of the scientific method and quantitative, structured approaches to measurement. This approach is based on positivism, which assumes that social phenomena can be measured objectively and analysed following the principles of the scientific method in the same way as natural sciences.

Some social scientists view positivism as misleading. They argue that human behaviour cannot be measured quantitatively, and that 'reality' is socially constructed through the interaction of individuals and their interpretations of events; thus the investigator must understand individuals' interpretations and experiences. They adhere to the philosophy of phenomenology and belong to the 'interpretive' school of thought. This includes branches of social science known as ethnomethodology, social or symbolic interactionism, labelling, deviance and reactions theory. They are collectively known as social action theory (see Chapter 6). The research methods favoured are qualitative; for example, unstructured, in-depth interviews and observation. Thus, in social science, theoretical perspectives influence the choice of research method (qualitative or quantitative). Discussion of key concepts in sociology, and medical sociology, can be found in Cockerham and Scambler (2010).

2.1 Health and illness

The bio-medical model

In the West, the dominant model of disease is the bio-medical model. This is based on the assumption that disease is generated by specific aetiological agents which lead to changes in the body's structure and function. The medical view of the body is based on the Cartesian philosophy of the body as a machine. Hence, if a part malfunctions, it can be repaired or replaced: the disease is treated, but not the illness, which is the subjective experience of dysfunction. It sees the mind and body as functioning independently, and while disease may lead to psychological disturbances, it does not have psychological causes. The model is based on an assumption of scientific rationality, an emphasis on objective, numerical measurement and an emphasis on physical and chemical data. With the medical model, health is seen in terms of the absence of disease (Jones 1994).

There have been challenges to the traditional medical model (e.g. Illich 1976; Navarro 1976), which have pointed to its inability to capture all factors pertinent to health status. It has been argued that it focuses too narrowly on the body and on technology, rather than on people in the social context in which they live. These challenges have been made mainly by social scientists in health psychology and medical sociology who view ill health as being caused by a *combination* of biological (e.g. genetic predisposition), social (e.g. poverty) and psychological factors, and predispositions.

In recognition of the fact that bio-medical models of illness ignore personal and social contexts, and are unable to explain much reported illness, Wade and Halligan (2004) proposed a new, less biologically dependent, model of illness, which is centred on the 'ill' person who does not necessarily need to consider themselves to be ill. Among their assumptions are that people are influenced by personal context and personal choice (e.g. beliefs, attitudes, expectations, values), and that people interact between different contexts (e.g. the physical and the social). This 'systems model' implies that abnormalities in one system can occur without adversely affecting its components, and may be dependent on other parts of the system (and thus a person can be ill without discernible pathology). Wade and Halligan's model is consistent with rehabilitation programmes whereby the condition is not removed, but intervention is required to facilitate coping.

The psychological model

Classic psychological theory holds that an individual's cognitive beliefs and expectations about their self-efficacy, control, mastery or ability, are related to their perceptions, motivations and actions, including health behaviours, self-management of their health and illness, and coping behaviour.

Control over life

Slagsvold and Sørensen (2008) described how a sense of personal control has been defined and measured variously in the literature, using overlapping concepts and measures (Pearlin and Pioli 2003). These include mastery (Pearlin *et al.* 1981), personal autonomy (the ability to shape one's own affairs and activities) (Reed and McCormack 2012) and independence (the freedom to determine one's own actions and judgements, free from the controlling influences of other people or circumstances) (Seeman 1983; Reed and McCormack 2012), locus of control (Rotter 1966), self-efficacy (Bandura 1977, 1986), and learned helplessness (Seligman 1975).

A sense of personal control refers to one's beliefs that it is possible to influence one's environment, and that one is able to do so, labelled by Bandura (1977) as outcome expectancy and self-efficacy expectancy. Levels of perceived control have been found to be lower in women than men. This has been partly explained by education (Slagsvold and Sørensen 2008). Perceived control also declines among older adults (Gecas 1989). The decline of sense of control with increasing age is partly due to declining health, and retirement from work, and may also be due to cohort differences in life experiences (Slagsvold and Sørensen 2008). Studies of older people have documented the great value they place on maintaining their independence and control over their lives, being able to carry out their daily activities, remain in their own homes, and look after themselves (Bowling 2005c). Frail and functionally restricted people are able to perceive themselves as independent if support services facilitate them in maintaining their physical independence at home, and thus some control over their lives (Hayden *et al.* 1999). Control over daily life is one of older people's priorities as an outcome indicator of social care (Netten *et al.* 2002).

Self-efficacy

Self-efficacy, or mastery, is a personality construct, and refers to one's competency and capability of success in producing an intended goal. It is the ability to maintain some control over life, and of being able to preserve a sense of control in the face of the challenges, or changes which can accompany ageing (Blazer 2002). Self-efficacy is often operationalised in measurement scales used in health care as 'confidence' in one's ability to perform various tasks or activities (e.g. Humphriss *et al.* 2004). However, this deviates from Bandura's definition, who noted:

> [T]he construct of self-efficacy differs from the colloquial term 'confidence'. Confidence is a nondescript term that refers to strength of belief but does not necessarily specify what the certainty is about . . . Perceived self-efficacy refers to one's agentive capabilities, that one can produce given levels of attainment. A self-efficacy assessment, therefore, includes both an affirmation of a capability level and the strength of that belief. Confidence is a catchword rather than a construct embedded in a theoretical system ... Theory-based constructs pay dividends in understanding and operational guidance. The terms used to characterise personal agency, therefore, represent more than merely lexical preferences.
>
> (1997, p. 382)

In theory, an individual's cognitive beliefs and expectations about their self-efficacy, mastery or ability, are related to their motivations and actions (Bandura 1977). The extent to which people perceive that they, rather than others, determine what happens in their lives leads to a greater sense of internal control (Lefcourt 1982), which theoretically leads to greater self-esteem, to greater perceived self-efficacy, which influences intentions, coping, behaviour and ultimately well-being (Mirowsky and Ross 1991; Pearlin 1999; Eckenrode and Hamilton 2000; and see Bowling *et al.* 2007).

Self-efficacy is an important factor in the promotion of physical and mental health, and quality of life of older people, in the adaptation to, management of, and coping with, the challenges of ageing, including disability (Baltes and Baltes 1990; Blazer 2002; Lorig and Holman 2003; Marks *et al.* 2005). Albrecht and Devlieger (1999) and Bowling *et al.* (2007) reported that people who rated their health as 'good' or 'excellent', rather than fair or poor, despite their disabilities, held a 'can do' attitude, a strong sense of self-efficacy and control over their lives. Self-efficacy and feelings of being in control over one's life are important to feeling that one has a good quality of life (Abbey and Andrews 1985; Hyde *et al.* 2003; Bowling *et al.* 2007). It is also key to successful ageing (Baltes and Baltes 1990).

This theory has had fruitful applications in behavioural intervention and health promotion programmes aimed at increasing people's sense of mastery and ability to cope with problems (Eckenrode and Hamilton 2000). It is also central to patient programmes of self-management of chronic conditions; these are being actively promoted in the USA and Europe. It should be noted that there is no agreement on the definition of self-management, and approaches include a medical model (patients receive professional support and direction); a collaborative model (patients seek, and are actively involved in a relationship with professionals on choice of self-management approach); and a self-agency model (independent patient activities) (Koch *et al.* 2004).

The social model of health

Social scientists distinguish between the medical concept of *disease*, and subjective feelings and perceptions of *dis-ease*, often labelled as *illness* or *sickness* by lay people. Illness and sickness, unlike disease, are not necessarily detected by biochemical indicators. Research shows that some people can be diseased according to biochemical indicators, without actually feeling sick or ill (e.g. high blood pressure), and others can feel ill without any biochemical evidence of being diseased (e.g. chronic back pain). Health and ill health are viewed by social scientists as a continuum along which individuals progress and regress (see Ogden 1996).

The social model of health is best expressed with reference to the World Health Organization's (1947, 1948) definition that health is not merely the absence of disease, but a state of complete physical, psychological and social well-being. This definition has frequently been criticised as utopian (Seedhouse 1985), but it is useful as a broad working model.

Lay definitions of health

A wide range of different concepts of health and illness exist both within and between different societies (see Currer and Stacey 1986). Medical sociologists and anthropologists have concentrated on lay theories of health and illness. Frequently employed methodologies include surveys as well as unstructured, in-depth interviews to explore the complexity of people's beliefs and experiences. The analysis of these theories is important for helping to understand whether services will be taken up (e.g. mammography), consultation and service use patterns, adherence to prescribed medications and therapies (Bowling 1989) and how people generally respond to, and manage, particular symptoms.

Qualitative and quantitative interview studies and postal questionnaire surveys have reported that lay people perceive health in a variety of ways. For example, perceptions range from health as: the absence of disease (consistent with the medical model); a strength (e.g. feeling strong, getting on well: Herzlich 1973); being able to maintain normal role functioning (e.g. to carry out normal routines); being fit (e.g. exercise); being able to cope with crises and stress (Calnan 1987); having healthy habits and vitality, being socially active (Cox et al. 1987); hygiene, good living conditions and personal development (d'Houtard et al. 1990); and a state of good mental and physical equilibrium (d'Houtard and Field 1984). (See Box 2.1.) Many of the definitions centre on health as the ability to function in one's normal social roles. Blaxter (1990) identified nine discrete categories of health from a large population survey:

1 Not ill (or without disease).
2 In spite of disease (e.g. 'I am very healthy although I do have diabetes').
3 As a reserve (e.g. 'when ill I recover quickly').
4 As a behaviour or living a healthy life (e.g. being vegetarian, non-smoker, non-drinker).
5 Physical fitness.
6 Vitality (e.g. 'full of get up and go' or 'full of life').
7 Social relationships (e.g. relating well to other people).
8 Function (e.g. able to do things).
9 Psychosocial well-being (e.g. being mentally and spiritually as one).

Studies have also shown that perceptions of health vary as a function of socio-demographic factors. For example, people in higher socio-economic groups appear to be more likely to define their health in positive terms, while people in lower socio-economic groups are more likely to define health negatively (e.g. not being ill) (Blaxter and Patterson 1982), and as outside their control (Blaxter 1983; Pill and Stott

1985, 1988). Definitions of health also vary by age and gender. Jones (1994) reported that women were most likely to define health in terms of ability to cope with household tasks.

Box 2.1 A survey of health and attitudes in Britain

A good example of the value of survey methods and questionnaires in this area is Cox *et al.*'s (1987, 1993) national longitudinal survey of health and attitudes in Britain. This study was mainly based on structured scales and questions (e.g. of anxiety and depression, smoking behaviour, diet, feelings of control over health, personality, social support) because a national population data set was aimed for. However, it was also possible to incorporate some open-ended questions in order to obtain information about areas about which little was known. Examples include: 'What do you think causes people to be healthier *now* than in your parents' time?'; 'What do you think causes people to be less healthy *now* than in your parents' time?'; 'At times people are healthier than at other times. Describe what it's like when *you* are healthy.' They reported that women were more likely to link energy and vitality to the performance of household tasks, while men linked energy and fitness to participation in sports. This research also indicated that men and women aged 60 and over were more likely than younger people to define health in terms of 'being able to do a lot, work, get out and about'. This reflects the impact of their age and functional status (e.g. physical frailty) on their own lives, and supports research on the most important domains of health-related quality of life cited by older people (Bowling 1995, 1996a, 1996b; Farquhar 1995). Consequently, Wright (1990) has summarised lay definitions of health as health as *being*, health as *doing* and health as *having*.

The evaluation literature in health and social care continues to mirror the shift away from a disease model of health as the simple absence of disease and abnormality of functioning, and incorporates measurement of experiences of not just ill-health, but of health, fitness, quality of life and well-being as outcomes in health and social care interventions.

Lay theories of illness

As pointed out earlier, a person can feel ill or sick though there may not be any physical indications for this. Lay definitions of health and illness need to be seen in this broader context. Pill and Stott (1988) argued that a person's readiness to accept their responsibility for health (and, by implication, their responsiveness to health promotion activities) partly depends on their beliefs about the causation of illness. In both the industrialised and non-industrialised worlds, there have been many attempts to classify lay theories of illness. Foster and Anderson (1978) differentiated between personalistic or purposeful action of an agent (e.g. spirits, germs) and naturalistic (e.g. cold, damp, disequilibrium within the individual or environment, such as yin–yang and humoral theories) systems. Theories of the body are generally based on the harmonious balance achieved by forces within the body, which is believed to be influenced by either internal forces (e.g. genes) or external forces (e.g. diet) (see Hunt 1976; Helman 1978, 1990; Young 1983).

Much of the research in the West has focused on socio-economic influences. For example, it has been reported by both qualitative and quantitative sociologists that people in the lower socio-economic groups are more likely to perceive health and ill health as caused by external factors outside their control (e.g. environment, germs). People in the higher social classes are apparently more likely to mention individual behavioural causes of health and illness (e.g. the effects of diet) (Pill and Stott 1985, 1988; Coulter 1987; Blaxter 1990).

Sociologists have used both qualitative and quantitative methods (from unstructured interviews to structured postal questionnaires) to explore and describe people's beliefs about illness. The richest data were obtained from the qualitative studies. Blaxter's (1983) qualitative research on women's beliefs about the causes of disease was based on one- to two-hour 'conversations' on health and illness with 46 working-class women. Blaxter carried out a content analysis of the transcripts and every mention of a named disease was extracted and analysed for attributed causes (by type). In the 587 examples of named diseases in her 46 transcripts, causes were imputed in 432 cases. Blaxter categorised 11 types of causes, and the most commonly occurring were infection, heredity and agents in the environment. She presented sections of her transcripts in illustration of these – for example (heredity), 'His mother, my husband's, her mother before that and further down the line, all had awful legs. They've all been bothered wi' their legs.' This is an example of qualitative research providing data that can be analysed in both a quantitative and a qualitative way.

A disability paradox?

One of the most commonly mentioned influences on quality of life by older people is health and functioning (Bowling 2001; Bowling et al. 2003). While poor health and functioning are widely reported to be associated with poor quality of life ratings, not everyone with poor health and functioning reports their lives to be less than optimum. Albrecht and Devlieger (1999), in their qualitative study of the quality of life with people with disabilities, reported that a 'disability paradox' existed whereby many respondents with severe disabilities, and with apparently poor quality of life to an outsider, nevertheless perceived their quality of life to be excellent or good. Koch (2000) pointed to other research which reported similar associations (National Organization on Disability 1994).

Albrecht and Devlieger suggested that this 'paradox' can be explained by balance theory, as their respondents perceived quality of life to be dependent on a balance between body, mind and spirit, and on maintaining harmony in their relationships. A further explanation proposed was that positive quality of life was due to secondary gain during the process of adaptation to disability, whereby people reinterpret their lives and meaning in their social roles. Supportive relationships could also act to enhance perceived life quality when people are ill. Indeed, there is a long, though inconclusive, literature on their association with emotional well-being, and potential buffering effects in the face of stress (see Bowling 1994; Lakey and Cohen 2000).

Koch (2000) criticised the concept of a 'disability paradox' on the grounds that self-perceived quality of life depends on several factors, not just health and ability, including people's coping styles, and accommodation to changes in physical status. In support of this, Bowling et al. (2007) found, in their population survey of quality of life in Britain among people aged 65+, over a third of respondents had fairly severe to very severe difficulties with daily activities and rated their quality of life as 'not good'; almost two-thirds had fairly to very severe difficulties and rated their quality of life as 'good'. The most powerful predictor of having a disability and rating one's life as good was self-efficacy. If people with a disability felt they had a lot of control over their lives, their odds of perceiving their quality of life as good, rather than not good, were five times that where respondents with a disability felt they had little or no control. These results indicated that psychological resources are the most powerful predictors of quality of life among people with disabilities.

Indeed, having a health problem is not always equated with poor perceived health or poor quality of life. For example, national survey data show that, in 2001, around 1 in 20 men and women in England and Wales considered themselves to be in good health despite reporting a long-term illness which restricted their daily activities. And among those aged 85+ who reported they were in good health, 33 per cent of men and 40 per cent of women reported a long-term illness which restricted their daily activities (Office for National Statistics 2004); on the other hand, having health is commonly prioritised by people as an important factor in life, as well as an essential component of quality of life in older age – even more so by people with health and functional problems (Bowling 2001; Bowling *et al.* 2003).

Variations in medical and lay perspectives

Variations in perspectives are not limited to the lay public. For example, uncertainty in modern medicine has led to situations where conditions are perceived as diseases in one country but not in others. For example, low blood pressure is treated in Germany but not usually treated in other countries. Variations in guidelines for treatment of blood pressure have also been found to vary between countries, and over time (Wolf-Maier *et al.* 2004).

Qualitative and quantitative investigations have reported clear cultural differences in diagnostic criteria and thresholds across the world. For example, Payer (1988) reported that Americans were more likely to possess an aggressive, interventionist 'do something' attitude (i.e. the body is viewed as a machine under attack, and the technology is available to keep it going), with high rates of surgery and diagnostic tests, stronger medications (including over-the-counter medications) and a popular lay worry about viruses. Britain was reported as having a less interventionist attitude, with less surgery, fewer tests, fewer medications (apart from antibiotics for minor illnesses) and more of a 'stiff upper lip' attitude to illness, though with a higher level of concern about bowels. Germany had higher medical consultation rates, a high use of medications, and diagnostic technology, and a popular worry about the circulation and emotional and spiritual elements of disease was recognised. French people apparently had more respect for the body as a biological organism and preferred gentle treatments: they were most likely to use homeopathy, for example, and to prescribe nutrients; there was a popular worry about the liver. As Laurence (2013) has summed up:

> Human beings may belong to the same species, but they experience sickness differently. Each nation has its favoured illnesses and its favoured explanations, which alter over time. A doctor in one country may label an illness as depression, while the identical symptoms may be labelled as low blood pressure in another, or as the effects of dental amalgam in yet another.
>
> (www.independent.co.uk, accessed 12 September 2013)

2.2 Social factors in illness and responses to illness

Social variations in health: structural inequalities

Socio-economic status (SES) is frequently implicated as a contributor to health inequalities in populations (Graham 2000; Shavers 2007). Investigators have concentrated largely on the health effects of social stratification, generally measured with indicators of socio-economic group or social class. Research on social stratification has a long history in sociology: both Karl Marx ([1933] 1967) and Max Weber (1946, 1964, 1978, 1979) saw class as the main vehicle of social stratification in industrialist, capitalist societies. Education, occupational status, and income are the most widely used indicators of socio-economic status internationally. Each of these captures different aspects of socio-economic position, but can interact with other socio-demographic variables (e.g. age, sex, ethnicity).

In the USA, education is a commonly used indicator of social position, particularly in epidemiology and demography (Liberatos *et al.* 1988), especially as its measurement can be attempted in all respondents, unlike occupation (which is problematic in relation to those not in paid work). However, there is inconsistent use of measures of socio-economic position in the USA (e.g. in public health) (see review by Krieger *et al.* 1997).

Occupational classifications have been consistently and successfully employed in Britain to analyse inequalities in health status between the higher and lower social classes (Townsend 1979; Townsend and Davidson 1982; Whitehead 1987; Townsend *et al.* 1988). This has inspired similar research across the world (Lahelma *et al.* 1996). The British *Classification of Occupations* was traditionally used as a measure of social class (Office of Population Censuses and Surveys 1980). This has been replaced with the *Standard Occupational Classification*, based on aggregation of occupations in terms of similarity of qualification, training, skills and experience associated with the performance of their constituent work tasks (Office of Population Censuses and Surveys 1990, 1991). The subsequent socio-economic classification, based on this, is the *National Statistics Socio-Economic Classification*, known as NS-SEC (Rose and Pevalin 2002). NS-SEC has been reported to be sensitive to differences in health status, in support of its construct validity (Chandola and Jenkinson 2000). However, such classifications do not include people who have never worked; in the past, women were traditionally classified by their husbands' occupations, which is an outmoded practice given the increase in women's employment in the labour market. Current practice is to record and analyse both partners' occupations. Measuring the socio-economic status of people not in paid work, especially retired people, presents particular difficulties for the use of classifications based on occupation. In addition, interpretation of analyses can be complex because the reasons for not being in paid work, or taking early retirement, may be associated with declining health – and poor health can lead to downward occupational and social mobility. As income is associated with employment, this is also a problematic indicator of socio-economic status in older people.

Grundy and Holt (2001), on the basis of secondary analyses of a national dataset, identified education qualification and social class, paired with an indicator of deprivation, as the best indicators of socio-economic status among older people (these were most sensitive to differences in self-reported health). However, even level of education presents difficulties as an indicator of the latter because most members of the older population left school at the minimum age with no academic qualifications. Thus, investigators aim to include indicators of level of education, wealth (e.g. number of rooms, consumables, car ownership, housing tenure), income, (un)employment status, as well as occupation. The standard methods of measuring these indicators have been presented by de Bruin *et al.* (1996), and recommendations about their optimal measurement have also been published (*International Journal of Health Science* 1996).

All measures of socio-economic status (SES) pose methodological problems. The use of different measures can lead to inconsistency in results of research on population health by socio-economic position. Shavers described the limitations of each in detail, and summarised the problem as:

> This [inconsistency in study results] is due in part to the: 1) lack of precision and reliability of measures; 2) difficulty with the collection of individual SES data; 3) the dynamic nature of SES over a lifetime; 4) the classification of women, children, retired and unemployed persons; 5) lack of or poor correlation between individual SES measures; and 6) inaccurate or misleading interpretation of study results. Choosing the best variable or approach for measuring SES is dependent in part on its relevance to the population and outcomes under study. Many of the commonly used compositional and contextual SES measures are limited in terms of their usefulness for examining the effect of SES on outcomes in analyses of data that include population subgroups known to experience health disparities.
>
> (2007, p. 1013)

Investigators of social variations subscribe to positivist theories of society, which emphasise the way in which society enables and constrains people (e.g. the distribution of power and resources in society affects employment and income opportunities, which in turn affect health). The studies are usually based on quantitative surveys or on the analysis of large routine datasets (e.g. mortality patterns by socio-economic group). The data are complex to interpret because people can be occupationally mobile, either upward or downward (Jones 1994). The two main explanations which attempt to account for social variations in health and mortality in developed nations are: the social causation hypothesis (Townsend and Davidson 1982), where factors associated with socio-economic status influence health; and the selection hypothesis, which takes a life course perspective, and argues, for example, that poor health in childhood and adolescence leads to lower socio-economic positions (Fox *et al.* 1982). Within the latter perspective, some argue that indirect selection is the cause, in which individual characteristics lead to both better socio-economic position and better health (Blane *et al.* 1993). One strong body of evidence indicates that longer-term unemployment leads to adverse health effects (Bartley *et al.* 1999).

Psycho-social stress and responses to stress

Psycho-social stress can be defined as a heightened mind–body reaction to fear or anxiety-arousing stimuli (e.g. illness). Some psychologists broaden this model and conceptualise stress as the product of the person's capacity for self-control, and include theories of self-efficacy (e.g. feeling of confidence in ability to undertake the behaviour), hardiness (e.g. personal feelings of control), and mastery (e.g. control over the response to stress) (see Ogden 1996). Brunner and Marmot (1999), in relation to the stress effects of position in the occupational hierarchy and effects on health, defined stress in relation to the biological response of the individual to the social environment acting upon him or her.

Several measurement scales have been developed by psychologists, which aim to measure the amount of stress that is experienced from life events, such as divorce, marriage, moving house, and so on (e.g. Holmes and Rahe 1967), as well as measures which attempt to evaluate the meaning of the stressful event to the individual (Pilkonis et al. 1985; see Leff 1991 and Cohen et al. 1998 for reviews). There is a large literature on the social, psychological, economic and cultural factors which influence response to stress, and also on lay models of stress (see Helman 1990). Most psychological approaches to the measurement of stress are quantitative.

Coping

Coping refers to the cognitive and behavioural efforts to manage the internal and external demands of the stressful situation (Folkman et al. 1986). In relation to health research, theories have been developed which relate to the immediate coping with the diagnosis (the stages of shock, an encounter reaction such as helplessness and despair, and temporary retreat such as denial of the problem before gradual reorientation towards, and adjustment to, the situation) (Shontz 1975), and the style of coping with the illness. Coping style is one hypothesised *mediating factor* in the link between stress and illness, and can be a moderating variable in relation to patients' health outcomes after treatment. Identified mediating factors relevant to coping include personality (e.g. dispositional optimism), material resources and social support. Most recent stress research is based on the model of cognitive appraisal as developed by Lazarus and Folkman (1984). This consists of primary appraisal (assessment of situation as irrelevant, positive or stressful), secondary appraisal (evaluation of coping resources and options) and reappraisal (which represents the fluid state of appraisal processes). It is argued that the extent to which a person experiences a situation as stressful depends on his or her personal (e.g. belief in control) and environmental (e.g. social support) *coping resources*, and previous experiences. Thus, the same life event will not produce the same effect in everyone (see Volkart 1951; Mechanic 1978; Cockerham 1995).

Psychologists have developed several structured batteries and scales for measuring coping and coping styles. A classic scale is Folkman and Lazarus's (1980, 1988) Ways of Coping Scale. This covers methods of coping based on managing emotion, problem-solving and the seeking of social support. For example, respondents tick 'yes' or 'no' to statements representing these domains in relation to a stressful situation they have experienced (e.g. 'Talk to someone who can do something concrete about the problem', 'I go over in my mind what I will say or do').

Crisis theory

Crisis theory, which relates to the impact of disruption on the individual, has been applied to coping abilities (Moos and Schaefer 1984). The theory holds that individuals strive towards homeostasis and equilibrium in their adjustment (Taylor 1983), and therefore crises are self-limiting. Moos and Schaefer (1984) argue that the coping process in illness comprises the cognitive appraisal of the seriousness and significance of the illness, adaptive tasks (e.g. treatment) and coping skills. Three types of coping skills were identified: appraisal-focused coping, problem-focused coping, and emotion-focused coping. Antonovsky's (1984) theory, which focuses on how people develop a sense of coherence in relation to their condition, emphasises the important role of the resources available to the person (he also developed a Sense of Coherence Scale in order to measure this). These models are consistent with the cognitive appraisal model.

Theory of planned behaviour

Both social structures and individual attitudes can influence behaviour. According to the theory of planned behaviour (TPB), it is not the disability that predicts what one can do, but one's attitude towards it (Ajzen 1988, 1991). Intention is the most important antecedent of behaviour, and is influenced by subjective norms (e.g. the influence of family and peers), attitudes, expectations of future health and ability, self-efficacy and perceived control over the situation (Bandura 1986). Low self-efficacy, for example, is associated with depression, anxiety, helplessness, low motivation and pessimism. The theory also includes components which assume that individuals do not always have complete control over their actions due to external influences, such as financial position and provision of ill-health retirement schemes.

While the evidence in support of the TPB is strong, there is still a gap between intent and behaviour. In order to address this, models of 'coping' based on the model of 'selection, optimisation and compensation' (SOC) may be fruitful. This model emphasises the success of coping by personal growth and positive outcomes by the substitution of activities in the face of losses at different stages in the life trajectory. Baltes and Baltes (1990) proposed that SOC explains how older individuals maintain performance in the face of stress such as illness. If a person is unable to do certain things, then they *compensate* by *selecting* things that they can do, thus *optimising* their social situation. It is a coping mechanism that theoretically predicts retention of social roles and control in life. Thus, for example, the response of older workers to health conditions which threaten their continued employment may be to select and implement those tasks at work in which they are better skilled. Important mediating variables of both SOC and the TPB may include individual levels of optimism and self-esteem. (See section on the theory of planned behaviour in Section 2.3.)

Other models

Other models include proactive coping strategies. In contrast to responsive action models, proactive coping models are oriented more towards the future (Greenglass 2002). They consist of efforts to build up resources to help cope with future challenges or stressors, achieving goals, personal growth. The proactive model holds that people are not passive actors, but they are capable of using effective problem-based strategies in the face of stress, though much is also dependent on the type of stressor and appraised amount of control over it.

Buffers to stress

Psychologists and sociologists have both contributed to theory and research in relation to social (e.g. social support), psychological and personality characteristics acting as *moderators* or *buffers* to reduce the impact of stress. The buffering hypothesis postulates that social support affects health by protecting the person against the negative impact of stress, through, for example, the potential for offering resources such as financial or practical assistance and/or emotional support. The cognitive appraisal model builds on these factors. Thus, availability of support influences the individual's appraisal of the stressor. The alternative theory is known as the main effect hypothesis, and holds that it is the social support itself which is beneficial and reduces the impact of the stressor, and its absence acts as a stressor. Social support has been variously defined, ranging from definitions emphasising the availability of someone who offers comfort, to those which emphasise satisfaction with available support (Sarason *et al.* 1983; Wallston *et al.* 1983; Wills 1985; Bowling 1994). There are several structured measurement scales for measuring social networks and social support (see Bowling 2005a), though there is little consensus over the domains of support which should be measured in relation to health and illness. Social support is encompassed within the broader concept of social capital. This can be defined as the community's reciprocal social support networks and resources, and is embodied in measures of social networks, social support and the availability of community resources (e.g. neighbourliness, recreational and leisure facilities, safety). Evidence to support the moderating effects of social capital on health is inconclusive (Lynch *et al.* 2000; Wilkinson 2000).

Sociology, stress and the management of illness

The focus of sociology differs from that of psychology in the study of social stress. In addition, different schools of thought focus on different aspects of stress. For example, positivist sociologists focus on the social system itself as a potential source of stress and consequent illness or even suicide patterns (e.g. during periods of economic booms and downturns) (Brenner 1987a, 1987b). In contrast, social interactionists concentrate on the concept of 'self', the stress arising from conflicting self-images (William I. Thomas (see Volkart 1951); Goffman 1959; Cooley 1964; and see Chapter 6) and the process of being discredited by others, with the risk of consequent lowered self-esteem (e.g. as in studies of social stigma and illness). These investigations focus on society's labelling of, and reactions to, the ill (deviant) person (known as labelling and deviance theory) (see Scambler and Hopkins 1986).

Research derived from social interactionist theories uses qualitative research methods and focuses more on how people *manage* their lives when suffering from illness (Charmaz 1983), and what they do when faced with illness (coping strategies and styles) (Bury 1991). (See Box 2.2.) Rich examples include Bury's (1988) study of the experience of arthritis (and see the collected volumes on experiencing illness edited by Anderson and Bury 1988 and Abel *et al.* 1993). Sociologists have reported that it is only when people are no longer able to carry out social roles normally that they reorganise their lives and reconstruct them to create for themselves a new normality (see Radley 1989; Sidell 1995).

Box 2.2 A study of the patient's experience of illness

In the late 1950s, a group of sociologists who were trained at the University of Chicago, began to examine illness from the patient's perspective, in contrast to the dominant 'Sick Role' model, that assumed the dominance of the medical perspective. Patients were seen as active agents, often with conflicting perspectives to doctors. The sociologists' emphasis was on the social and psychological experiences of people living with chronic illness, their 'illness trajectories', and how, despite their illness, these people managed to live as normal a life as possible (Strauss and Glaser 1975). From such work, the sociology of the experience of illness and its management in everyday life was developed (Conrad and Bury 1997).

Sociological research on the management of illness also focuses on the construction of dependency by society. For example, social handicaps are created by society not adapting or equipping itself to enable frail elderly people to get about outside their homes easily (see Phillips 1986; Grundy and Bowling 1991). This situation is known as the creation of structured dependency (Walker 1987), and is highly relevant to public policy-making.

Stigma, normalisation and adjustment

In relation to understanding the process of chronic illness, positivist sociologists have concentrated on the relationship of individuals with the social system, and have drawn on Parsons's (1951) theory of the Sick Role. Symbolic interactionists have focused on the meaning of illness to individuals, and the effects of being labelled as ill (or 'deviant') by society. The latter perspective has leant heavily on Goffman's (1968) work on stigma, on the sociology of deviance (Becker 1963; Lemert 1967) and on the effects on social interaction:

> Social groups create deviance by making the rules whose infraction constitutes deviance, and by applying those rules to particular people and labelling them as outsiders. From this point of view, deviance is not a quality of the act the person commits, but rather a consequence of the application by others of rules and sanctions to an 'offender'.
>
> (Becker 1963)

Thus, deviance occurs when people perceive, interpret and respond to the behaviour or appearance (e.g. a physical deformity) as deviant. (See Box 2.3.) Scambler (2009) re-emphasised the importance of Goffman's work in relation to understanding the stigma of HIV and epilepsy.

Box 2.3 The consequences of labelling: a study

One of the most important studies of the powerful nature and consequences of labelling was Rosenhan's (1973) 'On being sane in insane places'. This was a participant observation study in the USA, in which eight 'pseudo-patients', including the author (a psychology graduate student, three psychologists, a paediatrician, a psychiatrist, a painter and a housewife), feigned psychiatric symptoms (e.g. hearing voices) and were admitted to psychiatric wards in different hospitals. Immediately they were admitted, they stopped simulating any symptoms of abnormality and behaved 'normally'. When asked, they informed the staff that they no longer experienced any symptoms. All but one of the eight were diagnosed as schizophrenic on admission, and on discharge were labelled as having schizophrenia 'in remission' (i.e. the label had 'stuck'). Their length of hospitalisation ranged from 7 to 52 days (and discharge was not always easy for them to negotiate). As Rosenhan described, having been given the label of schizophrenic, there was nothing that the pseudo-patients could do to remove it, and it profoundly affected other people's perceptions of them. He clearly described the powerlessness and depersonalisation experienced, and the feeling that they were treated by staff as though they were 'invisible'. This is an example of the insights that can be obtained from covert participant observation.

Stigma and normalisation

One method of categorising *coping* and *adjustment* processes is in relation to the labelling of the person as ill and 'deviant', and the amount of *stigma* (the social reaction which leads to a spoilt identity and label of deviant) attached to the condition. Another area of research is the management strategies of people with illnesses (e.g. chronic illnesses) who try to present themselves as 'normal', rather than as deviants from societal norms (see Charmaz 1983). Social interactionists are interested in people's strategies for trying to minimise any social stigma associated with their illness and to reduce the likelihood of their identities being characterised with the condition. There may be several motives for this behaviour – fear of losing employment if the condition was discovered or thought to interfere with work, as well as the fear of social rejection and discrimination. Scambler (1984), on the basis of his qualitative interview study, described how people given a diagnosis of epilepsy tried to negotiate a change of diagnosis with their doctors in order to avoid the felt stigma associated with the diagnosis, and fear of discrimination due to cultural unacceptability.

Williams's (1990) research based on 70 people aged over 60 clearly demonstrated the value of qualitative interviews for exploring this topic. One of the themes of illness that occurred was 'illness as controlled by normal living'. He described the belief among elderly people with chronic illnesses that 'they could maintain their normal way of life against all odds by sheer moral effort'. His interviewees reported the need to normalise simply in order to cope: 'If I keep up my normal activity, I help myself to prevent or cope with illness'; 'If I do not keep up my normal activity, I make my condition worse.'

The concepts of 'passing', 'covering' (Goffman 1968) and 'secret adjustment' (Schneider and Conrad 1981) have been ascribed to individuals who manage their condition by concealing it. Pragmatic adjustment attempts to minimise the impact of the condition on life while being open about the condition when necessary (e.g. informing employers, family and friends). 'Quasi-liberated' adjustment is where the sufferer openly informs others of his or her condition in a manner which attempts to educate them (Schneider and Conrad 1981). Qualitative research has provided many rich insights in this area.

Adjustment

Social interactionists are critical of the concept of *adjustment*, in which people with illnesses are encouraged to accept themselves as 'normal', and work hard to fulfil role expectations, while simultaneously being told that they are 'different' – i.e. to be 'good deviants' (Goffman 1968; Williams 1987). The expectation of adjustment is viewed as unkind and unfair:

> The stigmatised individual is asked to act so as to imply neither that his burden is heavy nor that bearing it has made him different from us; at the same time he must keep himself at that remove from us which ensures our painlessly being able to confirm this belief about him.
>
> (Goffman 1968)

This concept of adjustment operates as a form of social control. For example, health professionals may attempt to help people to accept their problems and to make a 'good adjustment' to them (Williams 1987). Adjustment can create difficulties in longitudinal research designs, as well as in experiments with pre- and post-testing. If people change their standards and values as they adjust to their condition, then measures of perceptions (e.g. health status, quality of life) are affected by this (known as 'response-shift') (Sprangers and Schwartz 1999).

The Sick Role and illness behaviour

The Sick Role

The Sick Role is based on a functionalist theory of society which focuses on social systems as a whole, and analyses how each aspect is placed in the system, how it is related to other aspects of the system and what the consequences are (Parsons 1951). The Sick Role treats sickness as a form of social deviance, which has violated a norm of behaviour, and is dysfunctional to society. Norms are socially important because they help to define the boundaries of a social system. The Sick Role is conceptualised as a social 'niche' where people who are ill are given a chance to recover in order to return to their normal social roles. The doctor's role is to legitimise the status of sickness. Parsons was the first social scientist to describe this social control function of medicine within a social system. The Sick Role carries two rights and obligations for the sick person: there is exemption from normal social roles and responsibilities and no blame for failure to fulfil them. In return, the individual must want to return to normal roles and must cooperate with health professionals, with the aim of recovery. The Sick Role is functional for society because the individual is permitted to break the rules, but only if the obligations (which are functional for society) are met.

Criticisms of the concept of the Sick Role

Deviance theory (interactionism) disputes that there is an automatic response to the breaking of rules (deviant behaviour, in this case, illness). What happens next depends on how responsible people are perceived to be for their deviance. The absent worker is treated differently according to whether he or she has pneumonia or is thought to be lazy or evading work or responsibility. Despite the merits of this framework, it does not explain what causes the deviant behaviour itself, apart from other people's reaction to it, and societal reaction alone cannot be an adequate causative model.

Parsons's (1951) concept of the Sick Role has been criticised for failing to take account of the variation in human behaviour and cultural norms when confronted by illness, and for failing to take chronic illness into account. For example, the temporary exemption from normal responsibilities in exchange for the obligation to get well is absent in the case of chronic illnesses, which are not temporary conditions (Mechanic 1959). It has also been criticised for failing to take account of stigmatising conditions (e.g. psychiatric illness) where there may be concealment rather than help-seeking behaviour. Friedson (1970) attempted to adapt the model in the light of criticisms, but Gerhardt (1987) has argued that these criticisms are misplaced. She pointed out that the issue is one of approximation, and people with a chronic illness can be permanently, rather than temporarily, exempted from certain duties. The theory is meant to be one of approximation. As such, it should be seen as an 'ideal type' of the Sick Role – an abstraction, and a basis for comparing and differentiating behaviours in societies (Gerhardt 1987).

Illness behaviour

Kasl and Cobb (1966) defined illness behaviour as behaviour aimed at seeking treatment (e.g. consulting a doctor), and sick role behaviour as activity aimed at recovery (e.g. taking the medication). Health behaviour was defined in relation to action taken to maintain health and prevent ill health. Mechanic (1978) defined illness behaviour more broadly in relation to the perception and evaluation of symptoms, and action taken (or not) when experiencing ill health. How people perceive and react to illness depends on their perception of deviance from a standard of normality, which is established by their everyday experiences (Saunders 1954).

Numerous early classic structured surveys and qualitative accounts documented how the amount of morbidity reported to doctors represented just the tip of the clinical iceberg of disease in the community (e.g. Koos 1954; Wadsworth et al. 1971; Dunnell and Cartwright 1972). This inspired subsequent research on why people do or do not consult doctors over health problems.

Social and structural influences on illness behaviour

There are two main approaches to the study of illness behaviour in the literature:

- those which focus on social and structural influences (e.g. social class, age, gender) on the decisions people make about health and illness;
- those which concentrate on the psychological characteristics of people, their learned coping responses and skills, and triggers to action.

Such a distinction is often blurred, and the models overlap, though the difference in emphasis within the models tends to lead to competing, rather than complementary, explanations.

Socio-demographic influences on behaviour

Medical sociology has focused on illness and health behaviour, and the influences of socio-demographic variables (e.g. age, sex, ethnicity, income, level of education, socio-economic group, people's network of social relationships and their support and referral functions). Research is based on both quantitative and qualitative methods.

Gender

Numerous quantitative surveys in Europe and North America have shown that women report more illness and have higher rates of medical consultations than men. However, men have higher mortality patterns than women in every age group. Theories of illness behaviour postulate that it is culturally more acceptable for women to admit to feeling ill, to report distress and to seek help (Nathanson 1975, 1977). There are several feminist critiques of the conventional interpretations of higher morbidity and consultation rates among women, as well as of medical accounts of the biological weaknesses and dependence of women, and of the inclination of doctors to treat problems presented by women less seriously than those presented by men (see Jones 1994).

Socio-economic status

Because of the evidence that health varies according to socio-economic status, and people in the lower social classes are most at risk of ill health, but least likely to use preventive services and adopt healthier lifestyles, theory and research have focused on socio-economic factors. One theory employed by sociologists is the culture of poverty explanation (see Rundall and Wheeler 1979). According to this theory, communities that experience poverty and low status develop a response based on powerlessness, passivity and fatalism, and health is a low priority in the face of other life problems related to poverty (McKinlay and McKinlay 1972).

The concept suggests that poorer people do not have a positive image of society's organisations, including professional services, partly owing to their relative powerlessness within the social system; they develop a mistrust of modern medicine, and are therefore more reluctant than other social groups to use health and preventive services in relation to the volume as much as they need to. They are also less knowledgeable than middle-class patients about how to gain access to services and to communicate effectively with doctors (Bochner 1983). Such groups accept low levels of health and their culture is incompatible with a future-oriented, preventive view of health. The social and cultural distance between doctors and patients in lower socio-economic groups reinforces this reluctance (Friedson 1970). Poorer people are also more likely to have to continue functioning, rather than rest, due to loss of income if they take time off work. However, changes in the economy have blurred the distinctions between social groups (Parkin 1979), making such theories over-simplistic.

Another main theory is the cost–benefit approach (Le Grand 1982). This stresses the different costs and benefits involved in the use of services, as perceived by people from different social backgrounds. One such cost is time. For example, those on lower incomes are more likely to be dependent on public transport and have further to travel to health care facilities; they are more likely to be in manual occupations where they lose wages for time taken off work, and thus they incur greater costs than middle-class people, which acts as a disincentive to consultation. This theory was favoured by the Black Report on inequalities in health in Britain (Townsend and Davidson 1982).

A predictive model of help-seeking was developed by Anderson *et al.* (1975), based on the predisposing (e.g. socio-demographic variables, attitudes and beliefs), enabling (e.g. income in relation to private health services, availability of, and access to, services) and need components that are said to influence a person's decision to use services. Most research has reported that the need component of the model (e.g. perception of symptom severity) has the most predictive power. However, as Cockerham (1995) has pointed out, this is a predictive model, rather than one which develops an understanding of the actual processes of why behaviours occur.

Psychological influences on illness behaviour

The decision to seek professional help in the face of illness is the result of a complex series of psychological and social processes, depending on the person's values, models of health behaviour and culture. Mechanic's (1978) model lists ten heterogeneous variables, which, he hypothesised, affected the response to illness, based on the theory that illness behaviour is a culturally learned response. The variables are: visibility, recognisability or perceptual salience of symptoms; the perceived seriousness of symptoms; the extent to which symptoms disrupt family, work and social activities; the frequency of the appearance, or recurrence, of symptoms, and their persistence; the tolerance threshold of those exposed to the symptoms and those who evaluate them; available information, knowledge and cultural assumptions and understandings of the evaluator; perceptual needs which lead to autistic psychological processes (e.g. denial); needs competing with the response to illness; competing interpretations of the symptoms; availability of, and physical proximity to, treatment; and the psychological and financial costs of taking action.

While health may be a social goal felt in common by all groups, the salience of health to individuals needs to be assessed relative to other goals, depending on their values and beliefs. The place of health in a person's value system may be reflected in his or her definitions of health or illness, though these are often complex (see early research by Koos 1954 and Herzlich 1973, for insightful examples). Such definitions inevitably vary according to culture (i.e. a set of beliefs and behaviour shared by a specific group). There are many examples from qualitative interview and quantitative survey research in anthropology, psychology and sociology which illustrate cultural variations in relation to definitions and perceptions of, and actions towards, health and illness (Zborowski 1952; Zola 1966; Wolff and Langley 1977).

The interactionist approach

Critics of the positivist models presented here argue that socio-demographic and psychological variables explain a relatively small percentage of people's behaviour and attitudes. Instead, explanation must again be sought in the areas of social interaction and role (Wadsworth et al. 1971), and the meaning of situations to individuals. Robinson's (1971) work in this area was based on qualitative interviews and provided many insightful examples of how individual situations and interpretations influenced the course of action taken (also see earlier section on sociology, stress and the management of illness).

2.3 Models of health behaviour

Health lifestyles

There is increasing interest in ways of living that can affect health ('health lifestyles'). Health lifestyles can be defined as voluntary health behaviour based on making choices from the alternatives that are available in individual situations (Cockerham et al. 1993). Examples range from medical consultations to decisions about diet, smoking, alcohol intake, exercise and other disease-preventive and health-promoting activities, according to prevailing scientific paradigms. People aim for good health in order to use it, for example, for a longer life, sexual attractiveness, optimum functioning and quality of life (Cockerham 1995). This is consistent with research on people's definitions of health and perceptions of health as a means to an end (e.g. achievement of vitality, ability to work) (d'Houtard and Field 1984).

Those in the higher socio-economic groups are more likely to pursue healthy lifestyles than those in the lower groups. Lifestyles are partly determined by the person's access to financial resources to support the chosen lifestyle. A wide range of factors, over which individuals have relatively little control, also need to be drawn into the equation (e.g. pollution, food pricing, availability of sports facilities). There are critiques of society's emphasis on healthy lifestyles, on the grounds that this emphasis on individual responsibility for health excuses society as a whole from accountability and responsibility for health issues (Waitzkin 1983; Navarro 1986). Much of the research in this field has been quantitative, and based on structured survey techniques. The standard scales for measuring health behaviour and socio-demographic characteristics have been compiled by de Bruin *et al.* (1996). This research shows a great deal of inconsistency between different health behaviours and between attitudes and behaviour; for example, people may smoke cigarettes and exercise, or dislike cigarette smoke in public places and smoke themselves, and so on (Mechanic 1979; Stroebe 2000). Studies that have been based on semi-structured and unstructured, in-depth interview techniques have provided deeper insights into why people adopt unhealthy practices. For example, Graham's (1976) unstructured interviews with young working-class women, who were regular smokers and had children aged under 5, showed that smoking was important to them because it was the one thing they felt they could choose to do for themselves, as opposed to responding to the demands of their children (hence it was a response to social circumstances).

Adherence

Some bio-medical studies of health behaviour simply report associations between adherence to health advice and education, fear of illness and of side-effects. Few studies have been truly insightful of lay perspectives (Currer and Stacey 1986); most have assumed that adherence is 'rational' behaviour, without full exploration of lay reasonings; few have explored, in-depth, the perspectives of patients who have rejected medicines (Campbell *et al.* 2011).

Models of adherence can be complex. It should be noted that the term was changed to 'adherence' in a move away from the medical perspective of 'compliance' with advice or treatment from health professionals. However, some investigators have now moved on from 'adherence' and use the term 'concordance' instead. This can be problematic as the terms are not synonymous. Concordance is more concerned with the nature of interactions between patients and health professionals, than behaviour (Bell *et al.* 2007).

A major theory is that adherence is influenced by a person's perceptions of control over the condition and sense of self-efficacy (Mailbach *et al.* 1991; Patel and Taylor 2002). Models of behaviour and behaviour change, in relation to the literature on healthy lifestyles and health promotion, also need consideration (Ogden 1996; Stroebe and Stroebe 1995). Most relevant are models which not only focus on intention and motivations to behave, self-efficacy, perceived control, and the timeliness of cues to the behaviour, but include the individual's level of information, perceived skills for the behaviour, positive affect towards it, consistency of the behaviour with self-image, and environmental and societal barriers, including the role of social support and pressure (Elder *et al.* 1999). The use of a sound theoretical framework, which integrates relevant models, underpins rigorous research and policy, and increases understanding of health-related behaviour. It is essential for progress in the design of health promotion programmes (Skinner 1992) and such a partnership – between a social scientist, with expertise in investigating lay views, and professionals in public health and epidemiology – is ideally placed to make such progress.

Health behaviour

Promoting health and living healthily, as well as understanding people's illness behaviour, is an important area of investigation in medical sociology and health psychology. Kasl and Cobb (1966) distinguished health behaviour from illness and Sick Role behaviour, defining the former as an activity undertaken by a person who believes him or herself to be healthy for the purpose of preventing disease or detecting it at an asymptomatic stage. Other conceptualisations of health behaviour incorporate actions undertaken regardless of health status to prevent disease, actions undertaken to promote health, and both medically approved and lay actions, regardless of their effectiveness (see Bowling 1989; Edelmann 2000).

Although Kasl and Cobb defined health behaviour in terms of the intention of the individual, most researchers have interpreted this in relation to medically approved practices and use of health services. A lay perspective was incorporated into the model by Harris and Guten (1979). They defined 'health protective behaviour' as any behaviour performed by a person in order to protect, promote or maintain his or her health, regardless of his or her perceived health status, and regardless of whether the behaviour is effective. Other models include self-care within the concept, and distinguish between behaviour intended to reduce the risk of disease and behaviour intended to promote health (Berkanovic 1982; Stott and Pill 1983; Anderson 1989).

Models of health-related actions

The various models of behaviour used by psychologists in order to analyse how people view and react to health-related events have been critically reviewed and their implications discussed by Stroebe and Stroebe (1995) and Ogden (1996). They are briefly described here.

Apart from attribution theory and the health locus of control model, for which measurement scales have been developed (Wallston *et al.* 1976, 1978), the testing of other theories has relied on investigators selecting their own appropriate measurement items to include in questionnaires (e.g. symptom severity scales to measure the perceived severity of a condition). The approaches are generally quantitative and most instruments are untested. Research strategies in this area have been reviewed by Sheeran and Abraham (1995). The most widely used instrument is Wallston *et al.*'s (1976, 1978) multi-dimensional health locus of control scales. These are based on a six-point Likert-type response scale. Respondents indicate the extent of their agreement with a series of statements (e.g. 'If I get sick, it is my own behaviour which determines how soon I get well again'; 'No matter what I do, if I am going to get sick, I will get sick'). However, this scale does not reflect the revisions to the model (see below).

Partly due to the large body of inconsistent research results from studies aiming to explain and predict health-promoting behaviours and beliefs, psychologists increasingly prefer to measure perceived self-efficacy rather than perceived control over life. Self-efficacy represents the belief that one can change risky health behaviours by personal action (Scheirer and Carver 1985, 1987; Schwarzer and Fuchs 1995). The most well-used scales of self-efficacy are the Generalised Self-efficacy Scale (Jerusalem and Schwarzer 1992) and Scheirer and Carver's (1985) Self-efficacy Scale. A range of available measures is included in Schwarzer (1993) and Johnson *et al.* (1995).

Health belief model

The health belief model is one of the most influential theories of health-related actions. It postulates that people's behaviour in relation to health is related to their perceptions of the severity of an illness, their susceptibility to it and the costs and benefits incurred in following a particular course of action. Behaviour may also depend on a trigger, such as a symptom of ill health (Rosenstock 1966, 1974; Becker 1974). This model is used to understand people's use of preventive health measures and services, as well as their response to symptoms and adherence with prescribed therapies. The model holds that socio-demographic, social and psychological factors are likely to modify health beliefs.

The criticisms of the health belief model include its focus on rationality and the exclusion of emotions such as fear and denial (see Ogden 1996). Consequently, Becker and Rosenstock (1987) revised the model to include self-efficacy (i.e. beliefs in one's ability to perform the action).

Attribution theory

Attribution theory, which has been applied to health behaviours, holds that people try to view the social world as predictable and controllable. Kelley (1972) argued that attributions about causes of a phenomenon are made by individuals in relation to how specific the cause of the phenomenon is to the person, the extent to which the attribution is shared by others, the consistency of the attribution over time and in different settings. These criteria are argued to determine whether the cause of the phenomenon is perceived to be internal or external to the control of the individual.

Locus of control

Social learning theory proposed that the likelihood of a behaviour occurring in a specific situation is a function of an expectation that the behaviour will lead to a particular reinforcement, and the extent to which that reinforcement is valued (Rotter 1954).

One type of expectancy is the locus of control. Control can be categorised as internal (e.g. information, ability, urge) or external (e.g. opportunity, dependence on others) to the person (Ajzen 1988), and is influenced by the person's expectations of the outcome. With this theory a person's locus of control has the greatest explanatory power over whether a person will engage in preventive health behaviour (Wallston et al. 1976, 1978; Langlie 1977; Lau and Ware 1981; Wallston and Wallston 1981); internal locus of control in turn has been associated with self-esteem (Hallal 1982). Overall, however, results from research examining the relationship between locus of control and preventative health behaviours have been disappointing, partly due to the omission of assessing the value of health to respondents (Edelmann 2000).

Protection motivation theory

The protection motivation model postulates that the motivation or intention to engage in health-protecting behaviour depends on the multiplicative concepts of perceived severity of the ill health, the perceived probability of the occurrence of ill health and the likelihood of the protective behaviour to avert ill health (Rogers and Mewborn 1976).

Additional determinants of protection motivation have since been added to the theory, including the concept of self-efficacy (Rogers 1983; Rippetoe and Rogers 1987). The central hypothesis is that motivation to protect health stems from the linear function of the severity of the threat, personal vulnerability, the ability to carry out the behaviour, and the effectiveness of the behaviour in reducing the threat of ill health. It also incorporates the notion that motivation will be negatively influenced by the costs of the protective behaviour and the rewards associated with not undertaking it.

Theory of reasoned action

The theory of reasoned action is a general psychological theory of behaviour which assumes that the intention to undertake a behaviour is determined by the person's attitude towards it, which is determined by his or her beliefs about the consequences of the behaviour, and by subjective norms (e.g. important others' expectations about the person's behaviour) (see Eagly and Chaiken 1993). Several studies have reported that the prediction of behaviour is improved by including reported past behaviour in the model, and that this has greater explanatory power than intention (see Stroebe and Stroebe 1995, for a brief review). Debate has focused on the determinants of past behaviour (e.g. motivation) and the amount of control people have over their behaviour.

The theory of reasoned action is superior in its predictive power to the health belief model, but it has been criticised because it ignores the social nature of human behaviour, and the social and economic influences on it (Kippax and Crawford 1993; see review by Taylor et al. 2006).

Theory of planned behaviour

The theory of planned behaviour (TPB) is an extension of the theory of reasoned action (Ajzen 1988, 1991), derived from social cognition theory (Bandura 1977). It includes perceived control over the behaviour, as well as the attitude towards the behaviour (i.e. an evaluation about its outcome) and subjective norms (i.e. social norms and pressures to carry out the behaviour). This assumes that perceived control can affect intentions and thus affect behaviour, i.e. people adjust their intentions according to estimates of their likely achievement and therefore in relation to their ability. The theory also includes components which assume that individuals do not always have complete control over their actions due to external influences, such as financial position and provision of ill-health retirement schemes; however, it does not include a temporal element (Schwarzer 1992). Francis et al. (2004) have produced a manual outlining the stages of questionnaire construction based on the TPB.

Thus, in relation to health behaviour and reaction to illness or disability, according to the TPB, it is not the circumstances of the individual that predict what they can do, but their attitude towards these. Intention is the most important antecedent of behaviour, and is influenced by subjective norms (e.g. the influence of family and peers), attitudes, expectations of future health and ability, self-efficacy and perceived control over the situation (Bandura 1986). While the evidence in support of the predictive power of the TPB, as well as that in support of the theory of reasoned action, is superior to that of the health belief model, there are limitations (Taylor et al. 2006). There is still a gap between intent and behaviour. (See Box 2.4.).

> ## Box 2.4 A behaviour change wheel
>
> Mitchie *et al.* (2011) stated that improving the public's health depends on coordinated sets of activities, or interventions, aimed at changing patterns of behaviour (e.g. smoking cessation advice by health professionals). They argued that many are based on common-sense notions of behaviour, rather than theoretical models of mechanisms for action. Even the most commonly used models such as the theory of planned behaviour and the health belief model, do not address the roles of impulse, habit, self-control, associative learning and emotional processing (Mitchie *et al.* 2011). Consequently, Mitchie *et al.* undertook a systematic search of the literature, plus consultations with experts, in order to identify frameworks of behaviour change interventions. They were assessed in relation to comprehensiveness, coherence, and a clear link to a model of behaviour. They identified 19 frameworks, covering nine intervention functions and seven policy categories. None of the frameworks covered the full range of intervention functions or policies, and a minority met the criteria of coherence or linkage to a model of behaviour. They concluded that most designers of health behaviour interventions do not use existing frameworks to underpin their development, or to analyse why interventions fail or succeed. A possible reason is that existing frameworks did not meet their needs.
>
> Mitchie *et al.* then developed a new framework of behaviour, drawing on a unifying theory of motivation, involving three 'essential' conditions:
>
> 1 capability
> 2 opportunity
> 3 motivation.
>
> These formed the hub of their proposed 'behaviour change wheel'. This incorporated nine intervention functions and seven categories of policy that could enable the interventions to take place. It was initially tested for reliability, with satisfactory results, by classifying components of governmental tobacco control strategy and guidance on reduction of obesity. Developmental work is ongoing.

Health action process model

The health action process model was developed by Schwarzer (1992), who saw the need for a temporal element in understanding health beliefs and behaviour. This model also includes self-efficacy as a determinant of intended and actual behaviour, in addition to criteria from previous models. It incorporates a decision-making stage (motivational stage) and an action stage (plans to initiate and maintain the behaviour). The motivational stage includes self-efficacy (e.g. confidence in ability to carry out the behaviour), expectancy of outcome (e.g. benefits) and appraisal of threat (e.g. beliefs about the severity of an illness and personal vulnerability). The action stage comprises cognitive (volitional), situational and behavioural factors which determine the initiation and maintenance of the behaviour. This model omits consideration of irrationality and the external social world (see Ogden 1996).

Trans-theoretical model of behaviour change

The trans-theoretical model of behaviour change uses a temporal dimension (stages of change construct) to link together concepts drawn from a range of theories (Prochasksa and DiClemente 1992; Prochaska and Velicer 1997). It was developed in relation to understanding and promoting behaviour change in the context of smoking. The model consists of ten processes of change (consciousness raising, dramatic relief, environmental re-evaluation, self-re-evaluation, social liberation, self-liberation, counter-conditioning, helping relationships, reinforcement management, stimulus control), decisional balance (of the pros and the cons of problem behaviour), and self-efficacy for behaviour change (confidence, temptation) which influence six proposed stages of change (pre-contemplation, contemplation, preparation, action, maintenance, termination). The model has been popular in health promotion, though it has also attracted criticism about its ability to integrate social and economic factors and the validity of its construct of the stages of change. The limitations of the model, along with other models of behaviour change, have been described in detail by Taylor *et al.* (2006).

Spontaneous processing model

The spontaneous processing model is based on the absence of conscious thought. It is argued that spontaneity is influenced by (strong) attitudes towards the targets of the action. With this theory, once a person has accessed a strong attitude automatically, it is believed to exert a selective influence on his or her perception of the attitude object (Fazio 1990). This model is less developed than the others and Stroebe and Stroebe (1995) argued that it should be regarded as a supplement to existing models rather than an alternative.

Stainton Rogers (1993) has argued that these models are too simplistic as people use different explanations of health at different time periods, depending on the circumstances. This view has been confirmed in research by Backett and Davison (1992) and Blaxter (1990) which found, for example, that older people were less likely to be responsive to health promotion messages than younger people. This literature has been reviewed by Sidell (1995). However, the models (e.g. the health belief model) do generally take account of the variation in beliefs according to socio-demographic factors.

Summary of main points

- The aim of research on health is to understand how people become ill, their perceptions, behaviours and experiences in relation to health and the effects of illness.
- Sociologists have focused on variations in definitions of health and illness and the experience of illness in relation to the social system, and in particular by socio-economic group.
- Psychologists have focused on cognitive processes, psychological characteristics and personality.
- The decision to seek professional help once a health problem has been acknowledged is the result of a complex series of psychological and social processes.
- Health behaviour is an activity undertaken for the purpose of preventing disease, or detecting it at an asymptomatic stage, and to promote health.
- Models of health behaviour are variously based on a person's perceptions of the severity of the condition, costs and benefits of action, strength of attitudes, triggers to action, locus of control, expectations, past experiences, perceived success of possible action, confidence, and the perceived consequences of the behaviour.

Key questions

1 What is the difference between illness behaviour and health behaviour?
2 What is the health belief model and variants of it?
3 How can socio-economic status be measured?
4 Distinguish between the medical model of dis-ease and the social model of disease.
5 Why is it important for health services professionals to understand lay theories of health and illness and the influences on professional help-seeking?

Key terms

bio-medical model of disease
compensate, select, optimise
coping
functionalism
health behaviour
health belief model
health lifestyles
illness behaviour
locus of control

phenomenology
positivism
psycho-social stress
self-efficacy
self-management
Sick Role
social model of dis-ease
social stratification
stigma

Recommended reading

Cockerham, W.C. (1995) *Medical Sociology*, 6th edn. Englewood Cliffs, NJ: Prentice Hall.

Cockerham, W.C. and Scambler, G. (2010) Medical sociology and sociological theory, in W.C. Cockerham (ed.) *The New Blackwell Companion to Medical Sociology*. Chichester: Wiley-Blackwell, pp. 3–26.

Ogden, J. (1996) *Health Psychology: A Textbook*. Buckingham: Open University Press.

Scambler, G. (2009) Health-related stigma *Sociology of Health & Illness*, 31: 441–5.

CHAPTER 3

Quality of life: concepts, measurements and patient perception

Introduction

The emphasis on evidence-based practice, and patient-/client-based outcome measures, has led to an increase in the use of health-related, disease-/condition-specific, and generic (broader) measures of quality of life (QoL) in service evaluations. There has been much conceptual confusion between the distinct terms 'health-related quality of life' and the 'broader quality of life', and some investigators use the terms interchangeably. Others use the term 'quality of life' to refer to health status, or measure health status incorrectly with a quality of life measures. Lack of conceptual clarity has led to the widespread use of outcome measures that fail to match the aims of the study.

3.1 Health-related and broader quality of life

Health-related quality of life

It was pointed out in Chapter 1 that it is important to measure health-related quality of life when assessing health outcomes. Investigators have identified a wide range of domains of health-related quality of life, including emotional well-being (e.g. measured with indicators of life satisfaction and self-esteem), psychological well-being (e.g. measured with indicators of anxiety and depression), physical well-being (e.g. measured with measures of physical health status and physical functioning), and social well-being (e.g. measured with indicators of social network structure and support, community integration, functioning in social roles). The domains have been described elsewhere (Bowling 1996b, 1996c, 2005a). Some investigators prefer to use measures of quality of life that are specific to diseases/conditions, which may be more sensitive to the latter, though such use prevents comparisons being made across conditions.

Numerous measurement scales of psychological health, physical health status and physical functioning have been developed for the assessment of health outcomes. Generally, there is a large degree of overlap between the measures within each of these domains, though disagreement exists about content. A commonly used proxy indicator of health-related quality of life is the SF-36 (Ware *et al.* 1993, 1997a), which was developed to measure broader health status. A more recent instrument, developed across cultures, is the WHOQOL (WHOQOL Group 1998a, 1998b).

Most debate occurs in relation to the appropriate domains of emotional and social well-being which should be included in the measurement of health outcomes. For example, satisfaction with life has become a key variable in analyses of the emotional well-being of older, but not younger, people (see Bowling 2005a, for reviews). Related concepts which are often included in these investigations are happiness and morale (Bradburn 1969; Lawton 1972; Campbell *et al.* 1976), self-esteem (Wells and Marwell 1976), and control over life (Baltes and Baltes 1990; see Bowling 1993a). Measurement scales in relation to these concepts have been developed, mainly for use in social gerontology (see Bowling 2005a). Social well-being is also a key component of health-related quality of life, in relation to the availability of practical and emotional support that is perceived by the individual to be satisfying. The analysis of social outcomes in relation to the role of social support has received increasing attention as health and social care has increasingly shifted from hospital to community (Emerson and Hatton 1994). Again, a wide range of measurement scales has been developed that tap a range of domains, though there is little consensus over which are the most appropriate indicators in relation to health. Readers who are interested in pursuing the issue of the appropriate domains of measurement in psychological, physical, emotional and social areas of well-being are referred to Bowling (1994, 2005a). Caution is needed when interpreting longitudinal or experimental (with pre-/post-testing) datasets because follow-up measures can be contaminated by response shift, social desirability bias and cognitive dissonance reduction (Sprangers and Schwartz 1999).

Broader quality of life

The growing emphasis on evidence-based practice, and inclusion of patient- or client-based outcome indicators, has led to an increase in the use of health-related and disease-specific measures of QoL in service evaluations. However, few investigators have developed their measures truly 'bottom-up' with the population of interest, and most tend to focus on 'expert opinions'. Thus, most measures have unknown social relevance, and there is no certainty about whether they are measuring the right things. Moreover, definitions of broader QoL often vary by discipline of the investigator, though Lawton (1983, 1991) has developed a popular, multidimensional concept of QoL, represented by behavioural and social competence, perceived QoL, psychological and mental well-being, and the external environment, later expanded for older adults (Lawton 1983, 1994, 1997) to include: behavioural competence, positive and negative affect, objective environment and subjective well-being.

There is increasing recognition of the individual nature of QoL, summed up in the WHOQOL Group's (WHOQOL Group 1993, p. 153) definition:

> an individual's perception of their position in life in the context of the culture and value systems in which they live and in relation to their goals, expectations, and standards and concerns. It is a broad-ranging concept affected in a complex way by the person's physical health, psychological state, level of independence, social relationships, and their relationships to salient features of their environment.

Interventions that are expected to have a broader impact on a person's life, especially with an ageing population and increased longevity, include those that enable more independent living at home. These require broader, multidimensional measures of QoL, which are relevant to people's lives, for the evaluation of both health and socially relevant outcomes. Population – rather than disease – groups requiring broader outcome measures of QoL also include older people, and older recipients of social care. Given the amount of increasing service and research attention being given to quality of life in older age, recent developments in measurement are presented here.

Older people

Government policy is increasingly concerned with enabling older people to maintain their mobility, their independence, their active contribution to society, and to respond effectively to the physical, psychological and social challenges of older age – in effect, to add quality to years of life. This reflects a shift of emphasis away from a traditional view of structured dependency, in which the focus of research was on ill health, functional decline and poverty in older age. It moves towards a positive view of old age as a natural component of the life span, and development of personal fulfilment, though this can still be restricted by limited resources, ill-health or frailty. It also builds on the model of cognitive efficiency proposed by Baltes and Baltes (1990), with its emphasis on control over life, role functioning, cognitive competence, and adaptability to the challenges faced at older ages, consistent with the current focus on reablement in social care (Francis *et al.* 2011). Models of QoL have been heavily influenced by classic measures of life satisfaction, morale and well-being (Bradburn 1969; Lawton 1972; Andrews and Withey 1976; Campbell *et al.* 1976).

Measures of broader quality of life

Three measures of broader quality of life in older age have been developed and tested with good results and are given as examples of broader measurement here: (1) the CASP-19; (2) WHOQOL-OLD; and (3) OPQOL.

CASP-19

CASP-19 (Control, Autonomy, Self-realisation and Pleasure) was developed from the theory of human needs satisfaction, and tested with focus groups and a survey of people aged 65–75 (Hyde *et al.* 2003). It concentrates on four theoretically derived domains (19 items): Control (4 items), Autonomy (5 items), Pleasure (5 items), and Self-realisation (5 items), with four-point Likert response scales 'Often' to 'Never'. It was developed for use with an older population sample, but has also been used in several large population surveys, including the English Longitudinal Survey of Ageing (ELSA) (Blane *et al.* 2008).

Some of the items in CASP-19 are shown below:

My age prevents me from doing the things I would like to

Very often   Sometimes   Not very often   Never

I feel that what happens to me is out of my control

Very often   Sometimes   Not very often   Never

I feel free to plan for the future

Very often   Sometimes   Not very often   Never

WHOQOL-OLD

The WHOQOL-OLD was developed from the parent instrument: the World Health Organisation's WHOQOL Group's WHOQOL-100, and cross-cultural studies (see Power *et al.* 1999); and it was tested on convenience samples of older people across cultures (Power *et al.* 2005). It is a multi-faceted measure of QoL and comprises seven sub-scales (24 items): sensory abilities, autonomy, past, present and future activities, social participation, death and dying, and intimacy (4 items per sub-scale). Response scales are five-point Likert scales and vary in their wording ('Not at all' to 'An extreme amount'/'Completely'/'Extremely'; 'Very poor' to 'Very good'; 'Very dissatisfied' to 'Very satisfied'; 'Very unhappy' to 'Very happy'). The WHOQOL and WHOQOL-OLD have been used with different cultural groups across the world, see http://www.euro.who.int/ageing/quality.

Examples of some of the items in the WHOQOL-OLD are shown below:

How much freedom do you have to make your own decisions?

Not at all   A little   A moderate amount   Very much   An extreme amount

To what extent do you feel in control of your future?

Not at all   A little   A moderate amount   Very much   An extreme amount

How much do you feel that the people around you are respectful of your freedom?

Not at all   A little   A moderate amount   Very much   An extreme amount

OPQOL

The OPQOL – the Older People's Quality of Life questionnaire – is unique in being developed bottom-up from older people's responses to open-ended questioning about the 'good things' that gave life quality. Older people were interviewed about their quality of life in a national population survey, starting with open-ended questions which worked well to elicit people's perceptions of QoL (see Box 3.1) and a sub-sample were followed-up using in-depth interviews.

Box 3.1 Open-ended questions to elicit views of QoL

The questionnaire used a seven-point QoL self-rating scale ranging from 'QoL so good, could not be better' – 'QoL so bad, could not be worse'.

Thinking about your life as a whole, what is it that makes your life good – that is, the things that give your life quality? You may mention as many things as you like.

What is it that makes your life bad – that is the things that reduce the quality in your life? You may mention as many things as you like.

Thinking about all these good and bad things you have just mentioned, which one is the most important to you?

Again, thinking about the good and bad things you have mentioned that make up your quality of life, which of the answers on this card best describes the quality of your life as a whole?

Thinking about all these good and bad things you have just mentioned, which one is the most important to you?

And what single thing would improve the quality of your life?

And what single thing, in your opinion, would improve the overall quality of life for people of your age?

(Bowling (2005a); www.ilcuk.org.uk/files/pdf; accessed September 2013).

Responses were categorised into main themes by two researchers, independently. These were:

- social relationships
- social roles and activities
- activities/hobbies enjoyed alone
- health
- psychological outlook and well-being
- home and neighbourhood
- financial circumstances
- independence.

Detailed sub-themes were also categorised. Smaller numbers of people mentioned a wide range of other things. These responses were consistent with older people's views about what reduced quality of life. The themes and sub-themes are detailed in Bowling (2005a). The sub-scale domains in the OPQOL reflect this common core of main constituents of quality of life.

The full OPQOL is a 32–35 item QoL measure, with the longer version reflecting items also prioritised by ethnically diverse older people in England; it uses five-point Likert scales ranging from 'Strongly agree' to 'Strongly disagree', with 32 or 35 items, representing: life overall (4 items), health (4 items), social relationships and participation (7 items in the QoL follow-up survey, 8 items in the Omnibus surveys), independence, control over life, freedom (5 items), area: home and neighbourhood (4 items), psychological and emotional well-being (4 items), financial circumstances (4 items), religion/culture (2 items) (Bowling 2009a; Bowling and Stenner 2011). The measure has been used with geriatric out-patients, and was able to predict their outcomes (Bilotta *et al.* 2010, 2011, 2012). The OPQOL was shown to have better psychometric properties than two comparable measures of broader QoL for older people: the CASP-19 and the WHOQOL-OLD (Bowling and Stenner 2011). A shorter 13-item version – OPQOL-BRIEF – has also been developed (Bowling *et al.* 2013a). Some of the items are shown below:

I can please myself what I do

Strongly agree   Agree   Neither agree nor disagree   Disagree   Strongly disagree

I have a lot of control over the important things in my life

Strongly agree   Agree   Neither agree nor disagree   Disagree   Strongly disagree

I am healthy enough to have my independence

Strongly agree   Agree   Neither agree nor disagree   Disagree   Strongly disagree

Social care

Given the high costs of providing social care, and in the context of an ageing population, with increasing longevity, commissioners and providers of social care services face an increasing need to demonstrate the effectiveness of their services from the perspectives of the users. This is in addition to their standard quality targets. There is no simple definition of social care, though the term is generally used to describe services provided to people (clients) with assessed needs for social care, whether in their own homes, a day centre or in a care home. These vary widely by country. Services might include assistance with personal hygiene, dressing, going to the toilet, feeding, meals-on-wheels, home care and shopping. Clients include those with physical and/or sensory impairments, learning difficulties and mental health problems including dementia. Netten *et al.* (2012) argued that social care ultimately aims to improve people's QoL – i.e. to compensate people for the effect of their impairments on their QoL, in a way that is enabling, and allows people to make choices about how their needs are met. Measuring outcomes in a social care context, then, includes QoL rather than simply levels of ability, health, employment or housing status (see www.ccpscotland.org/assets; accessed

6 June 2013). Outcomes can be complex to measure in social care because several types of outcomes of both the client and any family carers may be relevant; these may also be affected by multiple factors. Moreover, interventions may require time to influence people's lives, and the appropriate timing of the administration of measurements is crucial in order to detect any changes.

In health research there has long been such pressure, and, as a consequence, a large industry devoted to the development and assessment of patient-based outcome measures (PROMS) has been established. In contrast, social care-specific outcome measures have been comparatively neglected. Most studies of social care outcomes have used a diverse range of outcome measures, including social, physical and mental functioning, life satisfaction, morale, well-being, and health status. The current lack of consensus on conceptualisation, best measurement, and the diversity of approaches used in social care, is problematic for the evaluation of services, and for evidence-synthesis of the cost-effectiveness of interventions. Homogenisation, or the pulling together, of diverse measures in combined datasets for comparative analysis is a time-consuming task, and not always possible when measures have different conceptual backgrounds, aims (e.g. questions about ability vs. performance in measures of functioning), question wording and response choices.

One example of the use of a battery of measures in social care is a prospective study to examine the success of a reablement intervention, designed to help people to re-learn the skills necessary for daily living (Francis *et al.* 2011). Apart from measures relating to changes in service use, which are important to include from a service outcome perspective, the authors also aimed to include measurement of the impact of reablement on people's well-being. They examined this aspect of the outcome of reablement using the following battery of measures: (1) a commonly used and adapted single-item question on perceived global health status on a five-point response scale from 'very good' to 'very bad'; (2) an adaptation of Bowling *et al.*'s (2003) single item on perceived global quality of life on a seven-point scale from 'so good could not be better' to 'so bad it could not be worse'; (3) the Euro-QoL (EQ-5D) (www.euroqol.org/about-eq-5d.html; accessed 6 June 2013); and (4) the Adult Social Care Outcomes Toolkit (ASCOT) (Netten *et al.* 2012).

A systematic review of nine randomised controlled trials of interventions targeting frail elderly people in the community reported that five of these used outcome measurements with unclear psychometric properties, and four used disease-specific measures (Eklund and Wilhelmson 2009). The ASCOT (see Box 3.2) was designed to address this gap in social care QoL outcomes measurement, though it was deliberately developed top-down.

Box 3.2 Adult Social Care Outcomes Toolkit for assessing social care-related QoL (ASCOT)

ASCOT was developed to fill an acknowledged gap in measurement tools, given the absence of dedicated social care outcome measures. The developers argued that studies in social care tend to use health outcome measures, such as the EQ-5D, to assess cost-effectiveness, but these focus on people's functional abilities (such as mobility) rather than the impact of support on their QoL, and are limited in the range of their outcome states. ASCOT was therefore developed to measure the full range of social care outcomes, and was envisaged to be more sensitive than the EQ-5D (Netten *et al.* 2012).

ASCOT was developed deliberately top-down, using an expert review with social care stakeholders to identify attributes and to ensure ASCOT's sensitivity to outcomes of interest to policy-makers and its relevance to the evaluation of social care interventions. It was also based on a literature review of service users' understanding of social care outcomes. Netten *et al.* (2012) and Malley *et al.* (2012) proposed that, in order to measure the value of social care services, a measure should reflect the compensatory activity of social care, be sensitive to client choice, and capture social care-related QoL. They argued that it should reflect those aspects of QoL that are the focus of social care support. Finally, cognitive interviews were conducted to check social care service users' understanding of terms in ASCOT, and clarify items where needed (Netten *et al.* 2012). ASCOT is a multi-attribute preference-weighted measure of social care-related (SCR) QoL. It includes eight distinct attributes: personal cleanliness and comfort, food and drink, control over daily life, personal safety, accommodation cleanliness and comfort, social participation and involvement, occupation, and dignity. ASCOT also includes a preference-weighted measure of social care-related QoL for use in economic evaluations. There is one item per attribute. Each attribute has four response options, reflecting four outcomes. The top two reflect states where outcomes are fully realised but differ in the extent to which respondents have choice over how the outcome is realised, or not. In order to generate a single score for use in cost-effectiveness analyses, it was designed to be preference-weighted to reflect the relative importance of the SCRQoL states (Netten *et al.* 2012). Some evidence for its construct validity has been published (Malley *et al.* 2012). The deliberate top-down development of this measure can be questioned, as while service relevance is important, so is user-relevance to ensure the measure asks the right question.

What are the criteria for a good QoL measure?

The US Food and Drug Administration and the European Medicines Agency have both released guidelines, specifying the minimum criteria for the scientific adequacy of scales used in clinical trials, though some controversies remain (Bottomley *et al.* 2009). The quality of research inferences is inevitably influenced by the appropriateness and robustness of the measurement scale used. Where a situation and intervention can affect life overall, a comprehensive service evaluation requires a broader QoL measurement with a validated measurement scale. While well-designed single-item questions have adequate levels of reliability and validity, none have as good psychometric properties as fuller measurement scales. The latter encompass multiple domains of relevance, and several items, or questions, can balance out people's natural inconsistencies.

Scientific rigour is also required in the development and testing of a measure, including:

- development of a clear conceptual basis underpinning the measure;
- rigour in the research methods used to develop and assess the measure;
- engagement with a diverse range of clients from the outset, to ensure social significance, as well as policy and practice relevance;
- use of adequate and generalisable sample sizes, coverage and types for psychometric testing, and provision of population norms;
- use of gold-standard psychometric testing;
- a convincing trade-off between scale length and levels of psychometric acceptability.

Psychometric testing of outcome measures

Whether a QoL outcome measure is useful or not depends on its psychometric properties. Psychometrics is a well-established scientific field that is concerned with the evaluation of the properties of measures of subjective judgements. A good measure has robust evidence of: (1) its validity (Does the instrument really measure what it purports to measure?); and (2) its reliability (Is the measure stable and internally consistent?). Types of reliability and validity, and factor structure, are described in Chapter 6, and summarised here in relation to QoL measurement; the same criteria apply to all subjective measurement scales, including health-related QoL.

In relation to QoL, the main challenge is that there is no universally accepted definition or conceptual model of QoL. The multiple definitions in existence largely reflect the interests of investigators, apparent experts' views, prevailing theoretical paradigms, and the multitudes of meanings attributed to QoL. A gold standard of QoL does not exist, against which the criterion validity of measures of QoL can be tested.

Other aspects of the validity of QoL measures can be assessed using psychometric gold standards, applied in a methodologically rigorous manner, and scale developers should describe the conceptual model they have used to underpin the measure. Psychometric properties should be examined using classic (or 'traditional') and modern psychometric methods, including the acceptability of the questions to respondents (including data quality such as number of missing items), scaling assumptions, reliability, validity, and responsiveness. These criteria underpin the US Food and Drug Administration's recommendations for patient-reported outcome instrument evaluation (see www.fda.gov/downloads/Drugs/Guidances/UCM193282.pdf; accessed 6 June 2013).

Fitzpatrick et al. (1998) also listed eight criteria that investigators should apply to evaluate patient-based outcome measures which are relevant here: (1) appropriateness (the match between the aims of the study and the instrument); (2) reliability (the instrument should be internally consistent and reproducible); (3) validity (the instrument should measure what it purports to measure); (4) responsiveness (the instrument should be sensitive to changes of importance to patients); (5) precision (the number and accuracy of distinctions made by an instrument); (6) interpretability (how meaningful the instrument's scores are); (7) acceptability (how acceptable respondents find its completion); and (8) feasibility (the amount of effort, burden and disruption to practitioners and services arising from the use of an instrument). The steps that need to be followed for the development of a QoL measure are summarised below and detailed in Table 3.1.

Validity

The logic, content and comprehensiveness of a measure can be assessed with face and content validity; and its burden on respondents requires examination (e.g. how long does it take to administer?). Construct validity can be ascertained by the extent to which a measure corresponds with theoretically relevant concepts. The predictive validity of the measure can be assessed using correlations between QoL and, for example, depression, and, for assessment of responsiveness – or sensitivity – to change, these associations can be examined longitudinally.

Convergent and discriminant validity can be assessed by correlations with the variables that QoL is expected to be associated with (e.g. depression) and the variables it is not expected to be associated with (e.g. income among people who are retired)

(Bowling 2005a). Its ability to distinguish between groups can be indicated with its correlations with, for example, severity of depression.

Reliability

Classical psychometric test theory aims to study the reliability of a measurement scale's variables. The reliability of measures can be discovered by assessing the internal consistency of the measure with item–item, item–total and split–half correlations, including Cronbach's alpha coefficients; and by examining the stability of scale scores over repeated administrations, during different time periods when no changes are expected, whether different interviewers of the same respondents obtain similar results, whether different modes of administration (e.g. paper questionnaires, telephone or computer-assisted questionnaire, face-to-face interview schedule) produce similar results, and whether it can be used, and is relevant, in different settings (e.g. residential care, clinic, home settings). Scale scores need interpreting, and cut-off points need justifying. For example, what does a severe score mean for users? How many scale points correlate with improvements or deterioration in other relevant areas (e.g. symptoms)?

Structure

The structure of a measure also needs to undergo statistical examination. Does it comprise multiple domains (e.g. sub-scales comprising either social relationships, activities, psychological well-being, independence, environmental) that can be scored separately and overall, or just one domain? To address this question, classic psychometric methods include principal components analysis, or exploratory and confirmatory factor analysis (for preference, see Tabachnick and Fidell 1996). (See the section on factor structure in Chapter 7.) These methods require item scores to be normally distributed and measured at the interval level, though they are commonly used with ordinal level data, which carries the risk of biased or inconsistent results. In such cases the methods should be used only as an approximate guide to factor structure.

The shortcomings of classic test theory approaches include the problem that each item may not contribute equally to the measure, and items may not have equal variance. It is only appropriate to apply statistical methods dependent on interval and normally distributed data, when scores are equally spaced. Item response theory is used in such issues. Non-parametric item response theory can be used to evaluate the unidimensionality of the measure, as indicated by scalability – a monotone homogeneity model (Mokken 1971; Sijtsma and Molenaar 2002; Sijtsma 2005; Bowling et al. 2013a). Non-parametric item response theory consists of a family of item response models for ordinal level data, e.g. Mokken's monotone homogeneity model and double monotonicity models, and Rasch's ([1960] 1980) analysis. As an example, Mokken's monotone homogeneity model is based on assumptions of unidimensionality, stochastic independence, and monotonicity in the latent attribute. It comprises an item selection phase, in which ordinal items measuring the same construct are clustered using an iterative procedure, followed by tests of the monotonic relationship between each item and the resulting scale. The summed scores of a set of items conforming to this model stochastically order respondents on a single dimension. The three approaches have been described and compared by Meijer and Sijtsma (1990). There is agreement in the literature that modern psychometric item response

Psychometric property	Criteria
Item generation and reduction	Potential questionnaire items should be generated from face-to-face interviews with a small sample of the target group, then the pool of items is examined conceptually, and by experts, and reduced using standard psychometric approaches. The generation of the item pool from a sample of the target group should be conducted alongside literature reviews and consultations with expert groups. The latter should not be used as a substitute for this exercise. Redundant items and those with weak measurement properties, floor and ceiling effects, as indicated by maximum endorsement frequencies (>80%), and high levels of missing data (>5%) can then be removed, and the resulting items grouped into scales using factor analysis, and then refined to form the intended measurement scale for testing for acceptability, reliability and validity, in a larger survey, before final refinement and final testing.
Acceptability	Assessed by data quality and targeting. Data quality: the completeness of item- and scale-level data, assessed by data completeness; criterion for missing data <5% (as above) (some use <10%, for example, with sensitive topics). Targeting: the extent to which the range of the variable measured by a scale matches the range of that variable in the study sample; assessed by maximum endorsement frequencies <80% (as above), aggregate endorsement frequencies >10%, skewness statistic −1 to +1, proximity of scale mean score to scale mid-point (closer matches = better), acceptable distribution of scores (closer to 100% indicates better targeting).
Scaling assumptions	Assessed by the extent to which it is legitimate to sum a set of items, without weighting or standardisation, to produce a single total score. Criterion is satisfied when items have adequate corrected-item total correlations ≥0.30, and grouping of items in subscales is correct. Assessed by principal components analysis (factor loadings >0.30, cross-loadings <0.20), item-convergent and discriminant validity (item-own scale correlations >0.30, magnitude >2 standard errors than other scales).
Reliability	Reliability: the extent to which scale scores are not associated with random error.
Internal consistency reliability	Precision of the scale based on the homogeneity (inter-correlations) of items at one point in time. Assessed by testing whether the items are inter-correlated, using tests of internal consistency (e.g. Cronbach's alpha coefficient ≥0.70; some use ≥0.80), mean item–item correlations (homogeneity coefficient) ≥0.30, and item–total correlations ≥0.30.
Test–retest reproducibility and inter-interviewer reliability	Agreement between respondent's scores at two short time intervals, expected to be stable; it estimates the stability of scales. Scale-level intra-class correlation coefficients ≥0.80, item-level intra-class correlation coefficients ≥0.50, should be achieved. Inter-interviewer reliability: reproducibility of the scale when administered to same respondents by different interviewers.
Validity	The extent to which a scale measures the construct that it purports to measure

Psychometric property	Criteria
Face validity	An estimate of whether a test appears to measure a certain criterion.
Content-related validity	The ability of the measure to reflect what is predicted by the conceptual framework for the measure – this can include tests for discriminant, convergent and known-groups validity (see separate listings below)
Validity (within scale)	Evidence that a scale measures a single construct, and that scale items can be combined to form a summary score. Assessed using internal consistency reliability (Cronbach's alpha ≥ 0.70, again, ≥ 0.80 is used by some) and factor analysis (factor loadings >0.30, cross-loadings <0.20).
Validity (correlations between scales)	Correlations between scales: moderate correlations (0.30–0.70) expected.
Discriminant validity	Evidence that a scale is not correlated with other measures of different constructs, hypothesised as not expected to be correlated with the scale.
Known-groups validity testing/ hypothesis tests	Ability of a scale to detect hypothesised differences between known sub-groups.

Source: Summarised from Cano *et al*. (2012) Tables 1 and 8 and Bowling (2009b).

Table 3.1 Summary of classic psychometric methods

theory (IRT) is a superior approach to techniques based on classic test theory, but there are advantages and disadvantages of both approaches.

Additional factors to consider

Additional issues in both health and social care include whether carer versions have been developed, to measure carers' QoL also, whether proxy measures can be used if individuals are too ill or unable to complete a measure, and whether these are reliable. While proxy measures are commonly used in research evaluating palliative and dementia care, they have been reported to have poor reliability (Addington-Hall and Kalra 2001). If a measure is to be used in other languages than that of the original design, then cultural equivalence needs to be established; standard and rigorous processes for these processes have been established.

In sum, the quality of research inferences is inevitably influenced by the appropriateness, relevance and psychometric robustness of the measurement scale used.

Methodological issues

As QoL reflects people's values, investigators also need to take account of changes in respondents' values in their analyses of QoL: perceived QoL can change over time with life experiences. Consciously or unconsciously people may accommodate, or adjust, to deteriorating circumstances, because they want to feel as good as possible about themselves, thereby leading to their perceptions of having a higher QoL when followed up (Diener *et al.* 1991). The roots of this process of adaptation are based on control theory, with response shift as a mediator which aims for homeostasis, and thus internal standards and values change – and hence perceptions of QoL (Sprangers and Schwartz 1999). Thus, all researchers using measures of QoL need to exercise caution when interpreting change data.

As the development of a QoL outcome measure in social care is in its infancy, there are several other methodological issues to consider when choosing a measure to use, including its relevance and appropriateness to the client group, as well as social policy, and relevance in different settings (see summary in Box 3.3).

Box 3.3 Summary of some key methodological issues

- There is a dearth of broader social care-related QoL measures.
- A broad approach to measuring QoL in social care is needed, as social needs and care can affect life as a whole.
- Measures need to be appropriate for younger and older people, different clients and types of services, and be sensitive to cultural differences.
- Measures need to be relevant to the target group, and applicable in a range of settings (e.g. community to residential care); they also need to be responsive to changes in individuals, resulting from interventions.
- Consideration of a generic core measure of QoL is needed, with additional domains for specific groups and settings.
- Partners may respond differently to other family carers – measures need to be appropriate for each type of respondent.
- Scale development needs to start 'bottom-up' by eliciting the perspectives of the target groups: only through their rigorous and sensitive involvement can outcome measures be developed which have social relevance.
- Response shift has enormous implications for the assessment of QoL, particularly in the interpretation of change and in shedding light on the paradoxical findings so often obtained.

No measurement scale is perfect. However, the principles of good practice in scale selection, including research where QoL is a target outcome, include following the steps outlined in Box 3.4.

Box 3.4 Principles of good research practice in scale selection

- Think about your research questions, the aims of interventions, and whether you need to use a single measurement scale or a battery of complementary measures within your questionnaire? What domains do you need to include?
- Examine the relevant literature in relation to the measurement of these domains, and consider the psychometric properties of potential measures. In particular, check the ability of the instrument to measure what it purports to (validity), its stability (reliability), and responsiveness to change over time. This depends upon the rigour of its development and testing. Also check whether target client groups were

involved in its development. Reviews of the measures of interest may have been published, which have the advantage of comparing measures and summarising their strengths and weaknesses.

■ Check which populations the measure was developed with, and in what settings: measures developed in community settings may not be appropriate for use in residential care settings.

■ Consider whether the measure is easy to use in your study setting. Think about how long it will take to complete, and how time-consuming it might be for the respondent and researcher.

■ If translated versions of the selected measure are required, search for published translations where semantic, idiomatic, experiential and conceptual equivalence has been established by standardised translation, back-translation, panel review, and pre-testing techniques.

■ Check whether the scale has been copyrighted, and whether permission is needed to use it. Some can be used without charge; others require consent plus a fee per copy used.

■ Consider whether you need to use expensive interview or more economical self-administered questionnaires. While many instruments can be administered in either mode, some may be too lengthy for self-administration (and lead to people giving up and not responding). Self-administration also depends on people being able to see and read, and comprehend, the questions; telephone administration may not be appropriate for people with hearing difficulties; internet questionnaires also assume everyone has access to the internet. There is a digital divide among several social groups, in particular among older people: only 37 per cent of households above the state pension age have internet access, compared to 79 per cent of households below the state pension age (Randall 2010; Berry 2011). The best response rates, and best quality data, are obtained with interviewer-administered questionnaires (Bowling 2005d).

■ Ask whether the measure is sensitive enough to detect changes in individuals over time as a result of interventions – and consider at what time periods it should be administered in order to detect any changes.

■ If unsure, then careful piloting of potential measures with the target group is needed.

Finally, if existing QoL measures might not capture all the relevant aspects of the situation, then the investigator can include open-ended questions for the respondent to add other issues important to them (e.g. see Bowling et al.'s open-ended generic QoL questions in Box 3.1). Their thematic categorisation and analysis, of course, while insightful, can be time-consuming.

Few measures satisfy all psychometric criteria perfectly; the design and testing of all measures are time-consuming and expensive. The body of knowledge about the adequacy and applicability of each measure in different settings, and with various populations, is cumulative and established over time; all researchers can contribute to this by publishing critical papers about the performance of the measures they have used, whether on basic assessments of reliability and validity, or more complex examination of scaling criteria. This section is intended to be an informative summary of the main steps involved in selecting a measurement scale, and to test them further.

Theoretical influences on measurement

Theoretical perspectives have had a clear influence on the development of measurement strategies in relation to health status and health-related quality of life scales, in particular in relation to scales of physical and role functioning. These influences are described next.

Functionalist approaches

Scales of health status and health-related quality of life are based on the assumption that social phenomena in relation to health and illness can be measured (in the positivist tradition), and most have adopted a functionalist perspective (a focus on interrelationships within the social system). For example, scales of physical functioning and ability, and their sub-domains in generic health status and quality of life scales, focus on the performance of activities of daily living (e.g. personal care, domestic roles, mobility) and on role functioning (e.g. work, finance, family, friends, social), which are necessary for the maintenance of society as well as the individual.

Popular measures of physical functioning have included the Barthel Index (Mahoney and Barthel 1965) (particularly for people with stroke), the Karnofsky Performance Index (Karnofsky *et al.* 1948), the Arthritis Impact Measurement Scales (Meenan *et al.* 1980) and the Health Assessment Questionnaire (Fries *et al.* 1982) (for rheumatism and arthritis). Typically, these scales focus on role performance in relation to daily activities, including personal and domestic chores and, in the case of the more extreme and negative Barthel Index, the need for help from others.

These approaches fit the functionalist model of ability to function in order to perform personal, social and economic roles (and contribute to the maintenance of society). Broader health status and health-related quality of life scales can also be seen to fit this model as they focus largely on physical functioning and mobility, and ability to perform social, recreational, domestic and, in some cases, work roles (e.g. the Sickness Impact Profile (Bergner *et al.* 1981), the Nottingham Health Profile (Hunt *et al.* 1986) and the Short Form-36 (Ware *et al.* 1993)).

Hermeneutic approaches

Phenomenologists would argue that health-related quality of life is dependent upon the interpretation and perceptions of the individual and that listing items in measurement scales is unsatisfactory because it is not known whether all the domains pertinent and meaningful to each respondent are included. It is also argued that this method does not capture the subjectivity of human beings and the processes of interpretation. This school of thought has partly influenced the development of the most recent measurement scales, which attempt to measure (still in a positivist manner) the meaning and significance of the illness state to individuals.

The approaches include the simple insertion of an item into lists of activities of daily living which aims to tap the individual's values (e.g. 'Which of these activities would you most like to be able to do without the pain or discomfort of your arthritis?'; Tugwell *et al.* 1987); open-ended questions on activities or areas of life affected by the respondents' medical condition (Guyatt *et al.* 1987a, 1987b, 1989a, 1989b; Ruta *et al.* 1994); and self-nomination of important areas of quality of life (O'Boyle *et al.* 1992). The Repertory

Grid technique, used by psychologists, also allows for the measurement of areas or things that are unique to the individual, and is being explored as a useful idiographic method of examining how an individual constructs subjective phenomena such as quality of life (Thunedborg *et al.* 1993).

These structured and semi-structured approaches would not satisfy phenomenologists who only value pure qualitative methodology, but they do attempt to recognise the importance of a hermeneutic approach. The essential nature of these approaches in the measurement of health-related quality of life was demonstrated in research based on a national population survey (Bowling 1995). Using open-ended questions, this research found that people mention different areas as important when asked about the five most important areas of life and the five most important areas of life affected by their medical conditions. Open-ended questions also led respondents to mention different areas of life affected by their condition, in comparison with pre-coded questions. Several areas of life which were prioritised by respondents were not included in the most popularly used scales of broader health status and health-related quality of life.

In sum, health status and health-related quality of life are usually assessed using nomothetic measurement instruments (i.e. they seek to measure traits based on preconceived assumptions of quality of life and their relevance to all individuals). In contrast, idiographic measures, which measure those things which are unique to individuals, are rarely used in health status and health-related quality of life measurement, though there is a slow but increasing trend to encompass these within the structure of traditional measurement scales.

3.2 Patients' perceptions

Interactions between health professionals and patients

Both sociologists and psychologists have focused on verbal and non-verbal interactions between doctors and patients in relation to consultation and treatment. Their methods have included qualitative and quantitative approaches. Ley's (1988) cognitive hypothesis of communication emphasised patients' understanding of the content of the consultation, recall of information provided during the consultation, and satisfaction with the consultation as essential for compliance with therapy and, hence, recovery from illness. The concept of concordance is now preferred to compliance, in an attempt to move away from the image of a compliant patient in relation to an expert health professional (Stanton 1987). Ogden (1996) has described Ley's theory and its limitations. For example, it assumes that health professionals behave objectively, and that compliance with therapy is seen as desirable, but ignores the health beliefs of professional and patient. However, adequate communication is important if health care is to be effective, not only in relation to adherence. For example, research has shown that the provision of information about what to expect before surgery can have the effect of reducing post-surgical pain (Hayward 1975; Boore 1979). Sociologists analyse interactions between health professionals and patients in relation to patients' socio-demographic characteristics, and in relation to the individual's understanding of the situation (see Cockerham 1995). Patients' evaluations of the communication process between doctor and patient are now recognised as an important component of evaluation of the process and outcome of health services.

Patients' evaluations of health care

An important contribution of social scientists to health and health services research is the assessment of patients' evaluations of their health and health services (Fitzpatrick 1990). Patients' assessments provide important information about both the results of health care (outcome) and the mode (process) of delivering that care.

Patients' satisfaction

Patients' reports of their experiences of health care, including satisfaction, are central to health care evaluation. Governments and regulatory bodies in many countries require health care providers to undertake surveys of patients' views (e.g. satisfaction). Patients' *satisfaction* with their care and its outcome is the most commonly used indicator in studies which aim to include their evaluations. Dictionary definitions of satisfaction focus on that which is adequate, suitable, acceptable, pleasing and the fulfilment of an objective. Few investigators have defined patient satisfaction, and it is therefore difficult to assess which dimension is being measured.

There is recognition of the importance of evaluating health services from a wide variety of perspectives, including the patient's. This has been developed, in particular in the 1990s, with the emphasis on consumerism and accountability. This in turn has led to a swing away from use of the term 'patient', and a fashion for the use of the term 'consumer' of health care. However, the term 'consumer' is of limited value in understanding the status and role of the recipient in an industry in which a service, and not a good, is produced (Stacey 1976).

Measurement of patients' evaluations

Patients' evaluations of health care have generally been assessed, in a positivist style, through patient satisfaction surveys. This method also suffers from limitations. Most research on patient satisfaction indicates that the majority of patients will report being satisfied with their care overall, though more specific questioning can yield higher levels of criticism (Cartwright 1964; Locker and Dunt 1978), particularly in relation to the amount of information provided (Hall and Dornan 1988).

Question wording as well as form can be influential (see Calnan 1988). For example, patients are more likely to report being satisfied in response to a general satisfaction question with a pre-coded Likert format response frame (e.g. 'How satisfied are you with the health service: very satisfied–very dissatisfied?'), than they are to more open-ended, direct questions (Cartwright and Anderson 1981). Cohen *et al.* (1996), in a comparison of three patient satisfaction surveys, reported that different results are obtained if patients are presented with negative statements about health care and asked to agree that something 'bad' happened, in comparison with presenting them with a positive statement and asking them to disagree that something 'good' happened (the latter achieved a substantially higher response, i.e. reported dissatisfaction). Moreover, simple 'yes/no' dichotomised pre-coded response choices, and codes ranging from 'very satisfied' to 'very dissatisfied', have the potential to lead to a response set (Cronbach 1946), and may account for the high number of 'yes' and 'satisfied' responses usually obtained. Where under-reporting of critical attitudes is expected, leading questions can be used, for example, 'What would you like to see improved in the health service?'

The aspects of care that have commonly been included in patient satisfaction questionnaires for hospital inpatients include the provision of information, cleanliness, the food, choice available, privacy, noise, manner of the staff, facilities, location of conveniences (from toilets to ability to reach the light switch or call button), visiting times, notice of admission and discharge, adequacy of assessment and preparation for discharge. Both inpatients and outpatients may be asked about waiting list and waiting times, courtesy of the staff, information given, and so on. A number of these areas are addressed in the CASPE patient satisfaction questionnaires (Clinical Accountability, Service Planning and Evaluation 1988). Less often included are more sensitive questions such as intention to return. It is useful to ask patients if they would be prepared to use the same service again if they needed to and if they had the choice (e.g. specific hospital, ward or clinic), and whether they would recommend it to a friend in need of the same care. For example: 'Would you be prepared to return to this ward in future if you needed similar treatment or care?'; 'Would you recommend this hospital to a friend who needed similar treatment or care?'

Some investigators have applied Anderson et al.'s (1975) model of help-seeking to patients' evaluations of care and analysed expressions of satisfaction and dissatisfaction in relation to predisposing, enabling and need factors. However, most investigators who have attempted to analyse the components of satisfaction have distinguished between the different dimensions of satisfaction. Ware and Snyder (1975), using factor analysis, reported finding 18 dimensions of patient satisfaction. The four main dimensions were access to care, continuity of care, availability of services and physician conduct. Ware and Hays (1988) later identified eight dimensions of patient satisfaction which should be included in questionnaires: the art of care, technical quality, accessibility, efficacy, cost, physical environment, availability and continuity. Also of importance are satisfaction with one's health status and ability, and outcome. John Ware has developed several satisfaction batteries (Ware and Hays 1988; Davies and Ware 1991; Rubin et al. 1993). This body of work has led to the identification of eight attributes of health care which Davies and Ware (1991) suggested should be included in a satisfaction instrument:

1 accessibility and availability of services and providers
2 choice and continuity
3 communication
4 financial arrangements
5 interpersonal aspects of care
6 outcomes of care
7 technical quality of care
8 time spent with providers.

It is important to conceptualise patients' evaluations in terms of what their priorities and expectations are of the service, and what they hope to achieve from the service; their need for an explanation of the condition; their need for curative treatment, or relief from symptoms; the choices open to them in relation to treatment/care and an explanation of the chances of the success of treatment and any side effects; and the process of the treatment/care. Bowling et al. (1995b), in their evaluation of specialists' clinics, used a battery of structured items on satisfaction (Rubin et al. 1993), as well as several open-ended questions about patients' expectations of the consultation, and whether these were met. The analysis of the open-ended questions indicated that people were keen to evaluate critically the medical aspects of their care if given the opportunity to do so.

However, Cartwright and Anderson's (1981) classic research indicated that, in response to open-ended questions, patients do not usually evaluate medical care in relation to competence – an acceptable level of competence is assumed – but make judgements based on human factors (attitudes and manner, provision of information, service factors). This bias is also reflected in satisfaction questionnaires, and it is difficult to assess whether the bias reflects patients' priorities or whether questionnaires contain an organisational bias which does not aim to explore the appropriateness and outcome of the treatment in a satisfaction questionnaire. This may also be because the developers of the questionnaires do not feel that patients have the expertise to judge the quality of clinical care, though the effectiveness of the care and the patients' perspective on this are one of the most important issues. Patient satisfaction surveys have proliferated in the British NHS since the 1980s, as a result of the impetus for 'management-led consumerism' (Griffiths 1983, 1988), and are popular among provider organisations in the USA, as indicators of quality in a competitive private market. Calnan (1988) has labelled this 'management-led consumerism' as 'managerial bias' – a domination of providers' interests and perspectives over those of the patients. This may change with the increasing contracting arrangements in health services across the world and the managerial focus on appropriateness and health outcomes.

Chalmers (1995) has called for lay involvement in the planning and promoting of research on health in order to provide evidence of health care that is relevant as well as reliable: 'Greater lay involvement in setting the research agenda would almost certainly lead to greater open-mindedness about which questions are worth addressing, which forms of health care merit assessment, and which treatment outcomes matter.'

The most economical way of assessing patients' evaluations is with survey methods. This approach is often criticised as superficial, however, and some organisations supplement survey methods with qualitative focus groups techniques (e.g. with existing patients' groups) and with in-depth interviews with small sub-samples of the population of interest in order to obtain more detailed information on sources of satisfaction and dissatisfaction.

In sum, conventional methods of eliciting patient satisfaction have been criticised for eliciting mainly favourable results and not having discriminatory ability, and for lacking a conceptual underpinning (Fitzpatrick and Hopkins 1983; Hall and Dornan 1988; Jenkinson *et al.* 2003). An alternative approach has thus been developed which aims to measure patients' experiences of health care instead of patient satisfaction, and provide more comprehensive and meaningful reports of patients' views (Jenkinson *et al.* 2003).

Patient choice and patients' expectations of health care

One paradigm shift in western health care is the health policy emphasis on 'informed choice', 'patient-centred medicine', or 'patient choice', which has been given impetus by the development of evidence-based medicine (Parker 2001). While this emphasis may have raised patients' expectations of health care, in practice, the choice may be limited. A telephone survey of Medicare beneficiaries who had undergone elective, high-risk procedures in the USA reported that, although all respondents stated that they could choose where to have surgery, only 55 per cent said there was an alternative hospital in their area where they could have gone for treatment (Schwartz *et al.* 2005). Moreover, the concept of patient choice assumes informed decision-making, though there are continuing reports of patients' misunderstanding of information given about risks and benefits of treatments and also clinical trials (including consent issues, randomisation and equipoise). Research has also shown that the way information is presented and framed can significantly influence understanding and decision-making among patients and clinicians (Edwards *et al.* 2001; Fuller *et al.* 2001; Robinson *et al.* 2005).

In contrast to most health economics models of utility, which are generally focused on outcomes (e.g. health states and effects of treatment), psychological models of expectancy include both outcome and process expectancies (Crow *et al.* 1999). It is generally acknowledged that health care planners need to understand the expectations underlying patients' views in order to interpret their satisfaction with, and feedback on, services. Understanding how expectations are formed is, in theory, crucial for furthering knowledge on a range of health topics from health and illness behaviour to patient-assessed outcomes.

The literature on patient expectations in health care appears to be characterised by diversity, lack of integration and a theoretical paucity of approach to both conceptualisation and measurement. This fragmentation and lack of integration of research partly reflect the multidimensionality of the concept, a characteristic shared with the concept of patient satisfaction. The largest body of literature on expectations appears to relate to patient satisfaction, reflecting its alleged theoretical underpinning of this concept. It is assumed that an excess of perceived delivery (e.g. of health care) over what is *hoped for, anticipated* or *expected* leads to increased satisfaction, and the converse of unmet expectations leads to increased dissatisfaction (Kravitz *et al.* 1996; Crow *et al.* 2002; McKinley *et al.* 2002; Dawn and Lee 2004). However, Bowling *et al.* (2012a, 2013b), in pre- and post-clinic visit surveys of 833 hospital out-patients and primary care patients reported no associations between their measures of ideal and realistic pre-visit expectations and post-visit patient satisfaction. Actual experiences during the consultation (especially indicators of communication with the doctor), having a sense of control over life, and socio-demographic characteristics were predictive of satisfaction, independently of prior expectations.

Several studies have indicated that treatment expectations (as 'beliefs') influence treatment outcomes (e.g. experience of severe nausea after chemotherapy – Roscoe *et al.* 2004). A systematic review of the placebo effect also concluded that expectancies are a mechanism by which placebos have their effects (Crow *et al.* 1999). However, a systematic review by Rao *et al.* (2000) in primary care settings reported that associations between expectations and health-related quality of life outcomes were inconsistent. This is likely to be due to weaknesses and variations in research design, as well as to the type of expectations measured. Although the concepts and measurement of patient satisfaction and health-related quality of life outcomes have been linked to the concept of patient expectations, there has been little attempt to support these links with conceptual development or a theoretical model. There is also little information on whether expectations can be modified, though it has been argued that high expectations should be encouraged and be used as a catalyst for improving health care (Coulter 2006).

Psychological theory holds that expectations are complex beliefs, or values, resulting from cognitive processes (Linder-Pelz 1982). The term 'expectancy' is used in psychology as a general concept, in contrast to the health literature which refers to 'expectations' in the real world (Janzen *et al.* 2006). Attitude theories are mainly based on expectancy–value theory, whereby attitudes (disposition to respond favourably or unfavourably towards an object) are related to beliefs (expectancies) that the object possesses certain attributes, and evaluations of those attributes (Ajzen 1988). Expectancy theory is regarded as particularly important in theories of behaviour. Role theory, for example, posits that human behaviour is guided by expectations, though there has been little analysis of their construction. Expectancy values – such as the value people place on processes and outcomes – have been used to explain relationships between attitudes and behaviour (Fishbein 1967), although empirical evidence is limited. Outcome expectancy and perceived competence to perform particular behaviours (self-efficacy) are held to be important predictors of behaviour (Bandura 1986). However, there is little evidence on how abstract theories might be used in empirical research in real-life patient settings. Many studies of expectations in the health field are ambiguous in their use of terminology, or have focused on different *types* of expectations.

Patients' preferences

A related topic is patients' preferences. Patients, particularly older people, may not always be presented with the range of treatment alternatives appropriate for the treatment of their condition. While patients may expect their doctors to act in their best interests, there is evidence that clinical judgements may be influenced by the socio-demographic characteristics of the patient, stereotyping and health care resource constraints (Bowling 1999). It could be hypothesised that, in general, doctors choose the treatment which is most likely to maximise life expectancy, except in the case of patients aged 75 and over where an age bias may operate and it is sometimes assumed, with little evidence, that older patients prefer to maximise their quality of life at the expense of quantity.

The ad hoc way in which treatment decisions are usually made by doctors contrasts strongly with the rigour of the research process, except where methods of Decision Analysis modelling are used, which can incorporate objectives, alternatives for action, possible outcomes and benefits, to inform decision-making. However, the evidence about the effectiveness of a therapy is rarely sufficient to eliminate uncertainty (Logan and Scott 1996). Clinicians' alleged failure to take patients' preferences into account has been blamed for some of the variation in clinical practice (e.g. Wennberg *et al.* 1988). On the other hand, it may have equitable or inequitable consequences if some patients (e.g. the more educated and affluent) are more aware of the choices being offered, and more adept at making more beneficial choices than others.

It is ethically desirable to take account of people's views before making policy or individual treatment decisions (termed evidence-informed (or evidence-based) patient choice). Where quality of life and life expectancy issues are an important consideration, people's informed preferences should be as important in health care decisions as the body of evidence on a procedure's clinical effectiveness and costs. This is essential for building up a more rounded body of knowledge on appropriateness. A powerful reason for asking sufferers about treatment preferences is that preference assessments are of value in building up a patient-based 'ethics of evidence', particularly when there is uncertainty about when to provide more or less intensive or invasive treatments to patients, and when issues of health service rationing are being debated and policies developed. However, there is limited information about patients' preferences for treatment, as opposed to health states (Say and Thomson 2003), even in situations of clinical equipoise, or where alternatives exist. Limited evidence suggests that older patients would be as prepared as younger patients to accept invasive clinical treatments where appropriate (Kennelly and Bowling 2001), a finding which challenges any age stereotypes among clinicians.

Research on preferences for treatment for prostate cancer in the USA has reported that 18 months after surgery 72 per cent of the men said they would choose the same treatment if necessary again and 7 per cent said they would not. This broader perspective on preferences for treatment, which is patient-based, along with any changes in preferences post treatment, provide real-world and broader information of value to policy-makers and to future patients (Stanford *et al.* 2000; Bowling and Ebrahim 2001).

The active participation of patients in shared decision-making about their health care is also an important dimension of contemporary models of patient-centred care and of doctor–patient decision-making. The gap between communication theory and practice has been highlighted by differences in decisions between doctors and older patients in relation to resuscitation orders (Ebrahim 2000; McShine *et al.* 2000). This participation requires doctors to share information, including that on uncertainties. It also requires health professionals to recognise the contribution that patients have a right to make. However, opinions vary about what aspects of participation are the most important indicators of the quality of the process of health care, and current measures may not capture the essential features of patient participation, requiring that new measures be developed within a clear theoretical framework (Bekker *et al.* 1999; O'Conner *et al.* 1999). The issue is complex. Models of doctor–patient relationships range from paternalistic (emphasising the doctor's authority) to informative (emphasising the patient's right to exercise their autonomy). Evidence indicates that most patients want to be informed about their conditions, a proportion want to participate in clinical decisions about their treatment, and some prefer to be passive and avoid receiving information. The latter style is preferred mainly by patients who are older and less educated, though such variables only account for up to 20 per cent of the variability in patients' preferences for involvement in clinical decision-making (Benbassat *et al.* 1998). In a review of models of doctor–patient interaction and communication styles, Gudagnol and Ward (1998) concluded that all models were limited because they assume patients are incapable of participating. Examples given were 'delayers' who consider options but this is perfunctory and immediately prefer one option; 'deferrers' who weigh the pros and cons and make a choice when satisfied; Type I ('You decide for me, doctor'); Type II ('I demand you do procedure x'); Type III ('I cannot decide'); and Type IV ('Given the options, your recommendation and my preference, I choose treatment x'). Further research is still needed on the optimum ways of presenting patients with information.

People's preferences and perceptions of risk

The topic of preferences has been fraught with methodological challenges. Methods of eliciting patients' preferences for treatment or health care are not standardised. Most publications of RCTs with patient preference arms do not even specify how patients' treatment preference was measured (King *et al.* 2005a, 2005b).

For research purposes, a preference is the expression of an act of deliberation – i.e. an attempt to weigh up, consider and express a value for alternative choices of action. It is more than the expression of 'want' and should be internally consistent. A study of people's preferences involves the assessment of their attitudes (preferences) towards specific options (e.g. treatments) which they would prefer for themselves, after informed deliberation on the risks and benefits. This then, in theory, provides information on acceptability in the light of people's own value systems. Detailed research on patients' preferences has been undertaken in oncology (McNeil et al. 1982; Chadwick et al. 1991; Singer et al. 1991; O'Conner et al. 1999), and in cardiology (Lambert et al. 2004; Rowe et al. 2005; Bowling et al. 2008). The valid measurement of risk perception, preferences, and the presentation of information to minimise framing effects has ethical implications, given that the framing of risks, both numerically and linguistically, has an effect on choices made (Wragg et al. 2000).

Risk assessment is about evaluating the chance of an undesired outcome. Knowledge about patients' understandings and perceptions of risk is essential for analysis of their preferences. While a generic body of literature exists which supports the beneficial effects of patient information on patient recovery and adherence (Schulman 1979; Webber 1990), research on patients' preferences for treatment, and perceptions of risk, has been largely confined to doctor–patient communication styles (see Edwards and Elwyn 1999) and little is known about patient outcomes in relation to their preferences for treatment. A valid body of evidence about patients' preferences and risk perception is pertinent to the health policy emphasis on patient choice. Moreover, the poor presentation of statistics on risk can lead to both doctors and patients making poor decisions about treatment; simple representation of risk can help both to make more fully informed decisions (Gigerenzer and Edwards 2003). While evidence-based patient choice has the potential to empower patients and develop further a patient-centred health care model, it has also been argued that the emphasis on the rights of the individual to choose is to the detriment of the interests of communities (Etzioni 1993). Parker (2001) has counter-argued that what is required is the establishment of a healthy balance between rights and responsibilities.

Methods of investigation

The dominant paradigm for the investigation of risk perception and preferences in psychology has been the study of laboratory gambles (e.g. driving behaviour in simulated studies) and lotteries, and in health research it has been largely limited to health behaviour and promotion survey questionnaires (especially in relation to smoking, alcohol intake and AIDS), and to utility analysis of health states to obtain measures of social values of health (using rating scales, standard gamble, time trade-off utility metrics) and obtaining reference utility scores (e.g. using the EuroQoL, see Chapter 5). Utility research has been valuable in relation to providing information on the wide range of acceptability of various health states, for example, it has pointed to the wide variation among patients with angina in their tolerance for their symptoms (Nease et al. 1995). But these approaches leave unexplored the social and cultural variations in the views expressed and the reasons and values underlying them, and the crude and/or complex nature of the measures employed across disciplines has led to unreliable results (Frogberg and Kane 1989).

It is unlikely that risk-taking and preferences measured under artificial circumstances can be generalised to everyday risk-taking (Yates 1992). However, a real methodological problem is the measurement of actual risk-taking and preferences, given the ethical concerns of exposing people to real or experimental laboratory situations, which may have negative consequences, and the limitations of hypothetical or retrospective self-report questionnaires on topics about behaviours which take place in an environmentally rich context. Also, people's preferences may be unduly influenced by recent experiences, and people who have not experienced the event in question may find it difficult to evaluate outcomes. Finally, perceptions of risk and patients' preferences are difficult to measure because of the large influence of question-framing effects (positive/ negative question wording biases), as McNeil *et al.* (1982) clearly showed in relation to treatment for lung cancer. Framing effects have also been documented among clinicians. A systematic review of 12 articles on the effects of framing on doctors' opinions or intended practices showed that doctors viewed results expressed in relative risk reduction or gain terms most positively (McGettigan *et al.* 1999). Hence the authors concluded that they preferred an intervention to be framed in gain rather than loss terms. Finally, there is the problem of recall bias. Research by Lloyd *et al.* (1999) suggested that patients' recall of information given to them about their risk associated with treatment options for carotid endarterectomy is limited.

The methods used in most research on preferences include single-item questions asking patients to state the option they would choose, Likert scales of the strength of the stated preference, utility measurements (e.g. rating scales, time trade-offs, standard gamble methods), and, less commonly, preferences have been explored using discrete choice analysis techniques (Ryan 1996; Ryan and Hughes 1997; Ryan and Farrar 2000; Ryan *et al.* 2006) (see Chapter 5). While this is less complex for respondents than traditional time trade-off and standard gamble techniques, it may still be a burdensome technique if several alternatives are under consideration. Other innovatory techniques include repertory grid techniques (Kelly 1955) as used in perceptions of risk in genetic manipulation of food (Frewer *et al.* 1998a), or preferences for type of treatment for cardiovascular disease (Rowe *et al.* 2005). Modified repertory grid methods were used to develop patient-relevant items to form the Patient Preferences Questionnaire for Angina Treatment, with good psychometric results (Bowling *et al.* 2008, 2010, 2012b).

It is well established that random assignment between experimental treatment and control arms is the gold standard in clinical trials to minimise differences between the groups being compared and to safeguard against bias. There is, however, a fear that such random allocation may not accord with patients' preferences for the intervention or treatment, thereby compromising trial validity. It is possible that patients may resent not receiving their treatment of choice, and their negative attitude may lead to non-adherence to treatment or affect outcomes in some other way. Consequently, one option for trial designers is to include patient preference arms, whereby patients with no treatment preference are randomly allocated to experimental and control arms. While there is little evidence of preferences biasing trial results, most reports of RCTs, which have included patient preference arms, do not specify how patients' treatment preferences were measured (King *et al.* 2005a, 2005b).

Surveys of older people's preferences for treatment for end-stage renal disease, using clinical vignettes, have indicated that older people would opt for dialysis when needed – in contrast to age-based rationing policies for renal dialysis in some countries (Ahmed *et al.* 1999). Some of these surveys have used measurement scales, though these are fairly crude, for example, the Autonomy Preference Index (Ende *et al.* 1989) simply asks patients to assign control for decisions on three health conditions to the doctor alone; mostly the doctor; both the patient and doctor equally; mostly the patient; or the patient alone (e.g. in relation to the decision, 'Does a patient with a sore throat, stuffy nose and a cough need an X-ray?'). More promising is Frewer's research on the public's attitudes to genetic engineering in food production, which was based on repertory grid techniques and internal preference mapping. The latter is a multivariate technique which produces a multidimensional map of items, showing how they are related in terms of scores given by respondents, with the application of a bootstrapping method to assess differences in perceptions. By repeatedly sampling (with replacement) from the respondents and recalculating the model, an empirical picture of the variation may be built up (Frewer *et al.* 1998a).

The conflicting nature of the health research evidence (see below) is unsurprising in view of the nature and range of measures employed. It may also partly relate to non-dynamic notions of preferences. Patients' needs for information vary with the stages of their diagnosis and condition. Leydon *et al.* (2000) reported that patients need 'faith, hope and charity', which limits their desire for information in relation to cancer.

Associations with preferences and perceptions of risk

Few of the studies which have examined patients' preferences or perceptions of risk have analysed or reported any socio-demographic differences in these attitudes, possibly because of the nature of most of the studies, which are largely either qualitative or based on small convenience samples. Sutton (1998, 1999), in his study of optimism–pessimism bias and perception of risk concerning smoking, reported that older smokers were the most optimistic about avoiding the health consequences of smoking, although no gender or social class differences were found. Frewer *et al.* (1998a) reported higher levels of perceived risk associated with different hazards among less affluent individuals and those in lower socio-economic groups, again probably due to their reduced level of control over risk management processes at an executive level, reduced levels of education, and poorer health and social circumstances (i.e. increased powerlessness in society).

An ICM poll funded by the Rowntree Reform Trust showed that two-thirds of women questioned wanted a lot of power, and one-third a little, over their medical treatment. The figures for men were 50:50. The gender difference was independent of age, class and region of residence (Hutton Commission 2000). It is unknown whether this reflects current levels of reduced power among women or men's greater reluctance to appear anxious about their health, or some other factor.

There is a large body of health literature demonstrating that older patients, and patients in the lower socio-economic groups, are less likely to be critical of their health care and to be more accepting of their doctors' decisions than other groups of patients (Cartwright and Anderson 1980; NHS Executive 1999). However, the literature on preferences and risk perception has yielded few or conflicting results, even on the issues of whether patients want to participate and on the effects of participation on patient health outcome. Gudagnol and Ward (1998) still concluded, on the basis of their review, and despite conflicting evidence, that, on the whole, patients want to be informed of treatment alternatives and to be involved in treatment decisions. Social, ethnic and educational differences are likely to exacerbate the imbalance of power in the patient–doctor relationship (due to the sick patient and the expert doctor) and hamper attempts to enable patients to participate.

The theoretical conceptionalisation of risk is currently located by psychologists within the individual (Ogden 1995). Many research results, which are based on variants of the Health Belief and Locus of Control models are, however, questionable, because of the widespread use of invalid and different indicators between studies (Champion 1984; Sheeran and Abraham 1995). Research has also under-emphasised the restrictions that the social structure can impose on behaviour (e.g. knowledge of limited health service resources; social and professional distance between patient and doctor). A combined individual–societal approach is required in the exploration of preferences for treatment and associated perceptions of risks.

Most research on health, perceived control and risk-taking has focused on primary prevention of risk factors for disease (e.g. smoking, obesity, alcohol), predictors of breast self-examination, take-up of screening services (e.g. mammography, cervical cytology) and practice of safe sexual behaviour in relation to HIV risk. A small amount of disease-specific risk research has examined adherence or concordance with antihypertensive, renal disease and diabetic regimens and is narrow in focus. This has indicated that, in general, people overestimate the frequency of rare causes of death, but also underestimate their personal vulnerability to health- and life-threatening problems ('unrealistic optimism'), particularly when events are perceived as more controllable (Slovic et al. 1977). Other research has supported the findings of individuals' sense of unique invulnerability (labelled 'optimistic bias' as well as 'unrealistic optimism') (Weinstein 1984; Gerrard and Warner 1991; Weinstein et al. 1998).

Frewer's research on the public's attitudes to genetic engineering in food production indicated that optimistic bias was present for all the food-related hazards investigated, although this was much reduced for those which were highly technologised. In addition, it was reported that initial attitudes were important determinants of post-intervention attitudes, and admission of risk uncertainty was influential in increasing acceptance of the technology (Frewer et al. 1998b). The implication for policy was that risk information campaigns may fail because individuals assume they are both invulnerable to risks and more knowledgeable about hazards relative to others: the more people feel they know about a hazard, the more they feel they have control over exposure (Frewer et al. 1998b). Frewer also reported a strong positive correlation between an individual's preference and trust in that option. Similarly, research on perceptions of risk among drivers (laboratory simulations) indicates that risk-taking behaviour can be influenced by perceptions of control over the activity (Horswill and McKenna 1998) – individuals who perceive personal control over a situation will take greater risks.

Optimism bias has been explained by the theory of 'illusion of control' whereby individuals believe that they have greater personal control over a potentially hazardous situation (and are thus at reduced risk from it) than a comparable other (McKenna 1993). However, not all findings are consistent with this, and a 'pessimism bias' among smokers in relation to their chances of getting heart disease has also been reported (Sutton 1999). Apart from optimism–pessimism bias, one's attitude to risk in life in general (high, neutral or low risk-takers), personality traits such as the need for control, beliefs about the nature of the doctor–patient relationship, risk-taking in health care and preferences for treatment may partly, but not universally, depend on anxiety/ depression, one's health status, age, level of education and ability to understand information provided, marital status, family responsibilities and many other factors (Weinstein and Fineberg 1980). An in-depth study of lay understandings of coronary heart disease by Emslie et al. (2000) reported that people's decisions about high-risk behaviours (i.e. which affect their risk) are complex and also take account of many aspects of their lives, including knowledge about the lives and health experiences of family members. For example, some people who thought that heart disease 'ran' in their family did not feel at increased personal risk of disease because they felt they differed in crucial ways from affected family members.

This indicates that culture also influences the individual perception and construction of risk, and, though not without criticism, cultural theory has a contribution to make to the emerging theories of deliberative processes. Various typologies of groups have been developed by social scientists, including indicators of 'high' and 'low' group cohesiveness, which influence the extent to which an individual is incorporated into a bounded unit (individualism, market competitiveness, libertarianism, fatalism, despotism, hierarchies, factionalism, egalitarianism) (see Tansey and O'Riordan 1999, for descriptions).

Finally, there is a limited, general literature suggesting that there are marked divergences between lay and expert perceptions of risk in coronary heart disease (Davison *et al.* 1991; Newman 1995). There is also research showing that doctors' and nurses' perceptions of the risk of a cardiovascular event among their own patients with hypertension correlated poorly (Montgomery *et al.* 1998). However, little is known about heart disease sufferers' own perceptions of the degree of personal risk to their quantity and quality of life imposed by the condition, the extent to which they can control the course of the disease, its likely course and alternatives for treatment, or likely effects of action vs inaction (Sheeran and Abraham 1995). Most research on perceived risk has been conducted on younger adults and college students – justified by investigators partly in terms of convenience, but mainly with reference to the belief that these are the people whose lifestyles are alterable before they experience illness events (Weinstein 1984).

Summary of main points

- Health-related quality of life generally encompasses physical, psychological and social domains of health. Generic quality of life is a broader, more multidimensional concept.
- The main theoretical influence on the construction of scales measuring health-related and broader quality of life is functionalism, which emphasises the ability to function in order to perform personal, social and economic roles in society.
- Hermeneutic approaches to measuring health-related quality of life aim to capture the subjectivity of human beings and the domains pertinent and meaningful to the individual.
- It is generally assumed, with little evidence, that an excess of perceived delivery (e.g. of health care) over what is *hoped for, anticipated* or *expected* leads to increased satisfaction.
- Patients' perceptions of risk, and preferences for treatment, can be influenced by framing effects.

Key questions

1 Define health-related and broader quality of life.
2 What are the main criteria to consider when selecting a measure of quality of life?
3 How are people's preferences for treatment influenced?
4 What are the different types of patients' expectations of health care?

Key terms

health-related quality of life
hermeneutic
patients' evaluations
patients' expectations
patients' experiences
patients' preferences

psychometrics
quality of life
reliability
response shift
validity

Recommended reading

Bowling, A. (2005) Measuring health outcomes from the patient's perspective, in A. Bowling and S. Ebrahim (eds) *Handbook of Health Research Methods: Investigation, Measurement and Analysis.* Maidenhead: Open University Press.

Bowling, A., Reeves, B. and Rowe, G. (2010) The Patients' Preferences Questionnaire for Angina treatment: results and psychometrics from 383 patients in primary care in England. *Quality and Safety in Health Care,* 19: 1–7.

Bowling, A., Rowe, G, Lambert, N., Waddington, M., *et al*. (2012) The measurement of patients' expectations for health care: a review and psychometric testing of a measure of patients' expectations. *Health Technology Assessment,* 16: 30.

Bowling, A. and Stenner, P. (2011) Which measure of quality of life performs best in older age? A comparison of the OPQOL, CASP-19 and WHOQOL-OLD. *Journal of Epidemiology and Community Health*, 65: 273–80.

Gigerenzer, G. and Edwards, A. (2003) Simple tools for understanding risks: from innumeracy to insight. *British Medical Journal*, 327: 741–4.

Harries, A. and Stiggelbout, A. (2005) Approaches to measuring patients' decision making, in A. Bowling and S. Ebrahim (eds) *Handbook of Health Research Methods: Investigation, Measurement and Analysis*. Maidenhead: Open University Press.

Harries, C. and Kostopoulou, O. (2005) Psychological approaches to measuring and modelling clinical decision-making, in A. Bowling and S. Ebrahim (eds) *Handbook of Health Research Methods: Investigation, Measurement and Analysis*. Maidenhead: Open University Press.

CHAPTER 4

Health needs and their assessment: demography and epidemiology

Chapter contents

Introduction

The relationship between public health and the assessment of need for health care can be traced back to the Acheson Report in the UK (Acheson 1988), which called for regular reviews of the nation's health, and health service reforms formalised this with splits between purchasers and providers of health care (Secretaries of State for

Health, Wales, Northern Ireland and Scotland 1989a, 1989b). The effect has been to place multidisciplinary research on health and effectiveness of health services, the development of evidence-based health care and the assessment of need for services firmly on international agendas of research and development (Peckham 1991; Department of Health 1993a). Health needs assessment is a tool which is now used internationally, including Europe and the USA. Part 4.1 of this chapter focuses on the concept of need and the practice of measuring needs for health services. Two main disciplines in this area are epidemiology and demography; their principal methods and techniques are described in Parts 4.2 and 4.3.

4.1 The assessment of health needs

Health needs

Health needs assessments have traditionally been undertaken by public health professionals in relation to their local populations, though the approach is relevant to all health care sectors, in all populations, and in all countries. As governments across Europe are also faced with rising demands for health care, limited resources and increasing inequalities in health, the World Health Organization (WHO) European Office published a tool describing the stages of community health needs assessment, at the level of families, communities and populations. It was aimed at family health nurses (nurses, midwives and public health nurses) (Rowe *et al.* 2001), to enable practitioners, managers and policy-makers to identify priority health needs, target health care resources to address inequalities, and involve local people, specifically in doing the following:

- to plan and deliver the most effective care to those in greatest need;
- to apply principles of equity and social justice in practice;
- to ensure that scarce resources are allocated where they give maximum health benefit;
- to work collaboratively with the community, other professionals and agencies to determine and prioritise the health issues that cause greatest concern and plan interventions to address them.

The assessment of health needs is a contentious area, and considerable confusion exists about the meaning of 'needs' (Frankel 1991). This stems from the different imperatives that influence the relationship between 'needs' and the provision of health care. The *public health imperative* is concerned with total population needs and the development of strategies based on prevention and health promotion. The *economic imperative* is concerned with marginal met needs and the most efficient ways of meeting needs. The *political imperative* has been one of reconciling a welfare system to the demands of the free market ideology (Jones 1995). The relationship between needs and welfare provision has received considerable critical attention, with the debate focusing on *absolute, normative* and *relative* definitions of need (Soper 1981; Wiggins and Dermen 1987; Doyal and Gough 1991).

Thus, there are multiple perspectives of need to incorporate: perceived and expressed needs of the profiled population; perceptions of professionals providing the services; perceptions and priorities of managers of commissioner/provider organisations (regarding national, regional or local priorities). Health needs assessment must balance these different perspectives when identifying priorities, and negiotiate with stakeholders to effect the changes required to improve health and reduce health inequalities.

Rowe *et al.* (2001), in their WHO guide to needs assessment, use a holistic model of health, emphasising the social, economic and cultural factors that affect health, plus individual behaviour. The concept of 'need' used incorporates those needs felt and expressed by local people as well as those defined by professionals. It moves beyond the concept of demand, and includes people's capacity to benefit from health care and public health initiatives.

However, the question of whether health needs assessment has actually helped to improve health or reduce inequalities, or whether changes would have happened anyway, remains unanswered.

The need for health and the need for health care

It is important to distinguish between the need for health and the need for health care. Health care is one way of satisfying the need for health. Arguments in the past have concentrated on the relationships between needs and the demand for, access to and use of services (Last 1963; Titmuss 1968; Hart 1971). In this sense, need is not an absolute concept, but is relative and dependent on socio-economic and cultural factors as well as supply-side factors. The need for health was perceived by Acheson (1978) as relief from the negative states of distress, discomfort, disability, handicap and the risk of mortality and morbidity. These concepts form the basis of, but do not wholly determine the need for, health services. This amounts to a bio-medical approach to health care needs that lends itself to the quantitative measurement of health status; the resulting health care needs reported fit conveniently with the bio-medical focus on the incidence and prevalence of disease.

Bradshaw (1972), on the other hand, constructed a paradigm of need in terms of: *expressed need* ('demand'), which is the expression in action of felt need; *comparative need*, which involves comparisons with the situation of others and considerations of equity; and *normative need*, such as experts' definitions, that change over time in response to knowledge. The expressions of need using these definitions are not necessarily consistent in relation to any individual. For many conditions, perceived need for care depends on the beliefs and knowledge of the person affected, and hence on value judgements (Buchan *et al.* 1990). In turn, these are influenced by psychological, socio-economic and cultural factors, not simply by the supply of services. Bradshaw (1994) later acknowledged the weaknesses of his original classification of need, but argued that it was never intended to form a hierarchy of needs. However, his paradigm forms a sociological approach that sets up a useful definitional matrix for needs.

Economists have consistently argued against the concept of objective need (Culyer 1995), seeing need as relative but at the same time recognising its practical importance and proposing concepts such as marginal met needs or, in relation to health care, the capacity to benefit from treatment. For example, Buchan *et al.* (1990) defined need as follows: 'People in need of a health service are defined as those for whom an intervention produces a benefit at reasonable risk and acceptable cost.' Culyer and Wagstaff (1991) considered the relationship between economic evaluation and need in detail, and proffered a precise definition of need that relates specifically to health care:

'A need for medical care is then said to exist so long as the marginal product of care is positive, i.e. so long as the individual's capacity to benefit from medical care is positive.' Economists have also emphasised the importance of health service priorities, given the scarcity of societal resources (Williams 1992). The debate has prompted some to argue that health care needs cannot be discussed in isolation from other needs (Seedhouse 1994), though in Britain, while national NHS policy recognises the importance of the views of the public in defining needs, there is less interest in the latter at local level, partly because health authorities do not know what to do with the results if they cannot clearly relate them to the need for effective services. As Fitzpatrick (1994) put it, 'From the health care provider's perspective, subjective health status problems are insufficiently specific to identify levels of medically determined need for particular health care interventions.'

Doyal and Gough (1991) constructed a theory of human needs based on the notion of basic needs being health and autonomy, an optimum level of which is fundamental to allow participation in social life. Thus, health care becomes a means of satisfying basic need. Soper (1993) sympathises with their argument but contests that their theory collapses when it is applied to specific needs. It is with this problematic specific level that health services researchers and planners have to deal. The orthodox response seems to be to follow the economic line and define needs in relation to supply. What is clear, however, is that if the meeting of needs is to be democratic, then they have to be debated openly. This means democratising the process of needs assessment so that individuals and communities are able to participate fully in decision-making about services. Such participation should extend beyond opinion polls and surveys to involvement in research and needs assessment itself.

Need for effective health care

Data from consumer consultation exercises, health surveys, mortality and morbidity statistics, and other information on the 'need for health' do not indicate to health planners what can be done to improve health (Stevens 1991). Thus, health planners prefer to base health need on a disease model and define it in relation to the need for *effective* health care and preventive services. Although a subsequent document produced by the NHS Management Executive (1991), and documents that followed it, modified this definition to include taking the views of interested parties into account in order to develop an overall understanding of need, and to be responsive to the views of local people about the patterns and delivery of services, the narrower definition has become that most widely used by health planners and public health specialists. Using this definition, need is linked to the appropriateness and effectiveness of the intervention in question. There is, however, considerable uncertainty about the appropriateness of different treatments, as reflected in variations in medical and surgical practice (Evans 1990). Any attempt to define health care needs is always open to criticisms of having a dual role of subjugating the individual or group being assessed to the needs of the system or professional interests within the system, while simultaneously constructing a picture of what that individual or group 'needs' (Jones 1995).

Social variations

While it is arguable that a health service agenda cannot take on the wider definition of need, which is affected by the social structure of a society, it should be concerned with tackling variations in health care provision to ensure equity, as well as understanding the contribution services can make to mitigating social variations in health, which are also related to the distribution of income and the degree of inequality in society (see Bradshaw 1994). As Popay and Williams (1994) stated, lay knowledge about health, illness and care is vital for understanding the experience of ill health and the processes and outcomes of health and social care. They pointed to 'the need to take seriously people's own views about their health and their health needs', which traditional epidemiological techniques are unable to make accessible, and to the increasing importance of the role of social scientists in research on people's health. Fitzpatrick (1994) also argued that the epidemiological techniques of documenting incidence and prevalence of illnesses and chronic conditions are not the same as identifying needs for health care. The issue of service effectiveness apart, he points to the vital role of the social sciences in developing an understanding of the patient's perspective regarding his or her illness, which should sensitise health professionals to his or her needs. The role of social science was described further in Chapter 2.

Local engagement

Some purchasers of health care do attempt to involve local people in the planning process by holding focus group meetings, or conducting surveys of their views and concerns, their health and their views for health priorities. Some undertake action research or rapid appraisal projects in local communities to achieve this end. Ong and Humphris (1994) argued that needs assessment requires a multidisciplinary approach and that

> The expertise held by users and communities has to be an integral part of needs assessment and to be considered alongside the public-health and clinical-needs assessments. The different inputs in the needs-assessment process offer specific and complementary insights on the complexity of needs as experienced by individuals and populations.

They recommend methods that combine a community perspective and a dialogue with decision-makers (e.g. rapid appraisal). Such techniques must be seen within a larger programme of the assessment of health needs, because they focus on felt and expressed need, rather than epidemiological or clinical assessments of need.

The narrow definition of health need as need for effective services also underpins the contracting process in health services. The underlying philosophy of this conception of need is related to prioritisation of health services and health service rationing, given that health needs are infinite and health care resources are limited. Ideal practice is to maximise the total amount of benefit within existing resources. This raises the problem of finding a method of prioritising health services, which is still unresolved (Bowling 1996a), though the QALY – or quality-adjusted life year – underpins treatments approved by some organisations (e.g. the National Institute for Health and Clinical Excellence, which is the independent organisation responsible for providing national guidance in England and Wales on health care, and the cost-effectiveness of new health technologies) (NICE 2004; http://www.nice.org.uk/pdf/CG011fullguideline.pdf; accessed September 2013).

The health services' research definition of need also makes the assumption that needs can only be met by a health service where adequate information exists about the cost-effectiveness of services. This has led to an active international research industry in systematic reviews and in health technology assessment (http://www.ncchta.org) (Oxman 1996).

Methods of assessing health needs

Cavanagh and Chadwick (2005) described health needs assessment as:

- a systematic method for reviewing the health issues facing a population – in an *ideal* world leading to agreed priorities and resource allocation to demonstrably improve health outcomes and reduce inequalities;
- a recommended public health tool for reviewing health issues;
- an opportunity to engage with specific populations;
- an opportunity for cross-sector partnership working.

A step-by-step guide to conducting needs assessment was produced by Cavanagh and Chadwick (2005). Rowe *et al.* (2001), in their WHO guide for nurses in Europe, also described the steps of community health needs assessment, referring to it as a developmental process, added to and amended over time. It describes the state of health of local people; enables the identification of the major risk factors and causes of ill health; and enables the identification of the actions needed to address these. The steps of community health needs assessment were listed as:

- profiling: the collection of relevant information about the state of health and health needs of the population;
- analysing this information to identify the major health issues;
- deciding on priorities for action;
- planning public health and health care to address the priority issues;
- implementing the planned activities;
- evaluation of health outcomes.

The authors emphasised the need to work in partnership with local people and collaborate with other professionals.

Information to collect

The measurement of need requires information about the level of morbidity (i.e. the size of the health problem) in a given population, the burden on that population and the impact the intervention is likely to have. The information required to address this includes data about the different types of treatments and services that are available in relation to the condition, their effectiveness and cost-effectiveness. This also raises the issue of how to measure burden and effectiveness (see Table 4.1).

The first decision to be made when assessing needs for health services in a particular area is which condition to start with. This will be influenced by local priorities, which in turn are influenced by mortality patterns and standardised mortality ratios (SMRs) in the area. For example, if there is a high rate of coronary heart disease, and a higher mortality rate than the adjusted average (as measured by the SMR), then this may be considered as a priority for action.

The range of techniques includes: calculation of existing health service activity levels and resource norms; calculation of rates of clinical procedures and treatments for specific conditions by population group; estimation of the prevalence of disease in the population and determination of appropriate intervention levels (i.e. the number in the population with a given set of indications for treatment); and application of social deprivation indicators to populations where social deprivation influences need. For some procedures, and in

Theory	Practice	Gap
Agree the disease/ condition for assessment and the diagnostic categories to be used.	Agree the disease/condition for assessment and the diagnostic categories to be used.	Medicalisation of needs. Definitions contested (e.g. disability, mental illness).
Define the population served.	Define the population served.	Populations are not static. Who is counted? Who is excluded? (e.g. non-random census undercounting).
Identify the range of treatments and services provided locally and elsewhere.	Identify the range of treatments and services provided locally.	
	Review the literature on incidence and prevalence of the disease, risk factors, mortality rates, the range of treatments and services offered, their effectiveness, cost-effectiveness and levels of appropriateness.	Burgeoning literature. Problems of meta-analysis. Importance of Cochrane reviews and databases.
Establish criteria of appropriateness for the health service intervention.	Apply this knowledge to the population of interest, taking local information into account.	
Establish the effectiveness and costs of each treatment and service.		Problems in obtaining accurate, reliable and comparable costing data.
Estimate the numbers in the target population, the numbers in the diagnostic group selected in that population, and the numbers likely to benefit from each type of intervention.	Build up neighbourhood profiles on health, mortality, socio-demographic characteristics, available services, access to, and use of, services. Local health surveys and rapid appraisal techniques, which involve the public and key professionals, might be used. Match this data, along with demographic and epidemiological disease profiles, to service availability.	Limitations of census data for particular populations. Local data sources (e.g. registers) may lack coverage. Routine data sources may be incomplete. Health surveys: expensive sampling problems response problems translation?

	Undertake comparative assessments of service type and level between districts.	Rapid appraisal: robust? reliable? generalisable?
	Identify gaps in routine information and research with a view to carrying out an epidemiological survey or apply data from elsewhere.	Selection of control districts. Norms-based approach. Problems of league tables and controlling for case-mix.
	Identify the strengths and weaknesses of providers (e.g. waiting lists, referral patterns, treatment delays, intervention rates, rehabilitation and prevention procedures); compare with providers of health care elsewhere.	
Set standards for monitoring and the level of resources required for effective provision of care.	Establish programmes to evaluate the outcome of services and treatments, and their costs, where existing information is inadequate, and calculate the proportion of people with the condition who would benefit from their supply.	Outcome data limited. Often not collected routinely.
	Establish mechanisms with clinicians at local levels to agree on thresholds for treatment and monitoring of contracts.	Consensus panel work difficult, local autonomy may be strong. Professional resistance.
	Monitor the impact of health service contracts with providers in relation to the needs of the population (e.g. number on the waiting list for a specific procedure, number of procedures performed).	Ownership of data may be a problem related to the tension between cooperation and market imperatives. Exclusion.
Community participation at all levels of needs assessment process.	Include the expertise of the public as (potential) users of health services (e.g. through rapid appraisal methods).	Public apathy. Barriers. Professional frustrations. Lack of accountability. Ethical and political objections. Democratic deficit.

Table 4.1 Assessment of health needs: comparison of ideal with practice

certain areas, an adjustment might need to be made for the proportion of the population absorbed by the private health sector. The assessment of health needs, then, involves a combination of the epidemiological assessment of disease prevalence, the evaluation of the effectiveness of treatment and care options, and their relative costs and effectiveness, analysis of existing activity and resource data, and the application of this knowledge to populations (in the case of health authorities to local populations, and in the case of general practitioners to their practice populations or catchment areas). It should also include the expertise of the public as (potential) users of health services (e.g. through rapid appraisal methods).

Because epidemiological surveys are expensive and time-consuming, one alternative is to apply the prevalence ratios and incidence rates reported in the literature to the population targeted (Purcell and Kish 1979; Wilcock 1979; Mackenzie et al. 1985). In some areas (e.g. heterogeneous inner-city populations), the level of inaccuracy with this approach will be too high to be acceptable. For example, variations in socio-economic group and the ethnic status of the population can affect the applicability of national data, or data from other areas, to local situations.

One approach that has been suggested is to compare existing service levels with those expected from the population covered, and to investigate further any specialties showing an unexpectedly high or low utilisation rate (Kirkup and Forster 1990). In some cases, it is certainly possible to compare existing service provision in districts with the number of cases that would be expected if national utilisation rates were applied. However, this is unlikely to lead to accurate estimates of need given that service use is affected by so many variables (e.g. resource allocation and supply, historical and political factors, and the patients' perceptions of health and level of knowledge).

In practice, it is unlikely that the information to do this will be available. The information that is available and currently used by health districts (departments of public health) to assess health needs in Britain falls short of the true epidemiological assessment of needs (Stevens 1991). Nevertheless, the information available includes national demographic statistics on mortality and fertility, small area statistics from census data and other sources on the social characteristics of areas which are relevant to health (e.g. unemployment rates, overcrowding rates, ethnic composition, age and sex structure), local health surveys and any available epidemiological data on incidence and prevalence rates, and morbidity statistics (e.g. cancer registration rates from the national cancer registry, and service use rates in order to assess supply and demand; Stevens 1991).

Some investigators have used action research, and, in particular, rapid appraisal methods to assess the needs of local communities with an emphasis on local people's views and involvement in defining need, priorities and evaluation (Ong et al. 1991; Ong and Humphris 1994; Murray and Graham 1995). This involves a collaborative, 'empowering', bottom-up approach to research, using triangulated research methods, for example, community meetings, interviews with key people, postal surveys, feedback of findings to key people and community members and joint development of a plan for action. This requires the use of social science methods to assess needs from a lay perspective, alongside traditional analyses of epidemiological and demographic trends (incidence and prevalence of disease, population trends, mortality patterns) (Fitzpatrick 1994). For example, a health needs assessment in the District of Columbia, USA, used mixed research methods including analysis of routine data, quantitative surveys, qualitative focus groups and assessment of national health areas of priority (Chandra et al. 2013). It was reported that multiple priority areas were identified (asthma, obesity, mental health, sexual health, stress-related disorders) and problems of general access to health services.

The role of epidemiological and demographic research

Epidemiology and demography can provide information on the need for health, though this has to be analysed together with evidence on the effectiveness of health care to be informative about the 'need for health care'. Where the service is of proven benefit (i.e. effectiveness), the demographic and epidemiological data are important *per se* because they are addressing the issue of whether the service is reaching all those who need it (e.g. is cervical cancer screening reaching all women?, are immunisation programmes reaching all children in predefined age groups?). Health services research is the focus for a number of disciplines, each of which plays a complementary role. The diversity of approaches has led to developments in the focus of epidemiological and demographic research as they are influenced by other disciplines and research paradigms. It is impossible to cover the contribution of each discipline to the assessment of needs in one chapter. In Parts 4.2 and 4.3 we concentrate on the main concepts and techniques of analysis within epidemiology and demography.

These disciplines operate within a positivist framework (see Chapter 6). This implies a belief in the scientist as a value-free observer and in the traditional scientific method, in which a hypothesis is generated, and data are gathered and tested objectively in relation to the hypothesis. Within this paradigm, disease in humans is an observable fact, the 'causes' and 'effects' of which are also subject to factual verification under the objective gaze of the investigator. The goal of such an approach is to search for universal explanation, derived from empirical regularities.

4.2 Epidemiology

The role of epidemiology

Traditionally, epidemiology has been concerned with the distribution of, specific causes (aetiology) of, and risk factors for diseases in populations. It is the study of the distribution, determinants and frequency of disease in human populations (Hennekens and Buring 1987). Epidemiology is also concerned with the broader causes of disease. For example, the epidemiological transition model suggests an association between national economic development and health using mortality data. However, this model has been hotly debated, as not all nations fit the model, patterns of mortality within nations change and mortality and health vary within countries by social group. It is also dependent on the way resources are distributed and targeted in societies (Wilkinson 1992).

Mainstream epidemiology examines data on levels of disease and risk factors for disease, while taking environmental factors into account. In contrast, materialist epidemiology is concerned with the role of underlying societal and structural factors. The latter is critical of the reductionist perspective of mainstream epidemiology, which focuses on individual, rather than societal, risk factors (reductionism). The focus on the biological make-up of the individual diminishes the importance of interactions between individuals and, more importantly, the idea that the whole is greater than the sum of its parts is lost. For the exploration of the latter, a more qualitative approach is needed. The limits of epidemiology can also be found in the way that disease classification is often taken for granted. Although epidemiologists are critical of the difficulties of categorising disease, it is too often assumed that medical classification is a valid research tool, forgetting that diseases, as physical phenomena, can be interpreted in different ways and the act of medical classification itself changes the way we look at and perceive disease. Types of epidemiology, including community, communicable disease, critical, environmental, occupational and social epidemiology, have been described by Moon *et al.* (2000). There is also an increasing focus in epidemiology on 'the life course' (the study of long-term effects on later health, and risk of disease, of physical or social exposures during gestation, childhood, adolescence, young and later adulthood; Ben-Shlomo and Kuh 2002), as well as the health effects of the accumulation of risk, and on genetic epidemiology (Lewis *et al.* 2005).

Epidemiological research

Epidemiological research includes both descriptive and analytical studies. Descriptive studies are concerned with describing the general distribution of diseases in space and time (examples include case series studies and cross-sectional surveys). Analytic studies are concerned with the cause and prevention of disease and are based on comparisons of population groups in relation to their disease status or exposure to disease (examples include case control studies, cohort studies, experimental and other types of intervention studies). However, these distinctions should be interpreted with some flexibility. Rothman (1986) pointed out in relation to epidemiologic research that its division into descriptive and analytic compartments, which either generate (descriptive research) or test (causal) hypotheses (analytic research), is derived from a mechanistic and rigid view of science which is inconsistent with current practice and philosophy. He pointed out that any study can be used to refute a hypothesis, whether descriptive (quantitative or qualitative) or analytic research methods are used.

Causal associations

Epidemiology is faced with difficulties when imputing causality. The difficulties of research design and interpretation of the results include temporal precedence in relation to the direction of cause and effect. This is the confidence that changes in X are followed by subsequent changes in Y, and elimination of the possibility of reverse causation – did depression lead to elderly people becoming housebound or did being housebound lead to depression? (See Chapters 9 and 10.) Experiments deal with reverse causation by the manipulation of the experimental (independent) variable, and measuring the dependent variable usually before and after this manipulation.

Longitudinal survey analyses use multivariable statistics, which can provide estimates for the strength of independent associations over time, where the variables of interest co-vary, and where a spurious association does not exist with other variables, and the hypothetical cause precedes, or occurs simultaneously with, the hypothesised effect in time (e.g. as indicated by the change in the causal variable occurring no later than the associated change in effect). Temporal regression analysis, for example, if carefully designed, can provide information suggesting that the second variable to change did not cause the first, though it is never possible to infer with absolute certainty that the first variable to change caused the second. Other longitudinal analysis techniques include structural equation modelling (e.g. cross-lagged and simultaneous model equations can be specified and estimated). This technique makes use of the inherent time-ordered data to address causal ordering. These analyses require careful formulation of hypotheses and models of the processes. The strength and duration of reciprocal relationships, and of hypothesised causal effects, are informative. No analysis yields trustworthy inferences about causal structures, due to the reciprocal nature of many potential influences (see Chapters 9 and 10). Difficulties include: chance results; study bias, which may influence the results; intervening variables or bias; and uncontrolled, extraneous variables which can confound the results.

Intervening variable

An intervening variable is an intermediate step in the causal pathway between the independent and dependent variables. In other words, the independent variable (e.g. the experimental or explanatory variable) affects the dependent variable (e.g. the outcome of interest) through the intervening variable. This is also referred to as *indirect* causation. An example is where consumption of fatty food can lead to narrowing of the arteries, which in turn can lead to coronary heart disease, so narrowing of the arteries is the intervening variable.

Confounding variable

A confounding variable is an extraneous factor (a factor *other* than the variables under study), *not controlled for*, which distorts the results. It is *not* an intervening variable (e.g. between exposure and disease). An extraneous factor only confounds when it is associated with the dependent variable (causing variation in it) *and* with the independent variable under investigation. The confounding and independent variables interact together to affect the outcome and their contributions cannot be disentangled. It makes the dependent and independent variables appear connected when their association may be *spurious* (see Figure 4.1).This raises the potential for extraneous variables to confound the results of research, leading to spurious (false) associations and obscuring true effects. If the confounding variable is allowed for, the spurious association disappears.

An example of confounding is where an association is found between cancer and use of hormone replacement therapy. If the cancer is associated with age, then age is a potential confounder; age should be allowed for in analyses (it might simply be that older age is responsible for the association with cancer). Another example relates to the hypothesis that the risk of myocardial infarction is increased among coffee drinkers, compared to non-coffee drinkers. Smoking may be a potential confounding variable in this association, as people who drink coffee also tend to smoke. In Figure 4.2, coffee appears to be associated with myocardial infarction. However, it is believed that smoking is a confounder because it is associated with

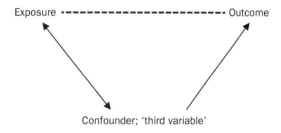

Figure 4.1: Confounders in research

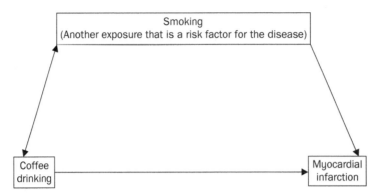

Figure 4.2: Coffee drinking as a confounder in myocardial infarction

both coffee drinking and with myocardial infarction. Smoking status is most likely confounding the association between coffee drinking and myocardial infarction, making it appear that there is a relationship when in fact there is none (see such examples in Varkevisser et al. 1991).

In ideal laboratory experiments in natural and biological science, one variable at a time is altered and observed, so that any effects that are observed can be attributed to that variable. This approach is not possible in research on people in their social environment, as human beings differ in many known and unknown ways. Other extraneous variables which are not associated with the independent variable can also lead to misleading results (systematic error or bias; see Chapters 7 and 8).

In epidemiology, the calculation of high relative risks may appear impressive, but important confounding variables may still be missed. A dose–response relationship gives added weight to imputations of causality between variables (e.g. there is a relationship between lung cancer and the number and strength of cigarettes smoked), but this still does not dismiss the possibility of confounding. Confounding is prevented by using randomisation in experimental designs, by restricting the eligibility criteria for entry into studies to a relatively homogeneous group and by matching (see Chapters 10 and 11).

A major research problem is how to decide whether a factor is causally related to an outcome, rather than simply being associated with the factor that is the true causal agent (see Davey Smith and Phillips 1992). This is important because a great deal of research is published which is based on descriptive studies that report associations between the risk of ill health and the exposure to particular factors. Examples include eating beef and risk of Creutzfeldt-Jakob disease, drinking coffee and risk of coronary heart disease, alcohol as a protective factor for coronary heart disease, not being breast fed being associated with low intelligence, use of babies' dummies being associated with low intelligence, use of oral contraceptives and risk of cervical cancer, use of oral contraceptives facilitating HIV transmission and the reverse – use of oral contraceptives protecting against HIV transmission.

It is important to be aware of potential extraneous variables which may confound results at the design stage of the study. These can then be measured and controlled for in the matching process (if used) and/or in the analyses. Age is a common confounding variable and so, to a lesser extent, is sex; most investigators routinely control for age and sex and analyse results separately for these groups. Randomised, experimental research designs are less likely to suffer from confounding (because of the random allocation to experimental and control groups), particularly if the number of participants is large.

The usual way to address confounding variables is to fit a regression model so that it is possible to examine the relationship between the variable of interest and the outcome while holding other variables constant. This is called 'adjusting' or 'controlling' for other variables. The limitation of this method is *residual confounding*, which arises because of the inadequacy of the measure representing the variable being controlled for (see Glynn 1993). For example, the apparent independent relationship between breast feeding and IQ (i.e. while controlling for social class) may be due to the inadequacy of using the father's occupation as a measure to control for social class effects. Biological plausibility is often appealed to in interpretation of epidemiological associations. However, it is possible to construct plausible mechanisms for many observed effects.

The way forward is for epidemiologists to use triangulated (e.g. multiple) research methods in order to minimise problems of interpretation in the study of the causes and process of disease. Causal arguments are strengthened by similar results being achieved by different studies and by different study designs, in different places and by different investigators. Epidemiologists should also work with social scientists to gather the information that lay people have about their health and lives, the causes of their health and ill health.

Methods of epidemiology

The range of epidemiological methods is described below, and those which are shared across disciplines are described in more detail in later chapters.

Case series and case studies

With the case series method a number (series) of cases with the condition of interest is observed, often using triangulated methods (e.g. questionnaires, data from records, observations) in order to determine whether they share any common features. The observations can be made retrospectively or prospectively, and they are relatively economical in terms of time and resources to carry out. They share the same weaknesses as survey methods, with the additional weakness that the sample is one of cases only, with no point of comparison. However, the method is useful for generating hypotheses. In-depth studies of single cases are known as *case studies*. These are also useful for developing a body of knowledge about a situation and for paving the way for future trials of interventions and cohort studies of conditions (Vandenbroucke 1999). They have a long tradition in medicine and are valuable for describing new diseases and new side-effects of treatment. The case study in relation to qualitative social research methods is described in Chapter 19.

Surveys

Descriptive cross-sectional surveys

Descriptive cross-sectional surveys are based on a representative sample or sub-sample of a population of interest who are questioned at one point in time (see Chapter 9). In epidemiology, the aim is usually to assess the prevalence of disease, associated factors and associations with service use. For the assessment of prevalence these studies are sometimes conducted in two phases, in which a screening instrument (e.g. a questionnaire measuring depressive symptoms) is used to identify people of potential interest, who are then followed up and assessed in more detail (e.g. with a psychiatric examination to confirm diagnosis). This is sometimes more economical than subjecting the whole sample to a full assessment.

Screening surveys and case finding

Cross-sectional screening and case finding surveys are conducted in relation to the detection of individuals or populations at high risk of disease in order that there can be a health care intervention or health promotion in order to protect them (e.g. as in cardiovascular disease). Population screening surveys have formed the basis for case finding, particularly in surveys of disability and psychiatric problems. Because of the high cost and time-consuming nature of population screens, case finding is now more commonly carried out in opportunistic screening exercises (e.g. detection of cases by questionnaire or record research among people attending a doctor's surgery for any other condition). The problems involved in screening relate to motivating health care professionals and the population to act, as well as ethical issues of invasion of privacy. Such methods are only ethical where the history of the condition is understood, there is a recognisable early symptomatic stage and there is an effective, safe, cost-effective and acceptable treatment available and agreed by policy-makers, clinicians and patients for predefined cases. Screening is generally confined to conditions which are recognised as common and perceived to be important.

Ecological studies

Ecological studies also aim to assess exposure (e.g. 'risk') and disease or mortality. With these, the unit of study is a group of people, rather than the individual (e.g. people in classrooms, hospitals, cities), in relation to the phenomenon of interest. In contrast to individual studies, the unit of analysis is a geographical area or organisation. The groups of interest are sometimes surveyed longitudinally to assess incidence (see Chapter 9). Data collection methods may include questionnaires and record research (e.g. medical records). Individual-level research can miss important area influences (e.g. on health), and hence the unit of analysis in ecological studies is the area level (geographical or organisational). A limitation is the assumption that the characteristics of populations (the study results) are applicable to the individuals within them: the *ecological fallacy* (Martin 2005; Moon *et al.* 2005).

Case control studies

At its most basic, a case control study (also known as a case-referent study) is a descriptive research method which involves comparing the characteristics of the group of interest, such as a group with a specific disease (e.g. ischaemic heart disease), or who have been exposed to a particular risk factor, such as radiation in a nuclear power plant incident (*cases*), with a comparison, or reference, group without the characteristic of interest, or the disease/condition (*controls*). The aim of the comparison is to identify factors which occur more or less often in the cases in comparison with the controls, in order to indicate the factors which increase or reduce the risk factors for the disease or phenomenon of interest. The analysis will lead to the calculation of an odds ratio, which is an estimate of the contribution of a factor to disease. The number of cases exposed is multiplied by the number of controls unexposed, and this figure is then divided by the product of the number of cases unexposed and the number of controls exposed. It is an approximation to the relative risk, which is a measure of how strongly associated the exposure is with the disease. The extent to which an exposure is more likely to occur in cases than controls is more accurately estimated in longitudinal surveys using relative risk, or rate ratio (the rate of the disease, being the number of cases occurring divided by the population at risk for a period of time). Thus, the case control study primarily aims to investigate cause and effect (see St Leger *et al.* 1992). The starting point is people who have the disease or condition, or who have been exposed to a risk factor. This is in contrast to the epidemiological longitudinal survey which starts with the potential risk factor of interest (e.g. smoking) and then follows up over time people who have and do not have the risk factor, and compares the number of events (e.g. cases of heart disease) in those with and without the risk factor.

In case control studies, then, people can be compared in relation to potentially relevant *existing* characteristics (risk factors) and/or retrospectively in relation to their reported *past* experiences (exposures). Data relating to more than one point in time are generally collected, making case control studies technically longitudinal rather than cross-sectional (longitudinal can relate to more than one point in time in the past – retrospective – as well as to more than one point in time in the future – prospective).

Many textbooks of epidemiology describe case control studies as retrospective. For example, when the group of cases of interest and an unaffected control group have been identified, their risk factors and past exposure to the potential aetiological factors of interest are compared (see Altman 1991). While case control studies are usually retrospective, they can be prospective (high- and low-risk groups are compared in relation to the incidence of disease over the passage of time). Case control studies can also be nested within a descriptive cross-sectional, or longitudinal, prospective study if the latter is sufficiently large to detect significant associations (see Mann 1991; Beaglehole *et al.* 1993). (See Box 4.1.)

Box 4.1 A study of injury amongst steelworkers

An example of a nested case control study is the study of injury in Brazilian steelworkers by Barreto *et al.* (1997). In their cohort study of 21,816 Brazilian steelworkers they found that mortality from motor vehicle injury was twice that in the state population. Therefore they undertook a nested case control study within their cohort to investigate possible socio-demographic, medical and occupational risk factors to explain this increased risk. For each case (all workers who died of motor vehicle injury while employed at the plant during a specific time period), four controls were selected randomly from workers within the cohort who were employed at the time of death of the case, and who were born in the same year as the case. Data for analysis in relation to risk of motor vehicle injury were collected from personnel, industrial hygiene and medical records.

Advantages and disadvantages of case control studies

The main advantages of case control studies are that they are relatively cheap in comparison with experimental designs, they are useful for the study of rarer conditions and they can provide relatively quick results. Case control studies, however, often require large numbers for study, they can suffer from the limitations of potential selection bias among participants, and extraneous, confounding variables (variables that are associated with both the presence of disease and the risk factor or exposure variables) may explain any observed differences between cases and controls.

Adjustment for confounding variables can be made by measuring them and adjusting for them in the data analyses (stratified analysis: the strata are the levels of the confounding variable). However, potential confounders may be unknown and unmeasured. It is also common to use matching techniques (see Chapter 11) in an attempt to limit the effects of extraneous confounding variables, though it is often difficult to match beyond common characteristics (e.g. age and sex). Case control studies suffer from a major limitation in that they are all, in effect, retrospective studies. Even if the cases and controls are followed up over time in order to observe the progress of the condition, the investigator is still starting with the disease or exposure and relating it to past behaviour and events. In particular, the cases may be more anxious to recall past behaviours (i.e. as possible causative agents) in comparison with controls and therefore questionnaire data may be subject to recall, or memory, bias.

A case control study is restricted to recruiting participants from the population *of interest*, and it is important that both groups of participants (cases and controls) should be representative of that population (see Chapter 8 on sample size and sampling). With case control studies, the control group is intended to provide an estimate of exposure to risk in the population from which the cases are drawn, and therefore they should be drawn from the same population – the difference between the two groups being the exposure (the exposed group form the cases). Appropriate controls can be difficult to find. As Altman (1991) has explained, people who do not have the outcome variable of interest may differ in other ways from the cases. It is also common in studies where the cases are hospital patients to use hospital patients with different medical conditions as controls. This can lead to bias because the conditions the controls are suffering from may also be influenced by the variable of interest, leading to underestimates of the effect of that variable in the cases (e.g. smoking is associated with several conditions). Ebrahim (1990) has described these problems, and pointed out that many investigators of hospital-based cases (e.g. stroke) now use two sources of controls: a community group (e.g. drawn from general practitioners' lists or local population register) and a hospital control group. As the rule for selecting controls is to ask whether cases and controls are equally likely to have been exposed to the variable of interest, then any doubt about this implies that the comparison of cases with controls may be biased.

One risk of the rigorous matching of multiple variables in case control studies is the 'controlling out' of the variable of interest. This is referred to as *over-matching*. This means having a control group that is so closely matched (and therefore similar) to the case group that the 'exposure distributions' differ very little. Rothman (1986) argued that this interpretation of over-matching is based on a faulty analysis which fails to correct for confounding variables – and is corrected if stratification by the matching factors is used in the analysis. He argued that the 'modern interpretation' of over-matching relates to 'study efficiency rather than validity'.

Research using documents

Epidemiologists use official statistics (which they call 'vital' statistics) on mortality (displayed by socio-demographic factors, area mortality and occupational mortality) and morbidity (e.g. on cancer registrations, congenital malformations and infectious disease surveillance). Their use plays a central role in disease surveillance. There are many problems with the use of official statistics because diagnostic criteria and disease classifications may change over time, and diagnostic definitions may also vary by area, making comparisons difficult. While data such as birth and death registrations are complete in the 'developed' world because it is a statutory duty to register them, other data may not be (e.g. routine patient administration data reporting types of procedures performed and disease classifications of patients discharged).

Prospective, longitudinal cohort surveys

These 'follow-up' studies are intended to assess the incidence of disease and the potential causative agents of disease in a population which divides itself 'naturally' into exposed and unexposed groups. The term 'natural' refers to the fact that they are not artificially manipulated by the research design as in experimental studies. There are two types of longitudinal study: panel and trend (see Chapter 9). With panel surveys there is no turnover of membership. However, account also needs to be taken of the time over which the survey members were observed (as well as the size of the population). With the fixed population in the panel survey, the population gradually diminishes in size as its members die and cease to be at risk of becoming 'a case'. Thus epidemiologists often use longitudinal trend surveys which are composed of dynamic populations (i.e. there is turnover of membership). 'Cohort' means the sample shares a common factor (e.g. age).

Life course approaches

Social science has long supported the analysis of processes that operate across a person's life in order to understand later outcomes of interest. Sociology of the life course is based on the assumptions that people's lives are embedded in, and shaped by, historical context; individuals construct their own lives through their choices and actions, and within the limitations of social and historical constraints; lives are intertwined via social relationships; and the meaning and impact of a life transition depend on when it occurs (see Clausen 1986). Data are collected from multiple sources, including longitudinal surveys, censuses, and life history interviews. The development of such life course approaches in epidemiology emerged later during the 1990s (Blane *et al.* 2007). Kuh *et al.* (2003, p .778) defined life course epidemiology as

> the study of long term effects on later health or disease risk of physical or social exposures during gestation, childhood, adolescence, young adulthood and later adult life. The aim is to elucidate biological, behavioural, and psychosocial processes that operate across an individual's life course, or across generations, to influence the development of disease risk.

A classic example of the value of life course approaches is analysis of a birth cohort from 1946 which demonstrated the importance of childhood illness (in turn influenced by parents' social class) to health in adult life (Wadsworth 1986).

Life course epidemiology involves building and testing theoretical models of pathways that link exposures across the life course to specific outcomes. The approach involves analysis of temporal ordering of exposures and their inter-relationships, and is complex, requiring time-related study designs. The ideal method uses birth cohort studies, in which data is collected from birth and throughout life. In practice, as with all longitudinal designs, the surveys rely on retrospective questioning at each follow-up phase, and are subject to recall bias.

The randomised controlled trial (RCT)

This is the ideal, true experimental method for the evaluation of the effectiveness of health services and interventions in relation to specific conditions. The method involves two or more groups who are treated differently, and random assignment to these groups. These features require the investigator to have control over the experimental treatment and over the process of random assignment between groups (see Chapters 10 and 11).

The natural experiment

At a basic level, the experiment is a situation in which the independent (experimental) variable is manipulated by the investigator or by natural occurrence. An investigation in a situation in which the experimental setting has been created naturally is known as the *natural experiment*. The classic and most popular example is John Snow's study of cholera in London in 1854, which established the foundations of modern epidemiology as a form of systematic analysis. (See Box 4.2.)

Box 4.2 Snow's study of cholera in London

At the time of the 1848 cholera outbreak in London several water companies supplied piped drinking water. Snow (1860) compared the mortality rates from cholera for the residents subscribing to two of the companies, one of which piped water from the River Thames near the point where large amounts of sewage were discharged, and the other which piped water from a point free of sewage. In effect, the natural experiment permitted Snow to obtain data on around 300,000 people, who spanned all socio-demographic groups, and who were divided naturally into two groups without their choice: one receiving water containing sewage and the other receiving water free from impurity. Snow used a map and plotted the location of the outbreak, having already noted the cases to be clustered around Soho in London. Snow discovered that people who had drunk water from the pump in Broad Street (now called Broadwick Street), supplied by the company drawing its water from the contaminated part of the Thames, were more likely to contract cholera than those who had not. Snow arranged for the removal of the handle to the pump and the outbreak stopped (though it had apparently already peaked). This is also a good example of how epidemiology is concerned with populations rather than individuals (see Lilienfeld 2000; Sandler 2000; Vandenbroucke 2000; Medical Research Council 2011).

Natural experiments worldwide include examination of whole population suicide rates in Sri Lanka in relation to the introduction of legal restrictions on pesticide imports (Gunnell *et al.* 2007); analysis of the use of health facilities to give birth, infant and child mortality in India, in relation to cash incentives to use health facilities to give birth (Lim *et al.* 2010);

and analysis of all-cause and cause-specific mortality in the population of Hong Kong in relation to the introduction of legislation to restrict the sulphur content in fuel (Hedley *et al.* 2002) (see Medical Research Council 2011).

Field experiments

Field experiments, or trials, are research studies in a natural setting in which one or more independent variables are manipulated by the investigator, under situations as controlled as possible within the setting. Field trials usually involve the study of healthy individuals in relation to the health outcome of preventive measures aimed at individuals (e.g. supplementation of diet with vitamins). With this method, large numbers of people have to be recruited in order to obtain an adequate proportion of them who will go on to contract the disease having received the intervention. This makes the method expensive. The difficulties of controlling intrinsic and extrinsic factors are also greater than in tightly controlled laboratory or clinical settings.

The *true* experiment, with the randomisation of participants to intervention or control group, and with pre- and post-testing, is the ideal model for this (see Chapter 10 for the distinction between the basic and the true experimental method). However, in practice, random allocation to the intervention is not generally feasible. Results are more difficult to interpret without random allocation of people to exposed and non-exposed (control) groups because of the potential for unknown extraneous variables which may confound the results (see Chapters 10 and 11).

Community intervention experiments

Community intervention experiments, or trials, involve a community-wide intervention on a collective (rather than individual) basis (e.g. in order to study the health outcome of water fluoridation, which is aimed at communities and not allocated to individuals). With this method, entire communities are selected and the exposure (e.g. the fluoridation) is assigned on a community basis. The community is defined either as a geographical community or as units in social groupings (e.g. hospital wards, school classrooms). Ideally, the *true* experimental method is adhered to, and the assignation of communities to the exposure or no exposure group is carried out randomly. With large numbers of people involved, this is rarely feasible and geographical comparisons are frequently made between areas exposed and not exposed (without randomisation), and the effects of the exposure. If there are no differences between the communities in their socio-demographic or other relevant characteristics, this non-random element may have little effect. Again, results are more difficult to interpret without random allocation of people to exposed and non-exposed groups (see Chapters 10 and 11). There can also be problems with sample size. An intervention community is commonly compared with one control community. This is a weak design, which is equivalent to a clinical trial with one patient in each treatment group, and no information can be provided on variation between communities (Hays and Bennett 1999).

Assessing morbidity, mortality, incidence and prevalence

Morbidity and mortality

The ideal first step when assessing the need for health care is the epidemiological survey of a defined population to establish the incidence (number of new cases) and prevalence (all existing cases) of morbidity in relation to the disease or condition of interest. Mortality patterns also require analysis. While figures on mortality by cause and by socio-demographic characteristics are available from official sources in the developed world, data on morbidity patterns (apart from cancer) are not routinely collected. In Britain, with a nationalised health service, some data are available centrally. These are collected from NHS hospitals, and cover numbers of patients discharged with their standard disease and operation coding. However, these data may be incomplete and subject to coding errors, and only represent people who are admitted to hospital (and who form the tip of the iceberg of illness in the community). Surveys of morbidity reported in general practice and comprehensive community health surveys are only carried out on an ad hoc basis. However, as noted earlier, it is sometimes possible to apply their findings to other populations if they are similar in structure. Except in relation to conditions where case-fatality is high and constant over time, and where the length of time with the condition is relatively short (e.g. as in some cancers), mortality statistics cannot be used as proxies for morbidity.

Information will also be required on the severity of disease and on current treatment patterns (in order to calculate the size of the gap between estimated need for a service and the expressed and satisfied demand for it), survival time and mortality rates. All this needs to be collected and analysed by age, sex, socio-economic group and ethnic status at minimum (where relevant), and an estimate should be made of the proportion of the population at risk and increased risk of the disease/condition. This requires precise definitions of the condition, rigorous assessments of health status in relation to the condition and agreement on clear and correct cutoff points for effective treatment (e.g. the level of high blood pressure which can be effectively treated). The last is essential in order to calculate the number of people who are likely to benefit from the service.

Incidence

Incident cases are new instances (of disease or death) which occur in a defined *time period*. *Incidence* refers to the number of new cases in a population in a defined time period. The *cumulative incidence* rate is the number of cases (the numerator) that occur (rate of occurrence) in a defined time period divided by the number of people in the population (the denominator) at the beginning of the period. It is more common to calculate the incidence rate of a disease over a specific period of time (e.g. a year); this is the number of *new* cases of the disease over the time period divided by the number in the population at risk (more specifically, the total time each member of the population remained at risk). Incidence is usually expressed as a percentage, or as number of cases per 1000 or per 100,000 people in the population.

Prevalence

The *prevalence* of a disease at a *specific point in time* is calculated by taking the *total number* of existing cases of the disease at that time divided by the number in the population at risk. With *point prevalence* (the number of cases at a certain point in time) a very short time period is examined (e.g. days or a few weeks). With *period prevalence* (the number of cases during a specified period of time) a longer time period is examined (e.g. weeks or months). *Lifetime prevalence* is measured by taking the number of people who have had the condition/disease at least once during their lifetime. Prevalence is usually expressed in terms of the number of cases (e.g. of disease) in a population at one point in time per 1000 or 100,000 population. The formulae for the calculation of incidence and prevalence ratios can be found in Rothman (1986).

Person time at risk

The person time at risk is the length of time each individual has been under observation without developing the disease. For a group of four people, one of whom was lost to follow-up after one year, one of whom developed the disease after two years and two of whom were still free of the disease after four years, the total person time at risk would be 11 years. Direct measures of the length of time a person is at risk are not available from routine ('vital') official statistics on mortality. Instead, the population at the mid-point of the time period of interest, multiplied by the length of the period (e.g. in years), is taken as an estimate of the person time at risk.

Case-fatality

This is a form of cumulative incidence and is related to the survival rate of the disease of interest. It measures the proportion of people with the disease who die within a defined period of diagnosis.

Odds ratio

While one way of comparing two groups (e.g. cases and controls) in relation to the disease of interest is to calculate the ratio of the proportions of those with the disease in the two groups, another method is to calculate the *odds ratio*: the ratio of the odds (loosely, a type of probability) of the disease ('event') in the two groups. This is an estimate of the contribution of a factor to disease. The calculation of odds has been clearly explained by Deeks (1996). The odds are calculated as the number of events divided by the number of non-events. More precisely, the number of cases exposed is multiplied by the number of controls unexposed. This figure is then divided by the product of the number of cases unexposed and the number of controls exposed. It is an approximation to the relative risk, which is a measure of how strongly associated the exposure is with the disease.

If the odds of an event are greater than 1, then the event is more likely to occur than not. If the odds are less than 1, the chances are that the event will not occur. The odds ratio is calculated by dividing the odds in the treated or exposed group by the odds in the control group. Epidemiologists attempt to identify factors that cause harm with an odds ratio of greater than 1. Clinical studies investigate treatments which reduce event rates, and which have an odds ratio of less than 1. The odds ratio can be used as an approximation of the relative risk in a case control study.

Measures of effect

In epidemiological terms, effect refers to the difference in disease occurrence between two groups of people who differ in relation to their exposure to the causal agent. There are three types of effect: *absolute effects* (differences in incidence, cumulative incidence or prevalence), *relative effects* (the ratio of the absolute effect to a baseline rate), and *attributable proportion* (the proportion of the diseased population for which the exposure to the causal characteristic was one of the causes of that disease). Measures of effect include relative risk, attributable risk and population attributable risk.

Relative risk

The relative risk, or rate ratio, is the incidence rate for the disease in the population exposed to a phenomenon relative to (divided by) the incidence rate of disease in the non-exposed population.

In other words, the relative risk indicates how much more likely a given disease or event is in one group compared with another. The relative risks of disease (e.g. lung cancer) in relation to the phenomenon under investigation (e.g. smoking) can be directly calculated if longitudinal survey methods are used, because the incidence and prevalence of the condition in the (exposed and unexposed) study population are known. It is also possible to calculate *confidence intervals* for relative risks. In a case control study with a sample of cases and a sample of controls, it is only possible to estimate relative risks indirectly (in the *odds ratio*). Only estimation is possible because a case control study does not include a sample of exposed and unexposed members (just a sample of cases and a sample of controls), and therefore the prevalence of disease is unknown.

Attributable risk

The attributable risk relates to the absolute effect of the exposure and is the difference between the incident rate in the exposed population and the incident rate in the non-exposed population. In other words, attributable risk indicates on an absolute scale how much greater the frequency of the disease or event is in one group compared with the other. This is an absolute measure of risk which is suited to the analysis of individuals, and not generalisable.

Population attributable risk

This gives a measure of the excess rate of disease in the whole population that can be attributed to the exposure of interest. It is calculated by multiplying the individual attributable risk by the proportion of exposed individuals in the population. It measures the population burden (*need*). The data are not generalisable.

Numbers needed to treat

Numbers needed to treat measures how many people need to receive the intervention (e.g. prescribed medication) for a given period in order that one more person will have the specified successful outcome, compared with the number who would have that outcome without the intervention. This is a meaningful way of expressing the benefit of the intervention. In a trial the number needed to treat is the inverse of the difference between the proportion of events in the control group and the proportion of events in the intervention group. An alternative model for the number needed to treat has been put forward as the inverse of the proportion of events in the control group multiplied by the reduction in relative risk (Chatellier *et al.* 1996). Rembold (1998) has proposed a formula for numbers needed to screen for use in evaluations of the efficacy of disease screening.

Comparisons of rates and standardisation

The comparison of rates across different populations can be misleading and therefore the standardisation of rates is essential in order to reduce any distortions. These methods are discussed, with demography, in Part 4.3.

4.3 The role of demography

Pure demography is the study of populations in terms of the numbers of people, and population dynamics in relation to fertility, mortality and migration; the broader area of population studies addresses the issues of *why* observed changes occur, and the consequences of these (Grundy 1996).

Changes in population structures are the result of changes over time in fertility, mortality and, to a lesser extent, international migration. Historically most countries had high levels of fertility and mortality. As major infectious diseases were controlled and declined, overall mortality levels declined and life expectancy at birth increased, while fertility remained high. One consequence was reduced infant mortality and a high percentage of children and young adults because younger age cohorts increase relative to older age cohorts. Populations begin to age when fertility falls and mortality rates continue to improve or remain low. Successive birth cohorts may become smaller. Countries that have low fertility and low mortality have completed what demographers call the 'demographic transition'. The term 'epidemiological transition' is used to describe the transition from relatively high to low mortality patterns, associated with changes in mortality by age and sex (Omran 1971); and the term 'health transition' refers to changes in the response of societies to health and disease (see Grundy 1996).

Demographical methods in relation to assessing need

The understanding of how populations change is vital to the assessment of needs for health services in order to plan services accurately (e.g. number of maternity beds and long-stay care places for elderly people that will be required). Demographic and social data (known as 'socio-demographic data') by definition provide information on the social and demographic characteristics of populations, and on areas of social deprivation. This information can be analysed in relation to mortality patterns, any existing data on morbidity for the populations of interest and service allocation. Such data have implications for 'need for health', though they cannot provide information on needs for effective health services.

Grundy (1996) has described how demography requires information about population 'stock' and 'flows' in and out of the population. The traditional demographic sources are population censuses and vital registration systems, supplemented with data from population surveys. National socio-demographic data are collected using the census, and local population data are derived from this. Interim profiles use the last census as the baseline and make adjustments (population estimates or informed guesses) for changes in the population since the last census was conducted. At the local level some further adjustments might be made in the light of local information. National data are available on births, marriages and deaths in populations, and also cancer registrations, as these are registered events. Similarly, information on immigrations and emigrations is available. From the information contained in the registrations it is possible to compile national figures on, for example, age and sex in relation to births and deaths. A wide range of analyses are carried out in relation to mortality (e.g. cause of death using International Classification of Disease codes, area, age, sex, socio-economic group, marital status). In Britain these analyses are carried out and published by the Office for National Statistics (formerly the Office of Population Censuses and Surveys). There are potential sources of bias and error in each of these sources. For example, certain sub-groups of the population may not be included in censuses (e.g. students, people temporarily away from home); there may be under-reporting of age in censuses; the cause of death recorded on death certificates may reflect changing knowledge or the training and perspective of the certifying doctor.

Using knowledge about current population structures, together with assumptions about future fertility, mortality and migration patterns, demographers can make predictions about future population structures. The method used for calculating population projections (estimates of future population numbers and socio-demographic characteristics, e.g. age and sex) is known as the *demographic component method*. Starting with a base (e.g. the census), assumptions are made about future birth, death and migration rates. Death rates are easier to predict than birth and migration rates as the latter can both be affected by economic, political and social circumstances. The range of demographic concepts, techniques, problems and methods of calculation has been described by Grundy (1996).

Rates: births and deaths

Population growth

This is a function of the balance of births and deaths, taking into account the extent of net migration. A common indicator of growth is the crude rate of natural increase (the difference between the crude birth rate and the crude death rate), taking migration into account (see Grundy 1996, for further details).

Crude birth rates

The crude birth rate is the number of births in a particular year divided by the total in the population and, at its simplest, multiplied by 100 (to express as a percentage). However, it is more usual to express birth and death rates per 1000 people in the population, and the multiplication is by 1000 instead.

Specific birth rates

Because it can be misleading to compare populations in relation to their crude birth rates (e.g. some populations may have higher proportions of males, which might explain their lower birth rates), it is necessary to use an estimate of the number of women of childbearing age in order to calculate the *general fertility rate*. This is calculated by the number of births divided by the number of women of childbearing age, multiplied by 1000.

Crude death rates

The crude death rate is the number of deaths in the population, expressed, for example, per 1000 total population. This is usually calculated, in relation to a particular year, by the number of deaths that year divided by the total population that year, multiplied by 1000.

It can be misleading to compare crude death rates of populations because they may have different age structures. For example, a country or geographical area may have a higher proportion of deaths (crude death rate) simply because it has more elderly people living in it or more males (and males have a shorter life expectancy than females). Therefore, it is essential to calculate *age-specific death rates for each sex* before comparisons can be made.

Age-specific death rates

The age-specific death rate is usually presented as so many deaths per 100,000 male or female population in the age group of interest per year. In relation to either males or females in a specific age group, for a particular year, the calculation is the number of men or women in a particular age group (e.g. 65–69 inclusive) dying that year, divided by all men or women in that age group, multiplied by 100,000.

Life expectancy

Age-specific death rates have the disadvantage of providing several figures for analyses, rather than just one. Therefore demographers and epidemiologists prefer to calculate and analyse life expectancy and standardised mortality ratios.

Life expectancy is a measure of the average (mean) length of life. Because the average length of life is affected by death rates in many different years, life expectancy is calculated from the average lifetime of a hypothetical group of people. This is based on the assumption that the age-specific death rates in the population of interest in a particular year would continue unchanged in all subsequent years. This allows hypothetical average life expectancy to be calculated and defined as the expectation of life at birth for a population born in a specific year. Although it differs from actual life expectancy in relation to individuals, because the latter do change over time, it does dispense with the requirement to wait until everyone who was born in a particular year has died before life expectancy rates can be calculated.

Standardisation

If the incidence or prevalence of disease or mortality is to be compared between populations, then it is necessary to ensure that the crude rates are calculated from data which are complete and accurate and not misleading. Crude rates are misleading. In theory, the age-specific rates should be compared, but it is cumbersome to deal with a large number of rates. The alternative is to calculate a single figure. In order to be reliable, the single figure must take account of different population structures. This is known as a standardised rate. For example, the standardised mortality rate refers to deaths per 1000 of the population, standardised for age.

Although it is common to standardise by age, and it is possible to analyse males and females separately, there are many other variables which are associated with mortality and morbidity in a population which are not taken into account (e.g. ethnic origin, socio-economic status). Thus analyses must always be interpreted with caution.

The two common methods of calculating standardised rates are direct standardisation and indirect standardisation. The indirect method is generally used. If sample sizes in the index population (population of interest in the area of interest) are small, there can be an increase in *precision* over the direct method, and the direct method can only be applied if the distribution of cases (of morbidity) or deaths in the index population is known. As these distributions are often unknown, the indirect method is generally used, though the direct method of standardisation is generally more consistent if sample sizes in the index population are large enough.

Direct standardisation

The direct method of standardisation has the advantage that it is relatively straightforward and likely to be more consistent than indirect standardisation. If one index population is to be compared with another, it is possible to take the ratio of the two directly standardised rates to yield the comparative incidence index or comparative mortality index. However, the sample sizes in the index population have to be sufficiently large, and the distribution of cases or deaths in the index population needs to be known for this method.

In order to overcome the problem of differences in the structures (e.g. age) of the populations to be compared, a standard population is selected (it may or may not be one of those under study), and the age-specific (or other relevant characteristic) rates (morbidity or mortality) of the index population are applied to the standard population. This provides the number of cases in each age group that would be expected if the index population rates applied in the standard population. The expected number of cases across the age groups is totalled to obtain the total number of expected cases. The standardised incidence *rate* for the index population is the total of these expected cases across the age groups, divided by the total in the standard population.

Indirect standardisation

Indirect methods of standardisation are often preferred because, unlike the direct method, the indirect method does not require knowledge of the age-specific rates in the index population and because the numbers of cases at each age may be small, and thus the age-specific rates of the index population used in the direct method may be subject to considerable sampling error.

The 'standardised incidence ratio' for morbidity and the 'standardised mortality ratio' for the study of mortality are derived using indirect methods of standardisation. The steps for the calculation of each are identical, except that the former is based on a set of standard age-specific incidence rates and the latter is based on a set of age-specific mortality rates (total or for the cause of death of interest).

Standardised incidence ratio

With the indirect method of standardisation for both incidence and mortality, a standard set of age-specific rates in relation to the variable of interest needs to be obtained (e.g. age-specific rates for breast cancer in the total population of females). These standard rates are applied to the index population (the predefined population in the area of interest) in order to determine the number of cases expected in each age group in the index population, on the assumption that the index population experiences incidence of the variable under investigation at the standard rates. These expected cases in the index population are totalled over the age groups to obtain the total number of expected cases in the index population. The total of the observed index cases is divided by the total number expected in order to obtain the standardised incidence ratio. The crude rate in the standard population is multiplied by the standardised incidence ratio to give the standardised incidence rate in the index population.

Standardised mortality ratio

In relation to mortality, the steps are the same as for the standardised incidence ratio (except that mortality, not disease incidence, is the variable of interest), and the ratio is called the standardised mortality ratio (SMR).

The SMR compares the standard mortality rate for the standard (whole) population with that of particular regions or groups (index population), and expresses this as a ratio. The standardised rate in the index population is obtained by multiplying the crude rate in the standard population by the SMR. The procedure for the calculation of the SMR is explained further below.

SMRs are a method of indirect standardisation and are calculated in order to be able to make comparisons of death rates from all causes and mortality from a single cause between geographical areas. They can be calculated for both sexes combined or for just males or females. For the SMR, the crude death rates for particular diseases are calculated (see earlier), often separately for each sex. In order to avoid using small numbers it is more usual to calculate crude death rates from specific causes per 100,000, or per 1,000,000, rather than per 1000. However, the age structure of the population must also be taken into account. As was previously pointed out, this can be done by calculating the age-specific death rates for the disease of interest for each index area and comparing them, though this has the disadvantage of providing several figures (for each age group). The alternative is to use *age standardisation*.

For age standardisation a standard population is selected as a reference point for the geographical area of interest (e.g. the population of a whole country). The SMR is then calculated by using the age-specific death rates for the standard population. A clear example of this has been provided by McConway (1994a):

> So to work out the SMR for male deaths from lung cancer in West Yorkshire, using England and Wales as the standard, the first step would be to find out the age-specific death rates for lung cancer for men in England and Wales. These can be used to work out how many men would have died of lung cancer in West Yorkshire if the impact of the disease on men of any given age there was the same as it was nationally.

The SMR for deaths from a particular disease is then calculated by expressing the actual number of deaths in the group of interest (e.g. number of female deaths from breast cancer) in the index area (geographical area of interest) as a percentage of the expected number of deaths from the standard population data. For example, if the actual number of female deaths from breast cancer in the index population (in the geographical area of interest in England) was 800, and if the application of national female breast cancer rates to the index population (in the geographical area of interest) yielded an expected figure of 700, then the SMR is calculated by expressing the actual number of deaths (800) as a percentage of the expected number of deaths (700). This gives an SMR of 114, and as this is over 100 it means that 14 per cent more females died of breast cancer in that area than would have been expected from national figures, allowing for differences in age structure. It is better to consider the upper and lower confidence limits for an SMR, as these tell us whether the mortality differs significantly from the national average.

Analyses of survival

Survival analysis and life tables

Survival analyses, leading to the estimation of survival rates (e.g. a five-year survival rate), can be carried out in relation to the period of time between a specific event (e.g. medical diagnosis) and death or in relation to a range of other *end-points* of interest (e.g. in relation to onset or diagnosis, recurrence of condition, readmission to hospital, success of therapy, and so on; or, in relation to marriage, divorce or widow(er)hood). The method of calculation and the formulae for the construction of life tables have been described by Bland (1995). Grundy (1996) has described the concept of *life tables*. Life tables are derived from age-specific mortality rates and show the probability of dying, and surviving, between specified ages. They permit life expectancy and various population projections to be calculated. To carry out the calculation for survival times for people with a specific cancer, for example, the investigator needs to set out, for each year, the number of people alive at the start, the number who withdrew during the year, the number at risk and the number who died. For each year, the probability of dying in that year for patients who have reached the beginning of it is calculated, and then the probability of surviving into the next year. Then the cumulative survival probability is calculated: for the first year this is the probability of surviving that year; for the third year it is the probability of surviving up to the start of the third year and so on. From this life table, the survival rate (e.g. five-year survival rate) can be estimated (Bland 1995).

Mortality compression

Where infant mortality is high but declining, as in developing countries, most of the improvements in life expectancy at birth result from the survival of infants. Once infant and child mortality are low, as in the developed world, the gains in life expectancy are greatest among the oldest members of the population. As mortality rates among elderly people decline, more people survive to older ages. Most of the common health problems in old age are chronic, rather than immediately life-threatening. There is evidence that physiological functioning is declining more slowly with age than was previously thought, though it appears that women can expect to spend more of their years in a disabled state than men, negating some of the benefits of longer life expectancy among females (Manton 1992; Kinsella 1996). With these trends (or epidemiological transitions), conventional indicators of the health of the population (e.g. life expectancy) are less useful. Thus, research in demography is also focusing not simply on the loss of healthy life years due to disability (e.g. the disability-adjusted life year), but on whether morbidity and functional disability in old age are compressed into a shorter and later time period than previously or whether it spans the whole range of later years (i.e. healthy life expectancy, often termed active life expectancy, quality-adjusted life expectancy and disability-free life expectancy).

Disability-free life expectancy (DFLE)

This is an indicator that aggregates mortality and morbidity data for a population into a single index (Sullivan 1971; European Concerted Action on Harmonization of Health Expectancy Calculation in Europe 1996). It represents the average number of years that a person of a given age may expect to live free of disability (Colvez 1996). Demographers have used a range of different survey and mortality tables for their calculations of DFLE (Jitapunkel *et al.* 2003), which creates difficulties in making comparisons across the world (Robine 1992).

The calculation of DFLE requires the availability of standard, current mortality tables (life tables), and data on the prevalence and incidence of morbidity from representative longitudinal survey data with valid and reliable measures of disability. However, longitudinal data on incidence are less often available and most investigators use data from cross-sectional surveys in their formulae. Calculation of DFLEs is usually based on the method of Sullivan (1971). With this method, a standard cross-sectional life table is taken which gives the number of person years between two ages. This is subdivided using cross-sectional survey data on age-related prevalence of permanent and temporary disability into years with and without disability. A new life expectancy is then calculated using only the years lived without disability. Thus, the rate of permanent and temporary disability is used to estimate the number of years free from disability: 'For example, if 1,000 person-years are lived between ages 75 and 79, and 30 per cent of the population aged 75–79 years suffer from disability, then the number of years free from disability is said to be 700' (Bisig *et al.* 1992).

This method, using cross-sectional data, is inevitably crude. In particular, the level of DFLE is influenced by the measures of disability used in the studies taken for the calculations. Further, as Colvez (1996) pointed out, data on the prevalence of disabilities derived from a series of cross-sectional surveys are not able to provide information on incidence or the probabilities of becoming disabled the *next* year. Cross-sectional surveys can only provide population profiles for a defined time period, and they cannot provide data showing the turnover of people from one category of health status to another.

Sullivan's (1971) method has been criticised by Newman (1988) and Péron (1992), as it does not take into account the reversibility of disabled states. Péron suggests that the correct method is to construct a table showing transitions into and out of states of disability and good health. This presupposes knowledge of the rates of transition from good health to disability and vice versa, and of the mortality rates of disabled and non-disabled people for the same period. Ideally, this requires robust and representative, systematically collected longitudinal survey data on disability, which are rarely available.

Developments include extending the method of potential gains in life expectancy to DFLE (Colvez and Blanchet 1983; Colvez 1996). The potential gain in life expectancy owing to the elimination of all deaths from specific causes is added to the potential gain in DFLE owing to eliminating disabilities due to the same cause.

Disability-adjusted life years (DALYs)

The World Bank (1993) adopted a slightly different approach with the development of DALYs. DALYs estimate the loss of healthy life using international mortality data. With this procedure, the number of years of life lost was estimated for each recorded death in 1990. This was then taken as the difference between actual age at death and the life expectancy at birth which would have characterised a country with a low mortality rate. The loss of healthy life owing to disability was estimated using information from morbidity surveys or expert opinion, and the typical duration of each disease was combined with a weighting to reflect its likely severity. Finally, death and disability losses of healthy life were combined to give the number of years of healthy life lost owing to death or disability (see Curtis and Taket 1996).

Potential years of life lost (PYLL)

The PYLL compares the life expectancy of the whole population with that of particular groups or geographical areas, and expresses it as a ratio.

Summary of main points

- Dictionary definitions of need focus on 'want', 'require' and 'necessity'. The definition of health needs varies between academic disciplines.
- Health policy-makers base health need on a disease model and define it in relation to the need for effective health care and preventive services.
- Lay knowledge is vital for the understanding of health and health care needs.
- The methods of epidemiology and demography can provide information on the need for health; this has to be analysed with other data on the effectiveness of health care to be informative on the need for health services.
- Epidemiology is concerned with the distribution of, causes of and risk factors for diseases in populations.
- Demography is the study of populations in terms of the numbers of people, and population dynamics in relation to fertility, mortality and migration. Population studies, a broader area of demography, addresses the issues of why changes occur and their consequences.

Key questions

1 Define the concept of need.
2 Distinguish between need for health and need for health services.
3 What are the ideal steps in the assessment of the need for health services?
4 What are the main research methods used by epidemiologists?
5 Define a confounding variable.
6 Explain the concept of over-matching in case control studies.
7 Distinguish between incidence and prevalence.

Key terms

attributable risk
case control study
case finding
case series study
cohort
community intervention experiments
confounding
cross-sectional study
demand
demography
disability-free life expectancy (DFLE)
ecological study
effect
epidemiology
extraneous variable

field experiments
health need
healthy life expectancy
incidence
intervening variable
life expectancy
life tables
mortality compression
natural experiment
need
needs assessment
population attributable risk
prevalence
prospective (longitudinal) survey
randomised controlled trial (RCT)

rate
ratio
relative risk
screening surveys
spurious association

standardisation
standardised incidence ratio
standardised mortality ratio
survival analysis

Recommended reading

Bland, M. (1995) *An Introduction to Medical Statistics.* Oxford: Oxford Medical Statistics.

Carneiro, I. and Howard, N. (2011) *Introduction to Epidemiology.* Maidenhead: Open University Press.

Deeks, J. (1996) What is an odds ratio? *Bandolier, Evidence-based Health Care*, 3: 6–7.

Grundy, E. (1996) Populations and population dynamics, in R. Detels, W. Holland, J. McEwan and G.S. Omenn (eds) *Oxford Textbook of Public Health*. Oxford: Oxford University Press.

Martin, R.A. (2005) Epidemiological study designs for health research and evaluation, in A. Bowling and S. Ebrahim (eds) *Handbook of Health Research Methods: Investigation, Measurement and Analysis.* Maidenhead: Open University Press.

Moon, G., Subramanian, S.V., Jones, K. *et al.* (2005) Area-based studies and the evaluation of multilevel influences on health outcomes, in A. Bowling and S. Ebrahim (eds) *Handbook of Health Research Methods: Investigation, Measurement and Analysis.* Maidenhead: Open University Press.

St Leger, A.S., Schnieden, H. and Wadsworth-Bell, J.P. (1992) *Evaluating Health Services' Effectiveness.* Buckingham: Open University Press.

CHAPTER 5

Costing health services: health economics

Chapter contents

Introduction

With the current emphasis on the purchase of health and social services that are effective and also cost-effective, there is an increasing need for policy-makers, health professionals and managers, and researchers to be aware of the basic concepts of health economics. There is a related need to be aware of the type of data that should be collected for economic analyses. This chapter describes the main concepts and techniques used by economists and the types of data that are required in relation to each. Cost data are complex to collect, and collaboration with a professional health economist is required in research projects which aim to evaluate the costs, as well as the health and social outcomes, of services. Useful introductions to costing health and also social services include those by Mooney (1992), Netten and Beecham (1993), Locket (1996), Drummond *et al.* (2005) and Brown (2005).

Health economics

Economic evaluation has its foundations in welfare economics (see Sculpher 2004, for a brief overview). The underlying assumption of economics is that the resources available to society as a whole are scarce, and thus decisions have to be made about their best use. For economists, resources are best employed when they maximise the benefit to society. This is as true for health care as any other resource area. Health economics, therefore, is about how health care resources are used in order to produce the greatest benefit to the population. This inevitably involves choosing between competing calls on scarce resources (e.g. should resources be spent on building another community clinic or on employing more nurses in existing clinics?). Decisions have to take account of what services have to be given up, or which planned services deferred, in order to pay for the alternative. In other words, the *opportunity cost* has to be assessed.

The basic assumption of economic analysis consists of 'rational' individuals or organisations operating in an 'ideal' market where goods and services are exchanged for resources. The 'ideal' market is where many buyers and sellers have free entry and exit, all organisations seek to maximise profits, maximum profit is made when the *marginal cost* of production is equal to the market price and there is a situation of *perfect knowledge*. Knowledge is necessary because individuals must be able to exercise informed choices which achieve a desirable outcome (their choice is, of course, limited to the opportunities presented to them, which are determined by price and income, which are related to the amount sold). They are said to have a preference for a good or service that gives satisfaction (utility), and they work towards maximising that utility, in a world in which financial resources are scarce. The 'ideal' market is not always achieved, and is threatened by monopolies, monopsonies and oligopolies. A monopoly is a situation in which there is only one producer, who has the power to influence price and can price goods and services discriminately, selling to different buyers at different prices. A monopsony is a situation in which there is a single purchaser. An oligopoly is a situation in which a few producers compete and output and prices are subject to the interrelationships between the producers.

In economics, idealised markets (the collection and interaction of buyers and sellers) operate according to the laws of supply and demand (see later). The aim of organisations (e.g. hospitals) is assumed to be the maximisation of profit (or its equivalent), and their constraints relate to the production process. Health economics, however, deals with an 'imperfect' market situation. The health care market is frequently referred to as the internal market or quasi-market. This is the application of rules to ensure an increase in efficiency and improved allocation of resources within the framework of the organisation (see Locket 1996, for examples of different methods of financing and organising health care).

The 'social good' is also relevant to economics, as expressed in the concepts of the *efficiency* of the distribution of resources and *equity* (which may conflict). Efficiency can be defined in relation to allocative efficiency (the allocation of resources to maximise the benefits to the population) and technical efficiency (the achievement of maximum benefits at minimum costs). Equity can be interpreted in a number of ways: for example, the fairness of the distribution of resources; entitlement to resources in relation to need or contribution; the production of the greatest good for the greatest number. Whitehead (1994) argued that equity related to everyone having a fair opportunity to attain their full health potential, and that no one should be disadvantaged from achieving this potential if it could be avoided.

Patient choice and equity

Most economic analyses involve the study of individuals making choices under constrained conditions (Le Grand 2003). This is because the availability of choice may lead to some patients choosing more expensive (though not necessarily more effective) health technologies and systems (Oliver 2003). Patient choice is arguably a feature of *equity of health care*. But the theoretical free will of individuals to make choices is constrained by the social system. It may have equitable or inequitable consequences if some patients (e.g. the more educated and affluent) are more aware of the choices being offered, and more adept at making more beneficial, though not necessarily more cost-effective, choices than others. In addition, the range of choices offered may vary depending on the geographic area and its characteristics.

Macro- and micro-level analyses

Health economists, then, are concerned with economic evaluations of health care in terms of costs and benefits. The costs and benefits of health care are analysed at the *macro* (the larger scale of organisations, communities and entire societies) and *micro* (the individual organisation, community and society) levels. Farrar and Donaldson (1996) have provided examples of the macro and micro levels in relation to care for elderly people. At the *macro level* one question is whether the ageing population is a growing burden that can be afforded by western societies. They break this question down into two issues. First, is an ageing population going to constitute an increasing economic burden? Second, what does 'affordability' in relation to health care mean? In relation to the first question, economists work with demographers and social scientists in order to assess trends in the age structure of the population, including information on morbidity rates and, in particular, on morbidity compression (the concentration of morbidity into the last years of life rather than spread out across older age groups). They then relate this to information on the costs of addressing these patterns of morbidity to provide estimates of trends in health care costs and expenditure for older populations. Regarding the second question, on affordability, the concept of opportunity cost is relevant: what has to be given up in order to provide the care in question, and is that what society wants? In other words, what proportion of society's scarce resources should be devoted, not just to health care, but to the health care of elderly people? At the *micro level*, economists are concerned with the costs and benefits of different ways of caring for elderly people *within* societies and ensuring that health care resources are spent in the best possible way. At this level it is essential to include the costs and benefits incurred by all relevant sectors, regardless of budget demarcations (e.g. primary and secondary health services, social services, voluntary sector), as well as the public (i.e. patients) and wider society (Farrar and Donaldson 1996).

Demand, utility and supply

Although health care markets operate differently from other markets, economists still use the concepts of demand, utility and supply in their analyses. *Demand* refers to consumers' willingness to pay for desired goods and services, in the context of limited resources. It assumes that the consumer is in the best and most knowledgeable position to decide what values should be attached to various goods and services, though this is less likely to be the case in relation to health services (Mooney 1992).

The demand curve for a good or service illustrates the relationship between its price and the quantity desired (holding other variables constant, such as income and the price of other goods). The curve usually indicates that the lower the price, the greater the quantity desired (sloping down from left to right). *Elasticity* refers to the degree to which demand responds to price.

The concept of *utility* underlies the concept of demand. It simply refers to consumers' satisfaction. Economists assume that the greater the utility (satisfaction) obtained from the good or service, the greater will be the price the consumer is willing to pay for it. Related to this are the concepts of marginal utility (the additional utility obtained from consuming one extra unit of the good or service) and diminishing marginal utility (as more units of the good or service are consumed, the utility obtained from each additional unit of consumption tends to fall).

Supply refers to how the costs of producing goods and services and the prices of the final product affect the quantity supplied. The supply curve illustrates the relationship between the price of the good or service and the quantity supplied, holding other variables constant (e.g. the price of other goods). The prices result in revenue, and the additional revenue for each extra unit produced is the marginal revenue. The curve reflects the incentives for the producer, in that the higher the price of the commodity, the more the producer will be prepared to devote resources to producing it because, if nothing else changes, profits can be increased (thus the curve slopes upwards from left to right). Maximum profit is earned when the output is set at the point where the marginal cost is equal to the marginal revenue.

The concept of *costs* is related to that of supply. In theory, the producer will supply goods only if costs can at least be covered. Producers have fixed and variable costs. Fixed costs are constant regardless of the volume of output; variable costs vary with the volume of output. The higher the price, the greater is the likelihood that costs will be met, and thus greater profits obtained; hence the supply curve is usually positive. In contrast, the consumer aims to maximise utility. This is where the notion of competition is relevant, because it refers to the negotiation between producers and consumers over prices.

The limits of economic analysis

Economists agree that the crude application of these concepts to health care is obviously inappropriate. Microeconomic methods of analysis are of limited value in situations where there is an agency relationship between the consumer and the provider, and where consumer choice is constrained by several factors – from lack of technical information for consumers to exercise informed choice to limitations in provision. A further danger of economic analysis is that the values given to individual and aggregate utilities become 'more real' than those of the individual or the groups they are said to represent (Ashmore et al. 1989). Locket (1996) pointed out that economic analysis should only be performed where there is information that a health care intervention works, is acceptable to patients (i.e. they will use it) and is accessible to those who need it.

Economic appraisal

Economic appraisal is the comparative analysis of alternatives in terms of their costs and consequences, and can take a variety of forms. It covers a range of techniques but the main approaches (which include cost minimisation, cost-effectiveness analysis, cost–benefit analysis and cost–utility analysis) are described in the following sections. Each involves systematic approaches to the identification and measurement of the costs and consequences of a particular service or intervention. These concepts have also been clearly described by Drummond (1994), who also points out that many economic evaluations do not fall neatly into one of these categories. For example, some investigators report a range of costs and consequences without attempting to aggregate the costs or the health benefits or calculate a cost-effectiveness ratio. This approach is labelled a cost–consequences analysis. The decision-maker (e.g. health care purchaser) then has to make the trade-offs.

With all costings it is important to collect up-to-date information, and each piece of cost information should relate to the same time period. The cost information must also be comparable between sampling units. The process is far from straightforward in relation to data collection, interpretation and analysis. For example, Kelly and Bebbington (1993) have described the considerable problems of reliability (the consistency of measures across location and time) of organisations' measures of unit costs and the caution required in interpreting and analysing these. Because of such inconsistencies, and because of the unavailability of data, economists are often forced to make assumptions about costs and organisational characteristics in their costing formulae. These assumptions are not always admitted to or made explicit but they should be, so that the reader can critically assess the validity of the exercises. Economics, while quantitative, is not an exact science, and many value judgements underpin costing analyses. Barendregt and Bonneux (1999) criticised the high level of arbitrariness and lack of transparency in economic evaluations of health care. They pointed out that standardisation would increase transparency, but not if the standard required researchers to make additional assumptions and use controversial methods of imputation. They argued that a modest standard would be a 'boon for transparency'.

Box 5.1 A review of health economics evaluations in RCTs

Barber and Thompson (1998) carried out a review of statistical methods used for health economics evaluations in RCTs published in 1995, identified from Medline. They found that information about the completeness of the cost data was given for only 24 (53 per cent) of the studies, there were major deficiencies in the way cost data in RCTs was analysed, and misleading conclusions about the costs of alternative therapies were often reported in the absence of supporting statistical evidence. They called for guidelines to improve practice.

The challenges involved in obtaining the prices of resources, the necessity of adopting a hybrid approach in many cases, as well as choosing estimates from the research data (with assessments of how typical they are) and nationally available statistics have been outlined by Drummond (1994).

Cost minimisation

Cost minimisation compares the costs of achieving a given outcome. This approach is used when the outcomes of the procedures being considered are known to be the same (e.g. two drugs whose efficiency and side-effects are the same). This makes it possible to focus on identifying the least cost option without having to worry about measuring and comparing outcomes. Cost minimisation should be undertaken *only* where there is a very high confidence that the outcomes are the same, because if they are, in reality, different, then the analysis will give misleading results. There are few cases in which health care interventions are identical in this way.

Cost-effectiveness

Because it is rare to find health interventions which are similar in effects to permit cost-minimalisation analyses, it is more usual to compare the difference in costs between interventions with the difference in their consequences. Where there is just one main parameter in this respect (e.g. cost per life year), cost-effectiveness analysis is used.

Cost-effectiveness analysis is an approach to the assessment of efficiency which is concerned with the measurement of outcomes in 'natural' units (e.g. improvement in health status), which are compared with the monetary costs of the health care. The cost-effectiveness of a health care intervention is defined as the ratio of the net change in health care costs to the net change in health outcomes. For example, if the total costs of the care have been calculated, and if a health status or health-related quality of life scale has been administered to a sample of the patient group of interest before and after exposure to the care under study, then the cost per change in health status/health-related quality of life can be calculated. An incremental analysis can examine the incremental change in effectiveness and costs of moving from one type of care to another (e.g. outpatient care to GP care). A decision will have to be made when the results are interpreted as to whether any observed increase or reduction in costs is enough to compensate for any increase or decrease in resulting health status/health-related quality of life.

With cost-effectiveness analysis, the costs are more narrowly defined than with cost–benefit analysis. They are generally confined to monetary measures of output (effectiveness) and are limited, as they have difficulties coping with more than one output.

Cost–benefit analysis

Cost–benefit analysis refers to approaches which assign a monetary value to the benefits of a project and compare this with the monetary costs of the project. This enables comparisons between alternative projects to be made in terms of efficiency.

Cost–benefit analysis values *all* costs and benefits in monetary units and enables the total service cost to be calculated (see Allen and Beecham 1993, for details). This is the broadest method. Once calculated, costs should be disaggregated to a unit of measurement that is as close as possible to client-level data in order to obtain a relevant unit cost for each service (e.g. hospital use is counted by the number of inpatient days or outpatient attendances) or to even more detailed levels (e.g. ward costs).

Cost–benefit analysis is used in decision-making about whether to introduce (or maintain) a particular programme (i.e. service). The principles underlying cost–benefit analysis are that programmes should be implemented only where benefits exceed costs, and they should not be implemented where costs exceed benefits (Mooney 1992). The point about cost–benefit analysis is that it allows *different* services to be compared (e.g. renal dialysis with rheumatology clinics). Because of the methodological complexities of measuring and including all health benefits in the analysis, some economists use 'willingness to pay' techniques instead.

Marginal cost

The marginal cost can be defined as the additional cost of producing one extra unit of output (e.g. of treating an extra patient), and includes staffing and treatment costs, but not buildings and large-scale capital equipment costs.

In *marginal analysis* the basic rules of cost–benefit analysis are applied at the margin (it is not to be confused with the use of the same term to refer to a method of asking groups of professionals to reach a consensus on where to spend or cut a given monetary amount of resources). The assumption is that a programme can be expanded or contracted to the point where marginal benefit equals marginal cost, except if there is budgetary constraint, when all programmes should operate at the level at which the ratio of marginal benefit to marginal cost is the same for all.

In relation to marginal costs, Allen and Beecham (1993) pointed out that short-run marginal costs are inappropriate for most costing exercises, as they do not include the full costs of, for example, creating new services. Long-run marginal costs enable analysis of the differences which the alternative service being studied will make to available resources. However, as knowledge of future events and costs is uncertain, the convention is to use short-run averages, which include both revenue and capital elements as an approximation for long-run marginal costs (on the assumption that *relative* price levels remain stable).

Complete costs

With cost–benefit analysis, all costs and benefits, from all sources (e.g. health and social services, voluntary sector and individuals as well as wider society) that arise from implementing the objective are relevant because the welfare of the whole society is regarded as important, and not just the health service. They are not confined to monetary measures of costs, but also encompass benefit valuations. Because costs are usually measured in monetary terms, economists want to make benefits commensurate with these and to measure them in monetary terms.

In addition, complete costings should include the costs to the individual patients and to any carers, as well as their opportunity costs (i.e. what they would have been doing instead and the costs of this). The economic costing of patients' and carers' time has not been resolved and is still fairly crude. The problem with costing people using a labour market cost, for example, is that not everyone works and this does not take leisure time into account. Some economists in the UK use the Department of Transport's (1994) estimate for the cost of leisure time, but this produces an embarrassingly low value of the cost of people's time (i.e. in relation to a few pence). It is good practice to carry out a *sensitivity analysis* using guestimates of the value of leisure time.

Where prices are charged (without a subsidy) for a health treatment, it is easier to set a monetary value on the services received. In socialist health care systems, however, there are, in the main, no charges for services. In such situations, economists sometimes consider the possibilities of public 'shadow prices'; that is, prices fixed by the state with the aim of reflecting the amount of resources that the community is willing to give up in return for a unit improvement in health. The attraction of shadow prices is that they can provide a practical approach to the problem of assigning monetary values, but they are a crude answer to a complex question.

In summary, time can be costed in relation to market activity (e.g. wages and salaries), leisure activities, meeting physiological needs (e.g. sleep) and productive, non-market activity (e.g. housework, caring for dependent people). Ideally, the impact of each type of activity that was forgone as a consequence of the service (or illness itself) would be costed separately. This is complex because of the lack of valid information on the cost of leisure time (based on the impact it has on market and non-market productivity). These issues have been discussed by Allen and Beecham (1993).

Intangible costs

When one is undertaking a cost–benefit analysis, an important issue is deciding which 'intangible costs' should be included. Intangible costs include things like work time and leisure time forgone (see above), the value of reassurance that accompanies a negative diagnostic test result and the reduction in stress gained by carers from respite care. In deciding which intangibles to include, it is useful to consider whether the gathering of more data on intangibles will change the results of the study significantly and whether the costs of gathering the data are prohibitive (Drummond *et al.* 1997).

Event pathways

The *Cochrane Collaboration Handbook* (1994) states that the following information is required for economic evaluations:

- identification of all main event pathways that have distinct resource implications or outcome values associated with them;
- estimation of the probabilities associated with the main event pathways;
- descriptive data to enable the resource consequences associated with each pathway to be measured;
- descriptive data to enable the outcomes associated with each pathway to be valued.

Event pathways are defined as a clinical event, details of its management and resources used for it, associated subsequent events and the cost of these resources.

Opportunity cost

The cost of spending resources in a particular way is not necessarily the monetary cost of the resource, but it is the opportunity lost (benefit forgone) by loss of its best alternative use. As described earlier, scarcity of resources implies choice, and this choice gives rise to the concept of opportunity cost. Given the scarcity of health care resources, it follows that the allocation and use of resources for one type of health care involves sacrifice of another. While the financial concept of cost simply relates to monetary outlays, the economist's concept of cost takes other considerations into account. Economists are interested in the health benefits that could be obtained by using the resources in a different way. Therefore, they measure costs in terms of the benefit that would be derived from the alternative use of the resource (*Cochrane Collaboration Handbook* 1994). In practice, money is a convenient yardstick against which to measure benefits and is generally used (Knapp 1993).

Problems with the calculation of opportunity costs

Opportunity costs are not straightforward to calculate. In particular, there is the issue of non-marketed items, on which economists attempt to put monetary values. These have been described by Knapp (1993), who points to three approaches to their valuation:

- the *human capital approach*;
- *implicit valuation methods*;
- clients' *willingness to pay*.

Human capital approach

With the human capital approach, earnings are used to value the effects. For example, the treatment may enable patients to return to work, or take less time off work, and this could be valued in societal terms of the extent of growth in national productivity. However, as some people are unemployed or retired or do not work for other reasons, there is little scope for using this approach. For the same reasons, loss of earnings is also problematic in relation to valuing the individual patient's opportunity costs. In addition, some people are salaried and do not necessarily lose earnings through time off work (e.g. to attend for treatment). In relation to predicting demand for health care, Torgerson *et al.* (1994) pointed to the importance of the private opportunity costs of time itself (i.e. the time taken to utilise health services) as a preferable measure to wages forgone.

Implicit valuation methods

Implicit valuation methods are based on the preferences for services that patients, clients and professionals reveal by their explicit behaviour. People are asked to put a price on the alternatives available in terms of how much they would be prepared to pay for them. This enables their expression of preference, and indirectly of satisfaction, to be calculated in financial units, which can then be directly compared with the actual financial cost. In theory, this facilitates policy decision-making about which alternative to purchase. It assumes an unproblematic relationship between price and cost. It is essential to be explicit about the assumptions and methods used.

Willingness to pay

Despite economic evaluation of health care being dominated by cost-effectiveness and cost per QALY comparisons between treatments, it has been argued that more use should be made of willingness to pay methods, especially in relation to cost–benefit analyses (Hanley *et al.* 2003). There are two main methods for setting a monetary value on a specific package of health or other benefits: '*contingent valuation method*' and '*choice experiments*' (previously called conjoint analysis, now referred to as discrete choice experiments).These methods have generally been used to set a monetary value on a package of health and/or non-health benefits in the context of a specific intervention. These methods have also been criticised as subject to bias and lack of sensitivity (Cookson 2003).

Gerard *et al.* (2008) described willingness to pay questioning, in which people are asked in surveys how much they are willing to pay for a good or service, as a contingent valuation method. This is because they are asked about their willingness to pay contingent on a hypothetical scenario and description of the good or service being valued. Willingness to pay is based on observed trade-offs between resources or states of health/ill health (Donaldson 1993; Drummond *et al.* 1997, 2005). In relation to health and social care, particularly in societies with government-controlled services, such exercises are often too hypothetical and difficult for many people to conceptualise: health care does not have an *explicit* monetary value. Some would also object, on ideological grounds, to asking people to consider the costs of health care when it is provided free at the point of consumption (see Ryan 1996).

Discrete choice experiments

Some economists have used *discrete choice experiments* to elicit people's values, in which preferences for scenarios (levels of attributes of the good or service) are obtained through surveys asking people to rank, rate or choose between scenarios. This provides a more realistic estimation of the relative importance of different attributes in the provision of a good or service, the trade-offs between the attributes, and the total satisfaction or utility the individual derives from the good or service with specific attributes (Ryan 1996) (see later section on discrete choice experiments).

Price stability

Knapp (1993) also outlined the problem of price stability. Even with valid information on market costs, does the economist take the initial or final price as the measure of opportunity cost? One example is that if a health authority, or other large health care purchaser, decided to increase greatly the number of elderly people discharged from hospital to the care of a hospital at home scheme (as an alternative to a longer hospital inpatient stay), then this would affect the supply price of the hospital at home scheme. So should the previous or the subsequent supply price of services be used? Knapp suggested using a formula that takes account of both.

Other problems with opportunity costs

Other complications include the issue of apportioning joint costs (e.g. where costs are met by social and health services, or social and health services and the individual), the issue of private costs (e.g. services provided within the organisation by external public or independent agencies), and costs to society, and price distortions. For example, in relation to price distortions, if the resources are supplied by a monopoly organisation, the price and cost will differ; indirect taxation distorts prices; if staff would otherwise be unemployed, they will have a zero shadow price (Knapp suggested setting their price as equal to forgone leisure time and the costs of travelling to and from work, although other complications, such as government policy, need to be taken into account). Knapp listed the following implications of an opportunity costing approach to social care, which can be applied to health care: the opportunity cost of using a resource in a particular way cannot be measured without knowing what alternative uses are available; costs are forgone benefits; opportunity costs are context-specific; some apparently costly items are costless; some apparently free items have non-zero costs.

Discounting

Discounting is designed to standardise different cost–time profiles, though the concept is untested. It is important to take into account the time period of the incurred costs and benefits. Future benefits are valued less than current benefits, regardless of inflationary effects (e.g. because desires may change). Discounting of the future is also based on the assumption that most people's real income increases over time. The UK Treasury sets a percentage discount rate for public sector projects. If discounting is employed, it is prudent to consider a range of discount rates as part of a sensitivity analysis. Mooney (1992) pointed out that this is particularly problematic in relation to health promotion services, where the benefits will not be obtained until the future.

Cost–utility analysis

Cost–utility analysis provides a fuller analysis of health care benefits than cost–benefit analysis, because it takes patients' quality of life into account. However, societal costs and benefits are generally still ignored. Different interventions often have several different health outcomes (e.g. efficiency versus side-effects of treatment; length versus quality of life). In such cases cost–utility analysis is used, where the different changes in health states are valued relative to each other. Cost–utility analysis is a technique that relates the cost of the project to a measure of its usefulness of outcome (utility). This produces an overall index of health gain, or health status in relation to output. The quality-adjusted life year (QALY) (see later section) is one index used, which attempts to combine quantity and quality of life into a single index, which gives it an advantage over single-dimensional measures of output (as in cost-effectiveness analysis).

This form of analysis requires the different impacts of the treatments on length and quality of life to be measured. It also requires a set of values for health states ('utilities'), in order that the different health states can be compared. These values can be derived from existing data, where available, and where relevant to the population of interest, or they may need to be derived as part of the specific study. Whether QALYs really are utilities is open to debate (Drummond *et al.* 1997).

Cost–utility analysis also provides one approach to addressing issues of *efficiency* of resource allocation in relation to the determination of *health* priorities. The advantage is that the approach is not solely monetary. However, it has several disadvantages in that it does not adequately address issues of equity in health care, or take account of objectives of health services other than the maximisation of health. It also follows the questionable assumption that it is based on an adequate measure of health.

Cost–utility analysis and summary health indices

Cost–utility analyses require outcome measures which combine quality of life and mortality outcomes. A *value of health states* is also necessary for cost–utility analysis. Economists have developed questionnaires that aim to measure quality of life with the advantage that the data derived can be applied to a pre-scaled matrix of health state preference values for use in cost–utility analysis (Drummond 1994). The values used are the expressed preferences for states of function on a scale anchored at the extremes by death and optimum functioning. The preference values can be derived from existing research data, where appropriate, or by undertaking direct utility measures within the study concerned. The measures can be used, in theory, as either health-related quality of life measures (if all domains are tapped) or as instruments in cost–utility analyses.

QALYs

Cost–utility analysis uses the QALY which claims to take account of quality of life and length of life. This is used for health care decision-making as it enables treatments for different conditions to be basically compared. The QALY is a form of health status measurement which places mortality and morbidity on the same measurement scale. The QALY figure reflects the change in survival (known as 'life years') with a weighting factor for quality of life. QALYs are used in making comparative assessments about the effectiveness of various treatments. Costs of the treatment per QALY are calculated and generally presented in QALY league tables (e.g. showing QALYs for hip replacements, bypass surgery, etc.). Caution is required in interpreting QALY league tables in view of the relatively crude methods underlying the calculation of QALYs, and the assumptions made.

The QALY takes one year of perfect health-life expectancy as worth a value of 1, and one year of less than perfect health-life expectancy as less than 1. Phillips (1996) explained the formula clearly as follows. An intervention which increases a patient's life expectancy by four extra years, rather than the patient dying within one year, but where quality of life falls from 1 to 0.6 on the continuum, generates the following value:

4 extra years of life at 0.6 quality of life values 2.4

Minus one year at reduced quality (1 – 0.6) 0.4

QALYs generated by the intervention 2.0

The assumptions underlying QALYs are open to criticism, as is their construction. Measures that include time as a dimension register fewer benefits for elderly people because of their shorter life expectancy, in comparison with younger people (Farrar and Donaldson 1996). Defenders of the QALY counter that it simply reflects the public's ageist attitudes, as the QALY values were developed from public surveys (Edgar *et al.* 1998).

QALYs can also be criticised on the grounds that they focus on cures rather than care, and are thus less appropriate for use in the priority setting of chronic care, in comparison with acute services. The fact that every QALY calculation places hip replacements over home or hospital dialysis in relation to value for money raises deep moral concerns (Lockwood 1988; Butler 1999). These limitations of the QALY are likely to result in treatment decisions which are inequitable and less than optimal. While various health economists have questioned the restrictive assumptions inherent in the QALY, and attempted to build in utility functions to address its shortcomings, their attempts remain inconclusive. There is also evidence that society expects broader benefits from health care than simply health and utility, including empowerment, social participation, feelings of safety, self-respect and dignity (Coast *et al.* 2008a, 2008b; Byrne *et al.* 2010).

QALYs have been reported to be less sensitive than other measures of physical functioning and emotional well-being when used to assess the health status of elderly people (Donaldson *et al.* 1988), suggesting that their use in priority setting might place elderly people lower down on the priority list than they ought to be. Oddly, however, as Farrar and Donaldson (1996) pointed out, the QALY league tables have ranked hip replacements and chiropody highly. There is undoubtedly a need for caution, particularly given the relative lack of robust evidence on costs and effectiveness of many treatments and procedures.

Decisions about priorities for health care interventions, owing to limited resources, entail making trade-offs between their estimated benefits and their estimated harms and costs. QALYs can be used in decision-making about health priorities, though this use is controversial. Different health care programmes can be compared in league tables in relation to their marginal costs per QALY obtained. The practice is that the programmes with the cheapest QALY are given the highest priority. This is based on the assumption that, with limited health care resources, the aim is to maximise the number of QALYs purchased within the budget (Mooney 1992). For example, in England and Wales, the National Institute for Health and Clinical Excellence (NICE), which was established in 1999, was charged with making decisions about whether treatments should be made available by the NHS, taking cost-effectiveness (or 'value for money') into account. NICE aims to purchase the greatest number of QALYs possible – i.e. to maximise health gain in relation to available funds. The QALY indicator is also used in other countries, including by the Pharmaceutical Benefits Advisory Committee in Australia, and the Canadian Agency for Drugs and Technologies in Health.

Eliciting values

Methods of eliciting values for specific health states include the *rating scale* (also called the *visual analogue scale*), *time trade-off* and the *standard gamble* (Torrance 1976, 1986). On the basis of their review of the literature of these techniques, Brazier *et al.* (1999) concluded that each was a practical method for use with most populations, though evidence on reliability and validity was generally lacking for each method. If anything, the rating scale appeared to be the most practical and acceptable technique. Other methods include the *magnitude estimation* and the *person trade-off*, though these two methods have little supportive evidence in favour of their psychometric properties or their practicality (Brazier *et al.* 1999).

UK economists (Kind et al. 1982; Williams and Kind 1992) developed an alternative method initially based on the Rosser Disability Index (Rosser and Watts 1972). However, this early method has long been criticised as limited, and of questionable reliability and validity. Brazier et al. (1999) argued that there is no place for this method of preferences in economic theory. The QALY formula now used in the UK is based on the utility value of a health state derived from the EuroQoL-5D (EQ-5D). In the USA, Kaplan and Bush (1982) and Kaplan et al. (1984) developed a slightly different approach using their more detailed Index of Well-being Scale. The Health Utilities Index, which is broader than the EuroQoL, is also increasingly popular (Feeny 2005), particularly in North America.

Alternatives scales to QALYs have been developed, such as the Time Without Symptoms and Toxicity scale (TWIST) (Gelber and Goldhirsh 1986; Gelber et al. 1989). It has been argued that a measure based on 'healthy years equivalent (HYE)' is more representative of people's preferences (Mehrez and Gafni 1989). The HYE also combines quality and quantity of life, and is regarded as an improvement on the QALY because it obtains the utility for the whole health profile (rather than each state separately), and therefore more fully represents the patient's preferences. It also allows attitudes towards risk to be incorporated. HYEs are calculated using two standard gamble questions and respondent burden is relatively high. Other alternatives to the QALY are the Saved Young Life Equivalent (Nord 1992), which compares treatment outcomes in terms of units of saving a young life and restoring the young life to full health; Quality-Adjusted Lives (Stevenson et al. 1991) (treatments are assessed in terms of number of lives saved rather than length of life); and Healthy Life Expectancy (Bone 1992) (an indicator of the health status of a population, combining morbidity and mortality into a single index used in epidemiological and demographic studies; there are three different methods for calculating this; Barendregt et al. 1994). Methods of eliciting utility values are time-consuming and complex, as well as imposing considerable respondent burden.

The rating scale (VAS)

The rating scale involves a horizontal line (a visual analogue scale or VAS) anchored at one end with 0 which is equal to death, and at the other with 1 or 100, which is equal to the best/most desirable state of health. It is used with a given health state. The scale is given to study members, in conjunction with a description of the given health state, who are asked to make judgements about where on the line various intermediate states of health lie. For example, if a particular state of (ill) health (e.g. diabetes) is judged to be 0.75 or 75, then the respondents perceived this state to reduce their health status by a quarter.

Torrance et al. (1982) specified attributes, which are graded, that should be included in a health state: physical function, emotional function, cognitive function, self-care and pain. The characteristics of the given health state include a description of these attributes either in written vignettes or shown on video. A technique known as multiple attribute theory is used to determine the value for each level of the attributes and the utility value of the associated health state (Torrance et al. 1982).

Time trade-off

This method involves asking respondents to establish equivalents. They are asked to consider an ill-health state that is to last for a fixed period of time. They are informed that a new health care procedure will give the individual normal health for a shorter period of time, but with the likelihood of death or severe disablement at the end of that time. The respondent is asked to 'trade off' the time with the ill-health state with normal health for a shorter period of time. The time spent in normal health is varied until the point of indifference is found. Variations include trading off the number of people helped by different treatments (e.g. how many people in state B must be helped to provide a benefit that is equivalent to helping one person in state A?). This method has been reported to be more reliable than the standard gamble technique (Dolan *et al*. 1993). Others have reported that the standard gamble has better construct validity than the time trade-off (Puhan *et al*. 2007).

Standard gamble

This asks the respondent to make a choice between remaining in a current state of ill health and the probability of being immediately restored to perfect health, with some chance of immediate death (e.g. in relation to a specific health care intervention). The respondent is asked to vary the level of probability until the point of indifference between choices is reached. As indicated above, the reliability and validity of these methods are debatable. Time trade-off and standard gamble techniques both suffer from a disjuncture between stated preferences and actual choices (Ryan *et al*. 2006).

The Rosser Index of Disability

The Rosser Index of Disability is an early measure, based on the concept of a health index, with people (or descriptions of health and ill-health states) being graded by respondents, recruited to make the assessments, into one of eight areas of disability, from no disability, to slight social disability, through to confined to bed, and unconscious. Each state is graded on a four-point distress scale: none, mild, moderate or severe. States are scored on a scale ranging from 0 at death to 1 for healthy (with negative values for states judged to be worse than death). Once these rankings have been completed, respondents are asked to undertake a series of complex priority ranking exercises in relation to the conditions assessed. For example, they are asked to place the conditions (or 'health states') on a scale in relation to 'how many times more ill is a person described as being in state 2 than state 1'; they are also asked to place a state of death on a scale of permanent states (e.g. vegetative state), and to assign a value to it (see Kind *et al*. 1982). There is no justification for this method as a measure of preferences in economic theory (Brazier *et al*. 1999). Results for inter-rater reliability and construct validity, including sensitivity to clinical outcomes, have been inconsistent (see Brazier *et al*. 1999).

Kaplan's Index of Well-being

The Quality of Well-being Scale provides an index value as well as quality of life descriptors. It is the best-known measure in this field. It was developed in order to operationalise 'wellness' for a general health policy model, in an attempt to develop an alternative to cost–benefit analysis for resource allocation (Kaplan *et al*. 1976, 1978, 1984; Kaplan and Anderson 2004). The instrument defines levels of wellness on a continuum between death and optimum function and integrates morbidity and mortality into the same number. It classifies respondents according to their level of functioning on three scales – mobility, physical activity and social activity – combined with their (most undesirable) problem/symptom. The level of function and the reported complaint (symptom) are weighted by preference on the scale of 0 (dead) to 1.0 (optimal functioning). The aim was to produce a point-in-time expression of well-being, so it has a fairly short-time reference ('preceding six days'). The scale is interviewer-administered, is lengthy and difficult to administer. It has been used extensively in clinical trials and population studies in the USA, and has good levels of construct validity when tested against other physical health status scales, but correlates poorly with measures of emotional well-being and psychological health (see review by Brazier *et al.* 1999). Its retest and inter-rater reliability is also unknown (Brazier *et al.* 1999). It has relatively few floor or ceiling effects. However, its widespread use has been hindered because it is complex to administer, although a self-completion version has also been developed (it is still 80 items and the time reference for reporting symptoms and difficulties functioning is either 'current' or scaled as 'no days/yesterday/2 days ago/3 days ago') (Andresen *et al.* 1998).

To derive a single utility score ('Kaplan's Index of Well-being'), Kaplan and his colleagues (Kaplan and Bush 1982; Kaplan *et al.* 1984) placed people with given health states into categories of mobility, physical activity and social activity, and then classified their symptoms and health problems on a given day. Case histories were compiled in order to illustrate the combinations of functional levels, symptoms or problems. The scale also includes death. Random samples of the public were asked to rate preferences to the descriptions, and weights were derived for each level of mobility, physical activity, social activity and symptom or problem. A utility value was assigned to each functional level, and questionnaire responses were used to assign the health states to one of a number of discrete function states. Kaplan's Index of Well-being, which provides a single score, developed out of this methodology (Kaplan *et al.* 1976, 1978; Bush 1984; Kaplan and Anderson 2004). The scale quantifies the health outcome of a treatment in terms of years of life, adjusted for changes in quality.

EuroQoL

The aim of the EuroQoL was to provide a self-administered, standardised, generic instrument for describing health-related quality of life and to generate a single index value for each health state. The EQ-5D, after revision, now contains five questions which can be used to generate a single summary index of health status, while still permitting analytical breakdown into its five domains, and a self-rating of health on a vertical visual analogue 'thermometer' scale from 0 (worst imaginable health state) to 100 (best imaginable health state) (EuroQoL Group 1990; Kind 1996; Dolan 1997; Kind *et al.* 1998). It measures current health on five domains: mobility, self-care, usual activities, pain/discomfort, anxiety/depression, and the items use three-point response categories. The EuroQoL was also later revised (middle values were added to increase sensitivity) and shortened. It does not cover broader health-related quality of life. A tariff, using time trade-off methods, derived from population samples in the UK, is then used to value the person's health state.

UK preference values for the EQ-5D were initially derived from time trade-off techniques, which is an accepted method for deriving preference values, with just over 3000 people (Dolan 1997; Gudex *et al.* 1997). The earlier version achieved adequate construct and convergent validity (Brazier *et al.* 1993a), there is evidence of its test–retest reliability (see review by Brazier *et al.* 1999), and there have been some design improvements. While research indicates it is less sensitive to changes in specific disease states (Wolf and Hawley 1997), it has been reported to be sensitive to variations in response to selected self-perceived health questions in a general population survey in Canada (Houle and Berthelot 2000) but with reduced sensitivity at the ceiling (i.e. at the lower levels of perceived health) (Brazier *et al.* 1993b). The EuroQoL has been reported not to be responsive to some conditions (e.g. vision – see Datta *et al.* 2008), and some items are so extreme that few people endorse them (see Wolfe and Hawley 1997).

Brazier *et al.* (1999), on the basis of their review of the literature, judged the EQ-5D, along with the Health Utilities Index (Mark III) to be superior to the other preference-based measures.

However, the instrument still contains several fundamental design flaws. It has also been criticised as being insensitive to changes in health status that are important to patients (Jenkinson *et al.* 1997; Jenkinson and McGee 1998). The item wording is inconsistent in parts which can increase response error (e.g. the self-care domain scale wording varies inconsistently from asking about problems with 'self-care' to more specifically 'wash or dress'). The mobility domain scale leaps from 'no' problems and 'some' problems walking about to 'confined to bed' (omitting the group of older people who are largely confined to chairs during the day). Also, neither the pain/discomfort domain or the anxiety/depression domain scaling make any provision for those who suffer 'a little' (both domain response scales leap from 'no' symptoms to 'moderate' and then to 'extreme' symptoms). The scoring is linear and additive. It is still relatively crude and produces skewed results (Brazier *et al.* 1992, 1993a, 1993b; Carr-Hill 1992), with variable response rates from moderate to good (Brazier *et al.* 1993b; Gudex *et al.* 1997; Bowling 1998; Kind *et al.* 1998). The aim of such instruments is to produce a point-in-time expression of health-related quality of life, and thus the time reference period is 'today'. The respondent is asked to rate statements which best describe their own health state 'today' by ticking 'at least one box in each group'. Short time frames, while most likely to produce the most accurate data (e.g. less prone to recall bias) do, however, increase the potential for regression to the mean in follow-up studies, as ratings for just one day are less stable than for longer periods of time.

Health Utilities Index (HUI-3)

Another single summary health utility index is the Health Utilities Index, version 3 (HUI-3), which contains 31 questions in eight dimensions (vision, hearing, speech, mobility, dexterity, emotion, cognition and pain) (Furlong *et al.* 1998). These attributes were selected for inclusion because members of the general population rated them as the most important dimensions of their health (Feeny *et al.* 1996). The HUI employs five- and six-point response choices and incorporates the full range of no, mild, moderate and severe problems. Preference values for the HUI-3 were derived from standard gamble techniques with 500 Canadians, and scoring is multiplicative (utilities).

The HUI-3 has been reported to have ceiling effects (Sung *et al.* 2003) and it carries modest study and respondent burden (Feeny 2005). There is only fragmentary evidence to support the scale's sensitivity to change (Feeny *et al.* 1995), although tests with the third version indicate that its responsiveness to change is similar to the EuroQoL (Houle and Berthelot 2000). As stated earlier, Brazier *et al.* (1999) judged the EQ-5D and the HUI-3 to be superior to the other preference-based measures. However, neither instrument is apparently as good at predicting changes in health status as a simple VAS of self-rating of health (0 'least desirable state' and 100 'perfect health') (Houle and Berthelot 2000). Results for the reliability and validity of earlier versions of the scale were poor (see Brazier *et al.* 1999). More recent results have been better and an improvement on the EQ-5D (Grootendorst *et al.* 2000; Fisk *et al.* 2005).

Discrete choice experiments

There is increasing interest in using discrete choice experiments, as well as other methods (e.g. ranking and scaling exercises), to estimate QALY values for cost–utility analysis. None are without problems (see Flynn 2010), as existing methods for generating preference weights are limited to changes in health states. Some health economists have adopted valuation methods used in other fields, in order to value processes of health care. Conjoint analysis is used in marketing, transport and environmental economics. In health care, the technique has been adapted (called 'stated preference discrete choice experiments') to predict service acceptance and utilisation, or option values. They are known as attribute-based approaches (Gerard et *al.* 2008).

This technique presents patients with hypothetical choices to make between services/treatments, and varies them with different attributes (components) that might underlie preferences for the choices. If cost is included as an attribute, then the aim is also to measure 'willingness to pay'. One example is the trade-offs people may be willing to make between location of treatment, or choice of hospital, and waiting times for treatment (Ryan and Farrar 2000; Burge *et al.* 2004). Statistical modelling of the results is used to provide estimates of the extent to which components of the service or treatment contribute to the preferences elicited.

It is essential to minimise measurement error and ensure that all attributes are included, and to check that respondents interpret the task accurately. As Lloyd (2003) has pointed out in his critical review, however, preference elicitation methods assume that people's preferences are stable and complete, and assume that they are consistent (Ryan *et al.* 2006). He suggested that little attempt has been made to apply psychological theories of judgement and decision-making which challenge the assumptions of the method. It is unknown to what extent preference elicitation is influenced by cognitive processing strategies and the employment of heuristics (cognitive strategies which result in shortcuts to simplify the cognitive functioning required for the task). Indeed, the measurement of human judgements, by both experts and lay people, is a highly specialised psychological subject (see Harries and Kostopoulou 2005; Harries and Stiggelbout 2005). As Harries and Stiggelbout concluded, preferences are prone to the inconsistencies inherent in making judgements, and are influenced by many external factors, including how information is presented, and time.

Disadvantages of methods

Each method has its limitations, and no gold standard exists. A major disadvantage of all these methods is their cost, owing to their time-consuming nature, the requirement for highly skilled interviewers and their complexity, leading to high respondent burden. The last point leads to a general reliance on convenience sampling, rather than random sampling, leading to results based on unrepresentative samples of the population.

One of the main debates surrounding the use of these techniques is whose values should be sought to provide utility values: those of the public, those of the health professionals, the patients and/or their families? Economists argue that patients' values would not be constant over the course of the illness, and thus the utility values would not be stable. The issue remains one for ethical and methodological debate. There is some evidence that the methods used to elicit values in economic analyses do not tap underlying true preferences (Kahneman and Tversky 1983).

Costing health services

This section provides some examples of the types of costs that are collected by economists in health service evaluations, which include cost–benefit studies. The economic costs of health care technically come under the umbrella of the structure of health services. However, health economists aim to incorporate costs into the assessment of outcomes of health care because clinical effectiveness needs to be interpreted in relation to economic, or cost, effectiveness. Decisions about priorities for health care interventions, owing to limited resources, entail making trade-offs between their estimated benefits and their estimated harms and costs.

Costings are rarely straightforward: there are many methodological obstacles when one is making cost comparisons, and costings often require assumptions to be made that are seldom applicable across settings (Wright 1993) and would probably be unacceptable in many other scientific disciplines. The implication is that costings and comparisons of costs must be interpreted with caution. When any cost comparisons are made, it is important to ensure that the same service is being costed, given the sometimes enormous variations in the organisation and quality of care within any one type of service in different places. This is often extremely difficult to achieve. The valuation of cost and benefit in economic terms inevitably involves elements of subjective judgement. When cost and benefit are presented in quantified form, this point is often, unfortunately, forgotten. While health professionals' time can be costed using their salaries and overhead costs, the costs of lay carers, for example, are difficult to value. Mooney (1992) pointed out that even when these intangible costs cannot be valued, it is important to note them to prevent them being ignored in decision-making processes.

Thus it is important that the data collected for economic evaluations are accurate and comprehensive, that assumptions underlying any categorisations are made explicit and that the time periods for follow-up in the data collection are carefully planned in order that they incorporate the 'subsequent events'.

Capital costs

Capital costs are building costs, equipment and land and other capital-intensive items (e.g. expenditure on structural alterations). There are two components of capital cost: opportunity cost of resources tied up in the asset, and depreciation over time of the asset itself. Building costs require information on the valuation of capital, and can be based on annual payments of capital, plus any charges for depreciation and interest, and then apportioned to the unit of interest. At a simple level, if the total is divided by the number of patients booked per clinic, then a building cost per consultation can be derived.

The costs of the buildings (annuitised over the lifespan of the buildings) used for the services need to be included in the total costs. This enables an estimate of the long-run *marginal (opportunity) costs* of services to be calculated. The capital costs are counted alongside revenue costs to enable the total costs of a service to be presented in one figure.

The opportunity costs of the capital (buildings and stock) also need calculation. Allen and Beecham (1993) explain that it is convention to calculate opportunity costs of capital by assuming that the best alternative use of the resources is investment. The value of the resources thus includes interest which could have been earned had the money not been tied up in buildings and equipment.

Allen and Beecham have described how, in the case of private sector care where information on the valuation of buildings and other capital-intensive items might not be accessible or easily available, an acceptable compromise is to take the fee charged, on the assumption that this (market price) approximates the real cost and includes the cost of the original capital investment.

Overhead costs

Overheads relate to those resources that service different programmes: for example, expenses related to the building (e.g. power, rates), staffing costs and other costs of providing the service (e.g. associated with administration, transport, catering, laundry, maintenance, cleaning, stationery). This information is obtained from accounts of expenditure and salaries. Overhead costs include direct and indirect overhead costs. Where individual programmes are being costed, these overheads should be shared out.

There are costs associated with the building and stock, such as power, water and sewage charges and building rates, repair and maintenance, cleaning and other operating costs. They also include day-to-day expenses for supplies and services, immediate line management, telephones, and so on. These can be difficult to calculate, and where information on total overhead costs is obtained from the organisations themselves, additional information on how costs were apportioned is required, and should be adjusted if necessary in order to ensure that like is being compared with like.

In order to calculate overhead costs, there are two options: to accept the organisation's figures on these costs and the costs of, for example, a clinic attendance, with information on how they apportioned costs in order to ensure the comparison of like with like across the study; or to measure the square footage of the space occupied by the clinic, ward or other unit under study and the square footage of the total building, collect all cost data and reapportion costs independently. Most investigators opt for the former, given the time and resource implications of the latter alternative.

Salaries and costs

The total salaries of staff members need to be obtained. Staff costs are calculated by multiplying the hourly rate of salaries at the appropriate grades. There are several other factors that will need to be included in staff costings, such as weighting factors for labour market variations, merit awards of consultants, employers' costs and contributions. In the British NHS, for example, employees who work in London are given a London weighting allowance. These need to be taken into account if the cost of services (e.g. clinics) in London is to be compared with that of clinics elsewhere in the country. Some costings take average salaries, or mid-points on the relevant scales (if the mid-point of the salary scale is used, then it needs to be adjusted for merit awards, e.g. the total value of distinction awards given to consultants in a specialty is divided by the number of consultants in that specialty; the average is then added to the consultant's salary).

The total costs for staff need to be calculated in relation to the unit under investigation (e.g. hospital outpatients' clinic) and will need to be allocated to that unit by dividing the total staff costs by the number of patients (e.g. booked to attend the clinic). This will give the cost per patient booked.

As before, the various staff costs should be spread over all the units of interest (e.g. patients booked into a clinic; appointment times) to give a cost per consultation.

Allen and Beecham (1993) describe the complexity of costing the time of staff employed in community and primary care. For example, in Britain the income of a GP is partly dependent on the type and amount of work done (e.g. certain minor surgical procedures for which additional payments are made) and the type of patients registered with their practices (there are higher capitation payments for older people).

Other costs may need to be taken into account. In evaluations of outreach clinics held by specialists in GP surgeries, for example, the travelling costs (e.g. a marginal cost mileage rate) of the specialist between sites also had to be included in the overall costings (see Gosden *et al.* 1997; Bond *et al.* 2000).

Apportioning to unit of study

As before, all costs need to be extracted and apportioned to the unit of study (e.g. clinics). They can be averaged, for example, in a costing of outpatients' clinics, by the number of patients booked per clinic. Annual overhead costs can be converted into an hourly rate by dividing by the average number of working weeks in a year and the average number of hours worked per week. The hourly rate is then equally apportioned between the clinics operating on the day on which the clinic is evaluated. Alternatively, overhead costs can be apportioned per hour to each type of clinic in a building by dividing total overhead cost by the total number of hours for which the practice or hospital departments were open.

Resource costs: patients' treatment costs to the health service

The allocation of treatment costs to individual patients involves tracking patients' use of investigations, including biochemistry (checking site of analysis in case costs vary), procedures, prescriptions, surgery, and so on. For this exercise the patients' notes are used, supplemented with reports from health professionals and patients themselves. The costs of each item have to be obtained. At the crudest and simplest level, the costs for diagnostic tests, procedures and operations can be obtained by reference to price lists compiled by the hospitals or community service units in the areas of the study, or to national cost sources, where held and accessible, by government departments. (See Box 5.2.) An example of the collection of cost data from individual health care sites and national sources, as well as patient-level data is found in Roderick *et al.* (2005). This is not without problems, as these costs may not always reflect true costs, and the higher prices of some procedures may be subsidising the lower prices of others. With prescriptions, the unit cost of items can be obtained from formularies (e.g. in Britain from the *British National Formulary*, which is published annually by the British Medical Association and the Royal Pharmaceutical Society of Great Britain). The information required for this is the name of

> ## Box 5.2 Example of use of records
>
> An example of medical and billing records being used to cost health care is the study of the costs and outcome of standardised psychiatric consultations in the USA by Smith *et al.* (1995). Their study was based on an RCT comparing an immediate with a delayed (for one year) standardised psychiatric consultation. The study was carried out with 56 somatising patients from 51 study doctors. The measures included the patient-completed Rand SF-36 to measure health status and analysis of medical and billing records. Smith *et al.* standardised the costs by costing all items according to Arkansas Blue Cross–Blue Shield charges, inflated at an annual compound rate of 7.3 per cent. There was a two-year follow-up period. This study reported that, using these methods, the intervention reduced annual medical charges by 33 per cent (particularly through a reduction in the number of hospital stays) and physical function was found to have improved slightly. The weakness of the study, however, is that it only focused on direct organisational costs, and did not take the intangible costs into account, nor those incurred by the patients and their families. Where intangible costs have not been included, this should be made clear.

the prescribed item, dose, form and duration. An alternative is to calculate defined daily doses (Maxwell *et al.* 1993), though this can be complicated and time-consuming.

Patients' costs

Patients' costs include their travel costs and other expenses (e.g. direct financial expenditure on goods and services, such as diet, prescriptions, equipment, aids; waged and non-waged time; care costs for dependants; future costs; and, in some cases, accommodation) in relation to their health care.

Patients also incur *opportunity costs*, which include forgone leisure time or time off work to attend hospital (e.g. clinics, day or inpatient stays). Having identified what patients have given up, one must then put a monetary value on it. Economists take society's valuation of the cost of time, rather than the individual's. However, the issues of estimating how much time a lay carer spends providing care and costing it, and costing the opportunity cost of carers' and patients' time, are complex and unresolved (see earlier).

Study methods used for costings

In relation to studies of costs and effectiveness, health economists use the full range of research methods and techniques to obtain cost data in relation to the unit of study. Gosden *et al.* (1997), in their study of the cost-effectiveness of specialists' outreach clinics in general practice, in comparison with specialists' hospital outpatient clinics, used a before–after study method, with cases (specialist outreach patients) and controls (hospital outpatients), and designed self-completion questionnaires as instruments for the collection of data from the patients, the doctors, the practices and hospital managers. In some cases, economists obtain their data by undertaking document research (e.g. they access and analyse billing records in private health care systems); but there is still the problem of how to standardise costs across providers to facilitate comparisons.

Summary of main points

- The underlying assumption of economics is that the resources available to society are scarce, and decisions have to be made about their best use.
- Health economists use the basic economic concepts of demand, supply and utility in their analyses.
- Cost-effectiveness is an approach to the assessment of efficiency that compares the monetary costs of different projects that produce the same kinds of non-monetary benefits.
- A cost–benefit analysis assigns a monetary value to the benefits of a project and compares this with the monetary costs of the project.
- The marginal cost is the additional cost of producing one extra unit of output.
- The opportunity cost refers to the opportunity lost (benefit forgone), when resources are spent, for spending them in their best alternative way.
- Discounting standardises different cost–time profiles (future benefits are valued less than current benefits).
- Cost–utility analysis relates the cost of the project to a measure of its usefulness of outcome (utility).
- Cost–utility analysis is based on an index of health status in relation to output (e.g. the QALY).
- The QALY attempts to combine quantity and quality of life into a single index, for use in making comparative assessments about the effectiveness of different treatments. Costs of the treatment per QALY are calculated and generally presented in QALY league tables.

Key questions

1 What are the underlying assumptions of economic analysis?
2 Distinguish between demand, supply and utility.
3 What are cost-effectiveness and cost–benefit studies?
4 Explain opportunity cost.
5 What is discounting?
6 Describe cost–utility analysis.
7 What is a QALY?
8 What are the main techniques used to develop QALYs?

Key terms

cost–benefit
cost-effectiveness
cost–utility
demand
discounting
economic appraisal
Index of Well-being Scale
marginal cost

opportunity cost
QALYs
rating scale
standard gamble
supply
time trade-off
utility

Recommended reading

Brown, J. (2005) Economic evaluation, in A. Bowling and S. Ebrahim (eds) *Handbook of Health Research Methods: Investigation, Measurement and Analysis*. Maidenhead: Open University Press.

Drummond, M. (1994) *Economic Analyses Alongside Controlled Trials*. Leeds: NHS Executive, Department of Health.

Fox-Rushby, J. and Cairns, J. (2005) *Economic Evaluation*. Maidenhead: Open University Press.

Locket, T. (1996) *Health Economics for the Uninitiated*. Oxford: Radcliffe Medical Press.

Mooney, G. (1992) *Economics, Medicine and Health Care*. London: Harvester Wheatsheaf.

Netten, A. and Beecham, J. (eds) (1993) *Costing Community Care: Theory and Practice*. Aldershot: Ashgate Publishing.

The philosophy, theory and practice of research

This section gives a brief introduction to some of the main concepts of the philosophy of scientific research and to the current principles of scientific research. The practice of science is based on a set of rules and processes which have evolved over time, although there is still active debate about their appropriateness across the disciplines. This debate is addressed in the next chapter. Chapter 6 focuses on the general principles of research and the steps that are necessary in designing a research study. Not all of these principles apply to qualitative research methods. The principles of qualitative research are specifically addressed in Section V. However, the qualitative investigator will still need to review the literature, justify the choice of research method, clarify aims and provide evidence of research rigour. These issues are all addressed in Chapter 7.

Section contents

The philosophical framework of measurement

Introduction

The history of ideas about the conduct of science (the philosophy of science) is long. The aim of this chapter is to introduce readers to the philosophy of science in order to enhance understanding of where current scientific practices and beliefs across all disciplines, and especially in the social sciences, are derived from. This is important because it has influenced the development of systematic and rigorous research practices and methods, and the choice of methods.

Scientific research methods involve the systematic study of the phenomena of interest by detailed observation using the senses (usually sight and hearing), often aided by technical instruments (e.g. in the natural, physical and medical sciences, using microscopes, X-rays, and so on), accurate measurement and ultimately experimentation involving the careful manipulation of an intervention in strictly controlled conditions and the observation and measurement of the outcome (Davey 1994). The important feature of the scientific method is that the process is *systematic*. This means that it should be based on an agreed set of rules and processes which are rigorously adhered to, and against which the research can be evaluated. The aim of scientific research is to minimise the contamination of the results by external factors (ranging from the effects of the equipment to the effects of questionnaires used, and even experimenter bias – see Chapters 7 and 10). The concept of *rigour* is also important in relation to minimising contamination and enhancing the accuracy of the research through the detailed documentation of the research process, the collection of data in an objective manner, the systematic collection, analysis and interpretation of the data, the careful maintenance of detailed research records, the use of additional research methods to check the validity of the findings, the repeated measurement of the phenomena of interest and the involvement of another trained investigator who could reproduce the research results using the same methods, measurement tools and techniques of analysis. The concepts of reliability (repeatability of the research) and validity (the extent to which the instruments measure what they purport to measure) are relevant in relation to rigour; these are described in Chapter 7.

The philosophy of science

The method of investigation chosen depends upon the investigator's assumptions about society. For example, the investigator may start with a general idea and develop a theory and testable hypotheses from it, to be tested by data (*deduction*), or start by collecting data and building up observations for testing from them (*induction*). The choice of approach has a long history of debate in the philosophy of science, and in the social sciences. *Positivism* is the dominant philosophy underlying quantitative scientific methods. It assumes that phenomena are measurable using the deductive principles of the scientific method. It also assumes that – like matter – human behaviour is a reaction to external stimuli and that it is possible to observe and measure it using the principles of the natural (e.g. biology) and physical (e.g. chemistry) sciences. A debate exists about the validity and appropriateness of this assumption. This debate will be outlined in this chapter.

Paradigms

Each branch of scientific enquiry is based on a set of theoretical perspectives, or paradigms. These consist of a set of assumptions on which the research questions are based – or a way of looking at the world. Theoretical perspectives are important because they direct attention and provide frameworks for interpreting observations. These in turn shape the paradigms through the reformulation of theories in which familiar premises are altered. Kuhn (1970) pointed out that what we see depends on what we look at and what 'previous visual–conceptual experiences' have taught us to see. While a sociologist and a psychologist may observe the same reality, the former may focus on the social structure and the latter may focus on interpersonal differences. It is important, therefore, for the investigator to be aware of his or her theoretical perspectives and assumptions about the research topic and to report these honestly when designing research and analysing data.

Objectivity and value freedom

Scientific research implies the exercise of objectivity in the inception of the research idea, the design of the study, the methods used, the process of carrying it out and the analysis and interpretation of the research results. Attempts to minimise the many sources of bias that threaten the validity and reliability of research aim to achieve this (see Chapters 7 and 10).

Although many scientists strive for value freedom, it is naïve to assume that this is actually achieved in any field of research. Critics of the idea that research should be governed by value-free neutrality argue that research, and social science in particular, are intrinsically value-laden. Values are inherent in natural and social science from the inception of an idea to its development as a viable research project, to the choice of research method and the synthesis of the whole research process and results, as well as in terms of the decision of a funding body to sponsor it, to the decision of journal editors to publish it. Chalmers (1995) cited Hilda Bastian (a consumer advocate) on this: 'Researchers cannot assume that their own values and priorities apply to others who do not share their world.'

Clear examples of value-laden approaches in biological and clinical research were given by Berridge (1996) in her history of the development of policy in relation to AIDS in the UK. She described the early scientific uncertainties surrounding AIDS and showed how 'The relation between "scientific" and "lay" concepts in this early period illuminates the relationship between dominant and popular concepts of disease. For high science was at this stage little distant from popular concepts of this syndrome.' She quoted Oppenheimer (1988) in relation to the multifactorial epidemiological model initially used by scientists to trace causation:

> Unlike the reductionist paradigm of the germ theory, the multicausal model embraces a variety of social and environmental factors. The model's strength, however, is also its weakness . . . Variables may be drawn in (or left out) as a function of the social values of the scientist, the working group, or the society. When included in the model, embraced by the professionals, and published in the scientific press, such value judgements appear to be objective, well-grounded scientific statements.

Scientists cannot divorce themselves from the cultural, social and political context of their work. (See Box 6.1.) What scientists can do is make their assumptions about their world explicit and strive to conduct their research as rigorously and objectively as possible. If scientific publications included a statement of the investigator's assumptions, the reader would be in a better position to appraise critically the values inherent in the research. One of the rare instances where this was done was in an article by Stacey (1986):

> My analyses [on concepts of health and illness] are predicated upon certain initial assumptions. The first is that for the purposes of investigation I take all value, belief and knowledge systems to be of equal importance and validity; initially they should be judged on their own terms and within their own logic. Such

a conceptual framework is essential for systematic analysis at both theoretical and empirical levels . . . variations in concepts of health and illness cannot be viewed merely as exotica of byegone [sic] or fading societies, or curious residual remains among eccentric groups or individuals in contemporary society, left over perhaps from the witches of old.

Box 6.1 Plato's cave

The importance of investigators evaluating their perceptions of situations critically, and aiming to achieve reflective understanding, is illustrated by Plato's (427–347 BC) allegory of the cave in which he described what is necessary to achieve reflective understanding (Plato 1987) (see also Bloom 1968). In the essence of this allegory, Plato was aware that people can think without any true awareness of 'form' – that moral and intellectual opinions often bear little resemblance to the truth. The concepts that we seemingly understand and name are not on the same level as the things we perceive: we name things that we cannot see, things that we can only grasp mentally. Plato likened people to prisoners chained up in a cave, who were unable to turn their heads at all. All they could see was the wall of the cave in front of them. Behind them a fire burnt, and between the fire and the prisoners there was a parapet. Puppeteers were behind the prisoners and were unseen by them. They held up puppets who walked along the parapet, and cast shadows on the wall of the cave in front of the prisoners. The prisoners, then, were unable to see the real objects (the puppets) that passed behind them. They only saw shadows, and mistook these for reality: they thought that the shadows on the wall were 'real', not knowing about their causes. When the prisoners spoke about what they could see, they were mistaken in their labels as they were only looking at shadows, and not at the actual things that cast the shadows. When the prisoners were released, and could turn their heads and see the real objects, they realised their error (and grasped the 'form' with their minds).

Deductive and inductive approaches

Deductive and inductive reasoning constitutes an important component of scientific reasoning and knowledge. With *deductive* reasoning, the investigator starts with general ideas and develops a theory and testable hypotheses from it. The hypotheses are then tested by gathering and analysing data. In contrast, *inductive* reasoning begins with the observations and builds up ideas and more general statements and testable hypotheses from them for further testing on the basis of further observations.

Scientific enquiry was initially built on a philosophical framework of deductive logic. The concept of inductive inference was later formalised by the seventeenth-century philosopher Francis Bacon, who demonstrated how deductive logic could not be predictive without the results of inductive inference, a view later contested by David Hume on the grounds of the incompleteness inherent in inductive logic (see Hughes 1990). However, John Locke popularised inductive methods and helped to establish *empiricism* (based on the importance of making observations, rather than theoretical statements) as the prevailing philosophy of science. *Probabilistic inductive logic* later became popular, as it was apparent that inductive logic was merely a method of making plausible guesses, and was unable to provide a method for proving 'cause and effect'. With probabilistic inductive logic what can only be suggested is a general explanation that there is a *high probability* that X causes Y, or that in a high percentage of cases X causes Y, rather than a universal law.

Falsification of hypotheses

Verification by this process of probabilistic logic was refuted by Karl Popper (1959), who denied that probability accrued to a theory by virtue of its survival of testing, and argued that statements of probabilistic confirmation are also scientific statements that require probability judgements. Popper accepted Hume's argument, and further proposed that knowledge accumulates only by the falsification of hypotheses, while rejecting the abandonment of causality. Popper argued, then, that scientific hypotheses can never be more than informed estimates about the universe, and since they cannot be proved to be true, scientists should concentrate on developing testable hypotheses, formulated in a way that allows predictions to be made, and then construct investigations which attempt to disprove their hypotheses. Thus knowledge accumulates only by falsification: for example, by setting up testable theories that can be potentially disproved by experiment, in deductive fashion. The surviving theory is the strongest (temporarily).

The ability of a theory to be disproved thus distinguished a scientific theory from a belief. This approach, which stresses the virtues of *falsification*, is known as the *hypothetico-deductive* method, and it underlies the contemporary scientific method. For example, a hypothesis is developed from existing theory, and consequences are deduced, which are then tested against empirical data. If the hypothesis is falsified, the investigator can develop another one. If not, other tests are used in further attempts at falsification. Therefore scientists aim to falsify rather than verify their theories, and scientific progress is a matter of eliminating falsehood rather than establishing truth.

Criticisms of the hypothetico-deductive method

The hypothetico-deductive method is not without criticism. For example, it may be argued that probability must accrue to hypotheses that survive testing, as otherwise it is irrational to rely on hypotheses that have survived testing to date; and that the research process is not as rigid in practice, and theories can acquire credibility in other ways. Brown (1977) argued that the refutation of hypotheses is not a certain process, as it is dependent on observations which may not be accurate owing to the problem of measurement; deductions may provide predictions from hypotheses, but there is no logical method for the comparison of predictions with observations; and the infrastructure of scientific laws from which new hypotheses emerge is falsifiable. The last point is consistent with Kuhn's (1972) argument that the acceptance and rejection of hypotheses come from the development of consensus within the scientific community and the prevailing view of science (see 'paradigm shifts', later). The first point on accuracy has always challenged investigators. One influential approach to tackling this by positivists, who believe that laws govern social phenomena, and that these can be measured following the principles of the scientific method (see later), was *operationalism*. This argues that the concepts employed in empirical research must be defined in terms of the indicators used to measure them (e.g. psychological health by a measurement scale of anxiety and depression). There is a long scientific debate about the inadequacy of operationalisation as a concept, and of how it can be limiting and misleading (see Blalock and Blalock 1971). This also leads to the problem of validity: is the measure measuring what it purports to? Today, however, operationalism is used flexibly, simply as a useful guide to the research process, rather than claiming that the concepts are synonymous with the indicators of measurement, though the investigator still has the problem of relating empirical concepts to theoretical concepts (see Hughes 1990).

Current practice

In theory, then, the current '*rational*' scientific method consists of a system of rules and processes on which research is based, following the principles of the hypothetico-deductive method, and against which it can be evaluated. In addition, research needs to be conducted rigorously and systematically. The investigator must record meticulously how the testing and measurements were carried out, collect valid, reliable and unbiased data, analyse the data with care and finally present clear conclusions based on the data and submit them to peer review (Russell and Wilson 1992).

In practice, science is based on a less rigid, and more haphazard, blend of the rules of deductive and inductive or probabilistic reasoning. It is a mixture of empirical conception and the certainties of deductive reasoning. Thus the theoretical logic and the practice of the scientific method do not necessarily coincide perfectly. For example, one has an idea for a theory (the hypothesis), and estimates its predictions, tests it against data, in deductive fashion. If the theory does not fit the data and is refuted, induction is used to construct a better theory, based on probability, and so on. In practice, hypotheses may also be developed at the same time as the data analysis (though stricter statisticians will argue that this is not an acceptable practice). Scientists sometimes develop their theoretical frameworks at the same time that preliminary results emerge, and in the process modify their hypotheses. In addition, hypotheses are not usually completely supported or refuted by the research data – some aspects are supported, and others rejected. The investigator will commonly refine and modify the hypothesis, in the light of the data, and again set out to test it.

The scientific method has frequently been interpreted liberally in order to avoid restricting hypotheses to testable predictions (which would seriously limit the scope of research). The steps of the scientific method, in ideal form, act as a guide, and as a framework within which scientific results are organised and presented (social scientists are more flexible and may adopt, in theory, the hypothetico-deductive method or may begin with data and develop theory later in inductive fashion – see later).

Prediction

More than these philosophies are required for the development of causal models in science, particularly in relation to human and social sciences where knowledge is frequently imperfect. However, *prediction* and understanding also constitute important components of research. The ability to make correct predictions is held to be the foremost quality of science. This is based on the belief that if knowledge is adequate, then prediction is possible: if it is known that X causes Y and that X is present, then the prediction that Y will occur can be made.

Hill (1965) cautiously suggested features for the assessment of causal associations: strength (the magnitude of the association), consistency (or reliability – the repeatability of the observation), specificity (a cause should lead to a single effect, and not multiple effects), temporality (the cause must precede the effect in time), biologic gradient (the presence of a dose–response or effect curve), plausibility of the hypothesis, coherence with information derived from elsewhere, experimental evidence and analogy. Rothman (1986) argued that weaknesses can be found in most of these features. For example, associations that are weak or inconsistent do not rule out causal connections; single events quite often have multiple effects, and experimental data in human life are not always available or possible to obtain. Rothman concluded that investigators need to recognise the *impossibility*, in theory, of proving causality and the incompleteness of scientific research in the light of advancing knowledge, and, in consequence, retain their scepticism.

The survival of hypotheses and paradigm shifts

The model of rational science holds that scientific knowledge – and consensus – reflect the survival of hypotheses after rigorous testing. However, Kuhn (1970, 1972) noted the transformation of scientific beliefs when revolutionary developments occurred. He labelled this transformation '*paradigm shifts*': over time, evidence accumulates and challenges the dominant paradigm, leading to a crisis among scientists and the gradual realisation of the inadequacy of that paradigm; pressure for change eventually occurs, leading to a 'scientific revolution', and the new paradigm becomes gradually accepted (until it, in turn, is challenged).

Prior to Kuhn's work, although there had been dissident voices, it had been taken for granted that scientific knowledge grew by the accumulation of demonstrated 'facts'. Kuhn noted that the prevailing, rational view of science – of a logically ordered accumulation of facts, leading to scientific laws – bore little relationship to historical scientific events. He argued that revolutionary science, or change in prevailing paradigms, was more likely to be the result of persuasion, personal influences and indirect influences from social change and propaganda. Only once the paradigm had shifted did scientific logic resume its lead, with the accumulation of scientific knowledge in relation to the new paradigm. The shift from an old paradigm to a new one is not necessarily without conflict. Kuhn noted that those who adhered to the old paradigm appeared to live in a different world from the adherents of the radical shift to a new paradigm. Established scientists have built their careers on the old paradigm and may not encourage its replacement with new ones. Developments in research methodology can also be interpreted in terms of paradigm shifts. The increasing use of evidence-based medicine, despite dissent by some clinicians who defend rigidly their right to complete clinical autonomy, has been described as marking a paradigm shift in clinical practice (Evidence-based Medicine Working Group 1992). Patient-centred medicine has similarly been described as a 'Copernican revolution' (Battista 1993; and see Parker 2001).

In theory, then, science develops by the accumulation of accredited 'facts'. In practice, however, not only is there greater flexibility, but investigators, rather than falsifying theory, attempt to extend and exploit it in many different ways. Changes in prevailing paradigms are more likely to be the result of external events.

Theoretical influences on social research methods

The study of humans and social life is more complex than the study of physical and natural phenomena. This is partly because ethical and practical considerations often preclude the controlled conditions and the use of the experimental method characteristic of the physical and natural sciences. There is an overall commitment among investigators of humans to the basic elements of the scientific method, in particular, in relation to the systematic collection of information, the replication of research results and the norms that govern the rigorous conduct of scientific research. Despite this, there has been a long history of debate in social science about the appropriateness of the traditional scientific method for the study of human life, given its complexity and the nature of individual behaviour, and about the interactions between scientific research and cultural beliefs which make a *value-free* science difficult to achieve. It is increasingly accepted that social science becomes scientific not by using the basic experimental method, but by adopting research methods that are appropriate to the topic of study, that are rigorous, critical and objective and that ensure the systematic collection, analysis and presentation of the data (Silverman 1993).

In contemporary social science, the importance of inductive, or probabilistic, *as well as* hypothetico-deductive logic is emphasised: one does not necessarily begin with a theory and set out to test it, but one can begin with a topic and allow what is relevant to that topic to emerge from analyses (this is known as grounded theory – see next section). Moreover, in social science in particular, associations are, at best, probabilistic (e.g. X tends to lead to Y), owing to the complexity of social phenomena and the difficulty of controlling for all confounding extraneous variables in natural settings.

Social science and grounded theory

In social science it is common to develop 'grounded theory'. This refers to a process of discovering theory from data that have been systematically gathered and analysed: 'generating a theory from data means that most hypotheses and concepts not only come from the data, but are systematically worked out in relation to the data during the course of research' (Glaser and Strauss 1967). It is a theory that is *inductively* derived from the study of the phenomena it represents. Thus data-gathering, analysis and theory have a reciprocal relationship. Moreover, theories do not have to be causal explanations. Descriptive questions can also form a testable hypothesis. However, in social science, where it is not always possible to control the conditions under which social phenomena are observed, there is a greater need to build theory inductively from several observations before a predictive, explanatory theory can be derived.

Grounded theory has been subject to critical theoretical and methodological debate (Bryant and Charmaz 2010). A main influence on current approaches is that of constructivist grounded theory, which emphasises multiple individual realities (Charmaz 2000). (See Box 6.2.)

> ## Box 6.2 Constructivist grounded theory
>
> Charmaz (2003) summarised the constructivist grounded theory approach as:
>
> - Simultaneous data collection and analysis.
> - Developing analytic codes and categories from the data, rather than *a priori* hypotheses.
> - Building inductive middle-range, rather than grand, social theories to explain processes and events through successive levels of data (e.g. theories such as resilience in relation to maintenance of health).
> - Writing analytic notes to explain behaviour and processes.
> - Comparing data with data, data with concepts, concepts with concepts.
> - Theoretical sampling to check and refine conceptual categories (rather than representative sampling).
> - Undertaking the literature review after the analysis.
>
> This is not without some controversy over whether it involves some artificial forcing of data (Puddephatt 2006), in contradiction of the original concept. Consequently it has been referred to as modified grounded theory. Some aspects of this approach are also unrealistic. Undertaking the literature review post analysis, however, is unlikely to attract research funding.

Positivism

The method of investigation used depends on the investigator's assumptions about society. A considerable body of social science is directed by research methods drawn from the natural sciences. This approach is known as *positivism*. The principles of scientific enquiry used by bio-medicine, for example, are rooted in positivism. Positivism aims to discover laws using quantitative methods and emphasises *positive facts*. Thus, positivism assumes that there is a single objective reality which can be ascertained by the senses, and tested subject to the laws of the scientific method. The positivist conception of science was advocated in the late eighteenth and nineteenth centuries and was developed in relation to sociology by the nineteenth-century philosopher Auguste Comte (for a brief history, see Keat 1979).

The natural scientist systematically observes and measures the behaviour of matter and the results of these investigations are regarded as 'facts'; these are believed to be undistorted by the value judgement of the scientist. This is owing to the availability, in theory (though not always in practice), of *objective* systems of measurement (e.g. of temperature). Positivism in social science assumes that human behaviour is a reaction to external stimuli and that it is possible to observe and measure social phenomena, using the principles of the natural scientist, and the hypothetico-deductive method, and thereby to establish a reliable and valid body of knowledge about its operation based on *empiricism* (actual evidence gathered through use of the senses, i.e. observed). It is argued that social science should concern itself only with what is observable and that theories should be built in a rigid, linear and methodical way on a base of verifiable fact. Positivists are not concerned with measuring the meaning of situations to people because they cannot be measured in a scientific and objective manner.

Most social science has developed adhering to this positivist philosophy, alongside the physical sciences. The most popular tools that are used are surveys and experimental methods, and statistical techniques of analysis. Similarly, positivist traditions shape many of the methods of research on health and health care, and the way the research instruments are administered. For example, interviews are standardised and structured in order to minimise the influence of the instrument and the interviewer on the respondent, and there has been an overemphasis on the experimental method, with little attempt to combine it with qualitative methods better able to provide rich insights into human behaviour and social processes. (See Box 6.3.)

Box 6.3 Distortion in Durkheim's study of suicide

A widely cited example of the distortion of reality by positivist methods is Durkheim's (1951) classic study of suicide. His hypothesis was that Catholic countries would have lower suicide rates than Protestant countries. This was based on the assumption that religious affiliation acted as an indicator of social integration, given the observation that Protestants were more likely than Catholics to emphasise personal autonomy, independence and achievement and hence have weaker social ties. Durkheim collected data on suicide rates, based on death certificates, across countries and argued that there was an association between religious affiliation and suicide rates. It was assumed that suicide statistics, based on death certificates, were correct and could be taken as 'social facts'. This was a false assumption, because for a death to be recorded as a suicide, the victim's motives and intentions have to be known or assumed and the society must be willing to accept the death as a suicide (otherwise a verdict of death by misadventure is more likely to be recorded). It is known that in the Catholic countries suicide was regarded as a religious sin, and was held to be taboo; hence death by misadventure, rather than suicide, was likely to be recorded on death certificates in these cases, leading to suicide rates falsely appearing to be lower in Catholic countries than elsewhere. Thus suicide statistics cannot simply be defined as observational data – they are not 'value-free'.

While this is a widely quoted example of the distortion of society by positivist methods, it should also be pointed out that Durkheim's perspective was in fact broader than this example suggests and was often contradictory. For example, Durkheim attempted to explain suicide rates on the basis of the relationship between the individual and society and the concepts of egoism, altruism, anomie and fatalism, which were not easily observable. In contrast, positivists would confine their analyses to observable elements of society (see Taylor and Ashworth 1987).

Functionalism

Functionalism is a positivist approach that focuses on the social system (and is part of the theory of social systems). Illness is conceptualised in relation to the impact on, and consequences for, the immediate social system (e.g. family, work and personal finance) and the wider social system (e.g. the wider socialisation and nurturing functions of families upon which law, order and stability in society are dependent, employment and the economy). Consequences that interfere with the system and its values are called *dysfunctional*, and those which contribute to its functioning are called *functional*.

This systems perspective can be termed *holistic* science, within which framework it is assumed that individual phenomena can only be understood if they are analysed in the context of the interactions and relationships with the wider social system. It is argued that social systems consist of networks that shape and constrain the individual's experience, attitudes and behaviour. It is a determinist mode of thought which implies that individuals have little control or free choice, and which assumes that everything is caused in a predictable way. This school of thought is known as 'determinism'.

Phenomenology

Although positivism has long been established and remains the dominant philosophy underlying scientific methodology, a number of social scientists have viewed it as misleading, as it encourages an emphasis on superficial facts without understanding the underlying mechanisms observed, or their meanings to individuals. The Popperian view of the process of science has also been strongly rejected by social scientists adhering to a phenomenological philosophy, who argue that research observation must precede theory because 'it initiates, it reformulates, it deflects, and it clarifies theory' (Merton 1968).

The philosophy of phenomenology, when applied to social science, emphasises that social 'facts' are characterised and recognised by their 'meaningfulness' to members of the social world (often termed 'actors') (Smart 1976). Social scientists following this philosophy argue that the investigator must aim to discover these social meanings. Phenomenology is based on the paradigm that 'reality' is multiple, and socially constructed through the interaction of individuals who use symbols to interpret each other and assign meaning to perceptions and experience; these are not imposed by external forces. Therefore, to use the tools of natural science distorts reality. The theory of social systems is thus rejected, as human action is not seen as a response to the system but a response to interaction with others and the meanings to the individual.

The phenomenological school of thought is broadly known as atomism: social systems are believed to be abstractions which do not exist apart from individuals interacting with each other. Thus it is the study of conscious human experience in everyday life. Readers interested in pursuing this school of thought further are referred to Berger and Luckman (1967) and Filmer *et al.* (1972). Other schools of social thought which are critical of the positivist perspective have been described by May (1993).

For phenomenologists, the research setting is accepted as unmanipulated and natural (studying people in their real, 'natural', settings), interactive and jointly participative by investigator and respondent. The vehicles are the open-ended, unstructured, in-depth interview or participant observation; the data are regarded as valid when a mutual understanding between investigator and respondent has been achieved (Denzin 1971). These methods are commonly called 'naturalistic research'.

Phenomenological approaches

Social scientists whose approaches are anchored in phenomenology are all concerned with *hermeneutics* and are known, depending on their precise focus, either as *humanists* or as *interpretive sociologists*.

Humanists aim for a meaningful understanding of the individual, human awareness and the whole context of the social situation. The approach carries the danger that common-sense assumptions about the validity of individuals' accounts of experiences are uncritically accepted (e.g. accounts obtained during unstructured, in-depth interviews).

Interpretive sociologists recognise that meaning emerges through interaction and is not standardised across social and cultural groups. Their approach differs from an uncritical humanist approach in that accounts and assumptions are investigated and analysed as research data, rather than as representations of the phenomenon of interest (Hammersley and Atkinson 1983; Silverman 1993). Weber (1964, 1979) argued that people are creative agents in society and do not simply respond according to its structure. He also argued that sociologists need to understand both how societies work and how people operate within them and construct their everyday realities of them. Weber (1979) termed the understanding or interpretation of meaning as *Verstehen* (empathy). This *interpretive* school of thought holds that social scientists should use research methods which respect hermeneutics. Interpretive sociology includes ethnomethodology, social or symbolic interactionism and labelling, deviance and reaction theory. Distinctions between different schools are summarized in Box 6.4:

Box 6.4 Different phenomenological approaches

■ Ethnomethodologists analyse how people see things, and how they use social interaction to maintain a sense of reality, mainly using *participant observational* studies.

■ Social or symbolic interactionists focus on the details of social behaviour and how we attach symbolic meanings to social interactions and experiences and create a sense of self. For example, words can be loaded with cultural meanings and even a piece of jewellery (e.g. earring, ring for a finger or badge) can convey a fashion or lifestyle statement, a personal or political message.

■ Labelling, deviance and reaction theorists draw on interactionism and analyse how people interpret, act upon and react to events and others, and the process by which members of a society are labelled (e.g. as deviants).

Social action theory

Weber

These different branches of interpretive sociology are collectively known as *social action theory*, which was initially developed by Max Weber (1964), and aims to explain social action by understanding the ideas, values, interpretations, meanings and the social world of individuals. The common criticism of these theorists is that they have ignored the social organisation of society and the effects of the distribution of resources and power on people's behaviour and attitudes. The former would argue that there is no social structure out there influencing behaviour, but everything can be socially negotiated.

Mead, Cooley and Goffman

The social action (interactionist) approach is reflected in the early work of G.H. Mead (1934), Erwin Goffman (1959) and C.H. Cooley (1964). This approach is based on Mead's

(1934) theory of the individual as a creative, thinking organism, who is able to exercise choice over social behaviour, instead of reacting mechanically to social phenomena. Both Mead and Cooley developed some of the early concepts central to social action theories, in particular in relation to socialisation processes among children. They postulated that children learn their concept of the self by means of negotiations between themselves, the immediate family and significant others. The child observes how other people act and respond to him or her and thereby learns patterns of social interaction. It was held by Cooley that the negotiation between the child's assertion of himself or herself as an individual and the creation of the social self through the reflected impressions described creates another dimension: the looking-glass self.

Along with Cooley's concept of the 'looking-glass self', Mead developed the concepts of *I*, *me* and *mind* to explain a person's ability to undertake social roles, to view and reflect on ourselves. Mead suggested that, as the unique meanings that a person attributes to situations cannot be fully shared with others, people learn to share symbols and attribute common meanings (see Volkart 1951, for developments of this).

Goffman (1959) held that information about others is required for social action to occur, and this information is obtained from appearances, previous experiences, the particular social setting, verbal and non-verbal action. The latter, in particular, is subject to an individual's control, and represents the impression he or she is trying to project about themselves (Goffman calls this process 'impression management'). He argued that people strive to project a certain self-image ('face'), and social interaction consists of people attempting to make their activities consistent with their projected self-image, deliberately manoeuvring for social gains. These perspectives necessitate a hermeneutic approach to investigation. Goffman is noted for the dramaturgical approach (or 'life as theatre').

In sum, debates about 'positivism' in the social sciences, about whether social science can be 'value-free', about whether it is a 'science' and about perspectives and choice of method have been rampant, particularly during the 1960s and 1970s (see Berger and Luckman 1967; Filmer *et al.* 1972; Giddens 1974; Keat 1979; Hughes 1990).

Choice of methods

Positivism and phenomenology appear diametrically opposed, are based on different perspectives of the social world and use different research methods. However, the question to be addressed should not be quantitative versus qualitative methodology, but how to identify innovative strategies to combine different perspectives and quantitative and qualitative methodologies in a single study, while at the same time respecting the distinct branches of philosophical thought from which they are derived. As a compromise, it could be said that people are influenced by their social situations, and they live in environments which do condition them, but at the same time they are never totally conditioned and constrained by these external factors and man 'can always make something out of what is made of him' (Sartre 1969).

In terms of the intensity of personal contact and numbers of people investigated, the large-scale survey and experiment are at one polar extreme (positivism and scientific methodology) and in-depth, qualitative interviews and observations are at the other (phenomenological and hermeneutic approaches). Both methods are valid if applied to appropriate research questions, and they should complement each other. Qualitative techniques are essential for exploring new topics and obtaining insightful and rich data on complex issues. They are essential in the initial stages of questionnaire design and scale construction. Quantitative techniques are appropriate if the issue is known about, relatively simple and unambiguous, and amenable to valid and reliable measurement. Even when the latter conditions are satisfied, there is always scope for using multiple (triangulated) methods (Webb *et al.* 1966) or supplementing quantitative methods with qualitative techniques in order to check the accuracy, content, validity and relevance (meaning) to the respondents of the quantitative data that have been collected. This has led to some blurring of the incompatibilities between qualitative and quantitative research paradigms, and the development of a middle way, in order to avoid the traditional clashes between quantitative versus qualitative paradigms (Morgan 2007; Cresswell 2009; Moriarty 2010).

Summary of main points

- Deductive reasoning: the investigator starts with general ideas and develops specific theories and hypotheses from them, which are then tested by collecting and analysing data.
- Inductive reasoning: begins with observations and builds up general statements and hypotheses from them for testing.
- Grounded theory: the process of generating theory from data that have been systematically gathered and analysed.
- The scientific method: a system of rules and processes on which research is based and against which it can be evaluated.
- Positivism assumes that human behaviour is a reaction to external stimuli; that it is possible to observe and measure social phenomena, using the principles of the natural scientist.
- Within a positivist perspective, functionalism focuses on the social system as a whole. Illness is conceptualised in relation to the impact on, and consequences for, the immediate and wider social system.
- The Popperian view of the process of science has been rejected by social scientists adhering to a phenomenological philosophy, who argue that research must precede theory because it initiates and clarifies theory.
- There has been a blurring of research approaches with the increasing use of mixed qualitative and quantitative approaches to investigate research questions.

Key questions

1 Select a research paper that reports an association between two or more variables indicating a causal link, and suggest rival explanations.
2 Distinguish between the deductive and inductive schools of thought.
3 Describe Popper's main argument on the falsifiability of hypotheses.
4 What is grounded theory?
5 Explain paradigm shifts.
6 How is illness perceived by functionalists?
7 What are the current principles of the 'rational' scientific method?

Key terms

deduction

empiricism

ethnomethodology

grounded theory

humanists

hypothetico-deductive method

induction

interpretive sociology

naturalistic enquiry

objectivity

operationalism

paradigm

paradigm shift

phenomenology

positivism

prediction

probabilistic inductive logic

rigour

scientific method

social action theory

social interactionists

symbolic interactionism

systematic

value freedom

Recommended reading

Bryant, A. and Charmaz, K.C. (2010) Grounded theory in historical perspective: an epistemological account, in K.C. Charmaz and A. Bryant (eds) *The SAGE Handbook of Grounded Theory*. London: Sage, pp. 31–57.

Glaser, B.G. and Strauss, A.L. (1967) *The Discovery of Grounded Theory: Strategies for Qualitative Research*. New York: Aldine Publishing.

Kuhn, T.S. (1970) *The Structure of Scientific Revolutions*, 2nd expanded edn. Chicago: University of Chicago Press.

May, T. (1993) *Social Research: Issues, Methods and Process*. Buckingham: Open University Press.

Morgan, D.L. (2007) Paradigms lost and pragmatisms regained: methodological implications of combining qualitative and quantitative methods. *Journal of Mixed Methods Research*, 1: 48–76.

Popper, K.R. (1959) *The Logic of Scientific Discovery*. London: Hutchinson.

Strauss, A. and Corbin, J. (1990) *Basics of Qualitative Research: Grounded Theory Procedures and Techniques*. Thousand Oaks, CA: Sage.

The principles of research

Introduction

This chapter covers the basic steps involved in carrying out a research project. These include: the review of the literature; the development of the aims, objectives and hypotheses of the research based on concepts and theories; the clarification of the independent and dependent variables; the selection of the methods of research and measurement instruments; the level of data; and the psychometric properties of the instruments selected. Many types of bias and error exist and these can threaten the reliability and validity of the research. The investigator has to strive constantly to eliminate or minimise these from the inception of the research idea to the design and process of the study. The various types of bias and error are also described in this chapter. Finally, issues relating to the ethics of the research and the dissemination of results are outlined.

Searching the published and unpublished literature

The first step in deciding on a topic for study is to search and review the published and also the unpublished 'grey' literature. Non-significant research findings are rarely accepted for publication, resulting in 'publication bias', which Chalmers (1990) has labelled as bordering on scientific misconduct. In drug trials with commercial sponsorship, a publication bias against negative findings is likely to exist. Some authors ignore non-significant findings and only publish those which attain statistical significance. In contrast, there may be dangers in including non-refereed papers, especially from those with conflicts of interest (e.g. commercial). It is possible that the English language publications are more likely to publish significant findings, and hence non-significant findings may be more likely to be in other language journals – hence the need to search all languages.

An analysis of 150 systematic reviews in conventional and alternative medicine by Moher et al. (2003) concluded that language-inclusive systematic reviews were a marker for better quality reviews. They reported that while language restriction did not bias the estimates of the effectiveness of conventional interventions, there was substantial bias in the estimates of the effectiveness of alternative medicine reviews. A systematic review of 159 meta-analyses by Egger et al. (2003) concluded that systematic reviews that were based on English language literature only, and which were accessible in the major bibliographic databases, tended to produce results close to those obtained from more comprehensive searches that are free of language restriction. However, they did find that trials which were unpublished showed less beneficial effects than published trials, whereas non-English language trials and trials not indexed in MEDLINE tended to show larger treatment effects. Trials that were difficult to locate were often of lower quality, and thus rather than their inclusion preventing bias, they could instead introduce bias. Egger et al. also reported that trials with inadequate or unclear concealment of allocation generally showed more beneficial effects than adequately concealed trials, and open trials were more beneficial than double-blind trials.

Non-significant research results tend to remain in internal departmental reports, known as 'the grey literature'. There is also some evidence of a peer reviewer bias in medicine, against publication of results of trials of unconventional forms of therapy (Resch et al. 2000). Thus investigators also need to network with other experts in the field, who will usually be aware of the 'grey literature'. This is done by contacting investigators who might know of relevant studies, attending professional conferences, and so on.

Subjective approaches to reviewing and synthesising the research literature in relation to health care have long been shown to be misleading, biased and even clinically dangerous (Antman et al. 1992). Consequently, systematic approaches to critical appraisal, evidence synthesis and review have been developed. Statistical methods of producing a single quantitative measure of the 'effect' have also been developed (meta-analyses). Meta-analyses are not always part of a systematic review, depending on the type of study and available data. Regardless of the method and topic of the research, or whether meta-analyses are included, reviews should always be conducted systematically following a written protocol and specified approach.

Computerised and other literature databases

Searching the literature has been facilitated by electronic databases in medical science (e.g. MEDLINE; BIDS (Bath Information and Data Service); EMBASE for pharmacological and biomedical journals), nursing (CINAHL: Cumulative Index to Nursing and Allied Health Database), social sciences (Sociological Abstracts; BIDS Social Science Citation Index; BIDS PsycINFO via the American Psychology Association), full indexes (British Library Information Index – BLII), Index to theses, web of science, and various other specialist database and citation indexes.

Manual searches through back numbers of relevant journals can also be valuable, as not all relevant articles will necessarily be indexed under the appropriate key words. It should not be assumed that all relevant articles will be indexed within one database. For example, many journals on ageing are indexed in sociology but not psychology or medical databases, and vice versa.

International interest in conducting rigorous, systematic reviews led to the development of the Cochrane Collaboration, which is an international group of subject and methodological specialists, who identify and synthesise the results of controlled trials, and maintain (update) their reviews. The Cochrane Collaboration developed a highly sensitive search strategy, given that failure to identify all relevant controlled trials for systematic reviews can result in bias. This strategy has since been improved upon by Robinson and Dickersin (2002), using a revised strategy. The Cochrane Centre was established to support the research and development programme of the British NHS, and to disseminate information (Cochrane Database of Systematic Reviews 1995).

Systematic literature reviews

Traditional, non-systematic, or narrative, reviews are limited by their subjectivity in terms of included publications and assessment of them. In contrast, systematic reviews aim to be systematic and comprehensive in the identification and evaluation of included literature, objective in their interpretation of this, and have reproducible conclusions. With a systematic review, the research question must be clearly defined and only studies addressing it can be included; *all* the relevant studies need to be included.

Details of the methods and results of studies included should be presented and appraised in a critical manner (O'Rourke 2005). Systematic reviews, critical appraisal, meta-analyses and economic modelling of the findings are key to evidence-based clinical practice and health care. They are increasing in volume in clinical medicine, though there is a dearth in other areas (e.g. veterinary medicine, laboratory and animal research; Pound *et al*. 2004).

Systematic reviews are prepared with a systematic approach, aiming to minimise the effect of biases and random errors in conclusions. They include information on materials and methods in relation to the published and unpublished literature (Chalmers and Altman 1995a). In quantitative research, they are usually based on RCTs but do include information derived from other research designs when appropriate (e.g. controlled study designs). Economic modelling of the costs of resulting optimum treatments is increasingly undertaken by investigators undertaking systematic reviews of treatment effectiveness.

Review criteria

Reviews should report the method and strategy of searching used (e.g. named database searches in relation to the topic (key words) and years searched). The references cited in all accepted studies should be reviewed for additional citations within the stated search period. References can be downloaded into bibliographic software packages. Flow charts showing the numbers of included and excluded papers should be presented. (See Box 7.1.)

Box 7.1 Holt Lunstad *et al.*'s (2010) systematic review

Holt Lunstad *et al.* (2010), in their systematic review of the influence of social support on mortality, included Dissertation Abstracts, HealthStar, Medline, Mental Health Abstracts, PsychINFO, Social Science Abstracts, Sociological Abstracts via Sociofile, Academic Search Premier, ERIC, Family and Society Studies Worldwide. In addition, they examined references from past reviews and references cited in identified papers which met their inclusion criteria. Figure 7.1 shows Holt-Lunstad *et al.*'s (2010) final results search tree (2010, p. 3).

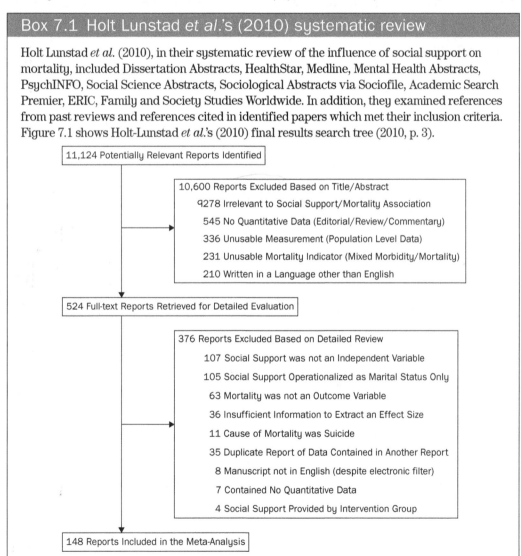

Figure 7.1: Holt-Lunstad *et al.*'s (2010) Final Results Search Tree

When reviewing literature, the investigator should assess publications in relation to rigorous research criteria, shown in Box 7.2. Guidance to enhance the quality of systematic reviews has been published (Pocock 1983; Grant 1989; Shea *et al.* 2007; Terwee *et al.* 2012). Updated checklists and quality assessment tools for primary reporting of RCTs and observational studies have been published, which should also facilitate their reviewing (Hopewell *et al.* 2008; Moher *et al.* 2010; Schulz *et al.* 2010; von Elm *et al.* 2007; Beller *et al.* 2013).

There are several guides on how to undertake literature reviews and systematic reviews (Light and Pillemar 1984; Roe 1993; Chalmers and Altman 1995b; Oxman 1995; Deeks *et al.* 1996). The necessary steps have been summarised by Cullinan (2005). The processes of undertaking a systematic review in health care and statistical approaches to meta-analysis have been described by Cullinan (2005) and techniques of critical appraisal in quantitative and qualitative research have been detailed by O'Rourke (2005).

Box 7.2 Detailed checklist of the points to be aware of when undertaking a critical appraisal of the scientific literature

- Are the aims and objectives of the study clearly stated?
- Are the hypotheses and research questions clearly specified?
- Are the dependent and independent variables clearly stated?
- Have the variables been adequately operationalised?
- Is the design of the study adequately described?
- Are the research methods appropriate?
- Were the instruments used appropriate and adequately tested for reliability and validity?
- Is there an adequate description of the source of the sample, inclusion and exclusion criteria, response rates, and (in the case of longitudinal research and post-tests in experiments) sample attrition?
- Was the statistical power of the study to detect or reject differences (types I and II error) discussed critically?
- Are ethical considerations presented?
- Was the study piloted?
- Were the statistical analyses appropriate and adequate?
- Are the results clear and adequately reported?
- Does the discussion of the results report them in the light of the hypotheses of the study and other relevant literature?
- Are the limitations of the research and its design presented?
- Does the discussion generalise and draw conclusions beyond the limits of the data and number and type of people studied?
- Can the findings be generalised to other relevant populations and time periods?
- Are the implications – practical or theoretical – of the research discussed?
- Who was the sponsor of the study, and was there a conflict of interest?
- Are the research data held on an accessible database, or are they otherwise available for scrutiny and re-analysis?

Data extraction and quality assessment

In relation to the process and quality of systematic reviews, a list of key questions needs to be generated, and standard data extraction and quality forms developed to enable recording of research data, and to rate the quality of the studies included. This is performed ideally by two independent raters. The forms needs to be piloted on a small selection of studies, and adjusted as necessary. Numerous guides and checklists of processes have been published (Chalmers and Altman 1995a; Khan *et al.* 2001). These include specification of the research question, the strategy for searching databases and other literature, methods of data extraction, study selection criteria, criteria of validity and quality to be applied to the studies selected for inclusion, data extraction and method of synthesis. Quality criteria apply mainly to experimental designs (e.g. RCTs) and include adequacy of blinding participants, comparability of groups at baseline and adequacy of intention to treat.

The systematic review needs to provide evidence of the sources used, the likely completeness and quality of the supporting evidence for each conclusion. Multiple publications of the same study findings by the included authors (duplicates) need identifying and removing. As Cullinan (2005) pointed out, the difficulty for the reviewer lies in establishing whether these are genuinely separate studies. Duplicate literature between database searches also needs to be identified. An examination of the quality of selected appraisals reported that over a fifth missed relevant articles to answer their questions (Coomarasamy *et al.* 2001). Various checklists exist for assessing the quality of systematic reviews, which overlap with those for critical appraisals. Data extraction proforma for empirical research reviews should include, at minimum:

- a clear statement of aims;
- a study design (experimental by type; observational by type);
- research quality criteria (e.g. type of/blinding in RCTs);
- appropriateness of methods and statistics;
- country and date of study;
- site of study (e.g. population/hospital/primary care);
- sample size, coverage and evidence of statistical power;
- response rates/sample attrition;
- sample characteristics, including condition;
- theoretical framework;
- predictors and outcomes assessed;
- measurement tools with evidence of reliability and validity;
- outcomes/results;
- generalisability.

Oxman (1996) recommended that those engaged in systematic reviews of trials should use the one criterion for which strong empirical evidence exists of a potential for bias: the adequate concealment of allocation (blinding). This is not always possible outside drug trials, and, as was pointed out earlier, the same treating professional may be required to provide two different types of care – one for the experimental and another for the control group (see Black 1996), with the potential for contamination.

Systematic qualitative reviews

The application of methods of systematic reviewing to qualitative research is more challenging (Campbell *et al.* 2003; Pope *et al.* 2007). The types of qualitative synthesis that have been proposed include numeric synthesis (e.g. converting qualitative data into quantitative formats), narrative synthesis (aggregation of findings for comparison based on narratives rather than numerical methods), and methods to develop an inductive and interpretive knowledge synthesis, which aims to go beyond individual studies and contribute to conceptual and theoretical development (see Campbell *et al.* 2007). Campbell *et al.*'s own synthesis of qualitative studies (2007) indicated that the interpretive, meta-ethnographic method was able to identify areas in which theoretical saturation had been reached. However, the method is still evolving and cannot be regarded currently as a standardised method for routine application. There is no general agreement within qualitative research on basic definitions or classifications, including qualitative research synthesis, although several methods have been suggested (see Mays and Pope 1996; Pope *et al.* 2007; Campbell *et al.* 2003, 2007). Where quantitative syntheses and meta-analyses of the data are not appropriate or possible, narrative syntheses, using framework analyses, to compile diverse evidence are generally used (Ritchie and Spencer 1994).

The difference between using meta-ethnography for a synthesis of the results of qualitative research, and traditional narrative or systematic literature reviews, is in the systematic identification and charting of the key concepts in papers undergoing synthesis (Britten *et al.* 2002). The latter authors provided a working example whereby the concepts of each study were compared one by one with the key concepts. This process assessed the extent to which they endorsed or contradicted them; and study conclusions were extracted in the form of explanations, interpretations or descriptions, which were then compared across all the studies. This approach does assume, however, that the study findings are not context-specific, and concepts are generalisable across settings, which could lead to objections by some qualitative researchers that this is methodologically inappropriate and ignores the richness of the data from each study, and that they are incommensurable. Britten *et al.* (2002) argued that the full contribution of qualitative research will not be realised if studies simply accumulate without synthesis of some type. Part of their example of synthesis of concepts, and second- and third- order interpretations is shown in Table 7.1.

A detailed framework for assessing the quality of qualitative health services research was given by Mays and Pope (1996, 2000) which includes:

- the appropriateness of the methodology;
- the clarity of the research question by the end of the research;
- the adequacy of descriptions of settings and context;
- the range of sampling for conceptual generalisations;
- systematic data collection and analysis and the existence of an audit trial to enable replication of each stage by an independent investigator;
- the incorporation of all observations into the analyses;
- the existence of unexplained variation;
- development of explanatory concepts and categories;
- clarity of the iteration between data and explanations;

Concepts	Second-order interpretations	Third-order interpretations
Adherence/compliance: stable adherence; correct behaviour and routine medicine taking Self-regulation: problematic adherence; levels of non-compliance; leaving off drugs; preference for not taking drugs; self-regulation Aversion: dislike of taking drugs; fear of side-effects; aversion to medicines; harmful effects of drugs Alternative coping strategies: range of alternative remedies; traditional remedies	(a) Patients weigh up perceived costs and risks, against the benefits, of each treatment (b) Medicine-taking is influenced by cultural meanings and cultural resources	(c) Self-regulation includes the use of alternative coping strategies

Source: Britten *et al.* (2002).

Table 7.1 Partial example of synthesis, second- and third-order interpretations

- evidence of seeking disconfirming cases;
- setting aside of investigators' preconceptions;
- assessment of the impact of the method on the data obtained;
- sufficient reporting of the data in the report;
- judgement as to whether the research was worth doing and its contribution to knowledge.

Elements of this framework, however, impose criteria of objective science onto qualitative research, which many qualitative researchers would find contentious. For example, a more relativist perspective in qualitative research is that reality is socially constructed and is unique to each person; thus ideographic accounts are presented and a synthesis of knowledge is not possible.

Meta-analyses

Technically, meta-analyses are categorised under quantitative literature reviews. They are observational studies of the body of evidence (Egger *et al.* 1997). Many clinical interventions have a weak evidence base, consisting of a small number of studies. Individual research studies are often small scale in design, and may lack the statistical power to demonstrate statistically significant effects. A meta-analysis, by pooling and analysing statistically the results from several combinable studies, can increase statistical power to detect small but clinically important treatment harms and benefits. (See Box 7.3.)

Meta-analyses are added to systematic reviews, where data permits, to obtain the best overall estimate of the effect of a treatment intervention. They depend on the quality of the initial systematic review. Only when it is certain that the search has been conducted systematically, comprehensively, and has met predefined, standardised criteria of quality,

Box 7.3 The implications of results of meta-analysis

An example of the potentially powerful implications of results of meta-analyses, as opposed to single studies, was the systematic review and meta-analysis of social support and mortality by Holt-Lunstad et al. (2010). They identified 148 prospective studies from North America, Europe, Asia, and Australia, which contained data on respondents' mortality as a function of social relationships. They extracted an 'effect size' from each study which quantified the size of a difference between two groups (i.e. the difference in the likelihood of death between groups differing by their social relationships). They reported that the average odds ratio was 1.5 – people with stronger social relationships had a 50% increased likelihood of survival, across age, sex, initial health status, cause of death, and follow-up period, compared with those with weaker social relationships. This led them to conclude with a strong public health message that the influence of social relationships on risk for mortality was comparable with well-established risk factors for mortality (Holt-Lunstad et al. 2010, p. 14):

> Cumulative empirical evidence across 148 independent studies indicates that individuals' experiences within social relationships significantly predict mortality. The overall effect size corresponds with a 50% increase in odds of survival as a function of social relationships. Multidimensional assessments of social integration yielded an even stronger association: a 91% increase in odds of survival. Thus, the magnitude of these findings may be considered quite large, rivaling that of well-established risk factors . . . Results also remained consistent across a number of factors, including age, sex, initial health status, follow-up period, and cause of death, suggesting that the association between social relationships and mortality may be generalized.

Such analyses are rarely straightforward. Apart from the need for adequate reporting of data in the studies included in meta-analyses (or access to original datasets), the complexity of the exercise is often increased by the use of different measures by investigators – in this case of social relationships. For example, Holt Lunstad et al. (2010) summarised the range of measures used in the studies they analysed:

- *functional, perceived to be provided by, or available from, social relationships:* received support; perception of social support; perception of loneliness;
- *structural, existence of interconnections between different social ties and roles:* marital status; social networks (e.g. density/size; number of social contacts); social integration (e.g. participation in broad range of social relationships, and active engagement in variety of social activities or relationships, sense of communality, identification with social roles); complex measures of social integration (e.g. multiple measures such as marital status, network size and network participation); living alone versus living with others; social isolation (e.g. lacks: contact, communication, activities, confidante);
- *combined, multifaceted measurement:* assessment of functional and structural measures, multiple measurement including more than one of above.

Careful comparisons between studies and the measures used, however, enabled the authors to report that social relationships were more predictive of risk of death in studies which used complex measurements of social integration than studies using simple measures such as marital status (Holt-Lunstad et al. 2010).

can the statistical analysis of pooled data be carried out. The number of interventions, the primary outcomes examined, and the heterogeneity of the research participants potentially undermine the conclusions drawn. Thus *sensitivity analyses*, which explore the ways main findings alter by varying the method of aggregation, are needed to explore the effects of such variations and assess the robustness of the combined estimates.

Statistical analysis

The meta-analysis is a technique using different statistical methods to combine pooled datasets (results) from different studies (overcoming effects of sample size and site-specific effects) and analysing them in order to reach a single observation for the aggregated data. Thus, by increasing the sample size, a meta-analysis can increase the power to detect true effects. Data are not simply pooled uncritically, but the statistical analysis is designed to recognise differing features between datasets. Studies also have to be selected critically and cautiously for entry. Statistical analysis can control for unit effects (site-specific and sample-specific effects) with regression procedures that permit the entry of one unit at a time and modelling for the unit-specific effects. Each study is treated as a component of one large study. The precision with which the size of an effect can be estimated depends on the methods of the study, the rigour of the research process and number of people included in the study.

There are many obstacles to performing a meta-analysis (see Egger and Davey Smith 1997). Patient allocation needs to be truly random in meta-analyses of RCTs. Individual results need to be expressed in a standardised, numerical format in order that studies can be compared and combined into a single estimate. If the primary end-point is continuous (e.g. weight), then the mean difference between treatment and control groups is used. Because the size of the difference can be influenced by the underlying population value, differences are often presented in units of standard deviation. If the primary end-point is binary (e.g. died or survived), then odds ratios or relative risks may be calculated. The odds ratio is more convenient for combining the data and testing its significance. The latter means that only those studies which are capable of resulting in a single estimate, when combined, can be included. One difficulty is in deciding which studies can be combined.

Different statistical methods exist for combining the data. The two main models in meta-analysis are fixed effects (which assume that variability of results between studies is due to random variation) and random effects (which assume a different underlying effect for each study – see Cullinan 2005, for a clear summary). There are also Bayesian methods of fixed and random effects models. These are based on prior specification of probability distribution before analysing the data, then updating the belief with posterior probability distribution (and see Egger *et al.* 1997, for a statistical overview). The choice of model depends on philosophy and the type of data.

Systematic reviews and meta-analyses also aim to examine evidence of bias. Funnel plots (or scatter plots, in which a trial-specific treatment effect is plotted against an indicator of its precision), and tests of heterogeneity between studies, are commonly used in attempts to detect publication bias. For example, when results are plotted, if publication bias is not present, it is often assumed that the funnel plot is symmetrical, and that publication bias is evident if the plot is not symmetrical. However, there can be several explanations for these patterns – the methods are flawed, and to be interpreted with caution.

However, as indicated earlier, there are many problems with meta-analyses, including the methods used by the studies included, the comparability of the samples and their inherent biases, which cannot be completely overcome. A representative sample of RCTs can provide valid estimates of the underlying effect of the same intervention, enhancing precision; in contrast, descriptive, comparative studies provide only estimates of association which may deviate from the true relationships being measured due to the effects of confounding variables (Egger *et al.* 1998). It is essential to use the technique critically and investigate sources of heterogeneity between studies (Thompson 1995). The methodological problems inherent in meta-analyses have been discussed by Lancaster *et al.* (1997).

Critical appraisal

Critical appraisal of the literature was referred to earlier, and key points to be aware of when undertaking critical appraisal were shown in Box 7.1. Critical appraisal is assessment of evidence by systematically reviewing its relevance, validity, and results in particular contexts (Chambers 1998). Important basic questions to ask are:

- Was the study question clear and focused?
- Was the study design valid? (Was it an RCT? Was the research design appropriate to address the study question?)
- Were the results reliable and valid?
- Can the study results be generalised to routine practice to inform care?

Critical appraisal is a skill essential to evidence-based practice. It is accepted that different research questions require different study designs. For example, randomised controlled trials address questions of clinical effectiveness, while to find out what living with a particular condition is like, qualitative research may be more appropriate. Critical appraisal skills enable people to identify the strengths and weaknesses of research, to assess the appropriateness of the method in relation to the research question, reliability and validity of results presented, to detect errors in research design and methods that influence the validity of the results, to develop a better understanding of methodology, to identify research biases and conflicts of interest, and, ideally, to facilitate the implementation of effective interventions in one's own practice.

There are several published guides for assessing the methodological quality of systematic reviews (e.g. Shea *et al.* 2007), for assessing the quality of papers included in systematic reviews (Terwee *et al.* 2012) (and see sections on systematic literature reviews and systematic qualitative reviews), standardised checklists for assessing randomised controlled trials, and criteria for assessing the quality of qualitative research. Questions to address in relation to trials were described by Guyatt *et al.* (1993), and include:

- Did the trial address a clearly focused issue in terms of the population studied, the intervention, the outcomes analysed?
- Was there concealment of allocation to intervention or control arms, and by what method (e.g. central allocation or use of sealed opaque envelopes)?
- Was the randomisation process described?
- Were patients/clients, workers and researchers all 'blind' to treatment?

- Were all those who entered the trial fully accounted for at its conclusion? Note the percentage who were followed up. Were they analysed in the groups to which they were randomised?
- Apart from the intervention, were the groups treated equally?
- Were the study intervention and control groups similar in their characteristics at the start of the trial?
- How large was the treatment effect? What outcomes were measured? Were all important outcomes considered? Was the number of people needed to treat to prevent one bad outcome provided?
- How precise was the estimate of treatment effect? What are the confidence limits? Were the statistical analyses appropriate?
- Can the results be applied to the local population, for example, given any differences in culture and region?
- Is any information on costs provided?
- Can it be accepted as Type II evidence?

Critical appraisal of qualitative research

In the section on qualitative reviews, the framework for assessing the quality of qualitative research by Mays and Pope (1996, 2000) was described. Using their framework, key questions to assist with the critical appraisal of a qualitative study include:

- Does the study address a clearly focused issue? Are the aims clear?
- Is the choice of qualitative method appropriate?
- Did the researcher state their perspective and examine their role for potential bias and influence?
- Was the sampling method clearly described and justified? Were the characteristics of those included described?
- Was there an adequate description of the method of data collection? What was the method and was it justified?
- Was the process of analysis and interpretation of data described and justified? Was there a description of how themes were identified in the data? Was the analysis performed by more than one researcher?
- What were the main findings? Did they address the research question? Were all important results considered?
- Are the results credible? Was a reasonable selection of original data presented in support of these? Is the data available for independent assessment? Are interpretations of the results plausible and are the results comparable with other studies?
- Can the results be applied locally, or are there differences between study and local populations which could affect the relevance of the research?
- Can it be accepted for use as qualitative research evidence?

Evidence-based practice

Evidence-based practice aims to improve the impact of health and social care practice. It aims to do this by assessing the strength of evidence of risks and benefits of interventions and by thorough and rigorous critical appraisals of current evidence, integrated with clinical expertise. Ideally patients' preferences are incorporated.

The processes of searching literature, systematic reviews, meta-analyses, qualitative reviews, and critical appraisal were addressed earlier. Evidence-based practice (EBP) has been applied in medicine, psychology, social work, nursing and allied disciplines, including physiotherapy, speech and occupational therapy. It originated in medicine (Guyatt *et al.* and the Evidence-Based Medicine Working Group 1993), and has since encompassed other health and social care disciplines. Its diffusion into clinical, health and social care practice reflects the health system's focus on cost-containment, quality assurance and the emergence of internal markets in health care.

Defining evidence-based practice

The most widely cited definition of EBP is still Sackett *et al.*'s early definition:

> Evidence-based medicine is the conscientious, explicit, and judicious use of current best evidence in making decisions about the care of individual patients. The practice of evidence-based medicine means integrating individual clinical expertise with the best available clinical evidence from systematic research.
>
> (1996, pp. 71–2)

This definition was later refined to include integration of patients' concerns, expectations and values (Sacket *et al.* 2000).

Evidence-based practice is based on the principles that practical decisions should be based on research evidence, and this evidence should be selected and interpreted according to specific criteria. The criteria are typically narrow, restrictive, and based on quantitative studies within a positivist framework, ideally large-scale randomised controlled trials and systematic reviews with meta-analyses, which are regarded as being at the top of a hierarchy of research methods for the generation of evidence. Such evidence is assumed to be objective, and reflect 'reality'.

Some social scientists view this approach with scepticism. Social constructionists hold that the foundations of knowledge are value-laden, negotiable and dependent on context, and that the distinction between objective and subjective knowledge is unclear (see Marks 2002). In social work too, the positivist approach has been criticised as entrapping social workers within a mechanistic form of technical rationality, and restricting social work to a narrow 'ends-means rationality' that only certain forms of action are legitimate (Webb and Kevern 2001). Moreover, causal chains in public health interventions are generally complex, making trial results subject to effect modification in different populations, and necessitating the additional use of observational studies to enhance internal and external validity (Victora *et al.* 2004). Other problems with the narrow definition of evidence-based practice are that systematic research is not always available, especially in nursing, other health professions, and social care, and it ignores the importance of patient involvement in their health care, though patients' values were incorporated into Sackett *et al.*'s (2000) later definition.

Muir Gray (1997) also suggested that evidence-based clinical care is an approach to decision-making in which the best available evidence is used, in consultation with the patient, to decide which option suits the patient best. In nursing, psychology and social care, evidence-based practice has also been defined as the conscientious and judicious use of current best evidence, but also in conjunction with clinical expertise and patient values, to guide health care decisions (Titler 2008). This gives *equal* emphasis to the best available research evidence, the patient's situation, values and wishes, and the expertise of the practitioner, and thus is the integration of:

■ the patient's preferences, including their wish to avoid risks associated with interventions;
■ the professional's judgement and expertise in assessing the patient/client and their potential responsiveness to possible interventions;
■ the best available evidence about the appropriateness of the interventions.

Models of evidence-based practice

While several models of evidence-based practice have been developed and used (Titler *et al*. 2001; Titler 2008), common elements of each (Dawes *et al*. 2004; DiCenso *et al*. 2005; Craig and Smyth 2007; Leufer and Cleary-Holdforth 2009) now include:

■ the development of a culture of enquiry;
■ selection of a practice topic, based on an important clinical, health or social care problem;
■ collection of the most relevant, valid and reliable articles relating to evidence;
■ critical appraisal and syntheses of evidence to determine if they come to similar conclusions, thus supporting an evidence-based practice or supporting change.

Selection of a topic

The topic should be based on an important clinical, health or social care problem. Examples of topics and questions that might be asked are suggested by Sackett *et al*. (2000), and might include:

■ how to identify the causes of a health or social care problem;
■ how to estimate the likely clinical progression of a condition/illness;
■ how to estimate any likely complications;
■ how to select interventions that do more good than harm;
■ how to reduce the chance of the problem reoccurring.

Rapid critical appraisal

Due to time constraints among practitioners, methods of rapid critical appraisal have often been advocated, using these important questions to evaluate a study's worth (Melnyk *et al*. 2010):

■ Are the results of the study valid? For example, were the research methods rigorous and appropriate? Were valid and reliable instruments used to measure key outcomes?
■ What are the results and are they important? Did the intervention work, what was the impact on outcomes, and the likelihood of obtaining similar results in other practice settings? For qualitative studies, this includes assessing whether the research approach was appropriate for the study, and whether results can be confirmed.
■ Will the results help me care for my patients? Were research participants similar to one's own patients or clients? Do benefits outweigh risks? What is the feasibility and cost-effectiveness of the intervention, and patients' values and preferences?
■ Was there integration of the evidence with one's clinical expertise and patient preferences to make a practice decision?
■ How was it implemented?
■ Was there evaluation of the outcomes of that decision, e.g. on impact on patient care and provider performance?

■   Did we monitor and evaluate any changes in outcomes so that positive effects can be supported and negative ones remedied? When results vary from those reported in the literature, monitoring can help to understand why. This may require consideration of the context/setting in which the practice is implemented.

Changing practice

Marks (2002) argued that if evidence-based practice is to be more widely adopted and to achieve genuine improvements in health care, it will be necessary: to broaden the evidence base; to create more inclusive methods for evidence synthesis; to clarify principles and assumptions to make them coherent and consistent with the evidence about decision-related behaviour from psychology and the social sciences; to differentiate more clearly between the dissemination of evidence and its implementation; to take into account the social, organisational and psychological barriers to behaviour change.

Research evidence alone is not sufficient to justify a change in practice (Melnyk et al. 2010). Clinical expertise, based on patient assessments, laboratory data, and data from outcomes management programs, as well as patients' preferences and values are important components of EBP. There is no magic formula for how to weigh each of these elements; implementation of EBP is highly influenced by institutional and clinical variables, including budgetary constraints. Leufer and Cleary-Holdforth (2009) summarised the work of several authors (Balas and Boren 2000; Ciliska 2005; DiCenso et al. 2005; Pravikoff et al. 2005; Craig and Smyth 2007) on barriers to EBP implementation that included:

■   tradition;
■   fear of inter-professional role erosion;
■   power imbalance;
■   funding sources;
■   influence of pharmaceutical companies;
■   poor critical appraisal skills;
■   poor access to quality information;
■   lack of leadership, motivation, vision, strategy or direction among managers

Implementation and subsequent evaluation are incorporated in translation research which is still an emerging area in terms of methods and effective strategies. Moreover, it is often claimed that 'lip service' is paid to the notion of evidence-based practice, and claims that it is being implemented do not stand up to scrutiny when examined in the context of what it actually is (Leufer and Cleary-Holdforth 2009).

Rigour in conducting research

The concept of rigour is relevant in relation to the reliability and validity of the data and the reduction of bias. Rigour refers to several essential features of the research process. These include: the systematic approach to research design, the awareness of the importance of interpretation and not perception or assumption, the systematic and thorough collection, analysis and interpretation of the data, the maintenance of meticulous and detailed records of interviews and observations, the use of triangulated (more than one) research methods as a check on the validity of the findings, and the ability of an independent, trained investigator to re-analyse the data using the same processes and methods and reach the same conclusions (see Section V).

Aims, objectives and hypotheses

One of the first stages of research design is to describe the aims (purposes) and more detailed objectives of the study. St Leger *et al.* (1992) provided a clear distinction between aims and objectives, which, as they pointed out, 'is a matter of degree rather than kind'. Objectives are simply 'at the level of operational tasks, which have to be accomplished in order to meet aims'.

The hypothesis (assumption) which the study is designed to test should also be clearly specified, unless the research is qualitative and based on inductive techniques and the use of grounded theory. It was pointed out before that, in scientific, deductive research, a hypothesis is proposed by the investigator, developed and tested. If it is rejected, then it is revised or another hypothesis is developed; if that is accepted, it is incorporated into the scientific body of knowledge (until it, in turn, is rejected). In practice, the process is more haphazard, but this is the logic underlying the scientific method. In contrast, in qualitative research a grounded theory approach is often adopted, whereby the hypothesis develops out of the research material, to be tested in subsequent data collection exercises or future research studies (see Chapter 6 and Section V).

It is insufficient to state in one's hypothesis simply that X is associated with Y. The association can be positive or negative, and may vary in differing social situations. For a hypothesis to be more specific, it is facilitated by being based on a concept or theory. A *hypothesis* is an assumption which is the expression of a tentative solution to a research question, phrased in the form of a conceptual relationship between the dependent and independent variables. This is known as a *substantive hypothesis*. A hypothesis is tentative because it is to be tested empirically by the research, and cannot be verified until then. A hypothesis is usually based upon theoretical assumptions (paradigms) about the way things work.

A causal hypothesis is a prediction that one phenomenon to be observed will be the result of one or more other phenomena that precede it in time (also to be observed in the study).

The issue of causal hypotheses and explanations is problematic when one is investigating human behaviour because the investigation of causality requires the use of an experimental analysis which is not always possible (see Chapter 10). The distinction between experimental and other types of research methods in relation to inferring causality should not be too rigid, because hypotheses can be developed, supported and refuted from any study, descriptive (quantitative or qualitative) or analytic (experimental or quasi-experimental) (Rothman 1986). Longitudinal survey analysis, while unable to establish causality, can estimate the strength of independent associations over time where the variables of interest are found to co-vary, and spurious associations are not found. Carefully designed temporal regression analyses can be conducted to analyse the timing of any changes in dependent and independent variables between waves of data collection. The strength and duration of the reciprocal relationships can be informative, especially if based on the careful formulation of explicit hypotheses, and models of the processes. The potential influence of social support on future health and mortality outcomes among population and cohort samples has a long history of research in social science and epidemiology. The direction of causality has long been an issue as these research hypotheses, summarised from several surveys, illustrate:

1 Social support has a direct effect on health by providing emotional comfort which can minimise the deleterious effects of stress on health.

2 Social support has a direct effect on health by leading to timely provision of help, which can prevent or reduce symptoms.

3 Social support has an indirect effect on health by mitigating (providing a buffer) against stress and its harmful effects on immune functioning and health.

4 Those in poor health simply fail to maintain social activities and contacts.

Value-free hypotheses

It was pointed out in Chapter 6 that *value-free* hypotheses are often difficult to achieve. Cultural beliefs affect the scientific research process. It is important for the investigator to be aware of his or her personal biases, to be honest and make these explicit, and to conduct the research as rigorously and objectively as possible. The investigator's values can influence the hypotheses selected for testing, the research design and method, the interpretation of the results and how the results are used. This issue was described earlier, and has been explored in more depth by May (1993) and Hammersley (1995).

Concepts and theories

It was pointed out earlier that hypotheses can be derived from *concepts* (i.e. abstract ideas) and formal *theories* (i.e. tentative explanations of relationships derived from interrelated concepts) in a deductive fashion, or directly from observations in an inductive fashion, or from a combination of these approaches. Conceptual and operational definitions will help to clarify the hypotheses:

1 *Operationalisation* refers to the development of proxy measures which enable a phenomenon to be measured. In order to test a hypothesis empirically, all the concepts contained within the hypothesis need to be defined and an explanation needs to be given about what can be used to measure (operationalise) them.

2 A *variable* is an indicator resulting from the operationalisation of a concept, and which is believed to represent the concept.

3 The *dependent variable* is the variable the investigator wishes to explain – the dependent variable is the expected outcome of the independent variable. The *independent variable* is the explanatory or predictor variable – the variable hypothesised to explain change in the dependent variable. It is sometimes called the intervention or exposure in the case of experimental designs.

4 *Theory* at the lowest level can be an ad hoc classification system, consisting of categories that organise and summarise empirical observations. It can be a taxonomy which is a descriptive categorical system constructed to fit the empirical observations in order to describe the relationships between categories (e.g. in a health care budget: spending on acute services, non-acute services, health promotion activities, and so on). The next, higher, level of theory is the conceptual framework in which categories are systematically placed within the structure of propositions. The propositions summarise and provide explanations and predictions for empirical observations. Theoretical systems combine taxonomies and conceptual frameworks by systematically relating descriptions, explanations and predictions. This is the most rigorous form of theory, in that a system of propositions is interrelated so that some can be derived from others, thus enabling the explanation and prediction of the phenomenon of interest. Acceptance of theoretical systems is dependent on whether their propositions have been empirically verified. Frankfort-Nachmias and Nachmias (1992) used Durkheim's (1951) study of suicide as a classic example of a theoretical system:

a   In any social grouping, the suicide rate varies directly with the degree of individualism (egoism).
b   The degree of individualism varies with the incidence of Protestantism.
c   Therefore, the suicide rate varies with the incidence of Protestantism.
d   The incidence of Protestantism in Spain is low.
e   Therefore, the suicide rate in Spain is low.

In this example, proposition (c) is deduced from propositions (a) and (b), and proposition (e) is deduced from (c) and (d). Furthermore, if, for example, one did not know what the suicide rate in Bulgaria was but did know that the incidence of Protestantism was low, this observation, together with proposition (c), would allow one to predict that the suicide rate there was also low. Thus the theoretical system provides both an explanation and a prediction of suicide rates (Frankfort-Nachmias and Nachmias 1992; derived from analyses by Homans 1964).

Finally, axiomatic theory contains a set of concepts and operational definitions, a set of statements describing the situations in which the theory can be applied, a set of relational statements divided into axioms (untestable statements) and theorems (propositions deduced from the axioms and which can be verified empirically) and a logical system which is used to relate all the concepts within the statements, and then to deduce theorems from the axioms, combinations of axioms and theorems. This level of theory is difficult to achieve because of difficulties in establishing the criteria for the selection of axioms. The main advantage of axiomatic theory is that it can provide a coordinated, parsimonious summary of *essential* actual and anticipated research, thus enhancing the plausibility of the theory. Further, because the propositions are interrelated, empirical support for any one proposition provides support for the theory as a whole. Interested readers are referred to Frankfort-Nachmias and Nachmias (1992) for further discussion.

It was pointed out in Chapter 6 that in social science one major school of thought believes that theory and hypotheses should be developed before research (deductive method). This follows Popper's (1959) belief that scientific knowledge makes more progress through the development of ideas followed by attempts to refute them with empirical research. The other major school of thought is that research should precede theory, and not be limited to a passive role of verifying and testing theory – it should help to shape the development of theory (Merton 1968). In practice, social science uses both strategies to advance knowledge. The need for theory-based research in population health, evaluation of 'post'-positive theory (in relation to logic, causality, falsification, scope and productivity), and a glossary of conceptual frameworks, theories and models can be found in Carpiano and Daley (2006).

Models

Models are often based on several theories, and used to make assumptions about the variables of interest, which can then be tested. They are closely related to theory. In the social sciences, models consist of symbols, rather than physical matter; they are abstract representations of the essential characteristics of phenomena of interest. They make the relationships between these characteristics explicit, leading to the formulation of empirically testable propositions about them. Sanderson *et al.* (1996) have provided a clear description of diagrammatic models. These typically consist of elements (usually represented by boxes), linked by relationships (usually with arrows). The common types of links are between cause and effect and between the stages in a sequence of activities. In the former type, the boxes usually contain variables, and the arrows indicate that variable A is likely to cause variable B, or that changes in A lead to changes in B. A connected set of *causal relationships* can be put together to form a causal model (or effects model). This could contain links that are hypothetical (A might affect B), theoretical or aspirational.

Mathematical modelling can test the diagrammatic model (Moser and Kalton 1971). A mathematical model consists of mathematical equations constructed to describe the relationships. They are useful in some situations where experimental study designs are not feasible (St Leger *et al.* 1992). There are many types of mathematical models used in health care. For example, simulation models have been developed to assess the costs and effectiveness of a range of interventions. Decision analysis modelling is also used as a systematic, quantitative method of assessing the relative value of different decision options. The types of modelling and their methods, along with the steps involved in building a mathematical model and its validation, have been described in detail by Biddulph (2005).

Research proposals

A well-structured research proposal (see Box 7.4) is a prerequisite of any investigation. The research proposal should clearly review the literature, justify the selection of the intended topic and state any hypotheses, together with the aims, objectives, overall study design, methods, sampling unit, sample type and size (with *power calculations* in the case of quantitative research), method of sampling, measurement tools and intended analyses. It should also include a plan for the dissemination of the results (e.g. meetings and conferences as well as journals to be targeted).

The overall design will require justification as the most appropriate in relation to the research question, and in relation to whether the investigator aims to adopt a positivist, *nomothetic* approach (a belief in general laws influencing behaviour or personality traits, and therefore an aim to generalise research findings) or an *idiographic* approach (an attempt to study and understand individuals and situations in relation to their uniqueness). The different methods are described in later chapters. More specifically, proposals should include an outline of the approach to be used to analyse the results (how hypotheses will be tested, and with what statistical techniques if appropriate), in what form they will be reported and disseminated (e.g. type of journals, conferences and meetings), the study timetable and the costs. Once completed, the proposal should cost the appropriate level of human and material resources to ensure that the timetable and aims are adhered to. It should be emphasised that high-quality research requires an adequate input of financial resources in order to ensure that appropriate sample sizes and methods of research are aimed for. This is no less true in the attempt to minimise non-response bias. No amount of sophistication in the data analysis can compensate for missing data or low response rates. A work plan and timetable showing when the stages of the study will be conducted and completed should be included in the proposal; grant-giving bodies will also require these details. These processes are incorporated into the next checklist (as before, not all the steps are appropriate for qualitative research, following inductionism).

Box 7.4 The research proposal

When the literature has been reviewed, the essential processes in the design of a study, which should be included in the proposal, are the clarification of:

- the research problem (question) to be addressed by the research, its feasibility, originality and importance, and the contribution of the research to a body of knowledge;
- the referenced literature and theory (e.g. conceptual framework) relevant to the research problem underlying the proposed study;
- evidence of multidisciplinary collaboration, where appropriate (including statistical advice);
- the aims and the specific objectives of the study;
- the hypotheses to be tested, based on the research problem;
- the definition and operationalisation of the concepts into items that can be measured, which is not circular (not referring back to the concept);
- the dependent variable(s);
- the independent variable(s);
- information about any potential extraneous, confounding variables that will need to be controlled for in order to test for spurious associations (false associations explained by the confounding variable);
- the population groups of interest to be sampled, selection criteria for inclusion in the study and their representativeness of the target population;
- justification of sample size in relation to statistical power;
- the method of sampling and method of allocation into groups where appropriate (e.g. experimental and control), appropriateness of identified control groups;
- the unit(s) of analysis (is the focus on individuals, groups, institutions, or societies?);
- the method (survey, RCT, and so on) and details of the rigour with which it will be applied;
- the measurement instruments, their validity and reliability and appropriateness for use with the study population and topic;
- the planned analyses, the level of the data to be generated (e.g. nominal, ordinal, interval, ratio), the appropriateness of the statistical tests to be used;
- the (realistic) time schedule (including any pilot phases) for the study and writing up of the results;
- justification of all costs;
- evidence of ethical approval, where appropriate;
- application of results (e.g. generalisability, relevance, implications for development, expected products, exploitability);
- plans for, and method of, dissemination.

Research design and research methods

The choice of appropriate research methods is also essential. Research design refers to the *overall structure* or plan of the research, for example, whether a descriptive or experimental study is to be conducted and with what target population. Once the study design has been decided upon, the *specific* methods of the study and of collecting the data have to be agreed. Research *methods* refer to: the practices and techniques used to collect, process and analyse the data (e.g. what type of experiment or survey); the sample size and methods of sampling and, in the case of experiments and analytical studies, of assignment to experimental and control groups; how the data will be collected (e.g. questionnaires, in-depth interviews, document searches); the choice of measurement instruments (or 'tools'); and how the data will be processed and analysed.

The research proposal will need to present and justify the appropriateness of the chosen research methods. If a positivist, empiricist perspective is adhered to, even with a critical stance, then the investigation will be carried out using quantitative, highly structured methods, including measurement scales which should have been tested for reliability, validity and their factor structure (see later), and with relatively large, representative populations. If a phenomenological or social action stance is adopted, or if the topic is exploratory and complex, then the methods of choice will be qualitative and based on smaller samples. These will not be discussed further here as they are the focus of other chapters.

Selection of measurement instruments

Research instruments or measurement scales are devices for measuring the variables of interest. They can be in the form of questionnaires comprising single items (questions), batteries of single items or scales of items which can be scored. They can also be in the form of observational schedules, structured diaries or logbooks, or standard forms for recording data from records. The measurement instruments should be carefully selected with a view to the type of statistical analyses that will be required (see sections on type of data: nominal, ordinal, interval and ratio).

Once a decision has been made about the type of measurement tool to use (i.e. a fully structured instrument and/or an instrument that also permits some measurement of meaning to the individual), there are several other criteria that need to be considered when selecting a measurement scale. These issues were addressed in relation to quality of life and similar measures in Chapter 3. Few scales satisfy all criteria, and many are still undergoing further development, but the investigator should be confident that they satisfy certain criteria of acceptability such as those shown in Box 7.5.

Box 7.5 Criteria of acceptability for measurement instruments

- What is it that the instrument measures (physical functioning, health perceptions, depression, and so on)?
- Does the instrument permit the measurement of the domains that are important to individual respondents?

- For what populations is the instrument appropriate (young, old, specific patient or cultural groups)?
- Do norms exist for comparative purposes?
- How acceptable is the instrument to the study population? (Frail people do not find long or self-administered questionnaires easy and an unacceptable scale will lead to higher total and item non-response.)
- What is the administrative burden of the instrument (office administration, printing costs, interviewer, coder, data entry and analysis)?
- Has the instrument been translated? If so, assess its conceptual and linguistic equivalence (wording, relevance and meaning).
- Is the instrument responsive to change within the study period, if required? Some domains are more likely to change over time than others (e.g. while feelings of happiness may change over time, personality, such as introversion–extraversion, is unlikely to change).
- Are the scores expressed in a way that will enable them to be correlated easily with other relevant variables?
- How have reliability and validity been tested, and on what types of populations?
- What level of data will the instruments relate to (e.g. most investigators aspire to use statistics appropriate for interval level data)?

Level of data and statistical techniques

The statistical techniques that are permitted for use with a quantitative set of data are dependent on the level of measurement achieved by the instruments used in the study. The best instruments are those that yield quantitative values and make fine distinctions among respondents. Quantification is the degree to which response categories can be accurately and meaningfully numbered. In research on health outcomes of interventions the investigator will want to know 'how much' patients have improved or deteriorated in comparison with controls. In order to be addressed, such questions require the use of the more sophisticated levels of data measurement. The four levels of data are:

1 nominal (numbers are used simply for classification, such as 'died' = 1, 'survived' = 0);
2 ordinal (scale items stand in some kind of relation to each other, such as 'very difficult' through to 'not very difficult');
3 interval (the characteristics of an ordinal scale, but the distances between any two numbers on the scale are of a known size, such as temperature); and
4 ratio (the characteristics of an interval scale with the addition of a true – not arbitrary as in interval scales – zero point, such as weight).

These levels of data are described in more detail below. Most measures of health status aspire to create at least interval scales, but rarely succeed. The more sophisticated the level of the data that have been collected (e.g. interval and ratio level data), the more powerful are the statistical analyses that can be employed (see Blalock 1972; Streiner and Norman 2008). For example, ordinal data must be treated as ranked, not scored, data – they must not be averaged or arithmetically manipulated. Consultations with a professional statistician are essential at the design stage of the research.

Levels of data, parametric and non-parametric statistics

Statistical methods were developed on the basis of a number of assumptions about the nature of the population from which the study results are drawn. Population values are known as parameters, and hence statistics with built-in assumptions about the population are known as *parametric*. For example, parametric statistics assume that the values obtained are based on a normal distribution in the population of interest. Thus, a study which yields skewed distributions of results could not use parametric statistics, and should use non-parametric statistics (these can also be used with normally distributed data). However, statistical methods do exist which can transform skewed data into a normal distribution. Guides to appropriate statistics for use with nominal-, ordinal- and interval-level data can be found in early and current statistical textbooks (e.g. Siegel 1956; Blalock 1972; Conover 1999; Swinscow and Campbell 2001). The levels of data are described below, with selected appropriate statistics. Katz (1999) described types of multivariable analysis appropriate for different levels of data, for example, multiple linear regression can be used with interval-level data (e.g. temperature); multiple logistic regression is appropriate for use with dichotomous (nominal-level) data (such as died = 1/survived = 0). There is a grey area between ordinal- and interval-level data. Investigators commonly use multiple linear regression, for example, to analyse outcome variables which are ordinal in level, though may superficially appear to function at interval level (e.g. patient ratings of their level of satisfaction with health care, or of their quality of life, using various numeric response scales such as rating their satisfaction from 1 (excellent) to 5 (poor), or their quality of life from 100 (best) to 5 (worst), or attitudes from 1 (strongly agree) to 5 (strongly disagree)). They are not true interval scales as the actual distance (interval) between response categories is unknown (e.g. on a Likert-type response scale of Excellent 1, Very good 2, Fair 3, Poor 3, the distance between ratings of 'Excellent' and 'Very good' may not be the same as that between 'Fair' and 'Poor'). As Katz (1999) indicates, when such variables are used as dependent variables in multiple linear regression, problems generally only occur where their relationship to the dependent variables do not fulfil the assumptions underlying multiple linear regression.

Nominal

Nominal, or categorical, data are data which have no underlying continuum, units or intervals that have equal or ordinal (ranking) properties, and hence cannot be scaled. Instead, there are a number of discrete categories into which responses can be classified or 'coded', but as they cannot be placed in any ordering, they have no numerical value or underlying continuum (observations are simply grouped and not ranked). Examples of nominal scales are dichotomous and descriptive responses (e.g. binary yes/no, descriptors of eye colour such as green, blue, brown, or of religion, such as Protestant, Catholic, Jewish, Muslim).

Appropriate statistics are non-parametric (e.g. descriptive frequency counts, comparisons of sub-samples by converting frequencies into percentages, analysis of differences between distributions in sub-samples using non-parametric techniques such as the chi-square test, which will compare observed and expected (by chance) raw frequency distributions). Nominal data cannot be added, averaged, multiplied or squared.

There are some other non-parametric techniques for testing associations and for the multivariate analysis of nominal or ordinal data (e.g. multidimensional scalogram analysis), though they are few in comparison to the wider range of parametric techniques available. Techniques which enable the investigator to correlate metric and non-metric nominal or ordinal data include the point-biserial correlation coefficient, in which each descriptor on a scale is expressed dichotomously (e.g. religion is expressed not as Protestant, Catholic, Jewish, etc. but as Protestant/non-Protestant, Catholic/non-Catholic, Jewish/non-Jewish), each dichotomy is related to the interval scale and a series of point-biserial correlation coefficients can be calculated. As this increases the number of statistical tests employed, this method also increases the likelihood of obtaining statistical significance by chance. Other techniques exist, such as a one-way analysis of variance and an *F*-test, but none will provide a single summary coefficient to describe the overall strength of the data (see Oppenheim 1992). They will indicate whether there is a statistically significant pattern of associations between variables, but nothing about their strength. Another technique is to transform the nominal data into an ordinal scale: for example, descriptors (groupings) of area of residence could be placed in a prestige hierarchy and used as an indicator of wealth or socio-economic background. These methods depend on making questionable assumptions. Some investigators allocate numerical values to each category, and wrongly assume equal intervals, to turn them into interval scales in order to use more powerful statistics.

Ordinal

Ordinal data are data in which observations are grouped and ranked. Likert scales are ordinal scales (e.g. very happy, fairly happy, neither happy nor unhappy, fairly unhappy, very unhappy). Non-parametric statistics have been developed for ranked data of ordinal level, such as Spearman's rank correlation and Kendall's tau. These techniques are less powerful than statistics developed for use with scaled or metric data – interval- and ratio-level data. Researchers often use parametric statistics on non-parametric data (e.g. ordinal data) – they assume their ordinal data have equal intervals between categories and calculate averages, or use *multivariable statistics* developed for parametric data, and so on. Strictly speaking, this is wrong, but it is common practice, as researchers hope that the statistical techniques are robust enough to withstand this.

Interval

Interval data are achieved where observations are grouped and their ranks considered to be of equal intervals. Guttman scales, which are hierarchical scales, claim to be interval scales (this is questionable; see Chapter 13). Parametric statistical techniques that are applicable to interval scales are more powerful, and can make fuller use of the data, than non-parametric techniques. Appropriate statistical tests include means, standard deviations, *t*-tests, *F*-tests, regression, analysis of variance and product moment correlation coefficients (which require all variables entered to be metric).

Ratio

Ratio data are achieved where observations are grouped, and of equal intervals with a true zero point (e.g. weight). The most powerful statistical tests are applicable. No rating scales achieve ratio scale levels.

Reliability and validity

The principles of psychometric assessment, in relation to QoL measurement, were described in Chapter 3. *Psychometric validation* is the process by which an instrument is assessed for reliability and validity through the mounting of a series of defined tests on the population group for whom the instrument is intended. Hobart *et al.* (2004) summarised the application of psychometric methods in health measurement and the work of Lamping and colleagues provides clear examples of the design and full psychometric testing of a wide range of patient questionnaires and health outcome measurement scales (Hobart *et al.* 2004; Guariano *et al.* 2005; Kahn *et al.* 2006; Smith *et al.* 2005).

Reliability refers to the reproducibility and consistency of the instrument. It refers to the homogeneity of the instrument and the degree to which it is free from random error. There are certain parameters, such as test–retest, inter-rater reliability and internal consistency, that need to be assessed before an instrument can be judged to be reliable.

Validity is an assessment of whether an instrument measures what it aims to measure. It should have face, content, concurrent, criterion, construct (convergent and discriminant) and predictive validity. It should also be responsive to actual changes. Reliability affects validity, and an unreliable scale inevitably has low validity. These concepts are described in detail by Streiner and Norman (2003).

Reliability

Tests of reliability assess the extent to which scale items measure the same construct, with freedom from random error (internal consistency) and repeatability. Item convergence and equivalence are assessed by split half, multiple form, item–item correlations and item–total correlations, and Cronbach's alpha for overall consistency. Repeatability is assessed by test–retest procedures (administering the instrument at different time periods when nothing else has changed), inter-rater administration of the instrument to the same person by different people, and comparing results, and alternate forms (interview or self-completion) of the measure and comparing results. It should be noted that the greater the number of response categories that items contain, the greater the scale resolution and thus their reliability (Andrews 1984).

Test–retest

This is a test of the stability of the measure (e.g. the reproducibility of the responses to the scale), over a period of time in which it is not expected to change, by making repeated administrations of it. Cohen's (1968) kappa coefficient is used to test nominal data, weighted kappa for ordinal data and Pearson's correlations for interval-level data. Kappa has a value of 0 if agreement is no better than chance, a negative value if worse than chance, and a value of unity (1) if there is perfect agreement. A low correlation can sometimes be difficult to interpret – it may reflect actual change rather than poor reliability of the measure. Some statisticians believe that correlations are a weak measure of test–retest reliability, and recommend the use of confidence intervals to assess the size of the difference between the scores (Bland and Altman 1986).

Inter-rater

This is the extent to which the results obtained by two or more raters or interviewers agree for similar or the same populations. As above, the kappa test or Pearson's correlations, Spearman's rho and Kendall's tau may be used for the analysis. Fleiss (1981) suggested that a kappa result of less than 0.40 indicates poor agreement, 0.40–0.59 is fair agreement, 0.60–0.74 is good agreement and 0.75–1.00 is excellent agreement. An intraclass correlation coefficient (e.g. between raters, or subjects at different time periods) of, for example, 0.80 or more indicates that the scale is highly reliable.

Alternate form

The distribution of responses to the alternate forms (modes of administration) of the questionnaire (self-administration and interviewer administration) are compared to assess whether they produce comparable responses (e.g. achieve correlations of at least rho 0.80).

Internal consistency

Internal consistency involves testing for homogeneity and is the extent to which the items (questions) relating to a particular dimension in a scale (e.g. physical ability) tap only this dimension and no other. The methods which should also be used are multiple form, split half, item–item and item–total correlations, and Cronbach's alpha (Cronbach 1951).

Multiple form

The correlations for the sub-domains of the scale are computed.

Split half

If the instrument is divided into two parts, the correlations between the two are computed (not always possible if the items are not homogeneous and cannot be divided, or the scale's sub-domains measure different constructs).

Item–item

This refers to the extent to which each item within a scale or sub-scale is correlated. Items should be moderately correlated with other scale items for homogeneity (i.e. internal consistency reliability): over-high item–item correlations (e.g. >0.70, but there is no conventional upper limit) indicate redundancy of one of the pair of items and one should be selected for removal (Streiner and Norman 2003). Over-low item–item correlations (<0.20) indicate failure to tap the attitude being measured by the other items; such items should be considered for removal. Briggs and Cheek (1986) recommended the optimal range for inter-item correlations of 0.20–0.40.

Item–total

Item–total reliability correlations refer to the extent to which each of the scale items, or items within a domain, is correlated with the total score, or total for that domain. The usual rule of thumb for item–total correlations is that items should correlate with the total scale score by more than 0.20 (some use 0.30), to satisfy reliability (homogeneity) and scaling assumptions. Lower values indicate that the item is measuring something different to the scale as a whole (Kline 1986; Streiner and Norman 2003). If items are dichotomous, then the point-biserial correlation is usually recommended; if there are more than two response categories, the product moment correlation is usually used (Havlicek and Peterson 1977; Streiner and Norman 2003). Item–total correlations are usually inflated in scales with few items, and thus methods of correlation for this have been developed (Howard and Forehand 1962).

Cronbach's alpha

This produces an estimate of reliability based on all possible correlations between all the items within the scale (for dichotomous responses, the Kuder Richardson test can be used). It is based on the average correlation among the items and the number of items in the instrument (values range from 0 to 1). It is an estimate of internal consistency.

There is no agreement over the minimum acceptable standards for Cronbach's alpha for scale reliability. Some regard 0.70 as the minimally acceptable level for internal consistency reliability (Nunnally 1994). Others accept 0.50 as an indicator of good internal consistency, especially for short sub-scales (as well as of test–retest reliability) (Cronbach 1951; Helmstater 1964). Cronbach's alpha is dependent on the magnitude of correlations among items as well as the number of items in the scale, with the effect that if the alpha is usually higher, the greater is the number of scale items. The range should usually be between 0.70 and 0.90 (Streiner and Norman 2003), but smaller alphas are acceptable with smaller sub-scales.

With shorter scales, it is appropriate to report also the inter-item correlations. If the alpha is too high, it suggests a high item of item redundancy. A reliability coefficient of 0.70 implies that 70 per cent of the measured variance is reliable and 30 per cent is owing to random error. A low coefficient alpha indicates that the item does not belong to the same conceptual domain. Where individual item alphas in the column are higher than the final scale alpha, this indicates that the item should be removed.

Factor structure

Exploratory and confirmatory factor analyses are distinct techniques that are used to examine the shared variance of variables thought to have an underlying factor (latent construct), and to identify a small number of factors to represent relationships among the sets of interrelated variables. This is a commonly used method of data reduction in the development of measurement scales. Exploratory factor analysis can be used to explore the dimensions underlying the questionnaire. Questions that deliberately tap different dimensions within a scale will not necessarily have high item–item or item–total correlations. Therefore, given the importance placed on high internal reliability, factor analysis has traditionally been used to define a small number of underlying dimensions, each of which contains items which group together in a consistent and coherent way (i.e. with sufficient consistency to each other).

Thus, factor analysis, like principal components analysis, is used in order to identify the separate factors (dimensions) that make up an instrument, and to describe how the items group together in order to form a more manageable set of variables (factors or principal components) (e.g. a health status instrument would be made up of the dimensions of physical functioning, mental health, social role functioning, and so on). These are assumed to reflect the underlying hypothetical constructs of the instrument (Streiner and Norman 2003, 2008). Orthogonal varimix rotation can then be used to choose the factors or principal components in such a way as to minimise their overlap (indicated by the amount of their shared variance) and thereby enhance interpretability of the instrument.

Exploratory and confirmatory factor analysis

In theory, exploratory factor analysis should be used in scale development in order to identify and discard items that are not correlated with the items of interest. Later on, confirmatory factor analysis is used to confirm that the scale items principally load onto that factor and correlate weakly with other factors. It is used, then, to test hypotheses about the structure underlying a set of variables. The number of cases available for analyses should exceed the required minimum of 300, and the 10 to 1 ratio (Nunnally 1994; Tabachnick and Fidell 1996). The number of factors to extract is determined by their eigenvalues, statistical criteria of interpretability (Cattell 1966), and congruity with other studies. A factor is considered as important, and its items worthy of retention in the scale, if its eigenvalue (a measure of its power to explain variation between subjects) exceeds a certain level. Eigenvalues should exceed the threshold of >1.0 to support the construct validity of the scale (some use the criteria of >1.5). In general, the criterion for acceptability is >0.30 for factor loading on the first unrotated factor with at least three items per factor (Nunnally 1994). More specifically, the correlation matrix should reveal many coefficients of 0.30 and above; the Kaiser-Meyer-Olkin Measure of Sampling Adequacy (KMO) should exceed the threshold of >0.60 (Kaiser 1970, 1974); and Bartlett's (1954) test of sphericity should be statistically significant ($p < 0.05$) for factor analysis to be appropriate. Another approach is to use Cattell's (1966) scree test, which involves plotting each of the eigenvalues of the factors to find the point at which the curve changes direction and becomes horizontal. Cattell advises retaining factors above the break in the plot, as these contribute most to the explained variance in the data.

Factor analysis encompasses several different techniques, in particular, principal components analysis (with this, the variables are transformed into a smaller set of linear combinations, and all of the variance in the variables is used), and factor analysis (where factors are estimated using a mathematical model, and only the shared variance is analysed) (Pallant 2007). While statisticians vary in their preferences, in general, factor analysis is recommended where a theoretical solution is required, which is uncontaminated by unique or error variability, and principal components analysis is recommended if an empirical summary of the data set is wanted (Tabachnick and Fidell 1996; Pallant 2007). However, it is important not to lose sight of the social and clinical significance of items. Where items are regarded as essential to the content validity of a measure, but they do not load onto a cluster of inter-related variables, their retention as separate items in a questionnaire should be considered on theoretical grounds, or the instrument developed and tested further. Scale items should therefore be included in a measure according to the information they contribute. The use of factor analysis can also lead to unexpected results, for example, where one dimension has been confirmed where two were hypothesised. Caution is needed in such cases as this may simply be due to the inappropriate use of factor analysis (e.g. where the data violates the assumptions of factor analysis; van Schuur and Kiers 1994). Kessler and Mroczek (1995) showed that undue emphasis on internal consistency can also result in considerable overlap and redundancy of scale items. They suggested replacing factor analytic methods with regression techniques to identify the items that capture most of the variance of an underlying construct. For example, a measure of quality of life is more valuable if it contains items that address the different components of quality of life, rather than items with high internal consistency but which address just particular components of this concept. Factor analysis, then, can lead to solutions that operate against more socially and clinically important items of measurement. Coste *et al.* (1997), on the basis of a review of the literature, reported that, most commonly, factor analysis of the longer versions of measurement scales, and statistical correlations between the longer and shorter versions of a measure, are used to finalise the content of an instrument. Less often is there any apparent check on whether the information content has been retained (with the risk of reduced content validity).

Validity

An instrument is assigned validity after it has been satisfactorily tested repeatedly in the populations for which it was designed. This type of validity is known as internal validity, as opposed to external validity, which refers to the generalisability of the research findings to the wider population of interest. The many different forms of validity are described below.

Face

Face validity is often confused with content validity, but it is more superficial. It simply refers to investigators' subjective assessments of the presentation and relevance of the questionnaire: do the questions appear to be relevant, reasonable, unambiguous and clear?

Content

This is also a theoretical concept, but is more systematic than face validity. It refers to judgements (usually made by a panel) about the extent to which the content of the instrument appears logically to examine and comprehensively include, in a *balanced way*, the *full scope* of the characteristic or domain it is intended to measure.

Criterion

This covers correlations of the measure with another *criterion* measure, which is accepted as valid (referred to as the 'gold standard'). This is not possible where there are no gold standards (e.g. of quality of life), and proxy measures are used instead. Criterion validity is usually divided into two types: *concurrent* and *predictive* validity:

- *Concurrent* validity is the independent corroboration that the instrument is measuring what it intends to measure (e.g. the corroboration of a physical functioning scale with observable criteria).
- *Predictive* validity asks whether the instrument is able to predict future changes in key variables, in expected directions, when measures are administered again at a later time.

Criteria identified by experts	Asthma symptoms scale Spearman Rank correlation coefficients	
	Concurrent validity (adverse occurrences 3 months pre-questionnaire completion)	Predictive validity (adverse occurrences 3 months post-questionnaire completion)
Number of asthma attacks	0.45	0.44
Chest infections	0.47	0.37
Routine consultations	0.53	0.57
Unplanned consultations	0.36	0.53
Impaired activity	0.56	0.53

Source: Steen and McColl (1996, p. 39) (partial reproduction).

Table 7.2 Concurrent and predictive validity of 10-item asthma symptom scale

Steen and McColl (1996) described in detail the process of developing and testing their asthma symptom-based outcome measure. Their assessments included examination of how well their measure correlated with criteria identified by a panel of experts to be appropriate for assessing concurrent and predictive validity, in a sample of 107 patients who responded to all questionnaire items. Some of their results are shown in Table 7.2 (all correlations were statistically significant at the 0.1 per cent level).

Construct (convergent and discriminant)

Construct validity is corroboration that the instrument is measuring the underlying concept it purports to measure. It involves testing a hypothesis about how the instrument is expected to perform and examining the data to assess whether the hypothesis is supported. Construct validity comprises two elements:

- *Convergent* validity requires that the scale should correlate with similar variables (e.g. correlations with measures of similar constructs, or with constructs hypothesised to be associated). Correlations will vary depending on the similarity of the measures.
- *Discriminant* validity requires that the construct should not correlate with dissimilar variables (e.g. low correlations between the measure and different constructs not expected to be correlated).

Additional tests of convergent validity are correlations between the scale and sub-scale scores. While it is not usual to specify in advance the precise correlations that would be acceptable to ascertain convergent validity, modest to strong correlations (e.g. around rho 0.40+) are generally judged to be acceptable for concepts that overlap but are not identical.

Inter-correlations from the multitrait-multimethod matrix are used to support convergence validity. The multitrait-multimethod matrix is a test of method effects (Campbell and Fiske 1959). The principle behind this technique of validation is that different methods of measuring the same construct should yield similar results, while measures of different constructs should produce different results, regardless of the measuring instrument. At least two constructs (variables), each measured by at least two different measures, are required for this technique which involves measuring different constructs with several different methods. The aim is to produce the set of correlations for each measure with every other measure – the multitrait-multimethod matrix. The expectation underlying its use is that a specified measure will correlate positively with other measures of the same construct, using different methods, supporting the claim that they measure the same variable (convergent validity). Conversely, the expectation is that a specified measure will not correlate with measures of different constructs (discriminant validity).

Precision

This is the ability of an instrument to detect *small* changes in an attribute.

Responsiveness to change

The instrument should also be responsive to actual changes which occur in an individual or population over a period of time, particularly changes of social and clinical importance. Responsiveness is a measure of the association between the *change* in the observed score and the change in the true value of the construct. There is an unresolved debate about whether responsiveness is an aspect of validity (Hays and Hadhorn 1992). The concepts of *responsiveness*, *sensitivity* and *specificity* are interrelated (see next sections; for methods of measuring and expressing an instrument's responsiveness to change, see Chapter 8).

Sensitivity

This refers to the proportion of actual cases (e.g. people who actually have clinical depression) who score as positive cases on a measurement tool (e.g. who score as depressed on a scale measuring depression), and the ability of the gradations in the scale's scores adequately to reflect actual changes.

Specificity

This is a measure of the probability of correctly identifying a non-affected person with the measure, and refers to the *discriminative* ability of the measure. Thus, it refers to the proportion of people who are not cases (e.g. do not actually suffer from clinical depression) and who test negative on the tool (e.g. who do not score as depressed on the scale measuring depression), and the ability of the gradations in the scale's scores adequately to reflect actual changes. We need to know how sensitive and specific measurement tools are.

When a measurement scale produces a continuous variable, the sensitivity and specificity of the scale can be altered by changing the cut-off point for detecting cases, though by raising the threshold for case detection, the danger is that fewer actual cases will be detected – and thus sensitivity is decreased. Bland (1995) has described the sample sizes required for reliable estimates of sensitivity and specificity, or positive predictive value (true positives) and negative predictive value (true negatives).

Sensitivity analysis

This is a method of estimating the robustness of the conclusions of the study or its assumptions. Sensitivity analysis involves making plausible assumptions about the margins of errors in the results in question and assessing whether they affect the implications of the results. The margins of errors can be calculated using the confidence intervals of the results or they can be guessed (St Leger *et al.* 1992).

Receiver operating characteristic (ROC) curves

The *discriminant* ability of a scale possessing continuous data can be investigated using receiver operating characteristic (ROC) curves (Hsiao *et al.* 1989). The ROC curve examines the degree of overlap of the distributions of the scale score for all cut-off points for defined groups, and the curve itself is a plot of the true positive rate against the false positive rate for each point on the scale (sensitivity plotted against one minus specificity). The degree of overlap between the defined groups is measured by calculating the area under the curve (AUC), and its associated *standard error* (Hanley and McNeil 1982). The greater the total area under a plotted curve from all cut-off points, the greater the instrument's responsiveness (see Chapter 9).

ROC curves can also be used to identify cut-off points for dichotomising continuous scales, though it should be noted that all cut-offs are essentially arbitrary. For a clear example, see Lindelow *et al.* (1997).

With item response theory, an item response curve assumes that the curve has a particular shape, which makes it possible to estimate from the respondents' responses to several scale items what their position is on the underlying scale dimension.

Item redundancy

Tests for scale item redundancy and elimination are based on missing data (the usual criterion is 5 per cent), endorsement frequencies (maximum endorsement frequency >80 per cent, maximum aggregate adjacent endorsement frequency <10 per cent), correlations (see later), exploratory factor analysis (loading <0.8 on all factors; cross-loading >0.8 on more than one factor, with a difference between loadings of <0.4).

Data quality, acceptability and scaling

- *Floor and ceiling effects.* Scaling requires avoidance of high scale values (maximum endorsement frequencies) at either extreme of the scale, in order to permit identification of changes at follow-up. Although there are no widely accepted criteria for maximum item floor and ceiling effects (calculated as the percentage of responses for the minimum and maximum scores), recommendations from published studies have reported that they should not exceed 15–20 per cent (see Hobart *et al.* 2004).
- *Spanning the full score range.* Sub-scale scores should ideally span the full range, and means should be close to the mid-point. The ideal is to achieve or approximate a normal distribution of the data. Some scales have short three- or four-point response scales. Shorter response categories, however, carry the risk of losing information, having floor and ceiling effects, and compromising sensitivity to change, especially in follow-up studies. In attitude measurement, five- or six-point response scales are recommended to ensure that respondents are not forced into inappropriate categories

(e.g. the five-point response scale 'strongly agree, agree, neither agree nor disagree, disagree, strongly disagree' is commonly used in attitude measurement). In contrast to the problem to scale floor and ceiling effects, one common experience in attitude measurement is that end values of response items are often so extreme or 'abnormal' that few people endorse them (an example is the EuroQoL; see Wolf and Hawley 1997). However, endorsement of extreme values by a small number of sample members may be an important social or clinical finding.

The even distributions of response scale endorsements can be difficult to achieve in relation to health-related and quality of life-related topics, with risks of social desirability biases (Diener 1994; Holtgraves 2004). It is also difficult to achieve in research on patient satisfaction and patient experiences, where mean item scores are similarly skewed towards the positive (Garratt et al. 2005). In real life, then, skewed distributions are often achieved (e.g. skewed towards the optimal health and functioning end in surveys of the general population and towards the negative, suboptimal end in patient populations).

In relation to skewness statistics, a result of 0 indicates a perfectly normal distribution, although this is rarely achieved in social science, especially on quality of life and life satisfaction topics, with known positive skews. An acceptability level of -1 to $+1.0$ is usually stipulated, though there are no widely accepted criteria (see Hobart et al. 2004). Data transformation procedures exist in data analysis packages to deal with non-normal distributions, to then permit statistical analysis.

Low levels of missing data. A high percentage of computable scale scores are also required for scale acceptability, indicating a low percentage of missing data – <5 per cent, or even <10 per cent – and missing responses are common standards (Hobart et al. 2004).

Summing criteria. In addition, if scale items are summed to produce a score, then it is assumed that item responses do not require weighting. This assumption is based on items having symmetrical item–response distributions, equivalent means and standard deviations. It is assumed that each item contains the same proportion of information about the construct being measured. This assumption is met if the item–total correlations are approximately equal. They are corrected for overlap so that estimates are not spuriously inflated (Hobart et al. 2004). Some investigators use >0.20 or >0.25, while others use >0.30 as the acceptability criterion for item–total correlations to satisfy scaling requirements (Ware et al. 1997b; Streiner and Norman 2003; Guariano et al. 2005). Scaling success is also judged when an item correlates more highly with its own (sub-)scale than with another (sub-)scale. Items which perform poorly should be eliminated.

Correlation criteria for item reduction

Tests of internal consistency (see reliability) also enable examination of item redundancy (assessed by over-high item–item correlations, e.g. the usual criterion is 0.70 (Streiner and Norman 2003), but there is no standardly used upper limit) and item elimination (assessed using the criterion that items with excessively low item–item correlations, e.g. <0.20, can be eliminated on the grounds that they fail to tap the attitude being measured by the other items). Other criteria used for item removal (item reduction) include the effect on alpha of item deletion (e.g. an increase above the sub-scale's final Cronbach's alpha with the item removed); and poorly performing corrected item–total correlation for the item (low values of 0.30 or less indicate that the item is measuring something outside the scale; Kline 1986, 1993).

Threats to reliability and validity

There are many threats to the reliability and validity of an investigation, apart from the questionnaire design and scale construction. These are known as biases and errors in the conceptualisation of the research idea, and the design, sampling and process of the study, which can lead to systematic deviations from the true value (Last 1988). Sackett (1979) reported 35 different types of study bias. Although it is known that many sources of bias and error can affect social research on human beings, contamination of results is also always a threat in laboratory research in natural science. Laboratory practice strives to reduce the risk that the sample under investigation might be contaminated by some other material, but there are occasional reports of the discovery of such material in routine testing of laboratory surfaces and equipment for contamination. This then leads to the questioning of the validity of the research results stemming from experiments conducted on those sites. Similar issues are occasionally reported owing to the deterioration of samples of fluids and matter. Thus the constant striving to eliminate and reduce very real sources of potential error and bias is not peculiar to the social sciences. The different types of bias, including potential biases at different stages of clinical trials, have been described by Delgado-Rodríguez and Llorca (2004).

Types of bias and error

Acquiescence response set ('yes-saying')

This refers to the fact that respondents will more frequently endorse a statement than disagree with its opposite.

Assumption (conceptual) bias

This is error arising from the faulty logic of the investigator, which can lead to faulty conceptualisation of the research problem, faulty interpretations and conclusions.

Bias in handling outliers

This can arise from a failure to discard an unusual value occurring in a small sample, or the exclusion of unusual values which should be included (Last 1988).

Design bias

This bias derives from studies which have faulty designs, methods, sampling procedures and/or group assignment procedures, and use inappropriate techniques of analysis. This can lead to a difference between the observed value and the true value.

Evaluation apprehension

This refers to the anxiety generated in people by virtue of being tested. This anxiety may lead people to try to give the responses they think are expected by the investigator, rather than their true responses.

Interviewer bias

The interviewer can subconsciously, or even consciously, bias respondents to answer in a certain way: for example, by appearing to hold certain values which can lead to a social desirability bias, or by asking leading questions.

Measurement decay

This refers to any changes in the measurement process over time.

Mood bias

People in low spirits (e.g. depressed) may underestimate their health status, level of functioning and amount of social activity and support (Jorm and Henderson 1992), thus biasing the study results.

Non-response bias

This is due to differences in the characteristics between the responders and non-responders to the study. Non-response is a major source of potential bias, as it reduces the effective sample size, resulting in loss of precision of the survey estimates. In addition, to the extent that differences in the characteristics of responders and non-responders are not properly accounted for in estimates, it may introduce bias into the results. Research results on the characteristics of non-responders are inconsistent. Non-response among successive waves of the study can be a problem in longitudinal research (known as withdrawal bias).

Observer bias

This is the difference between the true situation and that recorded by the observer owing to perceptual influences and observer variation.

Publication bias

It can be difficult for investigators to find a willing publisher for results which do not achieve statistical significance in relation to a hypothesised association. This results in publication bias – only studies indicating an association are likely to be published – and the potential of creating a false body of knowledge. There is also a tendency for investigators to bias their research reports by over-emphasising differences (Pocock et al. 1987). Turner et al. (2008) reviewed US Food and Drug Administration registered studies of antidepressant agents, and reported evidence of selective publication. Positive results from clinical trials were more likely to result in publication than negative results. As the authors concluded, it was unknown whether the publication bias was due to the failure of investigators to submit their negative results for publication, or due to a decision by journal editors and reviewers not to publish them. However, the implication of selective publication is that accurate data on the topic are then not available to researchers, practitioners and policy-makers and thus hinders the advancement of knowledge – as well as wasting resources, investigators' and participants' time.

Random measurement error

Random error simply means error due to chance. Measurement scales may contain a certain amount of random deviation, known as random measurement error, such as when respondents guess the answer rather than give a true 'don't know' reply, or give an unpredictably different response when interviewed on a different day or by a different interviewer. It is usually assumed that most measurement errors are in different directions and will cancel each other out in an overall scale score. It is important to use measurement scales which show a high level of reliability (repeatability), with minimal susceptibility to random error.

Reactive effects (awareness of being studied): Hawthorne ('guinea pig') effect

This refers to the effect of being studied upon those being studied. Their knowledge of the study may influence their behaviour (they may become more interested in the topic, pay more attention to it and become biased), or they may change their behaviour simply because someone (the investigator) is taking an interest in them. A 'guinea pig' effect occurs if, when people feel that they are being tested, they feel the need to create a good impression, or if the study stimulates interest not previously felt in the topic under investigation and the results are distorted. The term 'Hawthorne effect' derives from an early study where the people being studied were believed to have changed in some way owing to the research process (Roethlisberger and Dickson 1939). It is often referred to as a 'reactive (Hawthorne) effect' (see Chapter 10).

Recall (memory) bias

This relates to respondents' selective memories in recalling past events, experiences and behaviour.

Reporting bias

This refers to respondents' failure to reveal the information requested.

Response style bias

This refers to a person's manner of responding to questions, often known as 'yes-saying' to items regardless of their content. For example, if all responses to a set of negative attitude statements start with the same response category (e.g. 'strongly agree'), a response set may be created: the respondent who checks 'strongly agree' to the first few negative statements that they read will catch on that 'strongly agree' is the answer that is most appropriate for their responses. Thus they will not read subsequent items carefully, and may simply check 'strongly agree' all the way through. A response set can be avoided by varying the wording of statements so that some of them are positive and some are negative (taking care not to create a double negative statement that can confuse people). Some investigators also vary the direction of the response categories, depending on the length of the scale. If the wording is varied on the first few items, so that some are worded positively, and some negatively, the respondent is more likely to read each item carefully, and respond more thoughtfully. This is why it is important to alternate the wording of response choices so that the 'agree' or 'disagree' or the 'yes' or 'no' are not always scored in the same direction.

Response set

See above. One can avoid a response set by varying item wording and interspersing positive with negative items, so that some are worded positively and some negatively – without creating confusing double negatives between the item and response category. If this is done for the first few items, respondents will be more likely to read the items carefully before responding. This will break the response set.

Sampling bias

Bias is possible unless the sampling method ensures that all members of the population of interest have a calculable chance of being selected in the sample. The resulting bias means that the sampling procedure results in a sample that does not represent the population of interest.

Selection bias

If the characteristics of the sample differ from those of the wider population of interest, then a selection bias has occurred.

Social desirability bias

Social desirability bias may exert a small but pervasive effect (people wish to present themselves at their best) and lead to a *response set* (see above).

Systematic error

The term 'systematic error' refers to the various errors or biases inherent in a study. The errors result in an estimate being more likely to be either above or below the true value, depending upon the nature of the (systematic) error in any particular case. The errors usually stem from selection bias in the sample, information bias (e.g. misclassification of subjects' responses owing to error or bias) or the presence of extraneous variables, which have not been taken into account in the study design, and which intervene and confound the results.

Total survey error

This equals the sum of all errors from the sampling method and data collection procedures. It should equal the difference between the sample survey estimate and the true or population value, and needs to be estimated. Estimation, however, is often difficult and generally only attempted in relation to large population surveys and censuses.

Ethics and ethical committees

All research potentially raises ethical issues, and consent to proceed is required from relevant ethical committees before a research study can commence. While the organisational structure of research ethics approvals varies between countries, and specific guidance varies between the disciplines of funding bodies (e.g. biomedical, psychological or social), some basic principles are shared (e.g. see Carter *et al.* 2000). Ethical issues cover a wide range of concerns including the robustness of the research design, research honesty and transparency, whether the research will lead to distress or embarrassment among participants, the demands on people's time, guarantees of privacy, confidentiality and anonymity, data protection and security, or ensuring informed written consent. There can also be issues about the safety and security of research staff if they are exposed to any risks (e.g. when undertaking fieldwork). People who agree to take part in research studies need protection in relation to their privacy and protection from manipulation by the researcher. Also required is the protection of trust on which society and the research community depend; and the preservation of the good reputation of research.

The ethical principle governing research is that respondents should not be harmed as a result of participation, and they should give their signed, informed consent to participate after reading information about the study aims, confidentiality and anonymity, and what it involves. Participants should also be informed that they are free to withdraw at any time, and the investigator must answer any questions they may have about the study. This voluntary consent safeguards the freedom of the participant to choose to participate in the research or not, and reduces the legal liability of the researcher. The only exception to obtaining individuals' consent is with certain mass or crowd observational studies, conducted in social science (Punch 1986) (see Chapter 16). It has also been argued that such covert observational research is unethical, deceptive, invades personal privacy and harms public trust in research (Bulmer 1982), despite any attempts at justification by the enhancement of knowledge (Humphreys 1970). These issues have been discussed in more detail by Hornsby-Smith (1993). A detailed code of ethics for the social scientist, containing over 70 ethical principles, was compiled by Reynolds (1979). Updated ethical guidance is now available from funding bodies across disciplines. Ethical committees concerned with health care generally include population surveys within their jurisdiction, though not without controversy among social scientists:

> We do not think it is appropriate for [medical] ethical committees to concern themselves with surveys of people identified from public records. They are not the custodians of people's civil rights. People do not belong to their doctors and there should be no interference with people's liberty to make up their own minds about what questions they should answer and in what circumstances.
>
> (Cartwright and Seale 1990)

Ethical committees have closing dates for the submission of applications. Many proposals meet with queries and are returned for revision, or for the investigator to address the concerns of the committee. The resubmission is then reconsidered at the next committee meeting. The committee will want copies of study materials, including the proposed questionnaires, letters, information sheets and consent forms for participants. The provision of clear, information for lay people about the methods is essential, given that research indicates that many participants in clinical trials find the concept of randomisation difficult to understand, and they develop alternative lay explanations (Featherstone and Donovan 1998).

Dissemination

Investigators have a duty to ensure that the evidence, both positive and negative, produced by well-designed research projects is disseminated. Dissemination of research findings includes presentation at key meetings and conferences, and publication in sources likely to be accessed by the targeted audience. In relation to health services, the effective dissemination of the evidence produced by research is essential for service development. Information about the plans for, and methods of, dissemination is increasingly required in research grant proposals.

Effective dissemination requires that the research reports, papers and presentations are presented clearly and honestly. Written and verbal reports must provide the information for the target audience to understand how the conclusions were supported by the data, and the appropriateness of the study design and sample. End-of-project reports should also include a shorter summary, understandable to the lay person, and this should be available separately. There are several published texts offering guidance on presentation, report writing and writing for publication (British Medical Association 1985; Hall 1994; Chalmers and Altman 1995a; Dooley 1995). Basically, a well-structured research report will include an abstract, a statement of the aims, objectives and hypotheses of the research, a description of the design, methods and process of analysis of the study, the measurements used with reference to their psychometric properties, the results, conclusions and discussion. The discussion should contain a concise restatement of the main results, the interpretations of the data, the theoretical implications, any problems and limitations of the research design and process, and future proposals stemming from the research (e.g. policy implications, research questions).

Useful recommendations about the type of information that should be included in research reports of the results of RCTs have been made by Begg et al. (1996) and Altman (1996), using the structured headings common to most research reports and publications, of title, abstract, introduction, methods, results and discussion. The recommendations have been adopted by some medical journals in relation to papers, based on results from trials, submitted for publication. These include the description of the study method and study population, with sample inclusion and exclusion criteria, the hypotheses and objectives, the outcome measures and the minimally important differences, the calculation of sample size, all the statistical methods used in the analysis, stopping rules (where applicable), the unit of study (e.g. individual or cluster), the method of allocation and blinding, the intervention and its timing, details of the flow of participants through the study, any deviations from the protocol, sources of bias and threats to validity, and interpretation of the findings in the light of the available evidence. Most of these recommendations can be applied to the reporting of results from other research designs.

However, even with well-structured and targeted dissemination, there is no guarantee that professionals (e.g. doctors, nurses, other health professionals, managers) will change their practice as a result of the research. Several studies of the effects of clinical research findings on medical practice have reported negative results even ten years later (Office of Technology Assessment, US Congress 1983; Interstudy 1994).

Stocking (1992) reviewed the strategies which have been attempted to promote change in clinical practice: provision of information (research results and individual feedback on practice); vocational and continuing education; peer review and audit; personal contact by respected peers or opinion leaders; financial incentives. As she pointed out, the dissemination of research results alone is not enough to promote change, and even individual feedback requires audit to be effective. However, even education and audit have been shown to fail to induce clinical change; change presumably also requires the consensus of clinicians and peer group influence. Key sources of change appeared to be interpersonal contact with respected others, pressure from patients and financial incentives (Stocking 1992). In short, the promotion of change requires a fairly wide range of interventions, and simply disseminating information alone will not have the desired effect.

Dissemination is still one vital component of the process and should be undertaken, and it should include sources accessed by both professionals and the public. The latter group are potentially powerful in relation to their perceptions of need and subsequent demands for particular health services and interventions. Dissemination to the public, and particularly to participants in clinical trials, also needs to be handled sensitively and with care. It is possible that feedback to participants in trials can lead to feelings of distress on behalf of the group whose outcome was worst. For example, Snowdon et al. (1998) fed back the results of a neonatal trial (extracorporeal membrane oxygenation (experimental) versus conventional ventilatory support (control)) to participants (parents of children who survived), in qualitative interviews. The results showed the experimental treatment reduced the risk of early death. They reported that people wanted the feedback, even when it was emotionally exacting, and had expressed surprise that participant feedback was not a routine practice of researchers. However, some parents felt that the control group children had been at a disadvantage; some parents of the children in the control group found the results 'rather sobering' and they described themselves as 'lucky'.

Summary of main points

- Literature reviews should be comprehensive and include all the valid and pertinent papers, presented in a critical fashion.
- Systematic reviews are prepared with a systematic approach to minimising biases and random errors, and include components on materials and methods.
- One of the first stages of research design is to describe the aims, objectives and hypotheses, if appropriate, of the study.
- The concepts within the hypotheses need to be defined and also operationalised so that they can be measured.
- The level of data that the selected measurement instruments produce (nominal, ordinal, interval or ratio) determines the type of statistical analyses that are appropriate.
- Psychometric validation is the process by which an instrument is assessed for reliability and validity.
- Factor structure refers to the number of underlying dimensions within the scale (dimensions that account for a high proportion of the common variance of the items).

■ Threats to the reliability and validity of research are known as biases and errors in the conceptualisation of the research idea, and the design and process of the study, which can lead to systematic deviations from the true value.

■ One definition of evidence-based practice is the use of current best evidence, in conjunction with clinical expertise and patient values, to guide decisions.

Key questions

1 Distinguish between concepts and theories.
2 Define operationalisation.
3 What are the main threats to the reliability and validity of the research?
4 Distinguish between systematic error and random error.
5 What are the various levels of data?
6 How would you assess a measurement scale for reliability and validity?
7 Find a published research paper of interest to you and list all the possible sources of bias and error that it could suffer from.
8 What are the principles of evidence-based practice?

Key terms

bias	null hypothesis
concept	operationalisation
critical appraisal	ordinal data
dependent variable	paradigm
dissemination	parametric statistics
error	precision
ethics	psychometric
evidence-based practice	random error
factor structure	ratio data
grounded theory	reliability
hypothesis	responsiveness
idiographic	sensitivity
independent variable	specificity
interval data	statistical significance
level of data	systematic error
measurement scales	systematic qualitative review
meta-analyses	systematic review
models	theory
nominal data	validity
nomothetic	value freedom
non-parametric statistics	variable

Recommended reading

Biddulph, J. (2005) Mathematical models in health care, in A. Bowling and S. Ebrahim (eds) *Handbook of Health Research Methods: Investigation, Measurement and Analysis.* Maidenhead: Open University Press.

Chalmers, I. and Altman, D. (eds) (1995) *Systematic Reviews.* London: British Medical Journal Publishing Group.

Crombie, I. K. (1996) *Pocket Guide to Critical Appraisal.* London: BMJ Books.

Cullinan, P. (2005) Evidence-based health care: systematic reviews, in A. Bowling and S. Ebrahim (eds) *Handbook of Health Research Methods: Investigation, Measurement and Analysis.* Maidenhead: Open University Press.

Frankfort-Nachmias, C. and Nachmias, D. (1992) *Research Methods in the Social Sciences*, 4th edn. London: Edward Arnold.

O'Rourke, A. (2005) Critical appraisal, in A. Bowling and S. Ebrahim (eds) *Handbook of Health Research Methods: Investigation, Measurement and Analysis.* Maidenhead: Open University Press.

Pope, C., Mays, N. and Popay, J. (2007) *Synthesising Qualitative and Quantitative Health Evidence: A Guide to Methods.* Maidenhead: Open University Press.

Siegel, S. (1956) *Nonparametric Statistics for the Behavioural Sciences.* London: McGraw-Hill.

Quantitative research: sampling and research methods

This section includes chapters which describe issues of sampling and sampling methods in quantitative research. It also summarises the methods shared by quantitative and qualitative research where populations may be hard to reach. The later chapters include a description of survey methods, experiments and other analytic methods, as well as methods of group assignment (from randomisation to matching). The issue of sample size and sampling is crucial to the external validity of the results stemming from all methods, including experiments.

Section contents

CHAPTER 8

Sample size and sampling for quantitative and qualitative research

Introduction

This chapter describes issues surrounding the calculation of sample size and statistical power, sampling error and methods of sampling. Probability theory and statistical testing, type I and type II errors and the difference between statistical and social or clinical significance are addressed in Part 1, along with issues pertaining to sample size. Part 2 describes the methods of sampling.

8.1 Calculation of sample size, statistical significance and sampling

The sampling unit

A member of the sample population is known as a sampling unit. The sampling unit may be an individual, an organisation or a geographical area. The investigator will need to be clear about the sampling units of analysis in the proposed study and base the sampling procedures on those units. For example, is the study one of households or individual members within households or both? Is it a study of hospitals, hospital or primary care clinics, doctors or patients or all of these (i.e. multilevel)?

If the study is multilevel (comprising more than one of these units), then calculations have to be made of the number of units at each level to be included in the sample. For example, if the study aims to evaluate the outcome of providing specialist medical care in primary health care clinics in comparison with hospital clinics, then the study is multilevel and includes the clinics, doctors and patients. Thus the investigator must calculate how many clinics, doctors *and* patients are needed in the sample (see Mok 1995). Sampling based on clinics is important in order to ascertain the amount of natural variation between clinics, and to ensure the external validity (generalisability) of the results. The latter is required in order to decide whether any observed treatment effects are independent of this natural variation. For example, patients attending the same clinic (or doctor) may be more likely to receive the same treatment than patients attending other clinics (or doctors). The design and analysis of the study need to take account of these 'cluster effects'. The patients may also need to form a unit of analysis in order to ascertain important patient (personal) characteristics (e.g. associated with outcome); the doctors (see above) may also need to form a unit of analysis in order to examine between-doctor variation in practice, volume of procedures performed (pertinent to the study topic), level of qualification/grade and effects on patients' outcome. Hierarchical statistical techniques (multilevel models) have been developed for the analysis of multilevel studies. The different levels of data are referred to as 'nested'. Sample size calculations need to take account of each level, and these multilevel techniques of analysis are required (see Greenland 2000). There is usually a case for making the unit of analysis the same as the unit of randomisation. If clinics are randomised, then the results of the study (e.g. analyses of change) are analysed at the level of the clinic. Cornfield (1978) has labelled randomisation using the cluster as the unit, accompanied by analysis appropriate to the individual as the unit, as 'an exercise in self-deception'. Distortions will occur if relationships between variables are estimated at one level of analysis (e.g. the clinics) and then extrapolated to another (e.g. the individual patients). This is known as the *ecological fallacy*. The converse is known as the individualistic, or reductionist fallacy – where inferences about groups are drawn from individuals.

There is a strong case for working closely with statisticians in the design and analysis of such studies. Wood and Freemantle (1999) have published advice on how to choose an appropriate unit of analysis in trials evaluating an intervention.

Calculation of sample size and statistical power

The size of the sample aimed for should be calculated at the design stage of the study. The formula for calculating sample size and sampling error is usually given in statistical textbooks (e.g. Bland 1995), and there are several technical papers available (Altman 1980; Gore 1981).

The statistical approach to determining sample size in evaluation studies is the *power calculation*. Statistical power is a measure of how likely the study is to produce a statistically significant result for a difference between groups of a given magnitude (i.e. the ability to detect a true difference). The probability that a test will produce a significant difference at a given level of significance is called the *power* of the test. For a given test, this will depend on the true difference between the populations that are being compared by the investigator, the sample size and the level of significance selected (Bland 1995). It is important to ensure that the study is designed so that it has a good chance of detecting significant differences if they exist. If the statistical power of a study is low, the study results will be questionable (the study might have been too small to detect any differences). The 0.05 level of significance is usually taken, and the power should be greater than 0.8 (Crichton 1993).

Power calculations can also be calculated retrospectively for studies that have failed to justify their sample size – in order to assess how much chance the study results (once analysed) had of detecting a significant difference (Altman 1980).

There are many statistical packages available for the calculation of sample size, based on calculations of statistical power. All depend on some estimation of the likely differences between groups. For this, it is essential to have conducted a pilot study or to be able to extrapolate the information from other studies. For the calculation the investigator will need to estimate the type and amount of random variation (error) in the study, decide on the main measures to be used, decide on the smallest observed difference between the groups and sub-groups in the study that would be of interest (and, in the case of a mean, its standard deviation), assess the (real-life) consequences of making a type I or type II error (erroneous rejection or acceptance of the null hypothesis – see later) as the power of the study is determined from this, and consider the costs of the study in relation to required sample size. The size of the minimum difference to be detected, the significance level and the power can be entered into a computer package with a statistical formula for calculating the sample size based on the power (St Leger *et al.* 1992).

Confidence intervals are generally used in estimations of sample size for descriptive research (e.g. social, health and epidemiological surveys).

Considerations in determination of sample size

It is common for investigators to determine sample size and fail to consider the need for sub-group analysis (even if only cautious analyses are planned), issues of item and total non-response and sample attrition in the case of longitudinal designs, all of which will increase desired sample sizes (though this will not compensate for response bias, i.e. differences between responders and non-responders to a study which could affect the results). Pocock *et al.* (1987) argued that if a study has limited statistical power (i.e. too small a sample), then sub-group analyses should be avoided.

Some power calculations can produce relatively small target sample sizes, depending on the nature of the study, but researchers should also consider the limited generalisability of the data in such instances. Power calculations can also produce extremely large target sample sizes, which cannot be achieved (e.g. owing to the unavailability of people with the condition of interest or small existing numbers of specialised clinics). The calculation of statistical power varies with study design (e.g. follow-up studies require different power calculations from cross-sectional studies in order to allow for sample attrition). Sample size, the importance of suffcently large samples in clinical trials, and the contribution and appropriateness of smaller trials in relation to experimental design have been discussed in detail by Pocock (1983), Powell-Tuck et al. (1986) and Senn (1997). In sum, power calculations should be used realistically. Issues of sampling have been described in more detail by Moser and Kalton (1971), Blalock (1972), Pocock (1983) and Bland (1995).

Testing hypotheses, statistical significance, the null hypothesis

In relation to statistical inference, hypotheses are in the form of either a *substantive hypothesis*, which, as has been pointed out, represents the predicted association between variables, or a *null hypothesis*, which is a statistical artifice and always predicts the absence of a relationship between the variables. Hypothesis testing is based on the logic that the substantive hypothesis is tested by assuming that the null hypothesis is true. Testing the null hypothesis involves calculating how likely (the probability) the results were to have occurred if there really were no differences. Thus, the onus of proof rests with the substantive hypothesis that there is a change or difference. The null hypothesis is compared with the research observations and statistical tests are used to estimate the probability of the observations occurring by chance.

Probability theory

Statistical tests of significance apply probability theory to work out the chances of obtaining the observed result. The significance levels of 0.05, 0.01 and 0.001 are commonly used as indicators of statistically significant differences between variables. For example, if the P value for a test is less than 0.05, then one can state that the difference in percentages is statistically significant at the 5 per cent level. This means that there are less than five chances in 100 (or 1 in 20) that the result is a false positive (type I error). This 5 per cent level is conventionally taken as the level required to declare a positive result (i.e. a difference between groups) and to accept or reject the null hypothesis. The smaller the value of P (e.g. $P < 0.05$, $P < 0.01$, $P < 0.001$, $P < 0.0001$), the less likelihood there is of the observed *inferential statistic* having occurred by chance. The choice of 0.05 is arbitrary, though selecting a higher level will give too high a chance of a false positive result. If a P value of 0.001 (1 in 1000) was obtained in the statistical test, the obvious implication is that this probability is very small. The investigator could conclude that the evidence is incompatible with the assumption that the null hypothesis is true, and therefore reject the null hypothesis and accept the substantive hypothesis. There will be a probability of error in this decision which is reflected in the significance level. It should be noted that a smaller P value will require a larger sample size to be obtained.

Pocock (1983) and Tilling et al. (2005) have warned against the dogmatic acceptance or rejection of the null hypothesis, based on significance levels, and the misuse of P values. If the null hypothesis is not rejected, it cannot be concluded that there is no difference, only that the method of study did not detect any difference. Indeed, there is actually little difference between $P = 0.06$ and $P = 0.04$ (Pocock 1983). The confidence interval, and the magnitude of differences (statistics are sensitive to sample size and small differences can obtain statistical significance in large samples) should always be examined in addition to significance levels.

There are alternative inductive and deductive approaches to drawing inferences from statistical data, known as Bayesian theory and the more predominant frequentist approach. Bayesian theory is based on a principle which states that information arising from research should be based only on the actual data observed, and on induction of the probability of the true observation given the data. The Bayesian approach starts with the probability distribution of the existing data, and adds the new evidence (in a model) to produce a 'posterior probability distribution' (Lilford and Braunholtz 1996; Spiegelhalter *et al.* 2000). Frequentist theory involves the calculation of *P* values which take into account the probability of observations more extreme than the actual observations, and the deduction of the probability of the observation. Interested readers are referred to Berry (1996), Freedman (1996) and Lilford and Braunholtz (1996). The latter have called for a shift to Bayesian analysis and sensitivity analyses (a method of making plausible assumptions about the margins of errors in the results) in relation to public policy.

Type I and type II errors

Sample size is determined by balancing both statistical and practical considerations. There are two types of error to consider when making these decisions:

- a type I error (or alpha error) is the error of rejecting a true null hypothesis that there is no difference (and, by corollary, acceptance of a hypothesis that there are differences which is actually false);
- a type II error (or beta error) is the failure to reject a null hypothesis when it is actually false (i.e. the acceptance of no differences when they do exist).

These two types of error are inversely related: the smaller the risk of type I error, then the greater the risk of type II error. It is important to specify the significance level that is acceptable at the outset of the study, and whether one- or two-tailed significance tests will be used. If the investigator has valid reasons for not wishing to reject the null hypothesis (no differences), then he or she should consider using the 0.10 level of significance, thus reducing the risk of type II error. However, this level is rarely used, as investigators regard it as lacking credibility. The acceptable level of probability of making a type I error then determines the level at which statistical tests of differences between groups are conducted.

Sample size and type I and II errors

In general, the larger the sample, then the smaller will be the sampling error (other things being equal), and statistically significant results are more likely to be obtained in larger samples. Thus, with a very large sample, it is almost always possible to reject any null hypothesis (type I error) simply because statistics are sensitive to sample size; therefore the investigator must be careful not to report findings as highly significant (e.g. 0.001) with large sample sizes. For this reason, statistical tests of significance are usually omitted from analyses of large datasets (see Grundy *et al.* 1999, as an example). A factor large enough to produce statistically significant differences in a small sample is more worthy of attention than a factor which produces small differences that can be shown to be statistically significant with a very large sample. Moreover, the achievement of statistical significance does not necessarily imply that the observed differences are of social or clinical importance.

Also, a difference that is not statistically significant simply means that differences were not demonstrated *in the sample drawn*. This may also be due to lack of statistical power. Samples which are too small have a high risk of failing to demonstrate a real difference (type II error). Samples must be large enough to be representative of the population of interest, for the analysis of sub-groups (e.g. health status by age and sex group) and for the calculation of statistics. If the sample is large, there is also the problem of expense, as well as manageability, and large studies require careful planning and management. Target sample sizes also have to allow for non-response and, in longitudinal designs, for sample attrition (e.g. deaths, drop-outs) over time.

Pocock (1983) has reviewed evidence which has shown that many clinical trials have included too few patients. For example, one review he referred to reported that the median size of cancer trials was 50 patients – which makes meaningful analysis extremely difficult. Enrolment of patients into British cancer trials has been an ongoing problem (it has been estimated that only between 1 and <10 per cent of British cancer patients (at different sites) are entered into clinical trials). Pocock concluded that much research is futile, since it is not possible with small sample sizes to answer the question being posed. Thus, when planning research, it is important to consider the feasibility of collaborating in a multicentre study. This may be needed for recruitment of sufficient numbers of people, and in order to enhance the generalisability of the findings if correct sampling procedures are followed. Multicentre studies are much more difficult to organise, finance and manage (e.g. co-ordinators will be required in order to ensure that studies in each site conform to the same system of patient recruitment, follow-up, measurement process, data processing, analysis and reporting).

Multiple significance testing and type I error

Statisticians often argue that there is an overemphasis on hypothesis testing and the use of P values in research which casts doubt on their credibility (Gardner and Altman 1986). The inclusion of multiple endpoints in research increases the use of statistical testing and therefore increases the likelihood of chance differences and the risk of a type I error.

Appropriate use of significance tests

It is argued that research reports should just focus on a small number of primary hypotheses and end-points that are specified in advance, and that in relation to subsidiary, or secondary, hypotheses and end-points, the investigator should interpret significance tests with caution. Investigators should use as few tests of significance as possible in order to minimise the risk of a type I error being made. Similarly, it is argued that subgroup analyses should be confined to a limited number of hypotheses specified in advance and that statistical tests for interaction should be used, rather than sub-group P values; sub-group findings should also be interpreted cautiously in line with exploratory data analysis (Pocock 1985; Pocock *et al.* 1987). Because of the problems of interpreting P values, it is common when planning research to assign one of the end-points as the main criterion for assessing outcome, and the results of its significance test will accordingly be the main criterion in the assessment. This method also has disadvantages: for example, over-reliance on single indicators and, in particular, their statistical significance (and sometimes at the expense of their clinical significance).

Statisticians encourage investigators to report the actual significant *and* non-significant *P* values, rather than refer to arbitrary levels (e.g. $P < 0.05$), and to present the magnitude of observed differences and the confidence intervals of their data (Pocock 1985). The confidence intervals express the uncertainty inherent in the data by presenting the upper and lower limits for the true difference. For example, the confidence interval around a result from a clinical trial of treatment indicates the limits within which the 'real' difference between the treatments is likely to lie.

Statisticians often point out that statistical testing is really only appropriate for use with results derived from traditional experimental designs and that they are inappropriate, along with the use of confidence intervals, for use with other types of research methods because of the problem of bias and confounding variables which exists in the latter and confuses the issue of chance (Brennan and Croft 1994). Despite this caution, most investigators continue to emphasise *P* values in all forms of analytical descriptive research, and most journal editors will request them if they are missing from submitted publications, though there is an increasing awareness of their limitations.

One- or two-sided hypothesis testing

Decisions about sample size also require a decision to be made about whether the study will conduct one-sided or two-sided hypothesis tests. One-tailed (sided) tests examine a difference in one specified direction only, whereas two-tailed tests examine relationships in both directions. If a test is significant with a two-tailed test, it inevitably is with a one-tailed test. For example, in clinical research, a one-sided hypothesis only allows for the possibility that the new treatment is better than the standard treatment. A two-sided hypothesis allows assessment of whether the new treatment is simply different (better or worse) from the standard treatment. Although one-sided testing reduces the required sample size, it is sensible always to use two-sided tests, as one-sided testing rests on a subjective judgement that an observed difference in the opposite direction would be of no interest.

Statistical, social and clinical significance

It was pointed out earlier that there is often an over-reliance on the value of significance testing and the achievement of statistically significant results at the $P < 0.05$ level and beyond. Statisticians stress that *P* values should only be used as a *guideline* to the strength of evidence contradicting the null research hypothesis (of no difference between groups), rather than as proof, and that the emphasis should be shifted towards using confidence limits as methods of estimation.

The achievement of statistical significance does not necessarily imply differences that are of social or clinical importance. It is therefore important to differentiate between statistical and social and clinical significance, and ascertain the minimal clinically important differences. Statisticians argue that the overuse of arbitrary significance levels (e.g. $P < 0.05$) is detrimental to good scientific reporting, and that greater emphasis should be placed by investigators on the *magnitude* of differences observed and on estimation methods such as confidence intervals. This is particularly important in studies that involve multiple end-points, each of which is tested statistically, given that the increase in the statistical analyses increases the likelihood of finding statistical differences by chance (Pocock *et al.* 1987). It is also important to consider fully the *actual amount* of change from baseline scores when analysing statistically significant post-test or follow-up scores for experimental and control groups.

It is still relatively rare for medical investigators to report their intervention studies clearly in relation to what they consider to be a significant clinical effect. Mossad *et al.* (1996), in their report of a randomised controlled trial of zinc gluconate treatment for the common cold, reported at the outset that they considered a 50 per cent reduction in symptom duration to be a significant clinical effect. Their results could then be judged in relation to this statement, rather than reliance on the achievement of statistical significance.

Statistical significance, then, is not the same as social or clinical significance. The question should always be asked: is it meaningful? The larger the sample size, the greater chance there is of observing differences between groups (statistics are sensitive to sample size). For example, with a sample size of several thousands, a small difference between groups (even 1 per cent) would probably be significant at the 5 per cent level, while if the sample size is only 20 people in total, it is unlikely that even large observed differences between groups (e.g. 30 per cent) would be significant at the 5 per cent level. Social and clinical relevance must be assessed in relation to the actual size of the differences observed, and to confidence intervals, rather than reliance solely on *P* values (see Box 8.1).

Box 8.1 Example of statistical versus clinical significance

An illustration of statistical significance being over-emphasised and reported as having clinical significance is a study of the costs and outcome of standardised psychiatric consultations in the USA by Smith *et al.* (1995). Their study was based on an RCT comparing immediate with a delayed (for one year) standardised psychiatric consultation. The study was carried out with 56 somatising patients from 51 study doctors. The measures included the patient-completed Rand SF-36 to measure the sub-domains of health status, and analysis of medical and billing records. The study has been criticised for its reliance on statistically significant differences in physical functioning at one year after the intervention. Both treatment and control groups had low levels of physical functioning at baseline. The members of the treatment group improved their physical functioning score at follow-up by an average of seven units, which was statistically significant. However, they differed from the control group at baseline *too* by an average of seven units – and this was not statistically significant. Thus the significant increase among the treatment group was of the same magnitude as the insignificant difference between the groups at baseline. While the authors reported the improvement in the treatment group to be clinically significant, Bech (1995) disagreed; he also pointed to the lack of significant difference reported between groups in their social functioning, vitality, mental and general health at baseline and follow-up.

In addition, there are many examples of research studies in which statistical tests have been applied inappropriately, and where investigators have drawn conclusions from statistical testing of their data which are unwarranted. Many problems stem from the fact that the assumptions behind a statistical test (e.g. the level of the data, normal distributions, and so on) are not met by the investigator. These assumptions are dealt with in all statistical textbooks. A readable historical account of the 'abuse' of statistics by empiricists in the social sciences, and their appropriateness in comparison with alternative methods of statistical estimation, has been presented by Atkins and Jarrett (1979).

Sampling frames

The sampling frame is the list of population members (units) from which the sample is drawn. Ideally it should contain a complete listing of every element in the target population, and every element should be included only once. Commonly used sampling frames for national surveys in Britain include the register of electors and the postcode address files (for 'small users': private households). Both carry the problem of blanks (electors who no longer reside at the listed address, empty properties in the postcode file). There are methods of substitution in this case which are available, in order that target sample size is not adversely affected (see Moser and Kalton 1971). The electoral register may be incomplete (e.g. people who do not register to vote will not be listed on it) and biased (e.g. people in ethnic minority groups and inner-city populations may be less likely to register). This is a more serious problem as it will lead to a biased study. Many investigators use lists of patients, which can also suffer from duplicated entries, incomplete coverage of the population of interest and bias among those on the list, all of which can threaten external validity (generalisability of the data). Given that lists are rarely perfect, investigators should make checks of their lists against any other available lists of the study population where possible.

Postcode address files

In Britain, the Office for National Statistics carries out many national surveys. Before 1984 it used the electoral register as the sampling frame, and from 1984 it has used the British postcode address file of 'small users', stratified by region and socio-economic factors. This file includes all private household addresses. The postal sectors are selected with probability proportional to size. Within each sector a predetermined number of addresses are selected randomly with a target sample size of adults. Interviewers are given a formula for sampling the household to include if more than one household resides at the address sampled. All adults in the sampled household are interviewed up to a maximum of three (in cases where more than three adults reside in the household, the interviewer lists them systematically and randomly selects the required number for interview). The disadvantage here is the reliance on interviewers for the accuracy of the sampling in these instances.

Lists of patients

Where community health surveys are concerned, it is common for bona fide investigators to obtain permission to access the lists of patients registered with family doctors in the areas of the investigation. In Britain, these lists are more complete in terms of population coverage than many other population lists of individuals (about 98 per cent of the British population are registered with an NHS GP), though they also have the problem of blanks (out-of-date addresses where people have moved, people who have died and not been removed from the list). In one study of elderly people living at home, in order to minimise the problem of sampling out-of-date addresses and respondents who had died, respondents were sampled if they were on both the lists of GPs' patients for the area (held centrally by the district health authority) and the electoral register (Bowling *et al.* 1989). This is still not without problems, as any new addresses of respondents who might have moved since the lists were updated are not shown, leading to inadequate population coverage.

Studies focusing on specific diseases or institutional populations (e.g. hospitals, primary care centres) will generally take the lists of patients in the relevant sections as the sampling frame, but even these can be out of date (in relation to current addresses) and unrepresentative of the population of interest (not everyone with a disease or medical condition consults a doctor about it, or is referred to a specialist). Even lists of hospital inpatients contain problems. These lists are usually updated in the evening. If a survey using the lists as a sampling frame is carried out in the afternoon, patients who were discharged in the morning will still be on the list, and patients who were admitted that day will not yet be included on it. The extent of this problem was evident in an evaluation carried out by the author and her colleagues of hospital discharge procedures on medical wards (Houghton *et al.* 1996). The researchers updated their own admissions lists periodically throughout the day because the ward lists were out of date. This was necessary, as patients were interviewed by the researchers on admission. The result was that, as the researchers' admissions list was more up to date than the wards' lists, the hospital staff (especially the nurses) routinely consulted the researchers throughout the study to see who had been admitted and discharged for their reviews of their bed states and work allocation.

Sampling

In statistical terms, a population is an aggregate of people or objects. Since the population of interest to the researcher may contain too many members (e.g. people) to study conveniently, samples of the population are drawn. The advantages of sampling (i.e. smaller numbers) over complete population coverage are financial (sampling is cheaper in time, staff and resources), and better quality data are obtained (there is more time for checking and more elaborate information can be collected). See Moser and Kalton (1971), for history and examples.

Statistical sampling is recommended because when the estimates of the characteristics of the population are calculated at the analysis stage, the precision of the estimates can be determined from the results. A sample is selected, statistics are calculated (e.g. an average or proportion) and the statistics are used as an estimate of the population parameters. Since all sample results are liable to be affected by sampling errors, the estimates should be accompanied with information about their precision. This is the standard error.

Statements based on randomly selected samples are probability statements, based on inference because of sample non-response and potential bias in measurements. Sampling theory and estimation do not apply to samples selected by non-random methods. To enable inferences to be made about a study population, the relation between the sample and the population must be known. The selection procedure must be random and depend on chance, such as tossing a coin or the use of random numbers tables (see Armitage and Berry 1987, for an example of a random numbers table). A small sample, however random in selection, is likely to be less accurate in its representation of the total population than a large sample.

Sampling error

Any sample is just one of an almost infinite number that might have been selected, all of which can produce slightly different estimates. Sampling error is the probability that any one sample is not completely representative of the population from which it was drawn. Sampling errors show the amount by which a sample estimate can be expected to differ from the true value of that variable in the population. The concept has been clearly described, and the formula given, by the Office for National Statistics (2011). It points out the factors which determine the level of sampling error for a particular variable, which are: for a characteristic, the proportion of people who possess it; for a numeric variable (e.g. units of alcohol consumed), the distribution of the variable in the population; the sample design and the sample size. Sampling error cannot be eliminated but it should be reduced to an acceptable level. The existence of sampling error means that whenever a hypothesis is tested, there is a finite possibility of either rejecting a true hypothesis (type I error) or accepting it when it is false (type II error). The issue of sampling error is described further below in relation to the normal distribution.

Confidence intervals and the normal distribution

The normal distribution

Many variables are normally distributed, for example, the weights of all men between the ages of 60 and 70, the heights of all adult women and IQ scores of adults. The normal curve is simple in that there are only two constants in its formula: the mean and the standard deviation. If the mean and standard deviation (the latter is a measure of *dispersion*, based on the difference of values from the mean value: the square root of the arithmetic mean of the squared deviations from the mean) are specified, then the complete normal curve can be drawn, as is shown here:

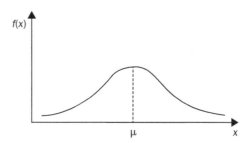

The curve of the normal distribution is symmetrical: it has a bell shape; and the average (mean) corresponds to the peak of the distribution. The equation of the curve is:

$$f(x) = \frac{1}{\sigma\sqrt{(2\pi)}} \exp\left(\frac{-(x-\mu)^2}{2\sigma^2}\right)$$

where μ is the mean and σ is the standard deviation.

In practice, if a sufficiently large number of observations or measurements are made, so that the shape of the distribution can be assessed, it will frequently transpire that the distribution does actually approximate closely to the normal distribution. Not all variables are normally distributed, however. For example, salaries are skewed towards the lower end of the scale.

The standard deviation (SD) is associated with the curve in the following way. Assume an upper limit of one SD above the mean and a lower limit of one SD below the mean. A certain proportion of the population will be contained within these limits. For the normal distribution this proportion is 68 per cent: that is, the middle 68 per cent of the scores in any normal distribution fall within the limits of one SD above and below the mean. If wider limits are considered – for example, two SDs above and below the mean – then the shape of the normal curve is such that 95.4 per cent of the scores fall within these limits. For plus and minus three SDs, the percentage increases to 99.73 per cent. As an example, if it is known that the mean IQ of a particular population is 100, the SD is 15 and IQ is normally distributed, then we know that 68 per cent of the population will be within limits of 100 ± 15 (85 and 115), 95.4 per cent within the limits 70 and 130, and 99.73 per cent within the limits 55 and 145.

What happens to these distributions if just a sample is drawn: for example, of all adult women? Does it matter what size the sample is? If a sample of the adult female population is taken, then the distribution of their heights may not be normal even though the distribution of the whole population is. Sampling errors may occur which means that the sample does not adequately reflect the population. The larger the sample size, the greater the chance that the sample represents the population and has a normal curve.

It is unlikely that a sample taken from a population which is not normally distributed will itself have a normal curve.

Sampling distributions of the means

What happens if many samples of the same size are taken from the population? What is the distribution of the average (mean) heights of all the samples (the *sampling distribution of the means*)? If all possible samples were drawn from a population, most sample means for the variable of interest would congregate near the middle of the distribution, with fewer sample means found at greater distances from the middle. (See Boxes 8.2 and 8.3.) The sampling distribution approaches normality as the number of samples increases. In mathematical terms, the *central limit theorem* states that the distribution of means of samples taken from any population will tend towards the normal distribution as the size of the samples taken increases. This applies whether or not the underlying population from which the samples are taken is itself normal. In practice, the distribution of the means takes the form of a normal distribution for sample sizes of 30 or more ($n \geq 30$). The mean of the new distribution (of means) is the same as the mean of the population but there is less variation. The standard deviation is smaller:

$$\frac{\sigma}{\sqrt{n}}$$

This (the standard deviation of the sampling distribution of means) is known as the standard error (SE). The larger the sample size, the smaller the SE. The more variation there is in the underlying population, the more variation there is in the sampling distribution of means, though there is less than in the population.

Box 8.2 Example of sampling distribution of means

The mean height of adult men is 179 centimetres (cm) and the SD is 5.8cm. This means that two-thirds of men are between 173.2 and 184.8cm tall. Suppose samples of size 400 are taken from the population and the mean heights of each sample calculated. The sampling distribution of means will be a normal distribution with mean 179cm and SE 0.29cm (5.8/($\sqrt{400}$)).

So two-thirds of the mean heights will lie between 178.71 and 179.29cm. If a much smaller size had been chosen, say 25, then the SE would be larger (1.16cm) and two-thirds of the mean heights would lie between wider limits (177.84 and 180.16cm).

Confidence intervals

We do not know the true population value for the variable of interest, so an estimate from the sample, its mean, is the best guess. Is there any way of telling how good this estimate is? A 95 per cent confidence interval (CI) for the population mean is an interval which, if calculated for each of many repeated samples of the same size and from the same population, would, for 19 out of 20 samples, be found to contain the true population mean. For 90 per cent CIs, fewer (nine out of ten samples) would yield an interval that contained the true mean. In practical terms, a CI calculated from a sample is interpreted as a range of values which contains the true population value with the probability specified. A greater degree of trust can be placed in a 95 per cent CI than a 90 per cent CI, but the drawback is that the limits may be too wide to be useful. Thus a CI for the desired degree of trust in the estimate can be specified and the sample size necessary for this degree of trust calculated. Conversely, for a given sample size, a measure of the confidence that can be placed in the estimate can be calculated. So it can be seen that sample size and CIs are closely related. As the sample size increases, the SE decreases and, as will be illustrated, the CI needed for the same degree of trust becomes narrower.

Thus, placing confidence intervals about an estimate will indicate the precision (loosely speaking, the degree of accuracy) of the estimate. In obtaining these interval estimates for parameters, we can determine the exact probability of error. The first step is to decide on the risk one is willing to accept in making the error of stating that the parameter is somewhere in the interval when it is not. If we are willing to be incorrect 0.05 of the time (one in 20 times), we use the 95 per cent CI. We can say that the sampling procedure is such that 95 per cent of intervals obtained would include the true parameter. Or (as described above) if repeated samples were drawn, 95 per cent of the CIs we calculated would contain the true mean. More strictly, if we are only willing to be incorrect once in 100 times, we use the 99 per cent CI. The 95 and 99 per cent CIs are conventionally used. The assumptions made for CIs are that random sampling was used, and that if a normal sampling distribution is used (as described here), we must assume a normal population or have a sufficiently large sample. A single confidence interval cannot be applied to all research problems, and the most appropriate method depends on whether or not the proportions are derived from independent samples and separate survey questions. The alternative methods have been described by Elliot (1994). The formulae for confidence intervals for means in single samples and two samples are given by Gardner and Altman (1986).

The standard deviation of a sample provides information on how much confidence can be placed in a sample estimate. It is known that about 95 per cent of all sample means fall within plus or minus 1.96 SEs of the population mean and that 99 per cent fall in the range of plus or minus 2.58 SEs.[1] These values are used in the calculation for obtaining CIs illustrated next. For a given degree of confidence, say 95 per cent, a smaller sample SD will yield narrower CIs.

Confidence intervals can be constructed for other estimates as well as the mean; for example, the proportion of people aged over 80 in the population, or the difference in the proportions of men and women aged over 80. The general formula for calculating 95 per cent CIs is:

$$\text{estimate} - 1.96 \times \text{SE and estimate} + 1.96 \times \text{SE}$$

and the formula for calculating the 95 per cent CIs for a proportion is:

$$p - 1.96 \times \sqrt{\{p(1-p)/n\}} \text{ and } p + 1.96 \times \sqrt{\{p(1-p)/n\}}$$

where p = the sample proportion
and n = the sample size

For the above formula it is important to make sure that the sample size is large enough to satisfy the statistical assumptions. As a rough guide, Bland (1995) suggests that $n \times p$ and $n(1 - p)$ should both be greater than 5.

Most statistical textbooks – Altman (1991) and Bland (1995), for example – give the SEs for the most commonly calculated estimates, with examples showing how to obtain the CIs.

Box 8.3 Example of sample size and CIs

Suppose in the previous example (Box 8.2) that it is considered necessary to have a 95 per cent CI of 177 to 181cm (with mean 179cm and SD 5.8cm). That is, in 19 out of 20 choices of sample the estimate should lie between 177 and 181cm. The calculation carried out to obtain the sample size is called a power calculation. In this case the sample size necessary is 33.[2] A more stringent CI with the same limits may be required, say 99 per cent. That is, the estimate from a larger proportion, 99 out of 100 choices of sample, should lie between 177 and 181cm. A larger sample size of 56 is needed. The reason that the sample sizes necessary in this example are small is that the SD (5.8cm) is small in relation to the mean (179cm) of the population.

Mathematical postscript on using estimates in confidence intervals

In practice, an estimation of the SD as well as the population mean is made, as the SD of the population is not usually known. The best estimate of the population mean that can be inferred from a sample is the mean of the sample. When estimating the SD, the denominator $n - 1$, rather than n, should be used. The standard error is therefore:

$$\frac{s}{\sqrt{n}}$$

where s is the SD of the sample.

Box 8.4 Example of calculation of a CI

In the examples given earlier, suppose that a sample of size 50 was taken from the population and the mean and SD of the sample were calculated as 180cm and 70cm. The estimates for the population mean and the SE would be 180cm and 1cm $(7/(\sqrt{(50-1)}))$. The 99 per cent CIs would be $180 \pm 2.58 \times$ 1cm, or 177.42 to 182.58cm. Notice the greater width of interval necessary to have the same amount of confidence: 5.6cm rather than 4cm (source: Joy Windsor, pers. comm., University College London).

Distribution of errors

It is relatively unlikely that the mean of a sample will be exactly the same as the population mean. The difference between the two is the error. The error in the example above is 1cm. Errors can occur for two reasons. One is that the sampling is not carried out properly, resulting in a biased sample. This is called *systematic error*. The other reason is the chance factors that influence the sampling process. For example, an unusually unrepresentative sample could be chosen. This is called *random error*. Just as the means of all possible samples have their own distribution, so do the errors of the samples. Theoretically the errors are normally distributed with a mean of 0, so the errors balance out over all samples.

External validity of the sample results

External validity relates to the generalisability of the research results to the wider population of interest. Internal validity was discussed earlier and refers to the properties of the measurement instrument. Sampling is concerned with sample selection in a manner that enhances the generalisability of the results.

Pocock (1983) has stated that it is unethical to conduct research which is badly designed and carried out. One common failure of research design is in using inadequate sampling techniques (which lead to sample bias and poor external validity) and inadequate sample sizes, which prevent investigators drawing a reliable conclusion. Small studies have a high risk of type II error. However, while trials which do not have sufficient power to detect real differences may be unethical, sometimes only a small trial can be run (e.g. in cases of rare conditions), and the development of meta-analysis means that small trials are more valuable as results across studies can be pooled and analysed (Powell-Tuck *et al.* 1986; Senn 1997).

A further problem stems from studies that achieve poor response rates, which limit the generalisability of the results. The journal *Evidence-Based Medicine* (1995) uses a minimum 80 per cent response rate, and minimum 80 per cent follow-up rate in post-tests, as two of the criteria for inclusion of research papers in its review and abstracting system.

There are several key questions to ask before sampling:

- What is the unit of study?
- What is the target population for the study?
- Will there be any difficulties in gaining access to them?
- Will ethical committee approval be needed?
- Whose permission will be needed to access the population?
- What type of sample will be needed? (If a survey is used, is stratification by geographical region, socio-economic group, etc. required? If experimental, what are the criteria for selecting the study and control groups?)
- What sample size is required?

8.2 Methods of sampling

This section describes the methods of random and non-random sampling commonly used in quantitative and qualitative research.

Random sampling

Sampling theory assumes random sampling. Random sampling gives each of the units in the population targeted a calculable (and non-zero) probability of being selected. Random samples are *not* necessarily equal probability samples whereby each unit has an equal chance of selection (both simple and unrestricted random sampling gives each unit an equal chance of being selected). The representativeness of the study population is enhanced by the use of methods of random sampling. Random sampling relates to the method of sampling – not to the resulting sample. By chance, a random method of selection can lead to an unrepresentative sample. The methods of random sampling are described below. For fuller details, interested readers are referred to Moser and Kalton (1971).

Unrestricted random sampling

Statistical theory generally relates to unrestricted random sampling. The members of the population (*N*) of interest are numbered and a number (*n*) of them are selected using random numbers. The sample units are *replaced* in the population before the next draw. Each unit can therefore be selected more than once. With this method, sampling is random, and each population member has an *equal* chance of selection.

Simple random sampling

The members of the population (*N*) of interest are numbered and a number (*n*) of them are selected using random numbers *without replacing them*. Therefore, each sample unit can only appear once in the sample. With this method, too, sampling is random, and each population member has an *equal* chance of selection. As this method results in more precise population estimates, it is preferred over unrestricted random sampling.

At its most basic, names can be pulled out of a hat. Alternatively, computer programs can be designed to sample randomly or to generate random number tables to facilitate manual random sampling. For example, with random number tables, the members of the population (*N*) are assigned a number and *n* numbers are selected from the tables, with a random starting point, in a way that is independent of human judgement. Random number tables are preferable to mixing numbered discs or cards in a 'hat', as with the latter it is difficult to ensure that they are adequately mixed to satisfy a random order. If a list of names is arranged in random order and every *n*th name is selected, this is also a simple random sample.

In sampling without replacement, the assumption underlying statistical methods of the independence of the sample has been violated, and a correction factor should, strictly, be applied to the formula to take account of this. Blalock (1972) describes the use of a correction factor for formulae involving the standard error of the mean.

Systematic random sampling

It is rare for lists to be in purely random order (e.g. they may be in alphabetical order, which means they are organised in a systematic way), so rarely is selection from such a list simple random sampling. Selection from lists is called systematic random sampling, as opposed to simple random sampling, as it does *not* give each sample member an equal chance of selection. Instead, the selection of one sample member is dependent on the selection of the previous one. Once the sampling fraction has been calculated, the random starting point determines the rest of the sample to be selected. If it is certain that the list is, in effect, arranged randomly, then the method is known as quasi-random sampling.

Systematic random sampling leads to a more even spread of the sample across the list than simple random sampling, except if the list really is randomly ordered (then the precision of the sample is the same). The method can lead to serious biases if the list is ordered so that a trend occurs, in which case the random starting position can affect the results (such as with lists ordered by seniority of position in an organisation). Such lists need reshuffling.

With systematic random sampling, then, there is a system to the sampling in order to select a smaller sample from a larger population. For example, if the target sample size is 100, and the total eligible population for inclusion totals 1000, then a 1 in 10 sampling ratio (sampling fraction) would be selected. The sampling would start at a random point between 1 and 10.

Stratified random sampling

A common method of guarding against obtaining, by chance, an unrepresentative (biased) sample which under- or over-represents certain groups of the population (e.g. women) is the use of stratified random sampling, which is a method of increasing the precision of the sample (dividing the population into strata and sampling from each stratum).

The population of interest is divided into layers (strata) – for example, doctors, nurses, physiotherapists, patients – and sampling from the strata is carried out using simple or systematic random sampling. If the sampling fraction is the same for each stratum (known as proportionate stratified sampling), then this method is an improvement on simple random sampling as it will ensure that the different groups in the population (strata) are correctly represented in the sample (e.g. age, sex, geographical area) in the proportions in which they appear in the total population.

If the sampling fractions vary for each stratum, the sampling procedure is known as *disproportionate stratified sampling*. A disproportionate stratified sample would be taken if some population strata are more heterogeneous than others, making them more difficult to represent in the sample (particularly in a smaller sample). Therefore, a larger sampling fraction is taken for the heterogeneous strata in order to provide results for special sub-groups of the population. For example, it is common to take a larger sampling fraction in areas where a range of ethnic minority groups reside in order to ensure that they are represented in the sample in sufficient numbers for analysis. This may lead to lower precision than a simple random sample, unlike proportionate stratified sampling. The different methods for calculating the standard error for proportionate and disproportionate stratified sampling are discussed by Moser and Kalton (1971).

Cluster sampling

With this method, the population can be divided into sub-populations. The units of interest are grouped together in clusters and the clusters are sampled randomly, using simple or systematic random sampling. The process of sampling complete groups of units is called *cluster sampling*. The reasons for doing this are economic. For example, rather than randomly sampling 200 individual households from a list of 200,000 in a particular city (which would lead to a sample spread across the city, with high travelling costs for interviewers), it would be more economical to select randomly a number of areas (clusters) in the city and then include all, or a sample of, the households in that area. The areas can be naturally occurring, or artificially created by placing grids on maps. The same procedure can be used in many situations: for example, for sampling patients in clinics or nurses in hospitals. This method is also advantageous when there is no sampling list. The disadvantage is that it is a less precise method of sampling, and therefore the standard error is likely to be higher.

Multistage sampling

The selection of clusters can be multistage (e.g. selecting districts – the primary sampling units, PSUs – within a region for the sample, and within these sample electoral wards and finally within these a sample of households). This is known as multistage sampling and can be more economical, as it results in a concentration of fieldwork.

Sampling with probability proportional to size

Sampling with probability proportional to size (PPS) is common in multistage samples, as they generally have different size units. If one PSU has a larger population than another, it should be given twice the chance of being selected. Equal probability sampling is inappropriate because if the units are selected with equal probability (i.e. the same sampling fraction), then a large unit may yield too many sample members and a small unit may yield too few. Instead, one could stratify the units by size and select a sample of them within each size group, with variable sampling fractions. Or one could sample the units with PPS, then the probability of selection for each person will be the same and the larger units cannot exert too great an effect on the total sample. The sizes of the primary sampling units must be known to carry out this method.

Non-random sampling: quota sampling

Quota sampling is a method favoured by market researchers for its convenience and speed of sample recruitment. It is a method of stratified sampling in which the selection within geographical strata is non-random, and it is this non-random element which is its weakness. The geographical areas of the study are usually sampled randomly, after stratification (e.g. for type of region, parliamentary constituencies, socio-demographic characteristics of the area), and the quotas of subjects for interview are calculated from available data (numbers (quota) of males, females, people in different age bands, and so on), in order to sample – and represent – these groups in the correct proportions, according to their distribution in the population. The choice of the sample members is left to the interviewers. Interviewers are allocated an assignment of interviews, with instructions on how many interviews are to be in each group (e.g. with men, women, specific age groups). They then usually stand in the street(s) allocated to them until they have reached their quota of passers-by willing to answer their questions.

It is unlikely that quota sampling results in representative samples of the population. There is potential for interviewer bias in the unconscious selection of specific types of respondents (such as people who appear to be in less of a hurry, or people who look friendlier). If street sampling is used, then people who are in work, ill or frail have less likelihood of inclusion. People who are housebound have no chance of inclusion. It is not possible to estimate sampling errors with quota sampling, because the method does not meet the basic requirement of randomness. Not all people within a stratum have an equal chance of being selected because not all have an equal chance of coming face to face with the interviewer.

Sampling for qualitative research

The following methods – convenience sampling, purposive sampling, snowballing and theoretical sampling – are generally restricted to qualitative research methods. They are summarised here because the first three sampling methods are often used by health economists in their quantitative utility studies, and by survey researchers of hard-to-reach populations. While these methods are non-random, the aim of all qualitative methods is to understand complex phenomena and to generate hypotheses, rather than to apply the findings to a wider population. Their sampling methods are presented here, together with other methods of sampling, for consistency, and also referred to in the section on qualitative methods. (See Chapter 4 on sampling.)

Convenience sampling

This is sampling of subjects for reasons of convenience (e.g. easy to recruit, near at hand, likely to respond). This method is usually used for exploring complex issues: for example, in economic evaluations, in complex valuations of health states (utility research). While the method does not aim to generate a random group of respondents, when used by health economists, the results are often aimed at health policy-makers but are of unknown generalisability. Opportunistic sampling is similar – the investigator seizes the opportunity to interview any respondent who is likely to have relevant information for the study.

Purposive sampling

This is a deliberately non-random method of sampling, which aims to sample a group of people, or settings, with a particular characteristic, usually in qualitative research designs. It is also used in order to pilot questionnaires or generate hypotheses for further study. This is sometimes called judgement sampling, where respondents are selected because they have knowledge that is valuable to the research process (e.g. senior managers in case studies of organisations).

However, purposive sampling is often used in experimental design for practical reasons. For example, a medical team might include all its current inpatients with breast cancer for an experimental design to test the effectiveness of a new treatment. The results are not generalisable to the wider population of interest unless random sampling from that population has been employed (though this is rarely possible).

Snowballing

This technique is used where no sampling frame exists and it cannot be created: for example, there may be no list of people with the condition of research interest, or they may be unlikely to respond to conventional approaches. Snowball sampling, while not providing representative samples, can be effective in the recruitment of members of vulnerable populations, including members of small social or cultural groups not easily reached by traditional sampling methods.

The snowballing technique involves the researcher asking an initial group of respondents to recruit others whom they know are in the target group (e.g. friends and family recruited by existing respondents; or specialists or members of relevant patients' groups may be asked if they know any patients in the relevant category). Anyone so identified is contacted, asked if he or she would be willing to participate in the study and, at interview, asked if he or she knows other people who could be included in the study and so on. The disadvantage of the method is that it includes only members of a specific network.

The adaptation of snowball sampling techniques by Sadler *et al.* (2010) helped the authors to gain access to each of the more vulnerable population groups of interest in several studies in California. They reported that sensitive recruitment, attention to good communications and identification of key sources from which to start the snowballing (e.g. within specific community groups), were effective in enlisting the involvement of members of vulnerable and minority populations. They provided a useful summary of their strategies and the types of populations the method was found to be successful with (e.g. illegal drug users; groups of bisexual, gay and lesbian people; people with AIDS; small ethnic groups with differing cultural values).

Theoretical sampling and saturation

With theoretical sampling, conceptual or theoretical categories are generated during the research process. The principle of this method is that the sampling aims to locate data to develop and challenge emerging hypotheses that have, in turn, been derived from previous interviews (Glaser and Strauss 1967). First, a small number of similar cases of interest are selected and interviewed in depth in order to develop an understanding of the particular phenomenon. Next, cases are sampled who might be exceptions in an attempt to challenge (refute) the emerging hypothesis. The sampling stops when no new analytical insights are forthcoming. This method necessitates the coding and analysis of data during the ongoing sampling process, owing to the interplay between the collection of the data and reflection on them. No attempt is made to undertake random sampling.

Sampling for telephone interviews

In order to conduct telephone interviews with the target population, the interviewer has to be able to access their telephone numbers. If the study is one of a specific population, such as people aged 65 years and over in a particular area, this can be problematic. Even if the rate of telephone ownership is high, people may not be listed in telephone directories ('ex-directory'). For some target populations (e.g. hospital outpatients) telephone numbers may be accessed through medical records, though ethical committees may prefer the investigator to offer the sample member the chance to decline to participate by post first.

Random digit dialling is a method which overcomes the problem of telephone owners not being listed in telephone directories. This is only suitable for general population and market research surveys. However, the method involves a prior formula and requires study of the distribution of exchanges and area codes. It requires the identification of all active telephone exchanges in the study area. A potential telephone number is created by randomly selecting an exchange followed by a random number between 0001 and 9999 (non-working and non-residential numbers are excluded from the sample). This method can substantially increase the cost (Webb *et al.* 1966). There is also the issue of who to select for interview: the interviewer will have to list all household members and randomly select the person to be sampled and interviewed; not an easy task over the telephone, especially if the required sample member is not the person who answered the telephone. Kingery (1989) compared different methods of sampling for telephone surveys of older people, and reported that random digit dialling was a very time-consuming method. For example, in the State of Georgia, USA, it took about 500 hours of calling to provide a maximum of 80 respondents aged over 65 who were willing to take part in a 20-minute telephone interview. It also took twice as long to contact eligible respondents aged over 55 as younger respondents, and response rates among older sample members were lower than with younger members.

Summary of main points

- The statistical approach to determining sample size is the power calculation. This is a measure of how likely the study is to produce a statistically significant result for a difference between groups of a given magnitude (i.e. the ability to detect a true difference).
- A type I error (or alpha error) is the error of rejecting a true null hypothesis that there is no difference (i.e. the acceptance of differences when none exist).
- A type II error (or beta error) is the failure to reject a null hypothesis when it is actually false (i.e. the acceptance of no differences when they do exist).
- With a very large sample it is almost always possible to reject any null hypothesis (type I error), as statistics are sensitive to sample size; samples which are too small have a risk of a failure to demonstrate a real difference (type II error).
- Sampling error is the probability that any one sample is not completely representative of the population from which it was drawn.
- External validity is the generalisability of the research results to the wider population of interest.
- Sampling is concerned with the sample selection in a manner that enhances the generalisability of the results.
- Random sampling gives each of the units in the population targeted a calculable (and non-zero) probability of being selected.
- Simple and unrestricted random sampling both give each population member an equal chance of selection.
- Systematic sampling leads to a more even spread of the sample across a list than simple random sampling.
- Stratified random sampling increases the precision of the sample by guarding against the chance of under- or over-representation of certain groups in the population.
- Cluster sampling is economical, and the method is advantageous when there is no sampling list for the units within the clusters (e.g. households within geographical areas).
- Cluster sampling can be multistage, which is more economical.
- Sampling with probability proportional to size gives the sampling unit with the larger population a proportionally greater chance of being selected.

- ■ Quota sampling is preferred by market researchers for practical reasons but the non-random element is a major weakness.
- ■ Qualitative research, and research on complex topics (such as economic valuations), tend to use convenience, purposive or theoretical sampling, and snowballing techniques.

Key questions

1 What is a sampling unit?
2 Explain a power calculation.
3 Distinguish between type I and type II errors.
4 What is a confidence interval?
5 What are the advantages of sampling over complete population coverage?
6 What are the main advantages of probability sampling?
7 When is it appropriate to use sampling with probability proportional to size?
8 Why do market researchers prefer quota sampling?
9 What are the weaknesses of non-random methods of sampling?

Key terms

clinical significance
cluster sampling
confidence intervals
convenience sampling
external validity
multistage sampling
normal distribution
null hypothesis
one- and two-sided hypothesis testing
population
power calculation
probability sampling
purposive sampling
quota sampling
random sampling
representative sample
sample size
sampling
sampling error

sampling frame
sampling unit
sampling with probability proportional
to size
simple random sampling
snowballing
social significance
standard error
statistical power
statistical significance
stratified sampling
substantive hypothesis
systematic random sampling
theoretical sampling
type I error
type II error
unit of analysis
unrestricted random sampling
weighting

Notes

1 Sixty-eight per cent of all sample means fall within ± 1 SE of the population mean; 90 per cent within ± 1.645 SEs; 95 per cent within ± 1.96 SEs; 99 per cent within ± 2.58 SEs.
2 Ninety-five per cent CIs are $\mu \pm 1.96$ SE; 99 per cent CIs are ± 2.58 SE. That is, $n = (1.96s/d)^2$ where d is the difference between n and the lower limit.

Recommended reading

Bland, M. (1995) *An Introduction to Medical Statistics*. Oxford: Oxford University Press.

Pocock, S.J. (1983) *Clinical Trials: A Practical Approach*. Chichester: Wiley.

Tilling, K., Peters, T. and Sterne, J. (2005) Key issues in the statistical analysis of quantitative data in research on health and health services, in A. Bowling and S. Ebrahim (eds) *Handbook of Health Research Methods: Investigation, Measurement and Analysis.* Maidenhead: Open University Press.

Quantitative research: surveys

Introduction

Quantitative research, by definition, deals with quantities and relationships between attributes; it involves the collection and analysis of highly structured data in the positivist tradition. Quantitative research is appropriate in situations in which there is pre-existing knowledge, which will permit the use of standardised data collection methods (e.g. the survey questionnaire), and in which it is aimed to document prevalence or test hypotheses.

Sociological observational research methods (see Chapter 16) are appropriate where the phenomenon of interest can be observed directly, but this is not always possible. One alternative is to ask people to describe and reconstruct events by using survey methods. With the survey, the investigator typically approaches a sample of the target group of interest and interviews them in person or by telephone, or asks them to complete a self-completion questionnaire (the latter is usually sent and returned by post). Surveys can be carried out at one point in time (cross-sectional or retrospective surveys) or at more than one point in time (longitudinal surveys). These types of surveys will be described in

Part 9.1 of this chapter, and issues in the analysis of change from longitudinal data will be addressed in Part 9.2.

9.1 Survey methods

The survey

The modern social survey originated in Victorian Britain, with the Victorians' enthusiasm for collection and enumeration, and the work of Victorian social reformers concerned with poverty and the collection of information about it (e.g. Booth 1899–1902; Rowntree 1902; see Moser and Kalton 1971, for an overview).

Social surveys aim to measure attitudes, knowledge and behaviour and to collect information as accurately and precisely as possible. Descriptive surveys are carried out in order to describe populations, to study associations between variables and to establish trends (e.g. as in regular opinion surveys). Longitudinal surveys are conducted at more than one point in time, and aim to analyse cause-and-effect relationships. Surveys try to do this in such a way that if they were repeated at another time or in another area, the results would be comparable.

The survey is a method of collecting information, from a *sample* of the population of interest, usually by personal interviews (face to face or telephone), postal or other self-completion questionnaire methods, or diaries. The survey is distinct from a census, which is a complete enumeration and gathering of information, as distinct from partial enumeration associated with a sample. Some investigators wrongly describe their sample surveys as sample censuses.

The unit of analysis in a survey is usually the individual, though it can also be an organisation if organisations were the sampling units (e.g. medical clinics), or both of these in multilevel studies. A major advantage of surveys is that they are carried out in natural settings, and random probability sampling is often easier to conduct than for experimental studies. This allows statistical inferences to be made in relation to the broader population of interest and thus allows generalisations to be made. This increases the external validity of the study.

Descriptive and analytic surveys

Surveys can be designed to measure certain phenomena (events, behaviour, attitudes) in the population of interest (e.g. the prevalence of certain symptoms, reported use of health services and the characteristics of health service users). These types of surveys are called *descriptive* surveys because the information is collected from a sample of the population of interest and descriptive measures are calculated (Moser and Kalton 1971). They are also known as cross-sectional because the data are collected from the population of interest at one point in time. The respondents are generally asked to report on events, feelings and behaviour retrospectively (e.g. within the last month), and thus the surveys are called retrospective.

A different type of survey aims to investigate *causal* associations between variables. These analytic surveys are known as longitudinal surveys and are carried out at more than one point in time. It should be pointed out that in all surveys, if seasonal influences on topics are expected, then, where possible, the data collection should be spread across the year.

There are two objectives of surveys. First, to estimate certain population parameters (e.g. levels of health status). The relevant statistics are calculated from the data derived from the sample studied, and these are used as an *estimate* of the population parameter of interest (and since all samples are subject to sampling errors, this estimate needs to be accompanied by a statement about its precision – the standard error). And, second, to test a statistical hypothesis about a population (e.g. people in the lowest socio-economic groups will be more likely to report poorer health status). Again, a measure of precision needs to be applied to the survey results (the standard error). It should also be remembered that statements based on samples of the population of interest, rather than the total population, are, at best, *probability* statements (based on inference).

In contrast to RCTs which can provide valid estimates of the underlying effect of the intervention being studied, surveys can only yield estimates of association, which may deviate from the true underlying relationships due to the effects of confounding variables.

Descriptive surveys

Statisticians often refer to descriptive, cross-sectional surveys as *observational research* because phenomena are observed rather than tested. This is a misleading description because observational methods are a specific method used by social scientists (see Chapter 16). These surveys are also sometimes referred to as correlation studies because it is not generally possible to draw conclusions about cause and effect from them.

In order to avoid confusion by using language reserved for specific techniques, in this chapter, cross-sectional surveys will be referred to as a type of descriptive study. Descriptive studies literally describe the phenomenon of interest and observed associations in order to estimate certain population parameters (e.g. the prevalence of falls among elderly people), for testing hypotheses (e.g. that falls are more common among people who live in homes which are poorly lit) and for generating hypotheses about possible cause and effect associations between variables. They can, in theory, range from the analysis of routine statistics to a cross-sectional, retrospective survey which describes the phenomenon of interest in the population and examines associations between the variables of interest. Descriptive studies cannot provide robust evidence about the direction of cause-and-effect relationships. However, the increasing sophistication of statistical techniques can help to minimise this limitation. The generated hypotheses can, if appropriate, be tested in experimental or analytic studies. However, distinctions between study methods in relation to their analytic abilities should not be too rigid (Rothman 1986).

Descriptive studies can still provide information about social change. For example, health services are increasingly encouraged to shift resources and services from the hospital sector to the primary care sector. Without surveys over time to document any shifts, the extent of any changes, the speed of change and any enabling factors or difficulties encountered will remain unknown. The range of surveys on health-related topics has been reviewed by Cartwright (1983).

Analytic surveys

Descriptive surveys contrast with analytic surveys. Longitudinal surveys are analytic, rather than descriptive, because they analyse events at more than one point in time rather than cross-sectionally, and, if the data collection points have been carefully timed, they can suggest the *direction* of cause and effect associations. Most longitudinal surveys collect data prospectively – over the forward passage of time. Longitudinal surveys can also be carried out retrospectively, for example, by collecting data (e.g. from records) about respondents from more than one time period in the past (in the same manner as most case control studies – see Chapter 4). However, this chapter is concerned with the more common prospective longitudinal survey.

Retrospective (*ex post facto*), cross-sectional surveys

These are descriptive studies (surveys) of a defined, random cross-section of the population at one particular point in time. Most cross-sectional studies are retrospective – they involve questioning respondents about past as well as current behaviour, attitudes and events. Cross-sectional surveys, using standardised methods, are a relatively economical method in relation to time and resources, as large numbers of people can be surveyed relatively quickly, and standardised data are easily coded.

The method is popularly used in the social sciences (e.g. psychology, sociology, economics) to investigate social phenomena and in epidemiology to investigate the prevalence (but not incidence) of disease (e.g. the population is surveyed at one point in time and the characteristics of those with disease are compared to those without disease in relation to their past exposure to a potential causative agent).

Retrospective studies are frequently criticised because they involve retrospective questioning (e.g. respondents may be asked questions about past diet and other lifestyle factors), and the potential for selectivity in recall and hence recall bias. Great care is needed with questionnaire design and the time reference periods asked about in order to minimise bias. However, even prospective studies involve questions about the past (between waves of the study) and retrospective studies can provide useful indications for future investigation.

As with all descriptive studies, because it is difficult to establish the direction of an association (cause and effect), cross-sectional surveys cannot be used to impute such causality. For example, an association found between being overweight and breast cancer could be interpreted either as that being overweight might cause breast cancer, or that having breast cancer might lead to being overweight; or some third unknown variable may lead to both. Cross-sectional studies can only point to statistical associations between variables; they cannot alone establish causality.

Prospective, longitudinal surveys

The prospective, longitudinal survey is an analytic survey that takes place over the forward passage of time (prospectively) with more than one period of data collection (longitudinal). It tends to be either panel (follow-up of the same population) or trend (different samples at each data collection period) in design. These types of studies are also known as follow-up studies. If the sample to be followed up in the future has a common characteristic, such as year of birth, it is called a prospective, longitudinal *cohort* study. The longitudinal survey is a method commonly employed by social scientists and also by epidemiologists (e.g. to measure the incidence of disease and cause-and-effect relationships).

Prospective, longitudinal studies require careful definitions of the groups for study and careful selection of variables for measurement. Data have to be collected at frequent time intervals (or they have the same disadvantages of memory bias as retrospective studies), and response rates need to be high. Results can be biased if there is high sample attrition through natural loss (such as death), geographical mobility (and untraced) or refusals over time. There should be a clear rationale to support the timing of repeated survey points (e.g. at periods when changes are anticipated), as well as the use of sensitive instruments with relevant items that will detect changes. Experimental and other analytic designs with follow-up periods over time are, in effect, longitudinal designs, and the same principles and difficulties apply.

This method is of value for studying the effects of new interventions (e.g. national health education and promotion programmes). It is also of use for studying trends in behaviour or attitudes, as greater precision will be obtained when measuring change than with a series of cross-sectional surveys. Responses to the same question on successive occasions in panel surveys will generally be positively correlated, and in such cases the variance of the change will be lower for a longitudinal survey than for surveys of independent samples. A further advantage of this method is that not only can trends be assessed, but the method can identify people who change their behaviour or attitudes, as well as other characteristics (e.g. health status).

These surveys are sometimes referred to as 'natural experiments' as interventions occurring in the course of events can be observed, and the sample is then 'naturally' divided into cases and controls. Thus, incidence rates can be calculated in exposed and unexposed groups, and possible causal factors can be documented.

Secondary data analyses

Secondary data refer to existing sources of data that could be used for research purposes. The sources include routinely collected statistics on hospital, primary care and community health service use, disease registers, population mortality, births, deaths, historical records (e.g. medical records), existing morbidity data and existing population research data that has been lodged in data archives. Secondary sources of data are usually very large datasets, however, they can be relatively economical to analyse in comparison with primary data collection.

There are many accessible, archived survey datasets in the USA, Europe and other countries, which may be relevant to address the research questions of interest (for examples, see Box 9.1). Archives generally store accessible details of the questionnaires used for each dataset, the variable list, and the downloadable, anonymised datasets. Longitudinal surveys are stored by wave and not often linked (due to the resulting size, given that users rarely need access to the whole dataset and each survey wave). Thus, the data handling and analyses can be complex, especially if record linkages and merges to produce longitudinal datasets are needed, and analyses of change over time are required. Missing data from various waves may also require imputation, and then modelling to assess the reliability of consequent results. Caution is always required when analysing secondary data in relation to its accuracy and completeness. Further information on accessing health care survey data can be found in Shaw (2005).

Box 9.1 Examples of accessible, large longitudinal survey datasets on ageing

The *Survey of Health, Ageing and Retirement in Europe (SHARE)* provides data from over 22,000 people aged 50+ in 11 European countries, using a longitudinal panel survey design. SHARE is harmonised with other large, national surveys of ageing such as the US

Health and Retirement Study and the English Longitudinal Study of Ageing. Data collected include health, biomarkers, psychological health and well-being, economic variables and social support. Eleven European countries have contributed data to the 2004 wave (wave 1), and several others have since joined in (waves 1–4 are available for analysis so far, and data are being collected for wave 5) (www.share-project.org; accessed September 2013).

The *English Longitudinal Survey of Ageing (ELSA)* is a multidisciplinary survey of the dynamics of ageing, and comprises a nationally representative sample of people aged 50 and over (born before 1 March 1952), living in private households in England at baseline. ELSA collects data on their economic circumstances, social support, psychological, physical and mental health, and biology. Many of the questions are harmonised with the US Health and Retirement Study. The sample was first interviewed in 2002, and included more than 11,000 participants. Five waves are available for analysis to date (www.esds.ac.uk, accessed September 2013).

The *US Health and Retirement Study (HRS)* is a longitudinal panel study that surveys a representative sample of over 26,000 Americans over the age of 50 about every two years. Topics include their economic circumstances, social support, psychological, physical and mental health, and insurance coverage. Twelve waves since 1992 are accessible so far (www.hrsonline.isr.umich.edu; accessed September 2013).

Difficulties of longitudinal studies

Prospective longitudinal surveys are expensive, take a long time and need a great amount of administration (e.g. to update and trace addresses, deaths or other losses of sample members), computing (e.g. merging of databases for different follow-up waves) and effort in order to minimise sample attrition.

However well conducted the survey, it is often difficult for epidemiologists to use longitudinal data to suggest a causal relationship between a variable and a disease for a number of reasons, for example, the long onset from exposure to the development of most diseases and the difficulties in timing the successive follow-up waves. In effect, they are often faced with the problem of reverse causation (the causal direction is the opposite to that hypothesised). Associations are also difficult to interpret owing to the multifactorial nature of many diseases, the interplay between genetic and environmental factors, and the difficulties involved in identifying the features of a particular variable that might have a role in disease. Even with diet, for example, the culprit might be the additives or contaminants in the diet, rather than the food itself. The problems of extraneous, confounding variables and intervening variables were described in Chapter 4. Longitudinal studies are often justified when cheaper, and less complex, cross-sectional data have suggested the appropriate variables to be measured.

Members of longitudinal samples can also become conditioned to the study, and even learn the responses that they believe are expected of them (as they become familiar with the questionnaire); they may remember, and repeat, their previous responses; they can become sensitised to the research topic and hence altered (biased) in some way; there can be a reactive effect of the research arrangements – the 'Hawthorne' effect – as people change in some way simply as a result of being studied (Roethlisberger and Dickson 1939).

Trend, panel and prospective cohort surveys are all types of longitudinal survey, and are described in more detail next.

Trend surveys

A trend survey aims to sample a representative sample of the population of interest at the outset of the study, and, in order to take account of changes in the wider population over time, to draw a new sample at each future measurement point. This method is popular in market research and polling (e.g. surveys of political attitudes over time). It is also used by epidemiologists in order to identify sample members with differing levels of exposure to a potential disease and to enable incidence rates to be calculated (the number of new cases of disease occurring in a defined time period); disease incidence rates are compared in the exposed and unexposed groups. Epidemiologists often call it a method of surveying a *dynamic* population, as opposed to a *fixed* population survey. The sample members should be derived from a random sample of the population. Information is sought from the members by post or by interview.

Panel surveys

A panel survey is the traditional form of longitudinal design. A sample of a defined population is followed up at more than one point in time (e.g. repeated questionnaires at intervals over time), and changes are recorded at intervals. Although the wider population may change over time, the same sample is interviewed repeatedly until the study terminates or the sample naturally dwindles as sample members have left (e.g. they have moved, dropped out of the study or died). Each person accumulates a number of units of months or years (known as 'person time') of observation. The aim is to study the sample's experiences and characteristics (e.g. attitudes, behaviours, illnesses) as the members enter successive time period and age groups, in order to study changes.

Again, the sample members should be derived from a random sample of the population. It can be based on a cohort sample (see next section). Information is sought from the members by post or by interview. This is a common method used by social scientists, and by market researchers and political pollsters, to measure trends (though the panel's selection is not usually random in poll and market research). Bowling et al.'s (1996) longitudinal interview surveys of older people are examples of panel surveys. These were based on two random samples of people aged 65–84 (and a census of everyone aged 85 and over in a defined geographical area). The samples were followed up over time, with the aim of examining the factors associated with positive ageing. This was done by analysing changes in emotional well-being, social networks and support, psychological morbidity, physical functioning and service use over time.

Cross-sectional and longitudinal cohort studies

It was pointed out earlier that if the population to be sampled has a common experience or characteristic which defines the sampling (e.g. all born in the same year), it is known as a *cohort* study. The key defining feature of a cohort is the sharing of the common characteristic. A birth cohort, for example, can be a sample of those born in a particular year, or in a particular period (such as a five- or ten-year period). A cohort study can be based on analyses of routine data, and/or on assessments and data collected for the study.

Technically, cohort studies can be cross-sectional and retrospective (collection of data at one point in time about the past, for example, as in a sample of hospital patients all undergoing the same procedure during the same time period, with retrospective analysis of their hospital casenotes relating to that period), longitudinal and retrospective (collection of data at more than one point in time about the past, for example, retrospective analysis of these patients' casenotes relating to more than one period in the past) or longitudinal and prospective (collection of data at more than one point over the forward passage of time, for example, collection of data from the patients' casenotes at future hospital episodes as they occur). However, even prospective studies include retrospective questioning about events that have occurred between waves of interviews. The prospective cohort study is one of the main methods used in epidemiological research to investigate aetiology (causes of disease).

Cohort sequential studies

Some longitudinal cohort designs involve taking cohorts at different points in time (e.g. a sample of 18- to 25-year-olds in different years) in order to allow for cohort effects (the sharing of common experiences which can lead to the unrepresentativeness of the cohort). These are known as cohort sequential studies, and cross-sectional, cohort and cohort sequential analyses can be carried out. However, they cannot properly control for period effects (e.g. changing economic, social or political circumstances over time which explain differing results). A well-known example of this method is the longitudinal study of people aged 70 years in Gothenberg, Sweden. The study commenced with one cohort born in 1901–2, which has been followed up for more than 20 years. The analyses indicated that there was some impact of the environment on health and functioning and so two more cohorts (born five and ten years after the first cohort) were added. In addition, in order to test hypotheses about the influence of lifestyle, environmental factors and the availability of health care on ageing and health, a broad socio-medical intervention was added to the third age cohort (Svanborg 1996).

Problems of cohort studies

As with longitudinal studies, cohort samples must be complete and the response rates at each wave of the study need to be high in order to avoid sample bias. In addition, a main problem with analysing data from cohort studies is the 'cohort effect'. This refers to the problem that each cohort experiences its society under unique historical conditions, and contributes to social change by reinterpreting cultural values, attitudes and beliefs and adjusting accordingly. For example, a cohort that grows up during times of economic depression or war may develop different socio-economic values from cohorts brought up in times of economic boom or peace.

Triangulated research methods and surveys

The most common quantitative descriptive method is the survey, although other methods exist. Just as Pope and Mays (1993) accuse medical doctors who undertake health services research of being blinkered by experimental methods and thus 'using a very limited tool box', Webb et al. (1966, 2000) lamented the over-dependence on survey methods in social science, whether by interview or self-completed questionnaire, and recommend the use of triangulated, unobtrusive (unreactive) methods (the use of three or more methods) to enhance the validity of the findings. No research method is without bias. Interviews and questionnaires must be supplemented by methods testing the same social variables but having *different* methodological weaknesses. Webb *et al.* (1966) gave several examples of less reactive alternatives:

> The floor tiles around the hatching chick exhibit at Chicago's Museum of Science and Industry must be replaced every six weeks. Tiles in other parts of the museum need not be replaced for years. The selective erosion of tiles, indexed by the replacement rate, is a measure of the relative popularity of exhibits . . . Chinese jade dealers have used the pupil dilation of their customers as a measure of the client's interest in particular stones.
>
> (1966, p. 2)

Each of these less reactive techniques is also subject to bias: for example, the siting of the entrance to the museum will consistently bias the path of visitors and confound the erosion measure, unless it can be controlled for. As the authors correctly point out, however, once a proposition has been confirmed by more than one independent measurement process, the level of uncertainty surrounding it is reduced: the most persuasive evidence comes through a *triangulation* of measurement processes, as well as through minimising the error contained within each instrument.

Webb *et al.*'s account of the types of unobtrusive methods available for research has been updated by Lee (2000) to include the internet, garbage and graffiti. For example, they give the example of research by Wales and Brewer (1976) of the graffiti in four high schools in a 'conservative Midwestern city' in the USA:

> Graffiti have been studied as clues to the social preoccupation of young people . . . Wales and Brewer found much more graffiti in women's toilets than in men's toilets. Graffiti produced by females tended to be 'romantic' in character as opposed to the sexual or scatological graffiti produced by males. However, for both males and females, sexually oriented graffiti increased as the socioeconomic level of the area served by the school rose.
>
> (Lee 2000, p. 24)

An increasingly popular archive for unobtrusive measurement is the internet, covering all aspects of life and behaviour. The anonymity provided by the internet can lead people to a frankness in chat rooms, question and discussion forums that they rarely show in interview or research situations. For example, Seale *et al.* (2010) compared data from internet discussion forums with face-to-face interviews. They illustrated the research advantages of unobtrusive online research, using the example of keyword analyses of the frank conversations which take place under anonymity in online health advice forum:

> We report a comparative keyword analysis of interviews and Internet postings involving people with breast and prostate cancer and discussion of sexual health. Interviewees produce retrospective accounts, their content guided by interviewers' questions, which might elicit rich biographical and contextual details. Internet exchanges concern participants' current experiences and contain detailed accounts of

disease processes, medical procedures, bodily processes, and, in the case of sexual health, sexual practices. They are used by participants to exchange information and support in a relatively anonymous context. Because of the ease with which large amounts of such archived Internet materials can be accessed and analyzed, this source has considerable potential for direct observation of illness experiences.

(2010, p. 595)

Disadvantages include the inevitable selectivity biases due to selective participation as well as selective key word searches.

This emphasis on the use of multiple (triangulated) research methods was echoed by Denzin (1989), who argued that triangulation elevates the researcher 'above the personal biases that stem from single methodologies. By combining methods and investigators in the same study, observers can partially overcome the deficiencies that flow from one investigator or one method'. Denzin (1970, 1978) proposed the use of data triangulation (the data should be collected at different times and places and from different people or groups), theory triangulation (the use of more than one theoretical approach to the analysis), and methodological triangulation (the use of multiple methods to collect the data and of multiple measurements within the same method).

9.2 Methods of analysing change in longitudinal studies

Analysing change

Care must be taken in the analysis of longitudinal data. For example, there can be longitudinal effects simply owing to the ageing of the sample (e.g. women may have more children as they get older because they are exposed to more opportunities to get pregnant; Johnson 1995). There can also be cohort effects – birth rates are also affected by changing social circumstances, as during the baby boom that followed the Second World War in Europe and North America, followed by the fertility decline of the 1960s onwards (see section on cohort studies earlier). A particular difficulty in the analysis of data from longitudinal surveys is known as 'response shift'. This refers to the scale of values which people use to make judgements, and the way in which it changes as changes in the variable of interest (e.g. health) occur (beta change). Occasionally, an individual's entire conceptualisation of the target variable might change (gamma change) (Sprangers and Schwartz 1999). Response shift is a problem for longitudinal research because changes that are detected (e.g. in self-reported health status) might not be 'real' changes (alpha changes), but reflect beta or gamma changes.

Moreover, in longitudinal designs, as in experimental designs with pre- and post-tests, it is misleading simply to compare total sample statistics at each point of data collection when one is assessing change (as opposed to the assessment of sample bias – see later), as these ignore the longitudinal nature of the data as well as sample dropout (and hence bias) and can mask underlying changes. For example, it might appear that the distributions of people with a scale score indicating depression are the same at each interval (e.g. 30 per cent score depressed at both baseline and follow-up assessment) – but are they the same people? Many of those categorised as depressed at baseline (interval 1) may have recovered by follow-up (interval 2) and a similar proportion of those categorised as not depressed at baseline may have become depressed by follow-up, with the result of producing similar overall distributions for depressed and not depressed sample members – but containing different sample members. 'Turnover tables' are needed, which provide a basic analysis of the percentage changes in all directions in a variable of interest (see Table 9.1 later).

Analyses of change can be complex where outcome measures produce more than one sub-score to reflect different dimensions of a concept (e.g. health-related quality of life, HRQoL), but not an overall score (e.g. Ware *et al.*'s 1993 SF-36). Statisticians prefer to compute simple summary measures of change for this reason, though this loses the complexity of the data. Billingham *et al.* (1999) suggest computing the maximum HRQoL score reached over time, or the change in HRQoL between two time points, or the slope representing the change over time for each individual. Withdrawn sample members may be included in the analyses in order to reduce bias if it is possible to impute appropriate quality of life values for them. Billingham *et al.* give the example of a quality of life measure on a 0–1 scale, with 0 representing a quality of life state equivalent to death, then withdrawals due to death could be allocated values of 0. One problem that they point out with such crude approaches is that the potential for change depends on the baseline value – and, arguably, the worse the respondent is at baseline, then the greater is the potential for improvement (e.g. patients who do not experience a symptom at baseline cannot improve). Quality of life measures usually result in more complex data, though the point about needing simple summary measures for the analysis to be manageable is important. Billingham *et al.* present examples of modelling techniques for longitudinal quality of life data from clinical trials.

Change scores

To assess the changes, a change score needs to be calculated for each sample member. These calculations can be complex in the case of multiple scale points when a new variable (change variable) needs to be created (e.g. to facilitate the use of certain analyses).

The issue of the best method of measuring change has not been resolved. Most commonly, the instrument's scores are compared before and after an intervention that is expected to affect the construct. As a check on validity, changes recorded by the instrument can also be compared with changes in other measures that are assumed to move in the same direction, and with patients' self-reported transition scores (e.g. better, same or worse in the case of health status). All scales require validated information indicating what the minimal important difference in scale scores is, in the assessment of change. This is a current issue in the interpretation of changes in scores on disease-specific and generic HRQoL scales and is still under investigation (e.g. Juniper *et al.* 1994).

Effect size and change scores

Effect size statistics test the relative magnitude of the differences between means, and describe the amount of total variance in the dependent variable that is predictable from information about the levels of the independent variable (Tabachnick and Fidell 1996). They provide an indication of the magnitude of differences between groups, or the magnitude of change (e.g. in health status) between assessment periods. They can also be used to judge the responsiveness to change of a measurement instrument – whether an instrument detects true change (see Chapter 7). Various methods of calculation are available. At the crudest level, in relation to the assessment of change, the 'after score' can be subtracted from the 'before score'. The use of such raw change or raw gain scores can be criticised primarily because such scores are systematically related to any random error of measurement (e.g. regression to the mean) (see Hemingway *et al.* 1997, for a method of calculation which takes regression to the mean into account).

This method also provides no information about the meaning of the change in score. For example, a loss of two supportive members from a social network between baseline and follow-up assessment would lead to a change score of −2. However, the meaning of this change to individuals is different depending on whether they started with only two supporters or whether they initially had four. Analyses of changes in continuous variables, computation and testing of average change scores and even significance testing for amount of change may provide little meaningful information if we do not take the baseline score into account.

The most commonly used method of calculating the effect size is to calculate the difference between mean scores at assessments, divided by the standard deviation of baseline scores. An effect size of 1.0 is equivalent to a change of one standard deviation in the study sample. Proposed benchmarks for assessing the relative magnitude of a change include: an effect size of 0.20 = small, 0.40–0.50 = medium and 0.80+ = large (Cohen 1977; Kazis *et al.* 1989). However, this method of calculating effect size has been criticised, and caution is needed when applying such cut-offs as it is possible for a sensitive instrument to obtain a large effect size for changes that can be subjectively interpreted as modest (Jenkinson and McGee 1998). Alternative measures of the responsiveness of an instrument, but which tap subtly different aspects of an instrument's change scores, have been proposed (Guyatt *et al.* 1987b; Liang *et al.* 1990; Juniper *et al.* 1994). These include standardised response mean (in contrast to the effect size calculation above, the denominator is the standard deviation of change scores rather than at baseline); modified standardised response mean (as with the above methods, the numerator is the mean group change score, but the denominator is the standard deviation of change scores for individuals who are identified independently as stable – this requires independent evidence, e.g. transition items of respondent-reported change at follow-up); relative efficiency (a comparison of the performance of different measures against a standard instrument in cases considered to have changed – in the case of health status, patients will have to complete several measures); sensitivity and specificity of change scores (assessment of the change in an instrument against an external standard of 'true' change in order to determine sensitivity and specificity); and receiver operating characteristic (ROC) curves. With the latter, information on sensitivity and specificity of an instrument as measured against an external standard is synthesised into ROC curves – a plot of the true positive rate (change) against the false positive rate for all cut-off points. The greater the total area under a plotted curve from all cut-off points, the greater the instrument's responsiveness (see Chapter 7). These different methods have been described clearly by Jenkinson and McGee (1998) and Fitzpatrick *et al.* (1998).

Transition items

Raw change scores should be supplemented with transition items as a validation check, in which respondents are asked directly about transitions. For example, they are asked to rate themselves as better, the same or worse in relation to the variable of interest (e.g. health), in comparison with their previous assessment. In this way, patient-based changes are assessed, though without three-way analyses the starting point is still unknown. One unresolved issue is whether patients should be provided with information about their previous assessments when making their assessments of change.

There is little information on the reliability and validity of transition indices, the extent of any regression to the mean (when comparing scores), the potential biasing effect of respondents' learning over time, becoming interested in the topic and learning from repeated tests.

Testing for change

At a basic level, the analysis of whether changes have occurred (turnover tables, see Table 9.1), the computation of change scores (mentioned earlier – the calculation of the difference between pre- and post-test scores) and the application of statistical tests to assess their significance are fairly straightforward. There are several parametric and non-parametric statistics available to test the significance of changes both within and between samples. There are also multivariate techniques of analysis, such as residualised change analysis, which are appropriate for estimating the effects of the independent variable on changes in the dependent variable between assessments/tests, as well as for testing for potential interactions between variables (see George *et al.* 1989).

However, as indicated earlier, it is important to understand the nature and meaning of any changes detected. Thus the complexity of longitudinal analyses is in the computation of meaningful change variables that can also be entered into bivariate and multivariate analyses. With dichotomous scores, or continuous scores with a cut-off point for 'caseness' (as with depression), it is relatively simple to create new variables on the

GHQ score	%	(no.)
Unchanged (non-cases[b]): non-cases in both years 0–5 in 1987 0–5 in 1990	60	(102)
Worsened non-case at baseline but case at follow-up 0–5 in 1987 6+ in 1990	13	(23)
Improved: case at baseline but non-case at follow-up 6+ in 1987 0–5 in 1990	12	(21)
Unchanged (persistent cases) 6+ at baseline 6+ at follow-up	15	(25)
No. of respondents		171

Source: The author's longitudinal survey on ageing (Bowling *et al.* 1996).
Notes: Wilcoxon matched pairs signed ranks test (two-tailed): no significant changes between 1987 and 1990.
[a]GHQ: Goldberg and Williams (1988).
[b]Case: psychological morbidity (mainly anxiety, depression).

Table 9.1 Turnover table. Changes in General Health Questionnaire (GHQ)[a] scores: 1987 and 1990 for the sample aged 85+ at baseline (survivors only)

computer which represent the meaning of the change (e.g. depressed at baseline and not depressed at follow-up). Other types of scores can be more complex to manage in relation to change analyses if they are not to appear superficial.

A typical turnover table is shown in Table 9.1. This study illustrated how a large sample size at the outset (over 600) can be substantially reduced by follow-up (in this case mainly through deaths), which is another factor to consider when deciding on sample sizes for longitudinal studies, particularly if the sample is initially one of older people. In the example given, the significance of the changes in the *raw scores* was tested using the Wilcoxon matched pairs signed ranks test (which is analogous to the paired *t*-test).

In the case of the author's study of people aged 85+, it was decided not to rely solely on the calculation of simple change scores (by subtracting the follow-up from the baseline score) as the resulting score provided no indication of respondents' starting point. The decision to create new variables with several 'change status' categories was worthwhile, as more meaningful and essential information was available about respondents' start and end-points on the variables of interest. Therefore, for the changes in continuous variables, without a single cut-off point, such as social support and network structure variables, changes across a range of defined scores were analysed separately using 'select if' procedures on SPSS (e.g. one network member at baseline and none by follow-up). Simpler change variables were also created for entry into bivariate and multivariate analyses, such as number of friends unchanged/increased/decreased (Bowling *et al.* 1996).

The next example is taken from the author's RCT of the evaluation of outcome of care of elderly people in nursing homes in comparison with long-stay hospital wards (Bowling *et al.* 1991). For this study, Mann–Whitney *U*-tests were used to test for simple differences in total confusion scores between respondents in each setting over four periods of assessment. This test is a non-parametric analogue of the two-sample *t*-tests. They were carried out on all respondents and repeated at each stage for the final survivor group only. They showed no significant differences between respondents in hospital and those in homes at each assessment period. However, using Wilcoxon matched pairs signed ranks tests, it was found that, when comparing change within each setting between each assessment period, significantly more of the nursing home respondents deteriorated than improved or remained the same over time (see Table 9.2).

Westermeyer (2013) reported predictors and characteristics of successful ageing among male students from a small Midwestern college, in the USA. Responding men were re-assessed by questionnaire at 32 years and 48 years follow-up. The authors reported on complete data for both years from 71 men, out of the 94 initially studied, in order to directly compare them at each follow-up, and assess changes. They presented direct comparisons of frequencies, means, standard deviations (SD) and correlations for both follow-up periods for the 71 men. A partial example is shown in Table 9.3.

There are a range of multivariate methods of longitudinal analysis, and authors adopt different approaches (for examples of traditional methods, see George *et al.* 1989; Kennedy *et al.* 1991a, 1991b; Miller and McFall 1991; Oxman *et al.* 1992; Bowling *et al.* 1996). Sophisticated methods exist for analysing longitudinal data in the social sciences and in epidemiology. For example, multi-level modelling (MLM) can be used to model *individual-level trends over time*, in which polynomial trends can be estimated for each respondent; this is referred to as *individual growth models.* Latent growth modelling (LGM) is another statistical technique, and used within the structural equation modelling (SEM) framework to estimate growth trajectory. It is a longitudinal analysis technique to estimate growth over a period

Comparison of assessment period	Mental confusion[a]	Hospital patients		Nursing home patients	
		No.	Mean rank	No.	Mean rank
1:2	Improved	10	9.20	4	6.13
	No change	10		6	
	Declined	12	13.42	24	15.90
	Total	32	ns	34	$Z = -4.064$ ($P < 0.001$)
1:3	Improved	11	12.41	7	10.00
	No change	1		8	
	Declined	16	15.09	14	11.50
	Total	28	ns	29	ns
1:4	Improved	8	8.13	2	5.00
	No change	11		9	
	Declined	11	11.36	16	10.06
	Total	30	ns	27	$Z = -3.288$ ($P < 0.001$)

Notes: Wilcoxon tests: two-tailed.
[a]Measured using the Crighton Royal Behavioural Rating Scale (Evans *et al.* 1981).
nsNot statistically significant.

Table 9.2 Change in mental confusion scores between assessments

of time. It is also called latent growth curve analysis. Latent growth modelling approaches are of value in identifying homogeneous sub-populations within the larger heterogeneous population, and for identifying meaningful groups or classes of individuals. Interested readers are referred to specialised explanations and examples of these methods (Bollen and Curran 2006; Jung and Wickrama 2008; Oi-Man Kwok *et al.* 2008).

Regression to the mean
It was pointed out earlier that the detection of any change in research participants as a result of an intervention, once intervening extraneous variables and any sampling biases

Outcome	32-year follow-up	48-year follow-up	
	Mean (SD)	Mean (SD)	*t*-statistic
Physical disability scale	1.90 (1.00)	2.90 (1.20)	6.10***
Overall social competence scale	6.80 (2.80)	6.32 (2.30)	1.79
Psychiatric symptoms scale	5.2 (4.10)	5.9 (5.10)	1.03

Note: *** $P < 0.001$.
Source: Westermeyer (2013, p. 332).

Table 9.3 Direct comparison of outcomes between 32- and 42-year follow-ups among 71 men (selective items shown)

have been ruled out, can always be due to *regression to the mean*. A regression artefact occurs when participants have an extreme measurement on a variable of interest, which is short-lived and may simply be owing to an unusual and temporary distraction. For example, an extremely poor depression score at pre-test may perhaps be entirely because of a sleepless night. On subsequent measurements, this value will tend to return to normal, and thus, in this example, the score appears to have improved at post-test but in fact has simply reverted to normal. Some respondents, then, may be at the upper or lower end of a measurement scale simply because of regular individual fluctuations. There may also be normal fluctuations in levels of the variable of interest, which makes the careful selection of measurement instruments, multiple data collection periods, the timing of data collection periods and comparison with control groups (natural controls in the case of longitudinal surveys and randomised control groups in the case of experiments) essential.

A good example is the measurement of blood pressure, as this varies hourly and daily. Thus, if some respondents are at the upper end when measured because of this fluctuation, then when they are measured again, they will have lower blood pressure. Similarly, if they were at the lower end when initially measured because of this fluctuation, when they are remeasured their blood pressure will be found to have increased. This is known as regressing to their mean levels (Yudkin and Stratton 1996). This is a common problem in other clinical studies of patients. Even the levels of various chemicals in the body can fluctuate naturally over time (e.g. chemicals which occur in response to malignant tumours), and any differences detected by measurements over time can reflect normal variations in levels rather than the hypothesised effects of the variable of interest (e.g. a new drug treatment).

Sample attrition and analysing change

In longitudinal study design there is the problem of sample attrition over time, leading to the 'healthy survivor effect' – the most vulnerable and ill members of a sample have died or dropped out, leaving the healthiest sample members for study, which will inevitably bias results. This can be an enormous problem with all topics (e.g. people who are depressed may be more likely to drop out, thus leaving the most psychologically healthy in the sample and thus artificially improving post-baseline psychological measurements; people who die by the time of follow-up in clinical trials thereby leave the healthiest remaining in the sample, again artificially improving follow-up results). Similar problems can occur where the least healthy members of the sample have not withdrawn but are more likely to have incomplete assessments (missing data). Either problem cannot be ignored in the analyses.

The rates of sample attrition may be affected by the length of the time period between survey waves, and the type of respondent included. This can be a sizeable problem in some longitudinal studies: for example, death will be a large source of attrition in longitudinal surveys of elderly people. The main reasons for withdrawal were summarised by Health (1995):

- respondents may move between waves and not be traced;
- elderly and ill people may drop out due to ill health or death;
- respondents who are uninterested in the study may not continue;
- some respondents will lack the cognitive skills required for some studies and drop out owing to the demands made on them;
- some respondents will drop out due to concerns over their invaded privacy or for a variety of other reasons.

Analyses dealing with missing data

Analyses of respondents with missing vital data are required, and comparisons made of those continuing in the study and those lost to it (at the latter's exit where possible) should be made in order to assess sample bias. Details of drop-outs (e.g. the reason and any further details) should be recorded with the date of withdrawal, and they should be included in the broader descriptive analyses where possible, along with their last reported health status. This will facilitate post-hoc analyses of the effects, for example, of impending death and frailty (where these are the reasons for the withdrawal) on the dependent variable of the study. Analyses should also be undertaken to assess whether respondents who withdrew from the study because they lost interest in it are different in any way to continuing respondents, thus biasing the results of the study (for examples of details of withdrawals and planned analyses, see Rabbitt *et al.* 1993).

In the case of withdrawal from the study due to death, methods of analysis which simultaneously assess quality of life and survival data need to be used. Billingham *et al.* (1999) have described their approaches to dealing with missing data on health-related quality of life (HRQoL) in cancer trials in detail. They described three methods for imputing missing data: (1) the last assessment value for HRQoL carried forward to the next data collection point (which assumes stable HRQoL status until date of death or withdrawal, whichever occurred first); (2) the worst value carried forward approach, which moves drop-outs into the poorest HRQoL state (which assumes withdrawal was due to the poorer state); and (3) linear decrease over time (which assumes HRQoL decreased linearly from drop-out date until death). They presented the problems inherent in each approach and suggested that the impact of different methods for imputation should be investigated in a sensitivity analysis; they selected the last value carried forward approach for their own study.

In the case of incomplete data from responding participants or missing data due to withdrawal from the study for reasons other than death, it may be possible to impute values from existing data (Little and Rubin 1987; Billingham *et al.* 1999).

Results should be compared over time for the *same* respondents who took part at each data collection stage (including the baseline stage), so that one is comparing 'like with like'. Respondents at each assessment period will be a subset of the original sample, with implications for sample bias. However, this approach will also have a biasing effect, in that the results will only relate to the healthy survivors. Thus, analyses should *also* (i.e. alongside) be carried out on those who dropped out at various stages in order to ascertain any differences between them and the remaining sample members, and in order to modify the potentially biasing effects of only analysing the survivors.

If sample attrition is small, and no biasing effects are detected, then a decision is occasionally made by investigators to include all respondents (at each stage) in the comparative analyses at each stage. If sample attrition is large, then comparisons at each stage must only be made using the same (surviving) members' earlier scores (excluding those who were lost to the study).

Descriptive analysis of longitudinal data should always be carried out first in order to gain insight into the data and inform further multivariate statistical analysis.

Cross-sectional comparisons of the sample sub-groups at each data collection point can be made to address relevant research questions (e.g. to what extent do treatment and control groups differ in relation to the variable of interest – e.g. HRQoL – at the specific assessment point?). These comparisons should be made cautiously as they are not the same as longitudinal assessments of change in the same individuals, and they ignore the longitudinal nature of the data. Care is also needed with the number of such analyses as multiple analyses undertaken may increase the likelihood of obtaining statistically significant differences due to chance (Billingham *et al.* 1999).

Rabbitt *et al.* (1993) collected data on the reasons for study members' withdrawal from their longitudinal study on cognitive performance and age, in addition to information on respondents' mortality rates and health status (provided by withdrawn respondents when they last participated in the study). This enabled them to carry out post-hoc analyses of the effects of impending death and increasing frailty on the amount and rate of cognitive change in older age. They could also analyse whether people who withdrew due to lack of interest in the study formed a significantly different sub-group to those who remained in the study. In Box 9.2 there is an example of how sample attrition was analysed and accounted for in the Rand Health Insurance Study, a longitudinal study involving the randomisation of respondents to different types of health insurance plans and effects on health outcome. It is often referred to as an experiment, along with its longitudinal survey approach, because it used the experimental method of random assignment between groups (insurance plans).

Box 9.2 The Rand Health Insurance Study: sample retention in the study

During the experiment, each plan lost some of its participants owing to voluntary withdrawal (including joining the military), involuntary factors (such as incarceration), health reasons (mainly by becoming eligible for disability Medicare), or death. The latter two health-related factors did not differ materially by plan . . . In all, 95 per cent of those on the free plan completed the experiment and exited normally by completing the MHQ and going through the final screening examination, as did 88 per cent of those on the individual deductible plan, 90 per cent on the intermediate plans, and 85 per cent on the catastrophic plans.

To test whether these differences affected our results, we collected data on general health measures and smoking behavior of people who had terminated for various reasons. Our findings were not altered by including or excluding these data, which were obtained from 73 per cent of those who withdrew voluntarily, 83 per cent of those who terminated for health reasons, 82 per cent of those who terminated for nonhealth reasons, and 78 per cent of those who were reported to have died. Thus, reported results include data from these individuals, and the final sample for the questionnaire-based analyses comprises 99 per cent of the participants on the free and intermediate plans, 97 per cent of those on the catastrophic plan, and 95 per cent of those on the individual deductible plan. The percentages with complete data on physiologic measures (as well as weight) are lower because no post-enrolment screening examination was administered to the participants who left the experiment early.

As a further check for possible bias, we examined the values for health status at enrolment in the actual sample used for each analysis. We detected no significant differences by plan.

(Brook *et al.* 1984)

Stopping rules and analysis of interim results

Finally, the debate on stopping rules includes philosophical and ethical issues (e.g. as in cases when longitudinal experimental trials of treatment are ended prematurely because of the adverse effects of the experimental treatment on patients). Some experiments continue without any formal aims or rules about when to stop collecting and analysing data. This is less of a problem with large longitudinal surveys as it is so expensive and difficult to mount each follow-up wave and each wave requires financial and theoretical justification.

Some studies are also published prematurely (e.g. interim results). The problem with such ongoing analyses is that investigators are usually tempted to publish results which show differences between groups; these results may simply be owing to a random 'high' in the population of interest, and subsequently there is regression to the mean which is reflected in later analyses showing a reduction in the magnitude of the differences between groups. For example, Rand were tempted to publish the initial results of their large-scale health insurance study experiment, which showed that people randomised to free health care plans appeared to have slightly improved health outcomes on a range of health status indicators. These results were not borne out in the main study, except among low income groups who had health problems on entry to the study (Brook *et al.* 1984; Lohr *et al.* 1986; Ware *et al.* 1987). A policy on publication should be stated at the outset of research, and adhered to unless exceptional circumstances dictate otherwise, in order to avoid publication of misleading results. The policy should include the rules for the reporting of interim results (e.g. taking into account the significance level required, and confirmation of results by triangulated methods).

There are a number of practical issues with premature publication, such as the biasing effect on ongoing participants in the study, and statistical issues, given that the more statistical tests that are conducted throughout the study, the greater the risk of chance differences being observed. The debates are described by Pocock (1983) and Sackett and Naylor (1993).

Summary of main points

- Surveys can be carried out cross-sectionally (at one point in time) or longitudinally (at more than one point in time).
- Cross-sectional surveys are appropriate for producing descriptive data, and longitudinal surveys, if the study periods are appropriately timed, are appropriate for addressing analytic questions of cause and effect.
- If a population has a common experience or characteristic which defines the sampling, it is known as a cohort study.
- It is misleading to compare total sample statistics at each point of data collection in longitudinal studies for the analysis of change, as these can mask underlying changes. Turnover tables are required.
- It is important to analyse the change in *magnitude* in the variable of interest in each group of interest between baseline and follow-up measurements, and compare it with the magnitude of the difference between groups on that measurement at baseline.
- The problem of regression to the mean occurs when participants have an extreme measurement on a variable of interest, which is short-lived and may simply be owing to an unusual and temporary distraction, or normal fluctuations.

■ In order to test for the 'healthy survivor effect', details of drop-outs (e.g. health status, deaths) should be recorded with the date, and included in the broader descriptive analyses. Analyses of respondents with missing vital data are also required.

Key questions

1 When are cross-sectional and longitudinal survey methods appropriate?
2 Distinguish between panel and trend surveys.
3 Define 'cohort'.
4 What is triangulation of research methods?
5 What are the main reasons for sample attrition?
6 What is regression to the mean?
7 Define effect size.
8 What are the main difficulties in analysing change in results from longitudinal surveys?
9 Explain the 'healthy survivor effect'.

Key terms

change score
cohort
cross-sectional survey
descriptive study
effect size
healthy survivor effect
longitudinal survey
magnitude of change
panel survey
prospective
regression to mean

retrospective
reverse causation
sample attrition
secondary data analysis
survey
transition score
trend survey
triangulated methods
turnover table
unobtrusive methods

Recommended reading

Billingham, L.J., Abrams, K.R. and Jones, D.R. (1999) Methods for the analysis of quality-of-life and survival data in health technology assessment, *Health Technology Assessment*, 3(10).

Fowler, F.J. (2009) *Survey Research Methods*. Thousand Oaks, CA: Sage.

Groves, R.M., Fowler, F.J., Couper, M.P. *et al.* (2009) *Survey Methodology*. Chichester: John Wiley.

Lee, R.M. (2000) *Unobtrusive Methods in Social Research*. Buckingham: Open University Press.

Pocock, S.J. (1983) *Clinical Trials: A Practical Approach*. Chichester: Wiley.

Shaw, M. (2005) Finding and using secondary data on the health and health care of populations, in A. Bowling and S. Ebrahim (eds) *Handbook of Health Research Methods: Investigation, Measurement and Analysis*. Maidenhead: Open University Press.

Webb, E.J., Campbell, D.T., Schwartz, R.D. and Sechrest, L. (1966) *Unobtrusive Measures: Nonreactive Research in the Social Sciences*. Chicago: Rand McNally College Publishing Company.

CHAPTER 10

Quantitative research: experiments and other analytic methods of investigation

Chapter contents

Introduction

The accurate assessment of the outcome, or effects, of an intervention necessitates the careful manipulation of that intervention (experimental variable), in controlled conditions, and a comparison of the group receiving the intervention with an equivalent control group. It is essential that systematic errors (bias) and random errors (chance) are minimised. This requirement necessitates carefully designed, rigorously carried out studies, using reliable and valid methods of measurement, and with sufficiently large samples of participants who are representative of the target population. This chapter describes the range of methods available, along with their strengths and weaknesses.

The experimental method

The experiment is a situation in which the *independent variable* (also known as the exposure, the intervention, the experimental or predictor variable) is carefully manipulated by the investigator under known, tightly defined and controlled conditions, or by natural occurrence.

At its most basic, the experiment consists of an *experimental group* which is exposed to the intervention under investigation and a control group which is not exposed. The experimental and control groups should be equivalent, and investigated systematically under conditions that are identical (apart from the exposure of the experimental group), in order to minimise variation between them.

Origins of the experimental method

The earliest recorded experiment is generally believed to be found in the Old Testament. The strict diet of meat and wine, which King Nebuchadnezzar II ordered to be followed for three years, was not adhered to by four royal children who ate pulses and drank water instead. The latter group remained healthy while others soon became ill. Trials of new therapies are commonly thought to have originated with Ambroise Paré in 1537, in which he mixed oil of rose, turpentine and egg yolk as a replacement formula for the treatment of wounds, and noted the new treatment to be more effective. Most people think of James Lind as the originator of more formal clinical trials as he was the first documented to have included control groups in his studies on board ships at sea in 1747. He observed that seamen who suffered from scurvy who were given a supplemented diet, including citrus fruits, recovered for duty, compared with those with scurvy on their usual diets who did not. Clinical trials using placebo treatments (an inactive or inert substance) in the control groups then began to emerge from 1800; and trials using techniques of randomising patients between treatment and control arms developed from the early twentieth century onwards (see documentation of developments on www.healthandage.com/html/res/clinical_trials/).

Dehue (2001) traced the later historical origins of psycho-social experimentation using randomised controlled designs. In a highly readable account, she placed the changing definition of social experiments firmly in the era of social reform, with the mid- to late-eighteenth- and early nineteenth-century concerns about child poverty, slum clearance, minimum wage bills and unemployment insurance in the USA and Europe. In this context, it was argued by free marketers that, if government or private money was to be spent on the public good, then there was a need to demonstrate proof of benefit and change of behaviour. This led to appeals by government administrations to the social sciences, who adapted to these demands, and moved away from their free reasoning, reflective approaches towards instrumental, standardised knowledge and objectivity (Porter 1986). Among the psychologists who became involved with administrative research was Thurstone (1952) who had developed scales for measuring attitudes. Strict methodological rigour became the norm and experiments were designed (typically with school children) which compared experimental and control groups of people (Dehue 2000). By the end of the 1920s in the USA, 'administrative' social scientists had a high level of political influence and social authority, and social science was flourishing. US researchers adopted Fisher's (1935) techniques of testing for statistical significance, and his emphasis that random allocation to groups was the valid application of his method. This culminated in Campbell's (1969) now classic publication on the need for an experimental approach to social reform. Despite increasing disquiet about the threats to validity in social experiments (Cook and Campbell 1979), and calls to include both value and facts in evaluations (Cronbach 1987), in the 1970s and 1980s, the Ford Foundation supported randomised controlled experiments with 65,000 recipients of welfare in 20 US states (see Dehue 2001, for further details and references).

The true experiment

Two features mark the *true* (or classic) experiment: two or more differently treated groups (*experimental* and *control*), and the *random (chance) assignment* ('randomisation') of participants to experimental and control groups (Moser and Kalton 1971; Dooley 1995). This requirement necessitates that the investigator has control over the independent variable as well as the power to place participants into the groups.

Ideally, the experiment will also include a *pre-test* (before the intervention, or manipulation of the independent variable) and a *post-test* (after the intervention) for the experimental and control groups. The testing may include the use of interviews, self-administered questionnaires, diaries, abstraction of data from medical records, bio-chemical testing, assessment (e.g. clinical), and so on. Observation of the participants can also be used. Pre- and post-testing are necessary in order to be able to measure the effects of the intervention on the experimental group and the direction of any associations.

There are also methods of improving the basic experimental design to control for the reactive effects of pre-testing (Solomon four group method) and to use all possible types of controls to increase the external validity of the research (complete factorial experiment). These are described in Chapter 11.

However, 'pre- and post-testing' are not always possible and 'post-test' only approaches are used in these circumstances. Some investigators use a pre-test retrospectively to ask people about their circumstances before the intervention in question (e.g. their health status before emergency surgery). However, it is common for retrospective pre-tests to be delayed in many cases, and recall bias then becomes a potential problem. For example, in studies of the effectiveness of emergency surgery, people may be too ill to be questioned until some time after the event (e.g. accident) or intervention. Griffiths *et al.* (1998) coined the term 'perioperative' to cover slightly delayed pre-testing in studies of the effectiveness of surgery.

Terminology in the social and clinical sciences

In relation to terminology, social scientists simply refer to the *true* experimental method. In research aiming to evaluate the effectiveness of health technologies, the true experimental method is conventionally referred to as the randomised controlled trial (RCT). 'Trial' simply means 'experiment'. Clinical scientists often refer to both randomised and non-randomised experiments evaluating new treatments as *clinical trials*, and their most rigorously conducted experiments are known as phase III trials (see Chapter 11 for definitions of phase I–IV trials). 'Clinical trial' simply means an experiment with patients as participants. Strictly, however, for clinical trials to qualify for the description of a true experiment, random allocation between experimental and control groups is required.

The advantages of random allocation

Random allocation between experimental and control groups means that study participants (or other unit – e.g. clinics) are allocated to the groups in such a way that each has an equal chance of being allocated to either group. Random allocation is not the same as random sampling (random sampling is the selection (sampling) of people (or other unit of interest – e.g. postal sectors, hospitals, clinics) from a defined population of interest in such a way that each person (unit) has the same chance of being selected).

Any sample of people is likely to be made up of more heterogeneous characteristics than can be taken into account in a study. If some extraneous variable which can confound the results (e.g. age of participants) happens to be unevenly distributed between experimental and control groups, then the study might produce results which would not be obtained if the study was repeated with another sample (i.e. differences between groups in the outcome measured). Extraneous, confounding variables can also mask 'true' differences in the target population (see also 'Epidemiology', Chapter 4).

Only random allocation between groups can safeguard against bias in these allocations and minimise differences between groups of people being compared (even for characteristics that the investigator has not considered), thereby facilitating comparisons. Random allocation will reduce the 'noise' effects of extraneous, confounding variables on the ability of the study to detect true differences, if any, between the study groups. It increases the probability that any differences observed between the groups are owing to the experimental variable.

By randomisation, true experiments will control not only for *group-related threats* (by randomisation to ensure similarity for valid comparisons), but also for *time-related threats* (e.g. effects of *history* – events unrelated to the study which might affect the results) and even participant *fatigue* (known as motivation effects) and the *internal validity* (truth of a study's conclusion that the observed effect is owing to the independent variable) of the results.

Overall advantages of true experiments

True experiments possess several advantages, which include the following:

- Through the random assignment of people to intervention and control groups (i.e. randomisation of extraneous variables) the risk of extraneous variables confounding the results is minimised.
- Control over the introduction and variation of the 'predictor' variables clarifies the direction of cause and effect.

- If both pre- and post-testing are conducted, this controls for time-related threats to validity.
- The modern design of experiments permits greater flexibility, efficiency and powerful statistical manipulation.
- The experiment is the only research design which can, in principle, yield causal relationships.

Overall disadvantages of true experiments

In relation to human beings, and the study of their circumstances, the experimental method also poses several difficulties, including the following:

- It is difficult to design experiments so as to represent a specified population.
- It is often difficult to choose the 'control' variables so as to exclude all confounding variables.
- With a large number of uncontrolled, extraneous variables it is impossible to isolate the one variable that is hypothesised as the cause of the other; hence, the possibility always exists of alternative explanations.
- Contriving the desired 'natural setting' in experiments is often not possible.
- The experiment is an unnatural social situation with a differentiation of roles; the participant's role involves obedience to the experimenter (an unusual role).
- Experiments cannot capture the diversity of goals, objectives and service inputs which may contribute to health care outcomes in natural settings (Nolan and Grant 1993).

An experiment can only be performed when the independent variable can be brought under the control of the experimenter in order that it can be manipulated, and when it is ethically acceptable for the experimenter to do this. Consequently, it is not possible to investigate most important social issues within the confines of experimental design. However, a range of other analytical designs are available, which are subject to known errors, and from which causal inferences may be made with a certain degree of certitude, and their external validity may be better than that of many pure experimental situations. Some of these were described in relation to epidemiological methods in Chapter 4, and others are described in this chapter.

Internal and external validity

The effect of these problems is that what the experimenter says is going on may not be going on. If the experimenter can validly infer that the results obtained were owing to the influence of the experimental variable (i.e. the independent variable affected the dependent variable), then the experiment has *internal validity*. Experiments, while they may isolate a variable which is necessary for an effect, do not necessarily isolate the sufficient conditions for the effect. The experimental variable may interact with other factors present in the experimental situation to produce the effect (see 'Epidemiology', Chapter 4). In a natural setting, those other factors may not be present. In relation to humans, the aim is to predict behaviour in natural settings over a wide range of populations, therefore experiments need to have ecological validity. When it is possible to *generalise* the results to this wider setting, then *external validity* is obtained. Campbell and Stanley (1963, 1966) have listed the common threats to internal and external validity.

Reactive effects

The study itself could have a reactive effect and the process of testing may change the phenomena being measured (e.g. attitudes, behaviour, feelings). Indeed, a classic law of physics is that the very fact of observation changes that which is being observed. People may become more interested in the study topic and change in some way. This is known as the 'Hawthorne effect', whereby the experimental group changes as an effect of being treated differently. (See Box 10.1.)

Box 10.1 Hawthorne's study

The Hawthorne effect is named after a study from 1924 to 1933 of the effects of physical and social conditions on workers' productivity in the Hawthorne plant of the Western Electricity Company in Chicago (Roethlisberger and Dickson 1939). The study involved a series of quasi-experiments on different groups of workers in different settings and undertaking different tasks. It was reported that workers increased their productivity in the illumination experiment after each experimental manipulation, regardless of whether the lighting was increased or decreased. It was believed that these odd increases in the Hawthorne workers' observed productivity were simply due to the attention they received from the researchers (reactive effects of being studied). Subsequent analyses of the data, however, showed associations in study outcomes to be associated with personnel changes and to external events such as the Great Depression (Franke and Kaul 1978). These associations have also been subject to criticism (Bloombaum 1983; see also Dooley 1995). Thus, despite Hawthorne and reactive effects being regarded as synonymous terms, there is no empirical support for the reactive effects in the well-known Hawthorne study on workers' productivity.

Despite the controversy surrounding the interpretation of the results from the Hawthorne study, pre-tests can affect the responsiveness of the experimental group to the treatment or intervention because they have been sensitised to the topic of interest. People may remember their pre-test answers on questionnaires used and try to repeat them at the post-test stage, or they may simply be improving owing to the experience of repeated tests. Intelligence tests and knowledge tests raise such problems (it is known that scores on intelligence tests improve the more tests people take and as they become accustomed to their format). The use of control groups allows this source of invalidity to be evaluated, as both groups have the experience.

Even when social behaviour (e.g. group cohesion) can be induced in a laboratory setting, the results from experiments may be subject to error owing to the use of inadequate measurement instruments or bias owing to the presence of the investigator. Participants may try to look good, normal or well. They may even feel suspicious. Human participants pick up clues from the experimenter and the experiment and attempt to work out the hypothesis. Then, perhaps owing to 'evaluation apprehension' (anxiety generated in subjects by virtue of being tested), they behave in a manner consistent with their perception of the hypothesis in an attempt to please the experimenter and cooperatively ensure that the hypothesis is confirmed. These biases are known as 'demand characteristics'.

There is also potential bias owing to the expectations of the experimenter ('experimenter bias' or 'experimenter expectancy effect') (Rosenthal 1976). Experimenters who are conscious of the effects they desire from individuals have been shown to communicate their expectations unintentionally to subjects (e.g. by showing relief or tension) and bias their responses in the direction of their desires (Rosenthal *et al*. 1963; Gracely *et al*. 1985). The result is that the effects observed are produced only partly, or not at all, by the experimental variable. These problems have been described by Rosenberg (1969). This experimenter bias, and how to control for it, are discussed later under 'Blind experiments'. There are further problems when individual methods are used to describe an experiment to potential participants in the same study, with unknown consequences for agreement to participate and bias. Jenkins *et al*. (1999) audiotaped the discussions between doctor and patient (*n* = 82) in which consent was being obtained in an RCT of cancer treatment. They reported that while, in most cases, doctors mentioned the uncertainty of treatment decisions, and in most cases this was raised in a general sense, in 15 per cent of cases, personal uncertainty was mentioned. The word randomisation was mentioned in 62 per cent of the consultations, and analogies were used in 34 per cent of cases to describe the randomisation process; treatments and side-effects were described in 83 per cent of cases, but information leaflets were not given to 28 per cent of patients. Patients were rarely told that they could leave the study at any time and still be treated. This variation could affect recruitment rates to trials.

Pre-testing and the direction of causal hypotheses

The aim of the experiment is to exclude, as far as possible, plausible rival hypotheses, and to be able to determine the direction of associations in order to make causal inferences.

To assess the effect of the intervention there should be one or more pre-tests (undertaken before the intervention) of both groups and one or more post-tests of both groups, taken after the experimental group has been exposed to the intervention. The measurement of the dependent variable before and after the independent variable has been 'fixed' deals with the problem of *reverse causation*. This relates to the difficulty of separating the direction of cause and effect, which is a major problem in the interpretation of cross-sectional data (collected at one point in time). If the resulting observations differ between groups, then it is inferred that the difference is caused by the intervention or exposure. Ideally the experiment will have multiple measurement points before and after the experimental intervention (a *time series* study). The advantage is the ability to distinguish between the regular and irregular, the temporary and persistent trends stemming from the experimental intervention.

The credibility of causal inferences also depends on: the adequate control of any extraneous variables which might have led to spurious associations and confounded the results; the soundness of the details of the study design; the demonstration that the intervention took place before the measured effect (thus the accurate timing of the measurements is vital); and the elimination of potential for *measurement decay* (changes in the way the measuring instruments were administered between groups and time periods). Caution still needs to be exercised in interpreting the study's results, as there may also be *regression to the mean*. This refers to statistical artefact. If individuals, by chance or owing to measurement error, have an extreme score on the dependent variable on pre-testing, it is likely that they will have a score at post-test which is closer to the population average. The discussion in Chapter 9 on this and other aspects of longitudinal methods also applies to experimental design with pre- and post-tests.

Timing of follow-up measures

As with longitudinal surveys, the timing of the post-test in experiments needs to be carefully planned in order to establish the direction of observed relationships and to detect expected changes at appropriate time periods: for example, one, three or six months, or one year. There is little point in administering a post-test to assess recovery at one month if the treatment is not anticipated to have any effect for three months (unless, for example, earlier toxic or other effects are being monitored). Post-test designs should adopt the same principles as longitudinal study design, and can suffer from the same difficulties (see Chapter 9).

It is also important to ensure that any early changes (e.g. adverse effects) owing to the experimental variable (e.g. a new medical treatment) are documented, as well as longer-term changes (e.g. recovery). Wasson *et al.* (1995) carried out an RCT comparing immediate transurethral prostatic resection (TURP) with watchful waiting in men with benign prostatic hyperplasia. Patients were initially followed up after six to eight weeks, and then half-yearly for three years. This example indicates that such study designs, with regular follow-ups, not only require careful planning but are likely to be expensive (see Chapter 9).

Sample attrition

Sample attrition refers to loss of sample members before the post-test phases, which can be a serious problem in the analysis of data from experiments. The similarity of experimental and control groups may be weakened if sample members drop out of the study before the post-tests, which affects the comparability of the groups.

The Diabetes Integrated Care Evaluation Team (Naji 1994) carried out an RCT to evaluate integrated care between GPs and hospitals in comparison with conventional hospital clinic care for patients with diabetes. This was a well-designed trial that still suffered from substantial, but probably not untypical, sample loss during the study. Patients were recruited for the trial when they attended for routine clinic appointments. Consenting patients were then stratified by treatment (insulin or other) and randomly allocated to conventional clinic care or to integrated care. Although their eventual sample size of 274 out of 311 patients considered for inclusion (27 were excluded by trial exclusion criteria and 10 refused to take part) still gave 80 per cent power of detecting, at the 5 per cent level of significance – a difference between the groups equivalent to 33 per cent of the standard deviation – there was yet more sample loss before the study was finished and just 235 patients completed the trial: A total of 135 patients were allocated to conventional care and 139 were allocated to integrated care. During the two years of the trial 21 patients died (10 in conventional care and 11 in integrated care). A total of 14 patients (10 per cent) in conventional care were lost to follow-up through repeated failure to attend. Sample attrition is discussed further in Chapters 9 and 11.

Reducing bias in participants and the investigating team

If the patient in a clinical trial is aware that he or she is receiving a new treatment, there may be a psychological benefit that affects his or her response. The reverse may be true if patients know they are receiving standard treatments and others are receiving new treatments. The treating team may also be biased by the treatments – for example, if patients are known to be receiving a new treatment then they may be observed by the clinical team more closely, and this can affect the patients' response to treatment, and hence the results of the trial may be biased.

Placebo (dummy) group

The word 'placebo' comes from the Latin meaning 'I shall please'. By the end of the eighteenth century it was being used to indicate a medicine, and from the beginning of the nineteenth century it was used to indicate a medicine intended to 'please' the patient rather than benefit them. From 1933, it was used to describe an inert treatment given to a control group, against which to measure the effectiveness of the active treatment given to the experimental group. Placebo groups, then, control for the psychological effects of treatment (as some people respond to placebo treatment). Psychological theories postulate that individuals expect the stimulus to be associated with a successful intervention and thus even inert substances have been reported to be associated with symptom relief. For example, in a drug trial the placebo effects derive from the participants' expectation that a pill will make them feel better (or different). However, a systematic review and analysis of 114 trials in 40 medical conditions, in which patients were randomised to placebo or no treatment, indicated that the evidence for a placebo effect was weak (Hröbjartsson and Gøtzsche 2001).

Ross and Olson (1981) summarised the placebo effect as: the direction of the placebo effects parallels the effects of the drug/intervention under investigation; the strength of the placebo effect is proportional to that of the active drug/treatment; the reported side-effects of the placebo and the active drug/treatment are often similar; and the times needed for both to become active are often similar. The placebo group, then, does not receive the experimental intervention (e.g. treatment), and instead receives an inert substance/intervention designed to appear the same, but which has no physiological effect. This is regarded as an important method of controlling for the psychological effect of being treated. It aims to make the participants' attitudes in each group as similar as possible. The investigator needs to demonstrate that the intervention (i.e. treatment) will lead to a greater response than would be expected if it was simply a placebo effect.

The type of control group used to make comparisons with the experimental group can raise ethical issues. It is often regarded as unethical to have a placebo group that receives a dummy treatment, or in effect no treatment, particularly when it is believed that an alternative treatment to the experimental treatment is likely to have some beneficial effect. Thus, in some trials the control group consists of a group receiving standard treatment and there is no real placebo (no treatment) group. It could also be argued that there is little *practical* benefit in comparing an experimental group with a placebo group when a standard treatment is available. An example of questionable ethical practice in the use of placebo treatments has been provided by an RCT in the USA for treatment of Parkinson's disease. The experimental treatment involves trepanning (drilling or boring holes) into the skulls of patients with Parkinson's disease, and the implantation of foetal brain cells through the holes. The aim was to promote the production of dopamine, in which sufferers of Parkinson's disease are deficient. The control group patients were also trepanned, but they did not receive the implantation of the cells through the holes in their skulls. Thus, the control patients received 'sham surgery', which would be regarded as unethical by some (Week 2001).

Some investigators in trials of medical interventions randomise patients to the treatment group or to the waiting list as the placebo. This is seen as ethical where long waiting lists exist. However, it is possible that the waiting list group might seek help for their problems elsewhere while on the waiting list (e.g. from psychotherapists, osteopaths, acupuncturists, herbalists) and thus they become non-comparable with the experimental group. The same problem can sometimes arise if patients are randomised to a no-treatment group, even if they are ignorant ('blind') about which group they have been assigned to: if they perceive the 'treatment' to be less effective than expected they may seek alternatives.

Blind experiments

It was pointed out earlier that bias owing to the expectancy of the patient, the treating professional and the investigator can contaminate results. There is likely to be an attachment to the hypothesis that the experimental treatment is more effective than the placebo treatment. It is known from studies in psychology that investigators (and also treating practitioners) can unconsciously influence the behaviour of the participants in the experiment (both human and animal) by, for example, paying more attention, or more positive attention (e.g. smiling), to the members of the experimental group. The methods for dealing with this are maintaining the ignorance of participants, professionals (e.g. treating practitioners) and assessors about which group the participant has been assigned to (known as 'blinding' or 'masking'), and assessors' effects are eliminated by excluding personal interaction with participants (e.g. they receive standardised letters, written or tape-recorded instructions and self-completion questionnaires).

Ideally, then, *each* participant is 'blind' and none of the directly involved parties knows which group the study members have been allocated to (study or control) in order to eliminate bias from assessments. This is known as a double-blind trial. If the investigator, but not the participant, knows the allocation, this is known as single-blind. When all parties are aware of the allocation the study is described as open. Blind studies are easier to organise for drug trials (where a pharmacist can arrange drug packages for a randomisation list; or sealed envelopes containing the drugs/prescriptions can be used) but they are obviously impossible in other more interventionist situations (e.g. open surgery versus keyhole surgery). The methodological processes have been described by Pocock (1983). Blinding in relation to RCTs is discussed further in the next section.

The RCT in health care evaluation

The discussion on the advantages and disadvantages of true experiments at the beginning of this chapter apply to the RCT, which is the classic experimental method. This section explores its use in relation to the evaluation of health care.

It was pointed out earlier that the RCT involves the *random* allocation of participants (e.g. patients) between experimental group(s), whose members receive the treatment or other intervention, and control group(s), whose members receive a standard or placebo (dummy) treatment. It is standard practice to use a random number table for the allocation (see Pocock 1983). The outcome of the groups is compared. It was also mentioned previously that, ideally, the investigators and participants do not know (are 'blind') to which group the participants have been allocated. Even if the study has to be open ('non-blind'), it is important that the investigator, and not any of the professionals involved in the care of the patient, conducts the randomisation in order to ensure that chance, rather than choice, determines the allocation procedure. However, there is evidence that relatively few published clinical trials which could have been double-blinded were carried out double-blind, that randomised clinical trials which are not double-blind can exaggerate the estimate of effectiveness by about 17 per cent and that non-randomised clinical studies can exaggerate the estimates of effectiveness by about 40 per cent (Schultz et al. 1995, 1996).

A distinction also needs to be made between pragmatic trials (in which patients are analysed according to the group to which they were randomised, regardless of their adherence to therapy – or 'intention to treat') and explanatory trials (in which patient adherence is taken into account by excluding non-adherers from analysis, or analysing the data according to the treatment actually received, but making allowance for the extent of adherence). The latter approach limits the external validity (generalisability) of the data when making inferences about the effectiveness of clinical practice in the real world. Thus pragmatic trials are designed to evaluate the effectiveness of interventions in real-life situations, and explanatory trials aim to test whether an intervention works under optimal conditions. As most results from exploratory trials fail to be broadly generalisable, the 'pragmatic design' has gained momentum. The generalisability of pragmatic trials can also be questioned as how comparable are clinical settings between populations and countries? Evidence of a treatment's effectiveness or ineffectiveness in a given setting does not guarantee that it will also be effective in a different one. Moreover, the distinction between an explanatory and a pragmatic trial in reality is not always straightforward as most trials have both explanatory and pragmatic aspects (Patsopoulos 2011).

Appropriateness of the paradigm of the true experiment (RCT) in health care evaluation

The true experiment is the paradigm of the scientific method (Campbell and Stanley 1966), and natural scientists have made rapid advances through its use. There has been a tendency in research on health and health services to follow as precisely as possible the paradigm developed for the natural sciences – i.e. one which proceeds by exposing the participant to various conditions and observing the differences in reaction. This also makes the implicit, positivist assumption that the active role of the participant in the experiment is a passive responder ('subject') to stimuli, which is difficult to justify in relation to conscious beings.

It should be noted that much of clinical and biological science is based not just on the methods of the true experiment, but on the simple observation of small (non-random) samples of material (e.g. analysis of blood samples from the patient group of interest), using non-randomised controls. Although its investigators are faced with problems of generalisability, over time a body of knowledge is gradually accumulated. Contrary to popular belief, the ability to meet the necessary requirements of *reproducibility* and *ecological validity* (realism of results outside the research setting) for meaningful experimentation is not just a problem in the social sciences and in research on health and health services. In theory, the true experiment is the method of choice for comparing the effectiveness of different interventions (e.g. health technologies). However, while other scientific disciplines routinely use and respect a wide range of research methods, from simple observation to the true experiment, investigators of health and health services increasingly strive single-mindedly to use the true experiment. It is not always possible to use this method in real-life settings, and investigators often fail to appreciate the value of data that can be obtained using other methods.

Problems with RCTs in evaluating health care

The general problems of experiments were discussed earlier. This section focuses specifically on those conducted in health care. Checklists and quality assessment tools for the structured reporting of RCTs have been published in order to enhance clarity and transparency. The Consolidated Standards of Reporting Trials Statement (CONSORT) (Moher *et al.* 2001) provided a checklist of items to include when reporting the results from trials, including the title and abstract of the study, the introduction and methods (including sampling, method of randomisation and statistical methods), the results (including recruitment and numbers analysed) and the comments (including interpretation and generalisability). The updated version of this is the CONSORT 2010 Statement, which consists of a 25-item checklist and participant flow diagram (Schulz *et al.* 2010; Moher *et al.* 2010). The checklist items focus on reporting how the trial was designed, analysed, and interpreted; the flow diagram displays the progress of all participants through the trial. The Statement has been translated into several languages. Numerous enhanced checklists have also been published (Hopewell *et al.* 2008; Beller *et al.* 2013). Checklists also exist to enhance reporting of epidemiological observational studies (von Elm *et al.* 2007). All checklists, however, have weaknesses.

Randomisation does not preclude the possibility that the population randomised between groups may be atypical of the wider population of interest. For this possibility to be minimised, the population to be randomised must first be randomly sampled from the population of interest, for example, by using equal probability sampling. In practice, this is rare, and in many cases impossible or highly impractical. While an ideal method for testing hypotheses, it is easy to find examples where randomisation is not a feasible method in the real world. Investigators tend to select the population for randomisation from easily accessible groups, potentially reducing the study's external validity (generalisability).

In addition, the health care professionals who are willing to participate in RCTs, and refer their patients to the study, may also be unrepresentative of the rest of their profession. The setting itself may also be atypical. For example, the setting might be composed of consultants performing surgery in teaching hospitals, whereas in real life the surgery is performed by doctors in training grades in both teaching and non-teaching hospitals (Black 1996).

RCTs are extremely difficult to set up in health care because there is often professional resistance to them. Professionals may be reluctant to offer the experimental treatment to their patients or to compare their service/treatment with those of others. There can be difficulties in obtaining ethical consent and there may be political and legal obstacles (Black 1996). The small numbers referred for treatment may make a trial impossible, and then unethical, in terms of the long and expensive trial period required (Greenfield 1989). This is where multicentre trials are advantageous, as patients can be pooled. Particularly large numbers will be required if the study aims to establish whether any rare, adverse effects of a particular treatment exist. For example, one RCT of non-steroid preparations in North America recruited almost 9000 men and women in almost 700 medical practices in order to assess potential complications (Silverstein *et al.* 1995). A common problem is the failure to recruit patients within the targeted time frame. Although the reasons for this are unclear, they may include constraints on clinical time, lack of available staff, impact on clinical autonomy, clinical commitment to, and understanding of, the trial, motivation, a sense of ownership, confidence about handling the clinical procedures, good management, communication and groundwork, flexibility and robustness within the trial to adapt to unexpected issues, the complexity of the trial procedures, the importance of the clinical question, and the esteem of the trialists (see review by Campbell *et al.* 2007).

As was indicated earlier in relation to experiments, randomised controlled trials are necessarily conducted under such controlled conditions (e.g. more careful observation of patients) that the conditions may bear little resemblance to common practice. A systematic review of randomised and non-randomised intervention studies, for a range of surgical, pharmacological, organisational and preventive interventions showed that, overall, they did not differ in relation to their estimates of treatment effects (Britton *et al.* 1998). However, a review of more basic follow-up studies has shown that complication rates of treatments reported can be three times the rates reported in RCTs (Brook 1992).

Black (1996) described a wide range of limitations with RCTs. He pointed to four situations in which RCTs may be inappropriate:

1 They are rarely large enough to measure accurately infrequent, adverse outcomes of medical treatment.
2 They are rarely able to evaluate interventions designed to prevent rare events, again owing to inadequate sample size.
3 They are rarely able to evaluate long-term outcomes of medical treatments (e.g. 10–15 years ahead).
4 They may be inappropriate because the random allocation into experimental and control groups itself may reduce the effectiveness of the intervention.

As he pointed out, patients' and clinicians' preferences are excluded, but the effectiveness of the treatment depends on the patient's active participation in the treatment, the degree of which may be influenced by preferences (e.g. preference for psychotherapy in a trial of psychotherapy in comparison with conventional therapy). The purpose of the RCT is to ensure equal distribution of all factors, and this is not necessarily achieved if the patient prefers one treatment over another. In illustration of this point, Muggah *et al.* (1987) described a trial in the USA of chorionic villus sampling (CVS) in comparison with amniocentesis in prenatal diagnosis of chromosomal abnormalities. They reported that while fear of an increased risk of foetal loss associated with CVS was the main reason for refusal to participate in the trial, most of the women who entered the trial accepted the rationale for randomisation, but were often disappointed when they were assigned to the amniocentesis group.

Preference arms

One alternative to randomisation against patient preferences is to ascertain patients' preferences and randomise only those with no preferences into X (experimental treatment) and Y (control), and include a separate control group consisting of those who chose X and another control group of those who did not want X. This can facilitate the estimation of the value of the intervention and the additional influence of motivational factors (Brewin and Bradley 1989; Torgerson *et al.* 1996; Black *et al.* 1998; McKee *et al.* 1999). While a systematic review of RCTs with preference arms reported there were no effects of preferences on outcomes, most studies reviewed did not specify how patients' treatment preferences were measured, and those that did used a mixture of unvalidated methods (e.g. standard gamble and single item questions) (King *et al.* 2005a, 2005b).

Differences between participants and non-participants

The effect of non-participation also differs between RCTs which evaluate clinical treatments and those which evaluate disease prevention programmes (Hunninghake *et al.* 1987). As McKee *et al.* (1999) pointed out in their review of single interventions evaluated by both RCTs and non-randomised studies, participants in RCTs of clinical treatment interventions tend to be less affluent, less educated and more seriously ill than non-participants. Participants in RCTs which evaluate preventive interventions, in contrast, are more likely to be more affluent, more educated and have healthier lifestyles than those who refuse to participate. Thus, the effect is to exaggerate treatment effects and to underestimate the effects of prevention.

Randomisation vs. non-randomisation

Bland (1995) argued, in relation to medical care: 'Without properly conducted controlled clinical trials to support it, each administration of a treatment to a patient becomes an uncontrolled experiment, whose outcome, good or bad, cannot be predicted.' However, as has been shown, RCTs are not always possible. Black (1996) argued that when trials cannot be conducted, other well-designed methods should be used; and they are also often of value as a complement to trials, given the limited external validity of the latter. Chalmers (1995) cited Stephen Evans (a medical statistician) as saying: 'It is better to measure imprecisely that which is relevant, than to measure precisely that which is irrelevant.' However, an evaluation of randomised and non-randomised intervention studies by Deeks *et al.* (2003) reported that the results of non-randomised and randomised studies sometimes, but not always, differed in relation to the same intervention, and that standard methods of adjustment for variations in the case mix of study patients did not guarantee the removal of selection bias. They concluded that non-randomised studies should only be undertaken when RCTs are infeasible or unethical.

Complex interventions

A potential source of heterogeneity is variation between trials in the way in which interventions are delivered (Herbert and BØ 2005), and difficulties in defining the components of the intervention (e.g. physical setting, skill mix, frequencies and timings of interventions). While this problem is least likely in simple interventions (e.g. drug trials), it is most likely in relation to multifaceted, complex individual or organisational therapies where social contexts can influence implementation and delivery (e.g. from physiotherapy and psychological therapy to specialised units such as stroke units, and programmes such as falls prevention). As Oakley (2006, p. 413) stated, such complex interventions 'combine different components in a whole that is more than the sum of its parts'.

In illustration of the issue in relation to systematic reviews and meta-analyses, Herbert and Bø (2005) identified four RCTs of pelvic floor training to prevent urinary incontinence during pregnancy. Two of the studies reported positive results, and in these each training session was supervised regularly by a physiotherapist. One study reported negative effects, but the women in this trial saw the physiotherapist only once. They concluded on the basis of their meta-analysis (albeit based on just four trials) that an uncritical synthesis of the data showed that the intervention was ineffective; a more accurate interpretation might have been that the intervention was effective only if administered effectively. The quality of interventions requires assessment in systematic reviews, and complex trials need more complex initial stages to ascertain how interventions should be administered, along with careful methods of evaluation. (See Box 10.2.)

Box 10.2 Phases of complex interventions

The UK's Medical Research Council (MRC) produced updated guidance for the evaluation of complex interventions (2000; 2008; Craig *et al.* 2008), which is used internationally. The MRC (2000) distinguished five phases:

1. *theory* (to explore relevant theory to inform choice of intervention and hypotheses, to predict confounders and design issues);
2. *modelling* (to identify components of the intervention and the mechanisms by which they influence outcomes);
3. *exploratory trial* (to describe the constant and variable components of an intervention, and feasible protocols for comparing the intervention with a feasible alternative);
4. *definitive RCT* (to compare a fully defined intervention to an appropriate alternative using a theoretically defensible, reproducible and adequately controlled protocol, with appropriate statistical power);
5. *long-term implementation* (long-term surveillance to assess real-life effectiveness and whether the intervention can be replicated reliably by others, in uncontrolled settings in the long term).

The MRC's (2008) updated guidance is broader in scope than the original version. It includes observational methods as well as randomised controlled trials; implementation as well as the development and evaluation of interventions; and has a broader definition of complex interventions beyond simply having multiple components (Anderson 2008). The guidance does refer to the need for a theoretical understanding of the intervention, for example, when selecting appropriate measures of outcome, though it has also been criticised for neglecting to detail the science of complex systems and theory-driven approaches to evaluation (e.g. of how and why interventions are thought to work, including realistic evaluation, and theories of change) (see Anderson 2008).

The MRC framework was applied in a Danish study aiming to evaluate a disease management programme for chronic obstructive pulmonary disease (COPD) (Smidth *et al.* 2013). First, the authors examined the literature. In phase I, the intervention was developed; in phases II and III it was tested in a block- and cluster-randomised study. In phase IV, the programme was evaluated for the feasibility for wider implementation. The authors concluded that the application of the model added transparency to the design phase, which helped to facilitate the implementation of the programme.

Process evaluation

Most randomised controlled trials focus on outcomes, rather than on the processes involved in the successful or unsuccessful implementation of an intervention (Oakley 2006). An important component in the evaluation of complex interventions, and insightful with all large effectiveness trials in real-life settings, is the inclusion of a process evaluation. Process evaluations are usually qualitative and aim to understand the circumstances in which interventions work or fail by exploring the implementation, delivery and receipt, and the setting of an intervention. They aid interpretation of results on outcomes by:

- identifying variations in the context and implementation of an intervention;
- identifying of barriers and facilitators to the intervention;
- relating such variations to variations in the impact of the intervention.

Other analytic methods of investigation

It is not always practical or ethically acceptable to conduct the true experimental method, with randomisation, in real-life settings. Instead causal inferences are often made *cautiously* on the basis of other types of non-randomised, analytic studies. Because of the difficulties involved with RCTs, a range of other analytic methods have been developed as alternatives. These depart from the ideal model of the true experiment, or RCT, but incorporate one or more of its elements. Usually the element of randomisation between experimental and control groups, or sometimes the pre-test stage, is missing. Causal associations may be inferred from data derived from these studies, particularly if matching of groups and adjustment in the analyses (see Chapter 11) have been used to try to eliminate extraneous variables which may confound the results. However, the conclusions will be more tentative. These methods are generally undervalued because of their weaknesses, but have much to offer if carefully used and interpreted.

Terminology

There is great variation in the terminology used to describe analytical studies which depart from the true experiment in relation to randomisation to experimental and control groups, but which have adopted one or more of its essential features. Moser and Kalton (1971) include after-only designs and before–after designs as experiments *only* if they include experimental and control groups *and* membership of the groups is based on random allocation. They described studies which do not qualify for the term 'experiment' as *investigations*, while acknowledging the wide range of other descriptors for them (e.g. *quasi-experiments*, *explanatory* surveys, *observational* studies) and their sources. Campbell and Stanley (1966) called studies which do not fit the ideal experimental model (e.g. the before–after study without a control group, the after-only study without randomisation) *pre-experimental*. Psychologists typically use the term *quasi-experiments* to refer to these investigations, which are defined as studies which involve the measurement of the impact of an intervention on the participants in the study (Dooley 1995). Statisticians tend to describe methods other than the true experiment as observational methods, but this is confusing, as social scientists use the term 'observational study' specifically to refer to methods of collecting data through use of the senses (sight and hearing). Others refer to both experimental (randomised) and non-randomised, controlled investigations as *intervention* studies (St Leger *et al.* 1992).

While a uniform language would be helpful, and avoid confusion, the choice of descriptor is relatively unimportant as long as it is used clearly and consistently and does not overlap with other methods (as does 'observation study'). The simple term *other analytic methods* is used here to describe the types of investigations in which the investigator cannot assume full control over the experimental setting and/or does not have the power to randomise between groups.

Limitations and strengths of other analytic methods

Analytic methods which depart from the ideal experimental model do have the potential for bias. Without non-randomised control groups for comparison, it is never really known whether any observed changes could have occurred without the intervention. There are statistical techniques for removing bias from non-randomised experimental designs, such as matching of participants in experimental groups with controls, and statistical techniques of covariance adjustment.

These methods of study need to be carefully designed, conducted and monitored. They need to take account of concurrent events and alternative explanations. If this care is taken, these alternative methods have much to offer in a research area where true experiments, or RCTs, are unethical, impractical or even impossible to conduct. For example, Houghton *et al.* (1996) rejected the RCT as a realistic method in their evaluation of the role of a discharge coordinator (the intervention) on medical wards. Instead they used a time series method, using different samples of inpatients over the different phases of the intervention period (historical controls; see later for description of method). They took external (historical) events into account by completing a diary of events and staff changes, which was later compared with trends in the data over time. As Houghton *et al.* explained:

> The ideal design for an intervention study of this kind would be a randomised controlled trial – that is, random allocation of patients into two groups in which one group would receive the intervention, in this case, the services of a discharge coordinator, and the other would not. However, we considered that there would be some serious and insurmountable problems associated with this approach. Firstly, the random selection of patients would mean that those receiving intervention would often be situated in the wards next to controls. With no control over contact between these patients and between controls and other ward staff, 'contamination' would be inevitable. Also, the presence of a discharge coordinator on the ward, a major part of whose job is to liaise with all staff involved with discharging patients, would undoubtedly result in a Hawthorne effect. In other words, discharge planning would improve generally during the period of the study.

In this example, the random assignment of wards to discharge planning or routine discharge practice was rejected because of wide variation in the organisation and standards of the wards, affecting comparability, in a single-site study. The investigators did not have the option of undertaking a wider study in which cluster randomisation could be carried out (e.g. all the individual inpatients in whole hospitals allocated to discharge planning or usual practice).

The analytic methods which use non-randomised control groups for comparison include investigations which may be before–after (studying the participants before and after exposure to the experimental (the intervention) variable) or after-only studies (studying the participants only after the exposure), preferably using control groups. The element of random assignment to experimental and control groups is missing. Studies using non-randomised control groups are usually cheaper than RCTs and are suited to services where matched controls can be found. For example, the *cases* are exposed to an intervention and their outcome is compared with a comparable (non-randomised) *control* group (matched or unmatched on key variables such as age and sex) who have not been exposed to the intervention. In social science, this is sometimes described as a *contrasted group* method. The experimental and control groups should be as similar as possible in relation to their characteristics. For example, in a study of a medical intervention, the experimental and control groups should be similar in relation to the severity and stage of their condition. The techniques used to achieve this, apart from randomisation, are matching and adjustment in the analyses. Without random allocation it will never be known whether any observed changes occurred as a result of an intervention or whether they would have occurred anyway. The range of other analytic studies is described next, along with their limitations (see Chapter 9 for longitudinal survey methods and Chapter 4 for specific epidemiological methods).

Before–after study with non-randomised control group

With this method, the experimental group is exposed to the experimental variable (independent variable), and the dependent variable (e.g. health status) is measured before and after the intervention to measure the effects of the independent variable. Comparisons are made with an appropriate control group, though the process of assignment to experimental and control groups is not random. The careful selection of controls is essential. Some studies of health care interventions make comparisons with patients on waiting lists for the treatment but this makes the assumption that patients on waiting lists simply wait patiently without seeking relief at the same time (as pointed out earlier, control patients might be more likely than the treatment group to be receiving help from complementary practitioners, over the counter medications, and so on).

Not all before–after studies employ control groups (e.g. the same participants are used as both experimental and control groups) but these are more seriously flawed, as it is unknown whether any detected changes would have occurred anyway (i.e. without the intervention in the experimental group). Many other events provide potential explanations for any changes in the dependent variable.

After-only study with non-randomised control group

With the after-only study, the effect of the experimental (independent) variable on the dependent variable is assessed by measuring it only after the experimental group has been exposed to it, and it is compared with an appropriate control group. If the allocation between experimental and control groups is not random, it is not possible to assume that any observed changes might be owing to the intervention without a measurement beforehand. There are several other weaknesses of post-test only comparisons, including the inability to calculate the amount of change between pre- and post-tests, and to take into account the starting point (baseline scores) of each group before meaningful interpretation of the results can be made.

Not all after-only studies employ control groups, but these are more seriously flawed, as it is unknown what other variables may intervene and explain any observed changes in the dependent variable.

Time series studies using different samples (historical controls)

With this method, a group of participants who are given a new procedure are compared with a group of participants previously given an alternative procedure. For example, patients receiving care or treatment before the new service or treatment is introduced act as the comparison group (historical controls) for patients subsequently receiving the new service or intervention. The difficulties with this method include selection bias (e.g. there may be less clear inclusion criteria (criteria for treatment) with the historical control group), changes in the way the data have been collected between the groups, changes in referral patterns to the service, in the service itself and even in patient expectations over time. There may also be experimental bias, as the previously recorded data available for the controls are likely to be inferior and subject to missing information.

Altman (1991) argued that the use of historical controls can only be justified in tightly controlled situations in relation to relatively rare conditions (as in evaluations of therapies for advanced cancer). One of the main problems relates to potential *historical* effects: events occurring at the time of the study might affect the participants and provide a rival explanation for changes observed. For example, an experimental design to evaluate the effectiveness of a health promotion campaign to reduce smoking levels in a local population will be spoiled if taxes on tobacco are increased markedly during the study period, which generally has the effect of reducing consumption.

Geographical comparisons

With geographical comparisons, people who live in an area without the service/ treatment, or with a different mix, act as the comparison group to people in the area with the experimental service/treatment. This is a method which is commonly used in studies of general practice. For example, a predefined group of patients who receive a particular service (e.g. in-house psychotherapy) in one general practice is compared with similar patients in a comparable practice which does not offer the service. This is cheaper than an RCT and suited to situations in which small numbers are being recruited to the experimental service. It is sometimes the only feasible method of study. However, it can be difficult to exclude other causes for differences between patients. It is common to find published reports of 'community intervention trials' in which an intervention community is compared with one control community. This is a weak design, as it is equivalent to a clinical trial with one patient in each treatment group, and no information can be provided on variation between communities (Hays and Bennett 1999).

People acting as own controls

Some investigators use the patients receiving the intervention to be evaluated as their own controls, and collect data about them both before and after an intervention. This is common in cases where there are no suitable controls, though such studies can only generate hypotheses to be tested in future rigorously designed trials when possible. The effects appear as a change between the pre- and post-test measures. This has the problem of contamination by historical events (unrelated to the study), and differences in the administration of the pre- and post-tests. It will not be known whether any observed differences between pre- and post-tests were owing to the experimental variable (intervention) under study.

Within-person, controlled site study

Other methods of matching do exist, but are rarely used. For example, there is the technique of within-patient design, which is possible if the patient has two sites (such as two eyes or two comparable areas of skin) for comparison. For example, one eye or area of skin would receive treatment A and the other eye or area would receive treatment B (with random selection of the eye/area of skin to receive the first (A) treatment). Fewer patients are needed for this type of design because there is less variation between individuals with matched sites than between different individuals. There are few opportunities to use this type of design, particularly as treatments may not be single site-specific and there is the risk of cross-site contamination (e.g. infection).

Threats to the validity of causal inferences in other analytic studies

It was pointed out earlier that alternative explanations often exist in relation to explanations of causality, particularly if ideal experimental methods are not used. It is rarely possible to design a study which excludes all sources of invalidity (Moser and Kalton 1971), and thus the aim is to try to exclude, as far as possible, rival explanations.

One of the most widely cited examples of a non-randomised trial leading to results which are probably biased is that of Smithells et al. (1980). In this study, women with a previous neural tube defect birth who were planning a future pregnancy were given multivitamin supplements, and then the outcome of pregnancy (incidence of neural tube defect infants) was compared to that of a control group who had not taken supplements. The potential for bias stems from the control group, which consisted of some women who had declined to take supplements, as well as women who were already pregnant, and a higher proportion of women from high-risk areas in comparison with the treated group. Thus, the groups were not comparable and the results, which indicated reduced incidence of neural tube defects after supplementation, were impossible to interpret.

Summary of main points

- The experiment is a scientific method used to test cause-and-effect relationships between the independent and dependent variables. The experimental method requires the investigator to have the power to manipulate the independent variable.
- The true experiment also requires the randomisation of participants to experimental and control groups.
- In order to assess the effect of the intervention, there should be a pre-test of both groups, undertaken before the experimental group has been exposed to the experimental (independent) variable, and a post-test of both groups, taken after exposure.
- External validity refers to the generalisability of the results to the wider target group. Randomisation does not preclude the possibility that the population randomised between groups may be atypical of the wider population of interest.
- The placebo effect refers to the expectation of the individual that the experimental stimulus will be associated with a successful intervention. A control group that receives an inert substance or intervention is used to control for this placebo effect.
- Bias owing to the expectancy of the patient, the treating professional and the investigator can contaminate results. Therefore, ideally each participant is blind about which group the members of the study have been allocated to.
- RCTs (experiments in medical and health care) are often extremely difficult to set up, and they are often conducted in such tightly controlled conditions that the conditions bear little resemblance to common practice.
- Other research methods can complement experiments (e.g. large-scale prospective case control studies of a particular cohort of interest can detect side-effects of particular treatments ten or more years ahead – which is beyond the scope of most experiments).
- Use of analytic methods which depart from the ideal experimental model has the potential for bias. Without non-randomised control groups for comparison, it is never really known whether any observed changes could have occurred without the intervention.

Key questions

1 Distinguish between internal and external validity.
2 Define a basic experiment.
3 State the essential features of a true experiment.
4 What are the advantages of randomisation of participants between experimental and control groups?
5 What is the placebo effect?
6 Explain the concept of blinding.
7 Why is pre- and post-testing important in experimental design?
8 Explain reverse causation.
9 Why are RCTs sometimes difficult to mount in real-life settings?

Key terms

after-only study
before–after study
blind study
complex intervention
confounding variable
control group
evaluation apprehension
experiment
experimenter apprehension
experimenter bias
explanatory trial
external validity
extraneous variable
geographical comparisons

historical controls
intention to treat
internal validity
people as own controls
placebo effect
placebo group
pragmatic trial
process evaluation
randomisation
randomised controlled trial (RCT)
reactive effects
sample attrition
time series
within-person study

Recommended reading

Black, N. (1996) Why we need observational studies to evaluate the effectiveness of health care, *British Medical Journal*, 312: 1215–18.

Bland, M. (1995) *An Introduction to Medical Statistics*. Oxford: Oxford University Press.

Campbell, T. and Stanley, J.C. (1966) *Experimental and Quasi-experimental Designs for Research*. Chicago: Rand McNally.

Dooley, D. (1995) *Social Research Methods*. Englewood Cliffs, NJ: Prentice Hall.

Pocock, S.J. (1983) *Clinical Trials: A Practical Approach*. Chichester: Wiley.

Tilling, K., Sterne, J., Brookes, S. and Peters, T. (2005) Features and designs of randomised controlled trials and non-randomised experimental designs, in A. Bowling and S. Ebrahim (eds) *Handbook of Health Research Methods: Investigation, Measurement and Analysis*. Maidenhead: Open University Press.

CHAPTER 11

Sample selection and group assignment methods in experiments and other analytic methods

Introduction

In theory, at the outset of a study the population to which the findings will apply should be identified, and the sample for study should be drawn randomly from it. This is not always possible owing to practical difficulties, but without this random selection the external validity of the research is likely to be reduced. However, with all sampling strategies, clear criteria for the selection of participants should be decided on and adhered to in all investigations. These issues and the methods of group assignment once the sample of participants has been drawn are described in this chapter.

Random sampling

Random sampling means that each member of the target population group has a non-zero and calculable chance of inclusion in the sample. This is essential for the study to have external validity: the external validity of the research is low if the study population is not representative of the wider population of interest because experimental investigators cannot then assume that their results can be generalised. Like descriptive surveys, experimental and other analytic investigations which aim to generalise their results to a larger target population should, in theory, adopt standard random sampling methods. The theories and principles of random sampling presented in Chapter 8 also apply, in theory, to experimental research.

In practice, random sampling from a comprehensive and representative sampling frame of the population of interest is more difficult to achieve in experimental designs: there can be difficulties obtaining or compiling sampling frames; there may be a high refusal rate among sample members; it may not be possible to obtain the cooperation of other centres (e.g. general practices or hospitals) to participate where this is necessary; and ethical concerns may emerge (particularly with medical treatments and health care services). The cost is the loss of external validity, which can render research results ungeneralisable. There might also be a bias in the recruitment of people for experimental research. For example, entry criteria to clinical trials of treatments are often restricted to patients with less severe conditions or most likely to benefit from the new treatment; this makes the findings of questionable generalisability. Pocock (1983) has given examples of inclusion criteria in trials.

Convenience and purposive sampling

Most investigators using experimental and analytic methods recruit participants (e.g. patients) from known, easily accessible populations (e.g. appropriate hospital outpatients are recruited consecutively as they attend). This has the advantages of ease of recruitment, easier monitoring and follow-up, generally good response rates and retention of sample members. However, if the treatment being evaluated is intended for patients treated in general practice, then a hospital-based population is inappropriate and will lead to results with poor external validity. There is often little information about the representativeness of samples in experimental studies. It is known from research in cancer that very few of the total pool of eligible patients are entered into trials, despite research showing that patients are either enthusiastic or uncertain, rather than negative, about entering trials (Slevin et al. 1995). It is essential for the investigator to estimate the extent to which the accessible population which has been included in the study deviates in important ways from the excluded, but relevant, population.

Volunteers

Some investigators, particularly in psychology and medical research, advertise for volunteer participants. This is not recommended because volunteers may be different in some way from non-volunteers, again leading to loss of external validity. For example, volunteers in medical trials of treatments may be healthier than the true population of interest, and thus bias the results. If volunteers are essential, then it is important to recruit them in such a way as to minimise bias. For example, advertising for volunteers in a health food magazine will lead to the recruitment of a select group of subjects (e.g. those with an interest in their diet, and their diet may differ from that of other members of the population).

While statisticians argue that participants in experimental and analytical research should be as representative of the target population as possible, and one should be wary of potential volunteer bias in studies of treatment effects (e.g. Bland 1995), it is usually acknowledged that such investigations are often limited, for real practical reasons, to participants who are easily accessible and willing to participate.

Type of investigation and type of sampling frame

Rothman (1986) pointed out that there are instances in which the experiment can legitimately be limited to any type of case of interest, regardless of representativeness of all such cases. This is particularly true where the investigator is only interested in a particular sub-group of a disease population (e.g. severely ill cases), and therefore there is no requirement to ensure that the sample members are representative of the wide spectrum of people with the disease in question. However, the aim should still be to aim for representativeness within the sub-group (e.g. representative of all severely ill cases with the condition) in order to enhance external validity. Findings can only apply to the population from which the sample was drawn (see Bland 1995).

The early stages of clinical research trials are known as *phase I* trials, such as experiments on drug safety, pharmacological action and optimum dose levels with volunteers, and *phase II* trials, such as small-scale experimental studies of the effectiveness and safety of a drug. In these early stages there is likely to be compromise in the experimental design, and an unrepresentative group of patients who are willing to cooperate is studied. Full *phase III* trials are the most rigorous and extensive types of scientific investigations of a new treatment (e.g. they include a substantial sample size and the careful comparison of the experimental group who receive a new treatment with the control group). With these it is important to aim to include a group of patients that represents the condition of interest, in order that the results are generalisable. This will often require a multicentre collaborative study. *Phase IV* trials are descriptive studies which survey morbidity and mortality rates once the treatment has been established (e.g. the drug has been licensed for clinical use).

Response rates: experiments and other analytic studies

Non-respondents

In all research it is important to document the characteristics of sample members who refused to take part. For example, are the people who refuse to participate in an experimental trial of a new treatment for a specific group of patients in some way more ill than those who agree to participate? Perhaps they felt too ill to summon the energy for participation, especially if the study involves additional bio-medical tests and the completion of lengthy questionnaires. If they are different in some way (e.g. severity indicators, length of time they have had their condition, mortality rates), then the implication is that the sample members who do agree to participate may not be representative of the target population, and external validity will be reduced (see Chapters 8 and 12).

Sample attrition

Sample attrition, once people have consented to participate, and been randomised or otherwise assigned to experimental and control groups, is problematic. There should be clear documentation throughout the study about not just those who drop out through refusals, but also the inclusion of any ineligible sample members, sample attrition during the study period through death, incomplete assessments (missing data) and people for whom the protocol was changed (e.g. with patients where it is deemed that continuation in the trial is not in their best interests). Sample attrition is discussed in Chapters 9 and 10.

In the RCT, as the randomisation procedure has produced comparable groups, the analysis must include an unbiased comparison of groups, based on *all* the people who were randomised wherever possible; this is known as analysis by 'intention to treat', rather than 'on treatment' analysis. This avoids systematic errors (biases). Some account also needs to be taken of people who refused to be randomised (e.g. analysis of their characteristics and health outcome where possible).

Of course, such analyses can only be carried out within the confines of the data actually collected, but assessment (e.g. of health status or biomedical markers in the medical notes) at any premature exit from the study is essential where the participant permits this (see Chapter 9).

Ensuring similarity in group characteristics: random allocation

The design of the selection of individuals, their randomisation to two or more intervention and control groups, followed by their exposure to the intervention (e.g. treatment), and assessment, is known as the *parallel group design*. It was pointed out in Chapter 10 that the comparison of two or more groups is a basic feature of the classic experiment. It is essential to try to control for any extraneous, confounding variables (see 'Epidemiology', Chapter 4). If the groups differ on some other variable, then this may explain the associations between independent and dependent variables. If the groups can be made equivalent on these other variables, then these cannot explain the association. There are potential biases in the control groups without random allocation.

Unrestricted random allocation

Random allocation was referred to under the heading 'The RCT in health care evaluation' in Chapter 10. This section describes the methods of carrying out this random assignment between groups. With an experiment – for example, a clinical RCT comparing a new medical treatment with standard treatment and/or a placebo treatment – it is usual practice to identify the population group of interest and assign the participants to either experimental or control groups using randomisation techniques.

The simplest method of allocating people to the experimental or control group, in such a way that each has an equal chance of either assignation, and ensuring that their assignation is only due to chance, is to toss a coin repeatedly. This is known as an *unrestricted* method of allocation. This is perfectly acceptable, though it is now routine practice to use computer-generated random numbers, allocating odd numbers for treatment A and even numbers for treatment B, or numbers within a specific range for treatment A and other numbers for treatment B; there are endless variations on this method (see Pocock 1983 and Altman 1991, for descriptions of the process). This procedure is usually carefully carried out with respect to the method of allocation and process of the research (e.g. as close as possible to the timing of the intervention in order to avoid sample loss before the intervention, through death or deterioration). It is important for the investigator to carry out the randomisation (and not, for example, a doctor caring for the patients in a clinical study), and it is important to log all patients on entry prior to randomisation in order to ensure that a complete list of all eligible patients is kept, regardless of whether they remain in the study. It can help to prevent investigators or health professionals 'cheating' over eligibility if they know that the patient has been registered beforehand. Randomisation processes, especially for multicentre studies, are major administrative undertakings. The randomisation procedure must be smooth, accurate, efficient and speedy. The person(s) conducting the randomisation must be easily and quickly contactable during the times when randomisation is required. Sometimes it is important to have out-of-hours randomisation procedures in place 24 hours a day, seven days a week (e.g. in settings where treatment decisions are made 24 hours a day as in accident and emergency departments, inpatient wards and general practice). This requires an automated service which either major telephone providers are able to arrange, or can be organised via the internet (though not all health service providers have access to the internet and so a dual, integrated telephone and internet system will need to be developed).

Cluster randomisation

It may be preferable, for reasons of cost or feasibility, to randomise the clusters containing individuals (e.g. clinics) rather than individuals themselves. The decision needs to be made in the light of likely experimental contamination (see Slymen and Hovell 1997, for guidance). The preferred design is always the assignment of individuals to experiment and control groups if it can be assumed that all individuals are independent, as individuals within the same cluster are likely to have correlated outcomes. However, independence cannot always be assumed, particularly with lifestyle or environmental health interventions (e.g. health promotion or water fluoridation interventions). Contamination may occur if members of the control group are exposed to the experimental intervention and/or the members of the experimental group are exposed to the control. This is likely to occur, for example, where control and experimental group members are in close proximity (e.g. clinic members) and they communicate information to each other. To overcome this problem, entire clusters of individuals (e.g. the clinics) can be randomised to the intervention or control group, though outcomes are still *measured* at the individual level. There are other situations in which cluster randomisation is preferable to individual randomisation. For example, contamination (experimenter bias) may occur if the same professional administers both experimental and control treatments to study participants. Blinding is the usual solution to this source of contamination, but if this is not possible, then a cluster design may be considered. An example of cluster randomisation is shown in Box 11.1.

Box 11.1 Example of a cluster RCT

An example of a cluster RCT is Orrell *et al.*'s (2007) intervention trial of the effect of a package to reduce unmet need in older people with dementia, living in residential care.

These authors conducted a single-blind, multicentre, cluster RCT, with assessments of unmet need pre- and post-intervention. They recruited 24 residential homes from three areas, as far as possible recruited in pairs, matched for size, locality and registering body. Homes were randomised to 'care as usual' or to the intervention package over 20 weeks. Inclusion criteria for the residents living in the homes included permanent residency, aged 60+, length of residence, gold standard diagnosis of dementia, and ability to give informed consent/assent in line with their level of cognitive ability. The residents who met the inclusion criteria (8–11 minimum from each home within each pair were randomly selected; remote randomisation by an independent person was used to determine intervention or control group allocation) led to 238 participants from the 24 homes. The investigators compared the outcome (unmet needs) of their experimental group with the outcome of a group allocated to 'care as usual' in their residential settings (analysis done on an intention to treat basis).

With cluster randomisation, then, the clusters (e.g. clusters of individuals, such as all individuals in whole geographical areas or all inpatients in hospitals) are randomised to the experimental or control group. For example, in an evaluation study of health promotion, health promotion material on alcohol consumption may be randomly assigned to intact clusters or communities (e.g. geographical areas, schools or other organisations) rather than to individuals; or, in a study evaluating the effect of psychotherapists on patients' mental health outcomes, clinics may be randomly assigned psychotherapists or conventional treatments (controls). Comparisons are made with the randomly assigned controls. The clusters may be stratified, if appropriate, before being randomised (see the section on stratified randomisation).

Correlated outcomes among individuals in the same cluster are measured by the intra-cluster correlation coefficient. Because of the problem of correlated outcomes among individuals in the same cluster, cluster randomisation (e.g. of clinics) leads to a reduction in statistical power compared with an individually randomised trial of the same size. Thus, in order to ensure statistical power (Kerry and Bland 1998a, 1998b), as well as external validity, the number of units in the sample has to be sufficiently large (Donner 1992; Donner and Klar 1994). There may also be large practical problems and problems in ensuring the comparability of the units. The sample size for the clusters depends on the estimated variation between clusters in relation to outcome measures, but large numbers of clusters who are willing to participate may be difficult to locate, and unwieldy to manage in a research study. Individual- (e.g. patient-) based RCTs assume that the outcome for an individual is independent of (i.e. unrelated to) that of any other patient in the study. This assumption is violated in cluster randomisation because individuals in any one cluster are more likely to respond in a similar way. For example, members of a particular cluster (e.g. patients attending the same clinic) are more likely to have similar outcomes, thus statistical power is weakened and sample size estimates have to be initiated to take account of the cluster design (Campbell and Grimshaw 1998). Thus, this lack of independence has implications for the design and analysis of these studies. For example, as cluster randomisation is less statistically efficient and has a lower statistical power than similar-sized individual-based RCTs, sample sizes have to be initiated and multilevel methods of analysis often need to be carried out. Hays and Bennett (1999) have provided simple formulae for sample size calculation for cluster trials. Donner and Klar (2000) and Kerry and Bland (1998a, 1998b) have also presented the factors relating to research design which need to be considered when estimating sample size for cluster randomisation. Ethical concerns have also been raised about cluster trials in relation to cluster members' informed consent – cluster trials affect whole clusters of people (e.g. health promotion campaigns on the media), and individuals cannot, in theory, decide to act independently. There is always a need for procedural safeguards appropriate to the risks of the intervention (Edwards *et al.* 1999). There are controversies surrounding the balance of benefits to the community versus risk of harm to the individual (Edwards *et al.* 1999; Donner and Klar 2000).

The complexity of cluster trials, moreover, can make them vulnerable to selection biases at both stages: biased allocation, that potentially affects outcome, can occur at the cluster level and at the recruitment of individuals into the study. The randomisation of clusters needs to be undertaken with care and by an independent person, and drop-outs need to be minimised. Unless complete identification and inclusion of individuals within the clusters are conducted, there is always danger of selection bias due to either the influence of existing knowledge or poor levels of consent to participate. Some of these problems have been discussed by Puffer *et al.* (2003), who reviewed 36 cluster randomised trials, published over five years in prestigious medical journals and reported that while they found little evidence of cluster bias, they found susceptibility to individual bias in 39 per cent of the studies.

Restricted random allocation for ensuring balance

There are also various methods of restricted randomisation which will ensure that approximately equal numbers of participants are allocated to each group. These are described below.

Stratified randomisation

The aim of the sampling process in experimental studies is to make the experimental and control groups as comparable as possible. In clinical research it is important to ensure that the participants are comparable on socio-demographic characteristics, and also in relation to diagnosis, severity and stage of disease, and other relevant clinical details. The groups should be as similar as possible except in relation to the independent variable (e.g. nature of the intervention).

Stratification of variables known to influence outcome is often carried out in experimental design (e.g. age, sex, comorbidity, disability, prognosis). Stratified randomisation procedures will take patient characteristics into account in order to equalise the groups on these variables. For example, to ensure the proper balance of both males and females in two groups the random allocation into the groups would be conducted separately for the males and then separately for the females. This is called stratification. As pointed out earlier, the stratification can also be carried out for clusters (e.g. clinics) and the clusters then randomised (Donner 1992).

A separate randomisation list has to be prepared for each of the strata, or combinations of strata. This technique is commonly used in clinical trials. The techniques of stratification have been described by Pocock (1983) and Altman (1991), though the latter points out that this more complex procedure is only suitable for very large trials, with adequate management resources, where there is certainty over the relevant variables for stratification. He argues that stratification is probably unnecessary in large trials, involving several hundred patients, where there is less likelihood of serious imbalances between groups.

Further, stratification can lead to too small numbers for meaningful analysis in sub-groups. For example, if it is decided to stratify by three potential prognostic factors, such as sex (in two categories, male and female), age (in three categories, such as under 45, 45–64, 65+), and functional ability (in three categories, such as poor, moderate and good), then this means 18 ($2 \times 3 \times 3 = 18$) sub-groups to take into account in the analyses. Pocock (1983) argues that it is often more profitable to use adjustments in the analysis for most trials ('stratified analysis'), such as adjustment for prognostic factors when analysing for treatment differences (see later).

The two main methods of stratified randomisation are *random permuted blocks within strata* and *minimisation*. These methods are described briefly next and have been described in more detail by Pocock (1983) and Altman (1991).

Random permuted blocks

With the block design the aim (e.g. in clinical research) is to ensure approximate equality of treatment *numbers* for every type of patient. A separate *block randomisation* list is produced for each sub-group (stratum). It is also important that stratified allocation of interventions (i.e. treatments) is based on block randomisation within each stratum rather than simple randomisation, or there will be no control of balance of interventions within strata and the aim of stratification will be defeated. Many investigators stratify by age and sex, although Altman (1991) argues that sex is not often prognostic and need not be used in clinical trials. When it is aimed to achieve similarity between groups for several variables, minimisation can be used.

With block randomisation, the blocks can be of any size, though using a multiple of the number of treatments is logical, and smaller blocks are preferable for maintaining balance. Altman (1991) gives the following example of this method:

> For example, if we consider people in blocks of four at a time, there are six ways in which we can allocate treatments so that two people get A and two get B:
>
> | | |
> |---|---|
> | 1 AABB | 4 BBAA |
> | 2 ABAB | 5 BABA |
> | 3 ABBA | 6 BAAB |

If we use combinations of only these six ways of allocating treatments then the numbers in the two groups at any time can never differ by more than two, and they will usually be the same or one apart. We choose blocks at random to create the allocation sequence.

Thus, in this example, of the first (block of) four patients (in their stratum), the first two patients receive treatment A (e.g. experimental), and the second two receive treatment B (e.g. control). This is block 1 in the example: AABB. The random permuted block method carries the disadvantage that at the end of each block it is possible for any member of the team to predict what the next treatment will be if he or she has kept account of the previous treatments in the blocks.

Armitage and Berry (1987) have described the approaches for ensuring equal numbers, including balancing using Latin square, in greater detail.

Minimisation

Minimisation is a valid alternative to simple randomisation and it will lead to experimental and control groups that will be more likely to have a similar balance in numbers regarding the defined variables than they would be if simple randomisation was used. With this procedure, the first participant (e.g. the first person to arrive for the experiment) is allocated to the experimental or control group at random. Subsequent participants are also allocated randomly, but at an early stage the investigator must take stock of the distribution of participants between treatments according to their characteristics (e.g. stratification for age, sex, stage of disease). For subsequent participants the investigator has to determine which group they should be allocated to in order to lead to a better balance between groups in relation to the variables of interest. The participant is then randomised using a defined weighting in favour of allocation to the group which would minimise the imbalance (e.g. a weighting of 4 to 1 leads to an 80 per cent chance of the subject being allocated to the group that minimises the imbalance). The weighting procedure can be as simple as the researcher choosing one of five sealed envelopes. If the weighting is 4 to 1 in favour of treatment A as opposed to treatment B, then four of the five sealed envelopes will contain the allocation to treatment A and one will contain allocation to treatment B. After the allocation, the numbers in each group are updated and the procedure is repeated for the next patient; if the totals for the groups are the same, then allocation can be made using simple (unweighted) randomisation as for the first participant (Altman 1991).

With minimisation, the aim is to ensure that the different experimental and control groups are similar in relation to the variables of interest for stratification, such as percentage aged under 40, percentage bed-bound, and so on: 'the purpose is to balance the marginal treatment totals for each level of each patient factor' (Pocock 1983). This requires keeping an up-to-date list of treatment assignment by patient stratification factors, and calculating which treatment should be given to each participant as he or she is entered into the study, based on the existing numbers in each pertinent factor. The procedure can be complex and is most suitable for smaller samples.

Randomisation with matching and matched analyses

Random allocation of participants between experimental and control group(s) will, in theory, equalise the groups on all extraneous variables. The sensitivity of the experiment can be improved further by using techniques of matching and/or adjustment alongside randomisation. For example, with this technique, and using *precision control matching* (see later), participants of the same age, sex and level of education could be matched in pairs, and then one member of each pair could be randomly allocated to the experimental group and the other assigned to the control group (paired comparison experiment). The technique could be extended if more than one control group is used. Matched pair analyses will then need to be conducted when the study has been completed.

Unequal randomisation

Generally, the aim is to randomise participants so that equal numbers are included in each group in the experiment. Sometimes, as when there is interest in finding out more about a new treatment, there is a case for randomising more (e.g. double) participants to the new treatment group than to the other groups, even though there may be a loss in statistical efficiency. An unequal randomisation list will need to be prepared for this. It is a little used method (see Pocock 1983, for further details).

Techniques for assigning treatments in the field

The techniques of randomisation in the field, if this cannot be conducted in the office (which requires the investigator to be at a telephone at all times eligible patients may be recruited), involve a variety of methods, from the use of sealed envelopes containing the name of the next treatment that the clinician is required to administer to the patient, to a sequence of drug packages (in drug trials) prepared by a pharmacist. With sealed drug packages, the clinician can remain 'blind' to the treatment (handing the package over to the patient or nurse), unlike with sealed envelopes.

Patients' preference arms

As pointed out in Chapter 3 (patients' preferences), when patients do not receive their preferred treatment in RCTs, for example, in unblinded trials, there may be problems in their recruitment, and consequently problems with sample bias, affecting representativeness. Patients who do receive their preferred treatment may also have high compliance rates, potentially changing treatment effects. An alternative is a *patient preference trial* (Torgerson and Sibbald 1998). Patients may be placed in groups according to their preference and willingness to be randomised. (See Box 11.2.)

Box 11.2 Patient preference trial groupings

Group A: patients who have no strong preferences and consent to randomisation

Group B: Patients with preferences and who consent to randomisation

Group C: Patients who refuse randomisation and opt for their treatment choice.

Patients with preferences are given their desired treatment, and those who do not are randomised in the usual way. In a trial of two interventions this leads to four groups:

Randomised to A

Prefer A

Randomised to B

Prefer B.

The example in Box 11.2 leads to a partly randomised design. Comparisons between the non-randomised groups are unreliable because of unknown, confounding factors. The two randomised groups are compared, and the non-randomised groups are treated as observational studies and adjusted for in the analysis. A more robust alternative, retaining full randomisation, is to elicit the strength and direction of preferences before randomisation, and to randomise all consenting patients (Torgerson and Sibbald 1998).

Zelen's (1979) design is an attempt to remove patient resentment due to not receiving the treatment of choice, and randomises patients to intervention or control arms before consent to participate has been sought (Adamson *et al.* 2006). Those participants allocated to the intervention group are then approached and offered the intervention, which they can decline or accept. Analysis is conducted with patients retaining their original assignment. However, there are ethical concerns relating to the use of the Zelen design (Torgerson and Roland 1998).

Other allocation methods: cross-over methods

Simple cross-over method

With cross-over methods (sometimes called change-over or repeated measure designs), each of the study participants (e.g. patients) receives sequences of the treatments which are under investigation, one after the other. The order in which the treatments are administered is *random*, as otherwise primacy effects may distort the results obtained. All participants should be pre-tested during a first phase of the study, before they receive any treatment at all, and then be reassessed at each treatment stage. The aim is to study differences between individual treatments.

The advantage of this method is that, as each patient acts as his or her own control, fewer patients are required to assess outcome because within-patient variability is less than between-patient variability, and it helps to control for observer variation. However, such designs are only possible with patients who have a stable (i.e. chronic) condition, as otherwise the condition of the patient may fluctuate naturally between treatments. There are a range of other difficulties with this method. The main problem is that there may be treatment order ('*carry-over*') effects. The first treatment may have residual long-term effects and therefore interact with, and affect, the response to the second treatment (unless a long interval between treatments can allow for this ('*wash-out period* '), with the greater risk of changes in the patient's condition over time which are independent of the treatment ('*period effects*') and also ethical implications). There is the danger that the effects of earlier treatments are falsely attributed to the final experimental treatment. Such effects need to be checked for in analyses, but can rarely be excluded as potentially biasing factors (Pocock

1983). Statisticians have sometimes treated cross-over trials with suspicion. This is partly because patients could be treated, for example, in three periods and allocated at random to one of the two sequences: ABB/BAA, or in four periods using the sequences AABB/BBAA: period effects, treatment effects and carry-over effects lead to the problems of too many variables to be examined on a within-patient basis (Senn 1995). Some conventional methods of analysis (e.g. two-stage analysis) are therefore inappropriate for use with cross-over trials (see Senn 1993, 1995, 1998, for elaboration and advice).

Latin square

The most common type of cross-over method uses the Latin square. This uses the block design for two factors, the levels of which are assigned to the rows and columns of a square. The cells of the square show the treatment levels. Assume that participants are randomly assigned to each of four treatment sequences. If this occurs on each of four days, blocks of four patients are randomly assigned to each sequence of treatments (giving a unique four-treatment by four-day matrix). Thus the order of the treatments is random and patients receive each one in (random) sequence. The treatments appear once in each period and in each sequence. There can be elaborations on this 'block' or 'cross-over' method (see Armitage and Berry 1987, for use of Latin square in 'balancing').

Stepped wedge trials

Stepped wedge trials (also called the pipeline approach) are randomised trials which involve sequential roll-out of an intervention to participants (individuals or clusters) over a number of time periods. The time at which the intervention is provided to each participant is randomised. By the end of the study, all participants will have received the intervention. A review by Brown and Lilford (2006) reported that this design was frequently used in developing countries, often in the context of HIV treatment interventions. The design involves extensive data collection. It is useful when RCTs are not possible, for example, when it is considered by health care providers that a control group would be unethical as sufficient evidence of effectiveness of an intervention exists, it is not realistic to provide the intervention to everyone at once, and to evaluate the effectiveness of interventions on a wider scale, where they have been shown to be effective in a more limited, research setting. It is also useful for modelling the effect of time and length of the intervention on the effectiveness of an intervention. A review of the design elements of stepped wedge trials can be found in Handley *et al.* (2011).

Methods of group design for improving the basic RCT

The strength of the RCT can be improved, in relation to *inferring* causality, the range of generalisations that can be made and generalisations to non-tested populations, by two variations of the classic experimental design: the Solomon four group method and the complete factorial experiment.

Solomon four group method

This design controls for the reactive effects of pre-testing, by including post-test only groups. The pre-test in an experiment provides an assessment of the time sequence and provides a basis for comparison. However, it can have a reactive effect by sensitising the study participants and so can affect post-test scores. Participants who have experienced a pre-test may react differently to the experimental variable from the way they would if they had never experienced the pre-test. The intervention (i.e. treatment) might have different effects depending on whether the groups have been pre-tested – and therefore sensitised and biased. The investigator will be uncertain about what produced the results: the pre-test or the experimental variable. The effects of the pre-test are known as potential reactive effects (i.e. they induce some reaction in participants).

To control for the reactive effects of the pre-test, the Solomon four group design can be used. This has the same features as the *true* experiment (e.g. random allocation), with the addition of an extra set of control and experimental groups that do not receive the pre-test. A minimum of four groups is used to compare the post-tests of the experimental and control groups in order to assess the impact of pre-testing without providing the intervention (i.e. treatment). The four groups are composed thus: one group is experimental, one group is experimental minus pre-test, one group is control, one group is control minus pre-test. The experimental groups can be compared to assess the effects of the pre-test, and so can the control groups.

Some investigators find this method too costly and impractical and instead use randomisation into experimental and control groups, omitting the pre-test stage altogether. However, without knowledge of pre-test measures, the *amount* of change due to the intervention can only be a cautious estimate based on the differences between experimental and control groups, because it is possible that the two groups, by chance, might have had different starting points (which would have been measured at pre-testing).

Complete factorial experiment

Many experimental designs are composed of one experimental group (exposed to the intervention) and one control group (unexposed). However, there are circumstances in which understanding can be enhanced by using more than one experimental or control group. In these cases, a factorial design is required. This still includes the same features as the *true* experiment (e.g. random allocation), but with the addition of more than one control or experimental group.

In some cases, more than one experimental group may be required, as well as the control group. For example, one might wish to study the immediate effects on health of different levels of exposure to cigarette smoke (e.g. symptoms such as sore throat, headache, eye and skin irritations). For this study, a control group would be needed (no exposure to cigarette smoke – placebo only), along with several experimental groups, each exposed to different, controlled levels of cigarette smoke. By comparing the groups, the way in which health symptoms vary according to the level of exposure to the smoke could be measured.

In other circumstances more than one control group can be used to make comparisons with the experimental group: for example, in the comparison of the effectiveness of a new treatment with standard treatment and no treatment. In this case the experimental group receives the new treatment, one control group receives the existing (standard) treatment and one control group receives the placebo (dummy) treatment. Factorial methods can be extended to take account of a range of alternatives against which to test interventions, and are not limited simply to a comparison of new versus standard and placebo interventions (see Cox 1958).

Another situation in which several groups may be used is in studies of the effects of more than one predictor variable. In contrast to the experimental versus control group model, several experimental groups are studied and the investigator deliberately varies more than one variable. For example, the Physician's Health Study in the USA was a randomised double-blind, placebo-controlled trial of aspirin and beta-carotine among 22,071 male physicians who were randomly assigned to aspirin alone, beta-carotine alone, aspirin plus beta-carotine or both placebos, using a 2 × 2 factorial design (Hennekens *et al.* 1996; Liu *et al.* 2000). To take another example, the hypothesis could be that small hospital wards have a more positive effect than larger wards on nursing staff's commitment to work. Other characteristics of the organisation, such as a decentralised structure, might also affect commitment, and these need to be taken into account. In this example, ward size and decentralisation are the independent variables to be studied in relation to their effects on staff commitment, which is the dependent variable. If each of the independent variables has just two dichotomous values, then four experimental groups will be needed in order to study each combination of them. For example, the combinations might be large wards and high decentralisation; small wards and high decentralisation; large wards and low decentralisation; and small wards and low decentralisation. The use of all possible combinations is known as a complete factorial experiment. The external validity (generalisability) of the results is enhanced by introducing variables at different levels. The investigator can infer whether the effect is the same or whether it varies at different levels of one or other of the variables (see Moser and Kalton 1971; Frankfort-Nachmias and Nachmias 1992, for fuller examples).

In summary, the method permits the examination of possible interactions between the independent variables. It also enables the investigator to base the research on an economical study size for the estimation of the main effects if interactions between variables are absent. The main advantage of factorial design is that it broadens the range of generalisations that can be made from the results and increases the external validity of the research.

Common methods of controlling to obtain equivalence in non-randomised studies

The use of non-randomly assigned experimental and control groups reduces the credibility of research results. When randomisation is not used, the most common ways by which extraneous variables can be controlled in order to obtain equivalence between groups are matching techniques (precision control and frequency distribution control), adjustments in the analyses or both. These techniques have been described by Moser and Kalton (1971) and are summarised below.

Matching: precision control and frequency distribution control

If the groups can be made equivalent on potential intervening (extraneous) variables (e.g. age, sex, level of education), then these cannot explain the association. There are two methods of matching for a combination of extraneous variables: precision control and frequency distribution control. Matching depends on the participants being available before the start of the trial, so that they can be matched at the outset – matching participants after they have already been allocated to experimental and control groups is not strictly a matched design and does not improve on the similarity of the two groups (e.g. desired pair may have already been allocated to the *same* group and therefore cannot be matched from different groups retrospectively).

Precision control refers to matching pairs – for each member of one group, a member with the same combination of the extraneous variables is selected for the other group(s) (e.g. a member of the same age group, same sex and same level of education). One-to-one matching is the norm, but it is acceptable to match more than one control group member to each experimental group member (i.e. when it is difficult to find members with the same combinations), though an equal number of members in one group should be matched with each member of the other. Difficulties arise when several extraneous variables are being controlled for, as it is increasingly difficult to find matching pairs. Many of the members of the other groups will not match and have to be discarded, which results in a decrease in external validity because of a restricted research population with limited generalisability to the total population group of interest. There is also the potential danger of over-matching. Over-matching occurs when a variable that is used for matching is associated with the intervention or exposure, but not with the variable of interest (e.g. disease).

Matching may reduce the power of a trial to address outcomes adequately (Martin et al. 1993). Thus, the gain in control over a number of variables carries considerable costs.

Frequency distribution control aims to equate the groups on each of the matching variables separately (not in combination), and thus results in fewer discarded subjects than with precision control. Thus, the age distributions would be equated for the groups, as would be sex and educational level. The combinations of age, sex and educational level would not necessarily be the same in each group. Thus, while this method eliminates the effects of these variables separately on any observed associations between the dependent and independent variables, it cannot eliminate the effects of them in combination with each other. Matching can introduce selection bias, regardless of the method of matching used. This is controlled for in the statistical analyses (matched analysis in studies using individual matching, and adjusting for the matching variables used in frequency matching).

Adjustments in the analyses

An alternative to matching is to make adjustments for the extraneous variables in the analyses. If they are measured, then these measurements can be used to adjust for differences between groups. This method is often known as control through measurement. The statistical methods for this include cross-tabulations (e.g. three-way cross-tabulations controlling for age, when cross-tabulating the independent and dependent variables), standardisation and regression techniques. Basic statistical techniques for these stratified analyses have been described by Moser and Kalton (1971).

The problem with techniques of matching and adjustment is that they can only control for a limited number out of a potentially unlimited number of extraneous, confounding variables. Furthermore, the investigator has to be knowledgeable about which are the potential confounding variables. Matching techniques also violate the assumption of statistical methods that samples are independent. This is an important assumption underlying statistical tests, though statisticians may argue that there is no simple way to make use of a statistical test which is efficient and which does not involve questionable assumptions (Blalock 1972).

Summary of main points

- In experiments, it is important to aim to include a group of people who are representative of the population of interest in order that the results are generalisable.
- There should be clear documentation throughout the study about those who drop out through refusals, the inclusion of any ineligible sample members, sample attrition through death, incomplete assessments (missing data) and people for whom the protocol was changed (e.g. with patients where it is deemed that continuation in the trial is not in their best interests).
- With cluster randomisation, the clusters (e.g. hospital clinic populations) are randomised to the experimental or control group. The clusters may be stratified beforehand.
- There are various methods of restricted randomisation which will ensure that approximately equal numbers of participants are allocated to each group.
- The sensitivity of an experiment can be improved by matching and/or adjustment alongside the randomisation.
- When randomisation is not used, the most common ways by which extraneous variables can be controlled in order to obtain equivalence are matching techniques (precision control and frequency distribution control), adjustments in the analyses or both.

Key questions

1 Describe the essential features of random sampling.
2 What are the threats to the external validity of the research in experimental design?
3 How can treatments be allocated in blind trials?
4 Why should participants in true experiments be randomised?
5 If a study reports a causal relationship between variables, what other explanations might account for it?
6 What is the appropriate study design to explore cause and effect relationships?
7 How can the strength of the RCT be improved by group allocation methods?
8 What is cluster randomisation?
9 What techniques ensure that approximately equal numbers of participants are allocated to the experimental and control groups?
10 Distinguish between the precision control and frequency distribution control methods of matching.
11 What are the difficulties of matching control and experimental groups?

Key terms

adjustments in the analysis
blind trial
causal relationship
complete factorial experiment
control group

cross-over methods
experimental design
experimental group
external validity
frequency distribution control

intention to treat
Latin square
matching
meta-analyses
minimisation
patient preference trial
placebo group
precision control
random permuted blocks
randomisation

randomisation with matching
randomised controlled trial (RCT)
restricted random allocation
Solomon four group method
stepped wedge trial
stratification
stratified randomisation
unrestricted random allocation
Zelen design

Recommended reading

Altman, D.G. (1991) *Practical Statistics for Medical Research*. London: Chapman & Hall.

Pocock, S.J. (1983) *Clinical Trials: A Practical Approach*. Chichester: Wiley.

Tilling, K., Sterne, J., Brookes, S. and Peters, T. (2005) Features and designs of randomised controlled trials and non-randomised experimental designs, in A. Bowling and S. Ebrahim (eds) *Handbook of Health Research Methods: Investigation, Measurement and Analysis*. Maidenhead: Open University Press.

The tools of quantitative research

This section covers the advantages and disadvantages of using questionnaires and interviews in quantitative research, along with methods of increasing response, questionnaire design, interviewing techniques and the preparation of the data for coding and analysis. Each method has its strengths and weaknesses and it is important to balance these when deciding upon which to use. Within different modes of questionnaire administration, there are also many potentially biasing influences on the responses obtained. These are greatest between different types of mode (e.g. self-administered versus interview modes), rather than within modes. It can be difficult to separate out the effects of the different influences, at different levels. Further, the response rate to the study and the types of responses obtained can be influenced by the method used, the nature of the approach made to the respondent, the design of the questionnaire and the interviewer (where used). These issues are described in the following chapters, along with techniques of reducing and checking for bias.

Section contents

Data collection methods in quantitative research: questionnaires, interviews and their response rates

Introduction

Whether the study is an analytic experiment or a descriptive survey, the method of collecting the data will need to be addressed. Some studies rely on data from records (e.g. medical records), though self-administered questionnaire and interview methods, perhaps within a triangulated approach, are probably the most common means of data collection. If an interview method is preferred, the issue of structured, semi-structured or in-depth needs to be addressed, as well as whether the interview is to be personal, electronic or by telephone. If the self-administered questionnaire is preferred, it has to be decided whether it should be given to sample members personally, with a pre-paid envelope to return it in once completed, or whether it is to be sent directly to sample members by post. Surveys, then, can be conducted in different settings, and with different questionnaire methods.

These modes differ in several ways at different levels. Within any mode of administration, there are many potential influences on responses. There are at least four steps involved in answering questionnaires, which make cognitive demands on respondents: comprehension of the question; recall of requested information from memory; evaluation of the link between the retrieved information and the question; and communication of the response. The channel of questionnaire presentation (e.g. auditory, oral, visual) is likely to affect the cognitive burden placed on respondents, especially the demand for literacy in the case of visual self-administration methods. And, as each mode inevitably imposes different cognitive requirements on respondents, and varies in the amount of privacy and anonymity it affords respondents, this can affect the process of responding to questions, and the quality of the data. Probably the least burdensome method is the personal, face-to-face interview (auditory channel) as this only requires the respondent to speak the same language in which the questions are asked, and to have basic verbal and listening skills. No reading skills are required (unless written materials for the respondent are contained within the interview). A friendly, motivating interviewer can increase response and item response rates. In contrast, telephone interviews make greater auditory demands and may be burdensome to respondents. The most burdensome modes are likely to be visual and written methods of self-administration, as these demand that respondents are literate in reading the language(s) of the survey, that they do not have visual impairments and have the dexterity (e.g. of wrist, fingers) to complete the questions. These differences, at different levels, can make it difficult to separate out the effects of each on the quality of the data obtained (Bowling 2005b). Even minor changes in question wording, question order or response format can result in differences in the type of response obtained, but can be difficult to separate out from other effects of different modes of administration. In addition to the traditional range of paper and pencil methods, there is increasing academic interest in the use of computer-assisted face-to-face interviewing, computer-assisted telephone interviewing, self-administered computer methods, audio computer-assisted self-administered interviewing, and interactive voice response telephone methods.

Thus, while each method has its advantages and disadvantages, each has implications for bias. These issues are discussed in this chapter, along with methods for increasing response rates.

Structured and semi-structured questionnaires

Questionnaires can be structured or semi-structured. Unstructured schedules (or 'exploratory', 'in-depth', 'free-style' interviews) can also be used and these are described in the chapter on qualitative methods (Chapter 17). Structured questionnaires involve the use of fixed (standardised) questions, batteries of questions, tests (e.g. psychological) and/or scales which are presented to respondents in the same way, with no variation in question wording, and with mainly pre-coded response choices. These are used in face-to-face, postal and telephone surveys. Semi-structured interview schedules include mainly fixed questions but with no, or few, response codes, and are used flexibly to allow the interviewer to probe and to enable respondents to raise other relevant issues not covered by the interview schedule. Some semi-structured schedules permit the interviewer to ask the questions out of order at appropriate opportunities during the interview.

Advantages of structured questionnaires

The strength of structured questionnaires is the ability to collect unambiguous and easy-to-count answers, leading to quantitative data for analysis. Because the method leads to greater ease of data collection and analysis, it is relatively economical and large samples of people can be included.

Routine information about medical conditions and major procedures experienced can be collected from patients by questionnaire, supplemented by information from medical notes where permission to access them has been obtained. There is generally a high level of reported concordance between medical record data and patients' reports of major conditions and types of treatment (e.g. diabetes, major medical conditions reported by people aged 65+; Bush *et al.* 1989; Midthjell *et al.* 1992). Concordance has also been reported to be good between medical records and relatives' reports of deceased people's episodes of hospitalisation and surgical operations undergone in the 12 months prior to death, though less good for other types of treatment received (e.g. physiotherapy, chemotherapy, drip feeding) (Cartwright and Seale 1990). Mothers' recall of their children's (aged 3–9) history of vaccinations and specific infections (e.g. measles) have been reported to be poor in comparison with medical records (McKinney *et al.* 1991). Recall will partly depend on the saliency and recency of the topic to people. In relation to medical conditions and procedures, it will also depend on their complexity, on the amount of information they were given by health professionals and on whether it was understood and remembered at the time.

Disadvantages of structured questionnaires

Their weakness is that the pre-coded response choices may not be sufficiently comprehensive and not all answers may be easily accommodated. Some respondents may therefore be 'forced' to choose inappropriate pre-coded answers that might not fully represent their views.

Structured interview and self-administered questionnaire methods rest on the assumption that questions can be worded and ordered in a way that will be understood by all respondents. This may not always be justified, as respondents may not all share the same perspective and the same words, terms and concepts may not elicit the same response from different respondents. The method relies on unstated 'general knowledge' about the group of interest, particularly concerning the perceptual and interpretive processes in the interviewer and participant. The method is best suited for obtaining factual data (e.g. family size, employment history), but can be subject to error in relation to the collection of information about attitudes, behaviour and social processes.

There is always scope for bias: for example, interviewer bias in interview studies, recall (memory) bias and framing, in which respondents' replies are influenced by the design (frame) of the pre-coded response choices. Many questions are about socially desirable attitudes, states and behaviour leading to potential social desirability bias (the respondent's desire to present a positive image).

Postal questionnaires and self-administration

The self-administered or postal questionnaire is less of a social encounter than interview methods and can be posted to people to minimise social desirability and interviewer bias. Bowling et al. (1999), in secondary analyses of three large British population survey datasets, reported that responses to a health status scale (the Short Form-36 Health Survey Questionnaire) during an interview survey produced inflated positive (good) health status scores in comparison with responses obtained by postal survey (suggesting that the interviews suffered from greater social desirability bias).

A common method of covering a large, geographically spread population relatively quickly and more economically than interview methods is to mail respondents a questionnaire to complete at home, with a reply-paid envelope for its return. A variation is to give the sample members a questionnaire in person and ask them to complete it at home, and return it to the investigator in a reply-paid envelope (e.g. patients in clinics can be approached in this way).

This method eliminates the problem of interviewer bias and is useful for sensitive topics, as there is more anonymity. However, the method is only suitable when the issues and questions are straightforward and simple, when the population is 100 per cent literate and speaks a common language, and when a sampling frame of addresses exists. It is less suitable for complex issues and long questionnaires, and it is inappropriate if spontaneous replies are required. The data obtained are generally less reliable than with face-to-face interviews, as interviewers are not present to clarify questions or to probe and hence the replies also have to be accepted as final. There is no control over who completes the questionnaire even if respondents are instructed not to pass the questionnaire on, or over the influence of other people on the participants' replies. Respondents can read all the questions before answering any one of them, and they can answer the questions in any order they wish – and question order, which can be controlled in interview situations, can affect the type of response. Response rates are generally lower for postal questionnaires than for personal interviews. Finally, there is no opportunity to supplement the questionnaire with observational data (brief descriptions by the interviewer at the end of the interview can be valuable, e.g. of the respondent and the setting, and interruptions and how the interview went). There is some evidence that postal questionnaires lead to an under-estimate of patients' health problems in comparison with personal interview techniques (Doll et al. 1991), or it may be that personal interviews can carry more social desirability bias and thus over-estimate health problems (Bowling et al. 1999; Bowling 2005b).

Structured and semi-structured interviews

Interviews involve the collection of data through talking to respondents (interviewees) and recording their responses. They may be carried out face to face or by telephone.

Face-to-face interviews

Face-to-face interview methods vary from in-depth, unstructured or semi-structured (i.e. structured questions without response codes) methods to highly structured, pre-coded response questionnaires, or they can involve a combination of the two (a structured, pre-coded questionnaire, but with open-ended questions to allow the respondent to reply in his or her own words, where the range of responses is unknown or cannot be easily categorised). Sometimes, measurement instruments are handed to the respondents (self-completion or self-administration scales) to complete themselves during face-to-face interviews (e.g. scales of depression where it is thought that the interviewer recording of the response may lead to social desirability bias).

The advantages of face-to-face interviews are: interviewers can probe fully for responses and clarify any ambiguities; more complicated and detailed questions can be asked; more information, of greater depth, can be obtained; inconsistencies and misinterpretations can be checked; there are no literacy requirements for respondents; questions in structured schedules can be asked in a predetermined order; response rates are generally higher with friendly interviewers than for questionnaires which are sent through the post or telephone interviews. With a well-trained interviewer, open-ended questions can be included in the questionnaire to enable respondents to give their opinions in full on more complex topics. They also provide rich and quotable material which enlivens research reports. Open-ended questions are used for topics which are largely unknown or complex, and for pilot studies.

The potential errors made by interviewers (e.g. by making incorrect skips of inapplicable questions and sub-questions) can be minimised by computer-assisted interviewing (use of laptop computers which display the questionnaire, which enable respondents' replies to be directly keyed in and which automatically display the next question, skips, errors, and so on).

The disadvantages are that interviews can be expensive and time-consuming, and there is the potential for interviewer bias, and additional bias if interpreters are used for some participants. Techniques for reducing potential bias include good interviewer training in methods of establishing rapport with people, putting them at ease and appearing non-judgemental. Interviewers can also be matched with participants in relation to their basic socio-demographic characteristics – though, in practice, the availability of potential interviewers rules out matching on a large scale, and there is little consistent information about reduction of response biases through matching. Structured and semi-structured interview questionnaires, if carefully designed for the topic, can yield highly accurate data. However, the topic has to be appropriate for this method; unstructured interview methods are more appropriate for complex and unknown issues (see Chapter 17). Despite the popularity of using face-to-face interview methods for health surveys, there is increasing evidence that these methods lead to under-reporting of health problems, in comparison with postal approaches, particularly for mental health topics, probably due to the operation of social desirability bias in the former situation (McHorney *et al.* 1994; Bowling *et al.* 1999; Lyons *et al.* 1999).

Telephone interviews

Interviews conducted by telephone appear to have equal accuracy rates to face-to-face interviews in relation to the collection of data on general health status and the prevalence of depressive symptoms. Their main *advantage* is that, in theory, the method is economic in relation to time (i.e. no travelling is involved for the interviewer) and resources (i.e. travelling and associated costs are not incurred). However, telephone interviewing is not necessarily a cheap option. At least three call-backs will be required, given estimates that 50 per cent of diallings are met with the engaged tone or there is no reply, and an increasing number of telephones have answering systems. Answering systems tend to be held by younger, unmarried people in higher socio-economic groups (Mishra *et al.* 1993). This necessitates repeated call-backs, which can be time-consuming, if sampling bias is to be minimised. There is the potential bias of over-representing people who are most likely to be at home (and who answer the telephone), who may be unrepresentative of the wider population.

One of the latest developments in telephone interviewing is computer-assisted telephone interviewing. The interviewer asks the questions from a computer screen and respondents' answers are typed and coded directly onto a disk. The advantage is the speed, and the minimisation of interviewer error when asking questions (e.g. the computer prompts the interviewer to ask the next question and only when the answer has been keyed in does the computer move on to the next question; skips are displayed; out of range codes are displayed).

Surveys using telephone interviews have been popular for many years in the USA, where levels of telephone ownership are high, and also among market researchers (e.g. random digit dialling or sampling from telephone directories or lists). They are slowly becoming more popular among social researchers in Europe, though they have the disadvantage that people in lower socio-economic groups have lower rates of telephone ownership, and consequently there is potential for sample bias owing to their being under-represented in the sample.

Apart from potential sample bias, the main disadvantage of the method is that it is only suitable for use with brief questionnaires and on non-sensitive topics. It has higher rates of total and item non-response in health surveys (Cannell *et al.* 1981), especially on more sensitive topics (see Wells *et al.* 1988) and results in less complete information and more 'don't know' responses (Körmendi and Noordhoek 1989). It also tends to suffer from a high rate of premature termination (the respondent does not wish to continue with the interview) (Frankfort-Nachmias and Nachmias 1992). However, there is also some evidence that there is more accurate reporting of health problems in telephone interviews in comparison with face-to-face interviews (Cannell *et al.* 1981) – that is, if over-reporting is assumed to be more accurate reporting.

Cartwright (1988) reported that most of her respondents to a survey on maternity services were willing to be contacted again about the study, and almost two-thirds provided their telephone number. However, though there were no differences with willingness to be recontacted and social class, the proportion who gave a telephone number declined from 85 per cent in social class I (professional) to 35 per cent in social class V (unskilled manual). There is some evidence that people prefer personal interviews to telephone interviews (Groves 1979).

Non-response

In telephone interviews, some telephones may be engaged or remain unanswered. In postal surveys some sample members will not return postal questionnaires. In interview surveys some people might not answer the door to the interviewer. In all types of study, some sample members will directly refuse to participate, will not be at home or will be away at the time of the study, or will have moved, died, have poor hearing or sight, be frail or mentally confused, or be too ill, and some will not speak/read the same language. These are all sources of non-response. In addition, non-coverage of the unit (e.g. where a household or person or clinic is missing from the sampling frame) is also a type of non-response. People who have died before the start of the study ('blanks') can be excluded from the sampling frame and from the calculation of the non-response rate.

The potential for survey bias from non-response highlights the importance of finding out more about the characteristics of non-responders, and potential resulting response bias. In cross-sectional and baseline surveys, where little or no information is available for non-respondents – unlike follow-up waves of longitudinal surveys – response bias can be difficult to estimate. At best, investigators compare the socio-demographic characteristics of responders with population census statistics to estimate likely differences due to non-response. In longitudinal research, sample dropouts can also compromise the validity of results from multiple time points, though pre-existing information can be used to compare future respondents and non-respondents to estimate bias.

In general, important groups to include in research are populations described as 'hard to reach' and thereby are more likely to be non-responders. These can include people in ethnic minority groups, frail people and people who live in socially disadvantaged areas (often labelled as 'socially excluded'). Their exclusion from the study can threaten its external validity (generalisability). In Britain, the proportion of ethnic minority groups in the total population is small, but concentrated in larger numbers in urban areas. A random, national population sample will only generate small numbers of people in ethnic minority groups, and usually insufficient numbers for analysis. In order to ensure that information is also collected about people in ethnic minority groups, survey organisations generally carry out *ethnic boost samples* in addition to random population sampling. For this, they sample in wards known to have high proportions of ethnic minorities.

Non-response is important because it affects the quality of the data collected by reducing the effective sample size, which results in a loss of precision in the survey estimates. Non-response also has the potential to introduce bias if the non-respondents differ in some way from the respondents.

Weighting for non-response

There are weighting procedures which can be used to compensate for unit non-response (e.g. weighting of the replies of males aged 16–24 if these have a particularly high non-response, on the assumption that the non-responders and responders do not differ). The method is aimed at reducing non-response bias, but it often leads to an increase in variance.

It is unwise to ignore non-response and assume that the responders and non-responders do not differ in relation to the estimates of population variables. If the survey estimates differ for respondents and non-respondents, then the survey results will consistently produce results which under- or over-estimate the true population values (response bias). If some information can be obtained about the non-respondents, and the survey estimates are different for the respondents and the non-respondents, then it may be possible to use statistical weighting methods which attach weight to the responding units in order to compensate for units not being included in the final sample.

The most commonly used weighting method is population-based weighting (which requires that the sample is divided into weighting classes where the population total within each class is known, e.g. from census data). Less commonly used because investigators do not have the required information is sample-based weighting (which requires that information in relation to key study variables is available for both responding and non-responding units). The principles and procedures for weighting for non-response have been outlined by Barton (1996), and described in more detail by Elliot (1991). However, weighting does make assumptions about the non-responders and it is preferable to minimise non-response at the outset of the study rather than to compensate for it by weighting sample results.

Response rate

The response rate is calculated from the number of eligible respondents successfully included in the study, as a percentage of the total eligible study population. Survey response rates have been in decline over the past two decades, as academic, policy and government survey researchers compete with market researchers, and with the various time pressures people experience in their daily lives.

There is no agreed standard for an acceptable minimum response rate, although it appears to be generally accepted that a response rate below 60 per cent is sub-optimal (Groves and Couper 1998), and a response rate of 75 per cent and above is good. This still leaves up to 25 per cent of a sample population who have not responded and who may differ in some important way from the responders (e.g. they may be older and more ill), and thus the survey results will be biased. Non-response can therefore affect the quality of research data as it reduces the effective sample size, resulting in loss of precision of the results (survey estimates).

Response rates are higher for interview than for postal and telephone surveys, and the difference can be in the range of 20 per cent (Cartwright 1988). The direction of the biasing of survey results will be largely unknown, but it is possible that non-respondents may be in some way different to respondents. For example, Cartwright (1988), on the basis of her national survey of maternity services, reported that Asian mothers were under-represented among those responding to the postal questionnaire, in comparison with her interview survey.

Methods for increasing response

The covering letter

There are several methods available for increasing response, including the content of the covering letter. This should include the aim and sponsorship of the survey, explain how respondents' names were obtained, the importance of their response and why a representative group is needed, emphasise the confidentiality of the results, and state how the results will be used. Each covering letter should include the name and address of the sample member, and be personally hand-signed, using blue ink (to avoid it looking like a photocopy). Extra care will be needed with covering letters if they are to be sent to respondents in advance. If they appear to be sent by commercial organisations some sample members will put them into the rubbish bin without opening them (Klepacz 1991). People are more likely to respond to a request from an attractive, legitimate body (Campanelli 1995).

Advance letters

Sending an advance letter to sample members in interview surveys can increase the response rate because it can increase the credibility of the study, explain its value, emphasise confidentiality and increase the interviewer's self-confidence. On the other hand, it can also give sample members time to plan their refusal and thus have a negative effect (Campanelli 1995). Sometimes local district ethical committees will insist that a postage-paid reply card, offering sample members a positive opportunity to opt out, is sent to all potential respondents before interview surveys. This can seriously reduce response. The Office of Population Censuses and Surveys reported that two local ethical committees in their survey areas insisted that advance reply cards must be sent to sample members, giving them the option of refusing to permit the interviewer to call. They adversely affected response and were received back from 22 per cent in one area and 48 per cent in the other (Dobbs and Breeze 1993).

In addition, local organisations (e.g. community organisations and health clinics) could be notified, where relevant and appropriate, that surveys are being conducted and asked to disseminate information (e.g. put leaflets in waiting and meeting areas) about the study in order to raise its profile and the community's awareness of the study.

Incentives

Market research companies often give sample members incentives such as money, gifts and lottery chances. In the USA it is increasingly common for academic investigators to offer sample members a small financial reward as an inducement to take part in research ($5–20). For example, Wells *et al.* (1988) offered randomly sampled members of households, who had taken part in an interview survey on the epidemiology of psychiatric disorder, $10 each for their participation in a subsequent telephone interview survey. This does increase response (Frankfort-Nachmias and Nachmias 1992).

Apart from certain invasive medical and psychological experiments where people (usually students) are offered a small sum (usually £5), financial inducements to take part in research are generally regarded as unethical in European research, and most research grant bodies disapprove of the practice. Exceptions are where professionals (e.g. doctors, nurses) are paid a fee to cover their time if the research necessitates them performing additional procedures which are likely to be time-consuming over a long time period. However, such incentives can be costly, and most grant-giving bodies will not pay these fees. Some surveys involving very long postal questionnaires offer respondents the opportunity to participate in a free prize draw if they return their questionnaires. However, this is a practice that is still more common in the USA than in other countries. For example, in one US study, which was an RCT of zinc treatment for the common cold, the investigators encouraged people to participate by entering respondents who completed the study into a raffle for one of two prizes (dinner for two or a holiday for two in the Bahamas) (Mossad *et al.* 1996).

While the issue of whether all research participants should be induced with a small fee continues to be debated in Europe, it is unlikely to become standard practice. The goodwill of the public, and the mutual respect of researcher and sample member, continue to be valued. Moreover, there is some evidence that offering incentives of a financial nature discourages responses from people in higher income brackets (Campanelli 1995). Research in the context of a postal health survey in the USA reported that offering financial incentives had no effect on response rates; non-monetary incentives (e.g. pencil and/or newspaper article about the study) also had no effect on response (Hoffman *et al.* 1998). Another study in the USA reported, however, that enclosing a free pencil with the reminder doubled the response rate among physicians, in comparison with mailing the questionnaire alone (Sallis *et al.* 1984).

Translations and interpreters

In areas where there are known members of ethnic groups who speak a range of languages, a short letter which has been translated carefully into the main languages spoken, and tested for meaning and cultural equivalence, should be sent out with the main covering letter. This should explain how help can be given by an interviewer/translator who speaks the same language, and provide a contact telephone number. In an interview study, interviewers should record details of sample members where an interpreter is required. Although interpretation may lead to interviewer and response bias, the alternative is a potentially greater loss of precision of the sample owing to the omission of key groups.

Appearance of the interviewer

The appearance of the interviewer in the case of personal interviews, and the layout of the questionnaire in the case of postal questionnaires, can affect response. The sex of an interviewer can also affect response. For example, elderly female respondents may feel more relaxed with a female interviewer. The way an interviewer dresses can also affect response. Interviewers with good persuasion skills, and who are motivated, will probably achieve higher response rates.

Call-backs in personal interview studies

In interview studies, interviewers are usually instructed to call back on sample members who are out on at least four different occasions, at different times and on different days, before a non-response is recorded. They should also write to the person if there is no answer on a number of occasions. They are instructed to arrange to call back on a more convenient date if respondents are busy. In the case of sample members who are too ill to be interviewed, interviewers can ask for their consent to interview a proxy (e.g. a carer). Interviewers should always inform respondents how long the interview will take. If it takes an hour and the respondent says that is too long, interviewers should ask if they can at least start the questionnaire and see how far they get in the time period allowed.

Postal reminders in postal surveys

With postal surveys, it is common to send two reminders after the initial mailing (enclosing further copies of the questionnaire and pre-paid envelope), at two- to three-week intervals, to non-responders. Each mailing should yield around a quarter to a third of responses.

Some investigators send a postcard or letter only as the first reminder, rather than sending the questionnaire again. However, resending the questionnaire plus a covering letter, rather than just a reminder postcard alone, might increase response. While in the British Health and Lifestyle Survey, the postcard reminder was as effective as the questionnaire reminder (Roberts and Pearson 1993), a study in the USA, comparing the two methods in a health survey, reported that this increased response from

10 per cent to 23 per cent at second mailing (Hoffman *et al.* 1998). As mailing additional questionnaires can be expensive, a compromise would be to send a postcard reminder initially, and then a second questionnaire to anyone who failed to respond to this.

There is slight evidence that a stamped, rather than a franked, reply and outgoing envelope in the case of postal surveys yields a better response rate. Time and cost considerations may preclude stamping, rather than franking, in the case of large surveys.

Recalling in telephone surveys

It was pointed out earlier that telephone surveys have high rates of premature termination where the respondent does not wish to continue with the interview. This will largely depend on the topic and the sponsoring organisation. In order to minimise non-response relating to no-reply/engaged tones, at least three call-backs will be required; and given the high no-reply/engaged tone rate, this is likely to be expensive. There is little that can be done about the increasingly high proportion of telephone answering machine ownership. This is disadvantageous to telephone surveys as, if messages are left about calling back, the respondent might be pre-warned and less willing to participate (given the high rates of premature termination anyway). In some cases the investigator might never get beyond the answerphone, and it is unlikely that he or she would have much success if messages were left asking sample members to telephone. As noted above, this source of non-response is of concern given the characteristics of people with answerphones (younger, unmarried, in higher socio-economic groups), which could lead to sample bias.

Response rates by length of questionnaire and sponsorship

Response rates vary widely, depending on the sponsorship and nature of the topic of study, its saliency and the length of the questionnaire. Cartwright (1988) reported that comparisons of response with a 1-page and a 3-page postal questionnaire showed that these yielded response rates of 90 and 73 per cent respectively. However, response rates were similar for 8-page and 16-page questionnaires. Hoffman *et al.* (1998) reported that, in the context of a health survey, response was similar for a 4-page (16-item) and 16-page (76-item) questionnaire. Jenkinson *et al.* (2003) reported results from an RCT of long versus short survey instruments in postal surveys of patients' experiences of health care. They found no differences in response rate or item completion between a 4-page (13 questions) and 12-page (108 questions) questionnaire format.

The sponsoring organisation of the survey can also affect results, with local universities likely to obtain a higher response rate in their area than an independent research institute based elsewhere (Cartwright 1983).

Response rates by saliency of topic

The saliency of the topic to the sample member can be more important than the length of the questionnaire. Cartwright (1978) reported that older doctors were more likely to respond to topics on death whereas female doctors were more likely to respond to topics on family planning. Response also varies with the perceived *threat* of the topic. Cartwright (1978) also reported obtaining a 76 per cent response rate for doctors on the topic of dying, but only 56 per cent on the topic of their prescribing behaviour. Dunne *et al.* (1997) reported results from a postal survey in Australia on the topic of sexuality, which sampled respondents from a national, longitudinal research register, and which enabled record linkage to provide information about the characteristics of responders and non-responders. They reported that people who consented to take part differed in several ways from non-responders, including being more likely to have higher levels of education and to have less conservative sexual attitudes. Such response bias can seriously distort survey estimates.

Response rates by type of respondent

Non-responders may be different in some way from responders. However, research evidence on the characteristics of non-responders is inconsistent, and is likely to be partly linked to the topic of the survey. Ann Cartwright's work has shown that response rates vary by area, and are related to the social class of the father's occupation (people in lower social classes are less likely to respond to interview, but not postal surveys), and response is lower among people in some ethnic groups (Cartwright 1983). Cartwright (1983) has also reported that response rates are higher among hospital patients than members of the general population, higher among nurses than doctors and lower in London than in other parts of the UK. The General Household Survey is able to link with census data for most of the households sampled, and analyses of the linked data show that the General Household Survey, and by comparison the Omnibus Survey, again slightly under-represents people who live in London (by <1 per cent) and people living in single person households in comparison with households with two or more people (the non-contact rate was 5.3 per cent in comparison with 2.6 per cent for the latter) (Foster *et al.* 1995).

Research has shown that, among older people, response rates increase with increasing age (Doll *et al.* 1991). With the General Household Survey (Foster *et al.* 1995), there is a very slight under-representation of people in the age bands under 30 years, but by less than 1 per cent in each band. Non-responders, especially very elderly people, have been reported to use significantly more medical services and have more, and longer, hospital admissions than responders (Rockwood *et al.* 1989). The implication is that non-responders are more ill than responders. However, research is contradictory, and Cartwright and Windsor (1989) reported no differences between attenders and non-attenders at hospital outpatient departments in response to a survey about outpatient attendance.

One puzzle in longitudinal and all follow-up research, and which is reliant on self-completion questionnaires, is the very small number of respondents who report a different gender at follow-up, compared with their baseline survey. It is assumed that the same named person will complete the questionnaire at follow-ups, but sometimes this might be completed by proxies if the sampled respondent is unwell or frail. This might explain the gender switch if the proxy respondents complete the demographic questions about themselves. Apart from the need to avoid repeating baseline demographic questions at follow-up, in order to reduce burden, there remains a need for verification of identity in the questionnaire.

Item non-response

Non-response to individual items on the questionnaire may also occur. Cartwright (1988) reported, on the basis of her early surveys in Britain, that inadequate responses to questions are three times more common on postal questionnaires than at interview (1.9 vs 0.6 per cent), particularly for questions requiring a single answer from multiple possibilities. There is little control over this with a postal questionnaire, though interviewers can attempt to minimise it. The well-trained interviewer will repeat the question or probe an ambiguous or irrelevant response until a full answer is given, and can document any instances where respondents feel the question is inappropriate or does not apply to them.

The longer health status questionnaires, such as the Sickness Impact Profile (Bergner *et al.* 1981), can suffer from high item non-response (McColl *et al.* 1995), and questionnaires with items that are not directly relevant to the population group targeted may also suffer high item non-response. For example, the Short Form-36 developed by Ware *et al.* (1993) has been reported to have high item non-response among elderly people (Brazier *et al.* 1992). It is possible that elderly people do not see the direct relevance of several of the items (e.g. difficulties walking a mile, activities with examples such as moving a table, playing golf) (see Hill *et al.* 1995).

Handling item non-response

There are documented methods for handling missing questionnaire data where it can be assumed that the items in question are missing at random (as opposed to consistent item non-response which suggests an inherent problem with the item such as its relevance to people or a problem with its wording). If an item response is missing (at random) from a scale which is scored, the researcher has the option of excluding the respondent from analyses of the whole scale, or using imputation methods for the missing item. The most common method is to assign the missing item the average value of the completed items in order to be able to include the respondent in the analyses of the total scale score. Most statistical packages for the computer have a procedure which will allow this. This is the recommended method for the Short Form-36 (Ware *et al.* 1993). However, the effects on the validity of the results have not been fully assessed. If missing values are not imputed, then the statistical analysis needs to allow for the number of items included in the scale scoring. For example, the use of means rather than summed scores allows for missing values (as the mean can be calculated for a reduced number of items); or the sum can be expressed as the percentage of the maximum achievable score (which also allows for the possibility of a reduced number of items); otherwise the global score should be recorded as missing (Billingham *et al.* 1999).

Imputation techniques, however, can miss uncertainty. One method of overcoming this is to use multiple random imputation – 'filling in' techniques – in which analyses are carried out on different formats of the randomly imputed dataset. In longitudinal surveys of ageing populations, the occurrence of missing data is likely to be related to mortality as well as frailty, thus distorting associations of interest and biasing inferential statements. Statistical analyses and modelling of only the survivors are thus misleading (as this depends on survival and the unknown data). Direct maximisation of the likelihood with missing data is complicated, and most methods use some form of data augmentation. Therefore, one approach is to carry out a series of sensitivity analyses (e.g. the use of multinomial modelling and inclusion of deaths as an outcome variable – deceased sample members will be known in flagged datasets). A similar approach can be attempted with other non-responders who are likely to be frail (using pre-exit study data), or where characteristics can be estimated. Multiple imputation techniques can be used, and the data can be analysed under a variety of non-response modes (i.e. sensitivity analyses).

An introduction to statistical methods for compensating for non-response is provided by Kalton (1983), and a more general text is by Lessler and Kalsbeek (1992). Billingham *et al.* (1999) have described methods of dealing with item non-response in relation to longitudinal quality of life data.

Summary of main points

- The strength of structured questionnaires is the ability to collect unambiguous and easy-to-count answers, leading to quantitative data for analysis.
- Structured questionnaires are economical and large samples of people can be included.
- The weakness of structured questionnaires is that pre-coded response choices may not be sufficiently comprehensive, and not all answers may be easily accommodated.
- Postal and other self-completion methods are only suitable when the issues and questions are straightforward and simple, when the population is 100 per cent literate, and speaks a common language, and when a sampling frame of addresses (e.g. postal or electronic) exists.
- The main advantages of face-to-face interviews are that the interviewers can probe fully for responses and clarify any ambiguities; more complicated and detailed questions can be asked.
- The main disadvantages of face-to-face interviews are their expense, and there is the potential of interviewer bias.
- Interviews conducted by telephone appear to have equal accuracy rates to face-to-face interviews in relation to the collection of data on health. They are only suitable for use with short, straightforward questionnaires and on non-sensitive topics.
- The main advantage of telephone interviews is that, in theory, the method is economic in relation to time and resources.
- The main disadvantage of telephone interviewing is that it is limited to people with telephones and those who are in to answer the telephone.
- Non-response potentially affects the quality of research data as it reduces the effective sample size, resulting in loss of precision of the survey estimates.

Key questions

1 Describe the advantages and disadvantages of telephone and postal questionnaire surveys in comparison with face-to-face interviews.
2 What are the essential features to be included in a covering letter for a survey?
3 What are the main types of non-response in telephone, postal and face-to-face interview surveys?
4 What are the methods for increasing response rates to postal, face-to-face and telephone interview surveys?
5 Why is non-response a potential source of sample bias?
6 What is known about the characteristics of non-responders?

Key terms

bias
computer-assisted interviewing
computer-assisted telephone interviewing
face-to-face interviews
interviews
item non-response
non-response
postal questionnaires

response rates
self-administered questionnaires
semi-structured questionnaires
structured questionnaires
telephone interviews
unstructured questionnaires
weighting

Recommended reading

Buckingham, A. and Saunders, P. (2004) *The Survey Methods Workbook: From Design to Analysis*. Cambridge: Polity.

Cartwright, A. (1983) *Health Surveys in Practice and in Potential*. London: King Edward's Hospital Fund for London.

Cartwright, A. (1988) Interviews or postal questionnaires? Comparisons of data about women's experiences with maternity services, *The Milbank Quarterly*, 66: 172–89.

Cartwright, A. and Seale, C. (1990) *The Natural History of a Survey: An Account of the Methodological Issues Encountered in a Study of Life Before Death*. London: King Edward's Hospital Fund for London.

Groves, R.M., Fowler, F.J., Couper, M.P. *et al.* (2009) *Survey Methodology*. Chichester: John Wiley.

Chapter contents

Introduction

A basic assumption underlying the use of structured questionnaires is that researchers and respondents share the same theoretical frame of reference and interpret the words, phrases and concepts used in the same way. Care is therefore needed when designing questionnaires; the emphasis is on simplicity and on following the basic rules of questionnaire design. It is important to remember that the question wording, form and order can all affect the type of responses obtained. The skill of questionnaire design is to minimise these influences and the subsequent biases in the results. The Centre for Applied

Social Surveys in the UK (a resource centre of the Economic and Social Research Council) has developed an online Social Survey Question Bank (now rebranded: surveynet.ac.uk/sqb; discover.ukdataservice.ac.uk/variables – links accessed 6 March 2014). This includes questions from large-scale surveys, including the various government surveys, on socio-demographic background, health, housing, the family, lifestyle, politics, and work. This is of value to investigators who wish to make their questionnaires comparable with major surveys covering the same topics. Harmonisation, development and easier availability of validated questionnaires for use in epidemiological research have been called for by the International Epidemiology Association European Questionnaire Group (Olsen 1998).

Planning

All research needs to be explicitly set in an appropriate theoretical and conceptual framework. Similarly, all measures selected for use need to be supported with their rationale, and a description of the concepts and domains that the measure intends to assess. In the case of existing measurement scales, these should be found in the published literature supporting a scale's psychometric properties. If this is lacking, then the measure is of questionable value.

The two important procedures at the outset of constructing a questionnaire are planning and piloting. In the planning of the questionnaire, it is important to list the topics of interest in relation to the aims of the study, collate appropriate and tested questions and scales, list additional items and response formats that need to be developed, and finally relate the questions back to the survey aims – and if a question is not essential, the rule is to leave it out. Appropriate and tested measurement scales should have been identified at the stage of the literature review for the proposed research. In addition, researchers could search for commonly used survey questions on databases that may exist in their field of study (e.g. Question Bank, see above). The British Office for National Statistics also displays online questions across its national social surveys (www.statistics.gov.uk/harmony/harmonfp.asp).

There are also many practical issues to be resolved at the planning stage, such as how frequently the measures are to be applied. If more than once, then should the follow-up period be one month, six weeks or six months? (The timing will depend on when changes are anticipated.) A further issue is the quality control of the research, and the methods by which it will be undertaken: strategies must be developed for dealing with, and minimising, poor compliance from sample members, missing data (respondents and/or interviewers forgetting to complete questions, or refusals by respondents to do so) and any suspect or inaccurate data which might have been collected.

Piloting

The research ideas and topics should be tested on colleagues and then pre-piloted with a small number of in-depth interviews (about 12) with the population of interest. The investigator should hold meetings with 'experts' in the field and group discussions with members of the target group in order to ensure the validity of the coverage. Then the questionnaire should be more formally developed and piloted. (See Box 13.1.)

Interpretations

The validity of questionnaire data depends on shared assumptions and understandings of the questions and response categories. Research has shown that respondents may interpret questions, including questions on health status, in different ways to the investigator (Tanur 1992; Mallinson 1998). Pre-testing of questions should therefore include asking people to describe what they are thinking of when they listen to, or read, each question, and about how they interpret it. This technique is known as 'think-aloud' testing (Suchman and Jordan 1992). The investigator thereby aims to discover whether or not the questions were understood, and responded to, as intended. Cognitive interviewing is a more intensive method of systematically developing and refining survey questions by intensively probing the thought processes of respondents who are presented with the study topic, and subsequently draft and final questionnaires (Willis 2005).

If the questionnaire contains new, previously untested items, then they will also need to be tested face to face on a sample of people from the target population (about 30–50, depending on the complexity of the items). Testing newly-developed scales for reliability and validity involves a great deal of time, effort and expense; therefore, there is a strong argument in favour of using existing scales.

Face-to-face piloting should continue with new sample members until the researchers are confident that the questionnaire requires no further changes. Respondents should be informed that they are being interviewed for a pilot study – most will be willing to help, and will then probably be more likely to admit any instances where they do not understand the questions or the response codes are not applicable to them. Piloting also acts as a check on potential interviewer errors (where face-to-face interview is the method of choice). As well as analysis of the returned questionnaires, the interviewers should be consulted (in a focus group forum) about any aspects of the questionnaire that they feel need revising.

Questionnaire layout

It is important that the questionnaire has been printed clearly and professionally, and that it is visually easy to read and comprehend. It is also important not to split the question, or question and response categories, between two pages. Lower-case letters, rather than capitals, should be used for text (capitals can have a dazzling effect). There should be space for verbatim comments where appropriate (and all respondents can be asked to record any additional comments in a space provided). Coloured paper may enliven a questionnaire, but the colour should not be dark (or the print will be more difficult to read), and dazzling colours should be avoided. Market research companies consult psychologists to advise on their product designs, and they use colour deliberately to package their products to imply a targeted image. For example, green is associated with 'healthy lifestyles', yellow with 'optimism', red with 'physical stimulation' and blue with 'freshness'. Thus the colour of the questionnaire pages can potentially influence the mood of respondents.

> ### Box 13.1 Issues to be addressed in the pilot study
>
> ■ Is each question measuring what it is intended to measure?
> ■ Is the wording understood by all respondents, and is the understanding (meaning) similar for all respondents?
> ■ Are the instructions on self-administered questionnaires understood by all respondents?
> ■ For closed (pre-coded) questions, is an appropriate response available for each respondent? Are all reasonable alternatives included?
> ■ Are any questions systematically or frequently missed, or do some questions regularly elicit uninterpretable answers?
> ■ Do the responses suggest that the researcher has included all the relevant issues in the questionnaire?
> ■ Do the questionnaire and covering letter motivate people to respond?
> ■ How do respondents feel about the questionnaire?

It is customary for the first few lines of a questionnaire to include the label 'Confidential', the respondent's serial (identification) number (to preserve anonymity), the title of the study and a brief introduction. The instructions for the respondent or interviewer should also be given clearly at the beginning, for example, whether answers are to be ticked, circled, written in or combinations (or entered directly onto the computer, if computer-assisted interviewing is used). Ensure that instructions for giving multiple, rather than single, answers where required, are given (e.g. 'Please tick all that apply.'). A thank you statement should be given at the end of the questionnaire.

Any filter questions for questions that do not apply to some respondents must be clearly labelled and all interviewers and respondents must understand which question to go to next. Instructions about filter questions and skips are usually printed for interviewers in the right-hand margin of the questionnaire. These need to be minimised and kept simple and obvious in self-administered questionnaires, as in Box 13.2.

> ### Box 13.2 Example of filter question and skip
>
> 1a. In the past three months, have you stayed overnight in hospital?
>
> Yes—
> No—GO TO QUESTION 2
>
> If you stayed overnight in hospital in the past three months:
>
> 1b. How many nights did you stay in hospital?
> write in number of nights: _____

Question numbering and topic ordering

Questions must be numbered (1, 2, etc.), and sub-questions clearly labelled (e.g. as 1a, 1b, etc.). A question and its response categories should never be split over two pages, as this can lead to confusion.

The order of questions is important (see later) and questions should not skip backwards and forwards between topics. Each section of the questionnaire should form a module and be topic based (e.g. questions should be grouped together by subject). This is more professional and less irritating for respondents. It is important to provide linking sentences when moving to new modules on the questionnaire: for example, 'The next questions ask about some personal details', 'These questions are about your health'. Questions should be simply worded, and double-barrelled questions (questions containing two questions), as well as questions containing double negatives, should be avoided, because they lead to confusion and ambiguity (see later). For examples of how to transform research questions into questionnaires, see Czaja and Blair (2005).

The covering letter

The importance of giving respondents a covering letter is explained in Chapter 12. Both interview and postal, or self-administration, questionnaire surveys should give all sample members a covering letter about the study to keep for reference and reassurance that the organisation and study are bona fide. The covering letter should be written on the organisation's headed notepaper, include the name and address of the sample member and the identification (serial) number, and address the recipient by name. The letter should explain how the person's name was obtained, outline the study aims and benefits (concisely), guarantee confidentiality and be signed in blue ink (so it is not confused with a photocopy) in order to personalise it (which increases response).

Question form, order and wording

The form, order and wording of the questions can all affect response. It is essential to be aware of this when designing questionnaires and selecting batteries of measurement scales.

Rules for form

'Question form' refers to the format of the question (closed or open-ended), and type of measuring instrument (e.g. single items, batteries of single items or scales). The format of the questionnaire can affect the answer. The comprehensiveness of response choices for closed questions is also important (to prevent responses being forced into inappropriate categories), though there appears to be little difference in type of response obtained between the various types of closed response scales.

Response formats (frames): open and closed questions

Response choices to questions can be left open (and the respondent or interviewer writes in the reply in the respondent's own words) or they can be closed or 'pre-coded': dichotomised (e.g. yes/no response choices), multiple response (no restriction on the number of responses that can be ticked) or scaled (with one response code per response frame permitted).

Structured questionnaires involve the use of fixed questions, batteries of questions and/or scales which are presented to respondents in the same way, with no variation in question wording and with closed questions (pre-coded response choices). It is assumed that each item means the same to each respondent. These are used in postal surveys and in personal interviews. With structured, pre-coded formats, the information obtained is limited by the questions asked and the response choices offered.

Some structured questionnaires will also include open-ended questions, to enable respondents to reply in their own words. Semi-structured interviews include fixed questions but with no, or few, response codes, and are used flexibly, often in no fixed order, to enable respondents to raise other relevant issues not covered by the interview schedule. These methods are discussed in Chapter 12. Unstructured interviews are comprised of a checklist of topics, rather than fixed questions, and there are no pre-codes. The more structured approach is only suitable for topics where sufficient knowledge exists for largely pre-coded response formats to be developed, as otherwise the responses will be distorted by inappropriate categories.

Open questions

Open-ended questions (without pre-coded response choices) are essential where replies are unknown, too complex or too numerous to pre-code. Open questions are also recommended for developing questionnaires and measurement scales. The information collected is only limited by the respondent's willingness to provide it, though open-ended questions do require more thought and are more taxing for respondents. Thus, it can be very informative as a method, but demanding for the respondent (the data gathered can range from rich to poor). Open questions also carry the disadvantage that replies can be distorted by the coding process back in the office (e.g. meaning may be lost, interviewers may have summarised the reply and led to some bias, and so on). They can be time-consuming and difficult to analyse, and require more skilled interviewers and coders.

Most interview questionnaires will include a combination of open and closed questions; self-administered (e.g. postal) questionnaires should be restricted to closed questions because most respondents will not bother to write their replies to open-ended questions.

Open questions following closed questions are useful for probing for clarification of reasons and explanations. Closed questions following open questions are of value on topics about which little is known (the closed question can be a useful summary of a narrative account) and where people are likely to be uncritical or influenced by social desirability bias if presented too soon with response choices (see Box 13.3).

Box 13.3 Examples of open questions, open questions following closed questions, and closed questions following open questions

What are the five most important areas of your life that have been affected by your illness?
(Bowling 1995a)

What are the qualities, the things about your GP, that you appreciate? Anything else?
(Cartwright and Anderson 1981)

Are there some occasions when you would prefer to see a doctor of a particular sex?

Yes . . . 1
No . . . 2

If YES: What sort of occasions?

(Cartwright and Anderson 1981)

Has there been any (other) occasion in the past 12 months when you think it would have been better if the general practitioner had sent you to hospital?

Yes . . . 3
No . . . 4

If YES (3): Could you tell me about that?

(Cartwright and Anderson 1981)

How do (or would) you feel about students or trainees being in the surgery with the doctor?

So do (would) you:
Not mind in the least . . . 4
Feel a little uneasy . . . 5
Prefer it if trainee/student left . . . 6
(Other) SPECIFY:

(Cartwright and Anderson 1981)

What do you think about the idea of a National Health Service?
So would you say you:

Approve . . . 4
Disapprove . . . 5
Have mixed feelings . . . 6

(Cartwright and Anderson 1981)

Closed questions

Closed questions with pre-coded response formats are preferable for topics about which much is known, and so suitable response codes can be developed, which are simple. They are also quicker and cheaper to analyse, as they do not involve the subsequent analysis of replies before a suitable coding frame can be developed for coding to take place. Pre-coded responses always carry the risk that respondents' replies are forced into inappropriate categories. However, while their design may be difficult because all possible replies need to be incorporated, there is a huge advantage if respondents' answers can be immediately coded into appropriate categories.

Care is needed when one is choosing the response choices for closed questions. There should be a category to fit every possible response, plus an 'other' category if it is felt that there may be some unknown responses. (See Box 13.4.) Unless the code is a multi-item response frame, whereby respondents can select more than one

> ## Box 13.4 Prompting effects of pre-codes
>
> Bowling (1995a), in a national survey of people's definitions of health-related quality of life (HRQoL), found that when respondents selected codes from a showcard to depict the most important effects of their illness or medical condition on their lives, they selected different areas to the areas previously mentioned in response to an open-ended question. The showcard obviously prompted replies. *In response to the showcard*, the most commonly mentioned first most important effects of their illness on their lives were, in order of frequency:
>
> - pain;
> - tiredness/lack of energy/lethargy;
> - social life/leisure activities;
> - availability of work/ability to work.
>
> In contrast, *the most common freely mentioned* first most important effects of illness were, in order of frequency:
>
> - ability to get out and about/stand/walk/go out shopping;
> - availability of work/ability to work;
> - effects on social life/leisure activities.

reply, or qualitative data are being categorised, whereby narratives can fit more than one concept or theme (see Section V), then each respondent's reply must only fit into one response category. Pre-coded numbers (such as financial information, age groups and time periods) need to be mutually exclusive, comprehensive and unambiguous. For example, use under 20, 20 but under 30, 30 but under 40 and so on rather than under 20, 20 to 30, 30 to 40. When choosing response categories for time periods it is advisable to be exact (e.g. daily, less than daily but more than weekly, weekly and so on, or ask how often the activity has been performed in a specific, recent time period, such as in the past seven days or four weeks, depending on the topic). Exact time periods are preferable to codes such as 'frequently–sometimes–rarely–never', which are vague and relative to the individual's interpretation, and make comparisons between respondents difficult.

Closed, or pre-coded, questions where the pre-coded responses are read out by interviewers, or are seen on self-administration questionnaires, supply the respondent with highly structured clues about their purpose and the answers expected. This can lead to different results in comparison with open-ended questions.

Form and prompts

Closed questions, by giving respondents a range of possible answers from which to choose, give them clues (prompts) about the types of answers expected, which they might not have thought of themselves. (See Box 13.5.) If it is decided that respondents should be given structured response choices from which to choose, then it is important

---

Box 13.5 Examples of closed questions

Do you think it was necessary for you to go to the hospital or do you think a GP could have done what they did?

Necessary to go to hospital . . . 1
GP could have done it . . . 2
Other: SPECIFY

(Cartwright and Anderson 1981)

Would you describe your health as:
Excellent __
Very good __
Good __
Fair __
Poor __

(Ware et al. 1993)

---

to ensure that all reasonable alternative answers are included, as otherwise they will be unreported. This may not be realistic if a complex area is being investigated, and therefore open-ended questions are preferable.

Form and under-reporting

Aided recall procedures (showcards displaying the pre-coded response choices which are handed to respondents) may be helpful if under-reporting is likely to be a problem. Again the list of alternatives must be comprehensive to prevent under-reporting. Open questions are better than closed questions for obtaining information about the frequency of undesirable behaviour, or asking threatening questions (card sorting and responses in sealed envelopes may also be worth considering where the range of likely responses is known).

Form and knowledge

With questions asking about knowledge, open-ended questions are preferable to the provision of response choices in order to minimise successful guessing. Postal questionnaires should also be avoided when asking questions about knowledge as they give respondents the opportunity to consult others, or to look up the answers.

Form and response sets

Form and acquiescence response set: 'yes-saying'

It is well established that respondents will more frequently endorse a statement than disagree with its opposite. This is not always straightforward to interpret. Cohen et al. (1996) reported that asking patients if they agreed with a negative description of their hospital experience produced a greater level of reported dissatisfaction than asking them if they agreed with a positive description. Generally the shared direction of the question wording enhances the association between two measures (see Webb *et al.* 1966). The standard rule is that the direction of question wording should therefore be varied.

Goldberg's General Health Questionnaire (GHQ) is a good example of the variation in the direction of the question wording and response categories (Goldberg and Williams 1988). There are several versions of this scale available (short to long), the items in each version of the scale vary from positive to negative wording, and the direction of the response categories also varies.

Form and stereotyped response set

Sequences of questions asked with similar response formats are also likely to produce stereotyped responses, such as a tendency to endorse the responses positioned on the far right-hand side or those on the far left-hand side of the questionnaire when they are displayed horizontally. This explains why scales alternate the direction of the response codes – to make people think about the question rather than automatically tick all the right-hand side response choices (see example from the GHQ in Box 13.6).

Box 13.6 Example of variations in response categories

Have you recently:
Spent time chatting with people?

| More time than usual | About the same as usual | Less time than usual | Much less than usual |

Been having restless, disturbed nights?

| Not at all | No more than usual | Rather more than usual | Much more than usual |

(GHQ-30, © David Goldberg 1978. Items reproduced by permission of the publishers, NFER-Nelson, Darville House, 2 Oxford Road East, Windsor SL4 1DF, England. All rights reserved.)

The same form of response scale should not be used too frequently throughout the questionnaire, as this can again lead to a response set (a tendency to answer all the questions in a specific direction regardless of their content). The wording and format of response categories should be varied to avoid this. The Short Form-36 questionnaire for measuring health status is a good example of this variation (see Ware *et al.* 1993).

The response formats vary in type and in direction throughout, from dichotomous formats (yes/no) to scaled (e.g. not at all/slightly/moderately/quite a bit/extremely; none/very mild/mild/moderate/severe/very severe; all of the time/most of the time/a good bit of the time/some of the time/a little of the time/none of the time). Examples of different response formats are shown in Box 13.7.

Box 13.7 Examples of questions with differing response formats

Dichotomous:

In the past six months, have you stayed overnight in a hospital?

Yes __
No __

Multiple choice:

Is your pain

Flickering __
Throbbing __
Tingling __
Intense __

Scaled:

During the past four weeks, how much of the time has your physical health interfered with your social activities?

All of the time __
Most of the time __
Some of the time __
A little of the time __
None of the time __

Question items, batteries and scales

Single item questions and social desirability bias

Single item measures use a single question to measure the concept of interest. Single item questions are imperfect indices of attitudes or behaviour, as responses to one question can only be partly reflective of the area of interest. A single item measure can include a question, such as:

Over the past 12 months, would you say your health on the whole has been:

Very good   ___
Good   ___
Fair   ___
Poor   ___
Very poor   ___

A single item can also form a scale, as in a visual analogue scale:

Here is a line which represents the quality of life. Place a cross on the line at the point which represents how good, or how bad, overall, you feel your quality of your life is:

So good, could not be better   I_____I So bad, could not be worse

Responses can be influenced by several factors, including question wording, social desirability bias and interviewer bias, all of which can lead to measurement error.

Social desirability bias exerts a small but pervasive influence in self-report measures. People may describe the variable (e.g. quality of life) of interest in a way they think the investigator wants to hear, and people want to present themselves in the best possible way. While psychologists have a range of scales of social desirability and lie scales to detect the extent of the influence of social desirability bias (Edwards 1957; Crowne and Marlowe 1960; Paulhus and Moore 1991), most investigators will not wish to employ these and lengthen their scales yet further. The solution is to use scales with several questions (items), rather than single items, then the internal consistency of the items forming the scale can be examined (for example, using item–item correlations, item–total correlations, Cronbach's alpha, split-half reliability). For example, if a person agrees to some extent, with the item: 'I feel good about my life', they should also be more likely to agree with the item: 'I feel that I am making a useful contribution to life'.

One should also train any interviewers to use VAS carefully, and emphasise careful question wording and other techniques of checking for social desirability bias such as comparing self-reports with observed behaviour, though not all responses can be checked in this way. Respondents could also be asked to rate how socially desirable the characteristic in question might be, though interpretation of absolute levels of bias is still difficult.

The range of techniques for assessing social desirability bias, most of which appear burdensome to respondents, was reviewed by Nancarrow and Brace (2000). Projective techniques have been used by psychologists in order to avoid the problem of social desirability bias in direct attitude measurement. Examples include Rorschach inkblot tests (the respondent is shown a series of ten irregular, symmetrical inkblots, and asked to explain what they see); thematic appreciation tests (the respondent is asked to view ambiguous scenes of people and to describe various aspects of the scene); and simple draw a person tasks. All are subject to criticisms of lack of objectivity, questionable validity, as well as ethical issues of deception as the respondent does not know that a specific attitude is being examined. Nederhof (1985) reviewed measures of social desirability bias and self-ratings of item desirability (which aim to detect it), and of methods of preventing or reducing it (including forced-choice items and self-administered questionnaires) and concluded that no method was judged to excel.

Single items are also more difficult to test. For example, they cannot be tested for split half or multiple form reliability, but they can be tested for face and content validity and against other measures. They can also be subjected to test–retest and inter-rater reliability.

It should be noted here that single items measuring self-rated health status or quality of life, for example, are used frequently in research on population health and health services. An example is: 'How would you describe your present health (in comparison with other people of your age): Excellent, very good, good, fair or poor?' Despite difficulties with bias and inconsistency of response, such single items have been reported to be predictive of future disease and mortality in longitudinal surveys (Idler and Angel 1990; Goldberg *et al.* 2001; Heistaro *et al.* 2001). Rating scales which ask people to rate themselves (e.g. their health) in comparison with other people (e.g. of their age) have just a small effect on the distribution of responses (Eriksson *et al.* 2001). However, the popular single item on 'self-reported long-standing illness, infirmity or disability' has been reported to capture medically diagnosed chronic disease, rather than 'illness, infirmity or disability' – non-diagnosed illnesses which people had normalised (Manderbacka 1998). Whether or not long-standing illness was reported by Manderbacka's respondents to restrict everyday activities was associated with severity of the condition, the life circumstances of respondents, and their level of adaptation to ill health. Thus such items reflect much subjectivity in response, and further questioning is desirable in order to aid interpretation.

Batteries

Batteries of questions are a series of single items (rather than a specially constructed scale where responses can be summed), each relating to the same variable of interest. Each item is analysed and presented individually, not summed together.

Scales

Scales involve a series of items about a specific domain that can be summed (sometimes weighted) to yield a score. If responses are averaged or summed across an appropriate set of questions, then a more valid measure than a single item question or battery of single items is obtained, because any individual item error or bias tends to be cancelled out across the items when averaged or summed. Therefore, items on the scale should differ considerably in content (i.e. they should all express a different belief about the area of interest, or different aspect of the behaviour) so that they will not all be limited by the same types of error or question bias. Scales also permit more rigorous statistical analysis.

Scores

Single scale scores

Many scale designers aim to provide a single score, partly because they are easier to analyse and apply. However, it is often preferable to analyse scores for sub-domains separately. An example is health status, which is more meaningfully analysed in relation to the sub-domains of physical functioning, mental health and social activity level. Single scores lead to loss of information: the same total score may arise from many different combinations of responses to the sub-domains of the scale, with unknown meaning (i.e. lack of information about precisely which sub-domain scores the strongest or the weakest), and hence unknown indications for action. Thus, if the scale items cover several different topics, then sub-scores will lead to more refined information than total scale scores.

Additive scores and weighting item scores

If the scale items lie on a single dimension, then it would be reasonable to suggest that they can be used to form a scale. The simplest, albeit crude, method of combining scale items is to add the item response scores to form a multi-item score. This is adequate for most purposes. For example, with knowledge questions (e.g. on scales measuring mental confusion), each correct answer can be given a value of 1 and each incorrect answer allocated 0, and the items added to form the score. With scaled responses, a numerical value can be attached to each class, such as strongly agree = 4, agree = 3, disagree = 2, strongly disagree = 1.

The crude addition (summing) of scores, which results in all items contributing equally to the multi-item scale score, makes the assumption that all items are of equal importance to people. This assumption can be questioned and may lead to the summing of scale scores which are not logically related (Jenkinson 1991). It is often dubious to assume that there are equal intervals between each score, particularly if statistics appropriate for interval-level data are then used. If some items are regarded as more important than others, they should be weighted accordingly (their scores are multiplied by X to enable them to count more). On the other hand, there is the difficulty that different sub-groups of people hold different priorities and values and it is unlikely that the same weighting would apply equally to all (Bowling 1995a, 1996b, 1996c).

Middle values

There is some debate in scaling about the appropriate value for middle scale values (e.g. 'neither agree nor disagree' or 'don't know' responses). If a value of 0 is assigned to these responses, it is assumed that there is 'no opinion' or 'no knowledge', which might not be true: people often select these categories as an easy option. The problematic scoring of these responses is one reason why some investigators omit them and force respondents to make a decision one way or another. Many investigators allocate a middle scale value to 'no opinion' (e.g. 'neither agree nor disagree') responses, as in Likert scales (see later). In this case, the scale values would be: strongly agree = 5, agree = 4, neither agree nor disagree = 3, disagree = 2, strongly disagree = 1.

Methods of weighting

The alternative is to weight responses. The statistical procedures that can be used to calculate appropriate weightings include factor analysis and principal components analysis, which identify the mathematical factors underlying the correlations between scale items, and can be used in the construction of appropriate sub-scales. Weighting the domain scores also requires robust evidence about how important one domain is over another to the population of interest (e.g. how much more important is physical over mental functioning, and so on). In psychology, a common method of deriving relative weights is to use Thurstone's method of paired comparisons, in which judges are used to sort scale items ('statements') into piles representing positive to negative evaluation continuums (Thurstone 1927). Jenkinson (1991) reviewed the weighting of items in the Nottingham Health Profile and reported that Thurstone's method was unsuccessful as the results were similar whether responses were scored (1/0) or weighted. Moreover, the score of someone with walking difficulties exceeded the score of those who were unable to walk at all. He suggested that this was because Thurstone's method was applied inappropriately. It was developed for the measurement of psychological variables (e.g. attitudes) and not the factual statements common in health status and functioning measures.

Weighting vs. simple summing of scores

However, there is increasing debate about the usefulness of weighting item scores. The literature comparing standardised weighted and unweighted cardinal (i.e. summed) scales – whether of life events, life satisfaction or health status – consistently reports no benefits of more complex weighted methods in relation to the proportion of explained variance or sensitivity to change over time. While this may simply be due to insufficient variance in weights, there is little support in the literature for complex weighting over simple summing of scores (Andrews and Crandall 1976; Jenkinson *et al.* 1991; Streiner and Norman 2003). Trauer and Mackinnon (2001) presented evidence that weighted scores in quality of life measurement scales present difficulties in interpretation, and that multiplicative composite scores (e.g. combining satisfaction with QoL and importance ratings of QoL domains) have little or no advantage over unweighted ratings. Relatively little experimental work has been carried out to test the different values which can be attached to weights, such as relative importance, satisfaction or goal achievement and gap ('expectancy') ratings of individuals.

Constructing additional items and scales

As previously indicated, given the complexity and expense of developing new scales, most investigators prefer to use existing scales, and adapt existing items where permissible. Not all scale developers will permit modifications, because even slight changes in question wording and order can affect responses and the reliability and validity of the instrument. However, some domains of interest to the investigator may be missing on existing instruments and will require development. Where additional items are required, they should be included in the broader questionnaire to be administered and not embedded within an existing scale, which should have been carefully developed and tested for question form, wording and order effects. It should be remembered that all measurement instruments require rigorous testing for reliability and validity, as well as for their factor structure.

Most scales for measuring health status, HRQoL, patients' and professionals' evaluations of health care and so on are based on the techniques used for developing attitude scales.

Attitude measurement scales

An attitude is the tendency to evaluate something (called the 'attitude object') in a particular way (i.e. with some degree of positivity or negativity). The attitude object can be any aspect of the physical or social environment, such as things (buildings), people (doctors), behaviour (smoking cigarettes) or abstract ideas (health status) (Stroebe and Stroebe 1995). This evaluative component is usually studied in relation to cognitive (people's beliefs), evaluative (feelings) and behavioural (action) components. The assessment of each of these aspects in relation to a specific 'attitude object' (e.g. health status) may produce results which are not consistent with each other (Stroebe and Stroebe 1995; Edelmann 1996). The rules of measurement have been most carefully developed by psychologists in relation to the measurement of attitudes, and these have usually been drawn on in the development and construction of scales measuring health beliefs and behaviours, and self-evaluations of health status and broader quality of life.

Most attitude measures assess attitudes by presenting respondents with sentences that state beliefs about the particular attitude being measured. The statements for inclusion in attitude scales should assess favourable or unfavourable sentiments. The four main scaling methods used to assess the evaluative component of attitudes are the Thurstone, Likert, Guttman and semantic-differential methods. Each method assumes that a person's attitude can be represented by a numerical score. These methods are all used in scales measuring self-evaluations of health status, symptoms (e.g. pain) and HRQoL. Likert scales are the most popular, and are often known as rating scales (better–same–worse; more–same–less; strongly agree–agree–neither agree nor disagree–disagree–strongly disagree).

The Thurstone scale

This was the first major method to be developed (Thurstone 1928). With the Thurstone method, attitudes are viewed as being ordered along a continuum ranging from favourable (complete endorsement) to unfavourable (complete opposition). An attitude scale is constructed by choosing an 'attitude object' (e.g. abortion). The next step in the development of a Thurstone scale involves collecting a wide range of 'belief statements' expressing favourable (e.g. 'abortion is a woman's right') or unfavourable (e.g. 'abortion is murder') sentiments. These are usually obtained from the literature, meetings with experts in the field or direct questioning of relevant populations, either in interviews or on panels. In order to obtain a spread of views about an issue, the resulting scale usually contains 20–40 statements (which have been derived from a larger pool of statements in the development of the scale).

Numerical values ('scale' values) are then derived for these statements on the evaluation continuum. For example, if the scale values selected by the investigator range from 1 to 11, then a panel of 'judges' (often about 300) are asked to sort the statements into 11 piles (categories) placed along a continuum according to the degree of favourable or unfavourable evaluation each one expresses. Each statement is given a numerical scale value that is an average of the ratings assigned by the judges. The level of the agreement between judges is also calculated, and items with poor agreement are discarded. From the resulting statements 20–40 are selected for inclusion in the final scale. The final statements selected for inclusion in the scale have to meet certain other criteria. They should be chosen to represent an evenly graduated scale from negative to positive attitudes. High scale values are traditionally associated with positive attitudes.

It is assumed, because of the method of construction, that the distance in numerical terms between any two statements is equal. When the scale is then used in the field, a respondent's attitude is usually represented by the average scale value of the statements he or she endorsed.

The drawback of this method if it is used to construct a scale from scratch is that it is time-consuming, though once constructed and made available for others to use, its advantage is the equal weighting between scores based on clear methodology (though whether the equal weighting is always achieved is still open to question). There are few scales using the Thurstone method because of the time-consuming nature of construction. However, similar techniques of creating categories using panels are in use in other areas of psychology (e.g. Q-sort).

The Thurstone technique has been used in the development of some health status measurement scales (e.g. the Nottingham Health Profile; Hunt et al. 1986). However, most scale developers have simply constructed scales on the basis of the literature – 'expert' opinion – only occasionally involving a panel of lay people or patients. In such cases, the content validity of the scale cannot be assured.

The Likert scale

This is the most popular scaling method used by sociologists and psychologists in both scale development and their final scales. The method is relatively quick and most questionnaires and scales use this scaling method within them. The method of construction is similar to that of Thurstone – an initial pool of statements is collected and edited. In contrast to Thurstone's method, there is no assumption of equal intervals and thus the exercise using 'judges' to order the statements is avoided.

The Likert scale (Likert 1932) contains a series of 'opinion' statements about an issue. The person's attitude is the extent to which he or she agrees or disagrees with each statement, usually on a five-point scale. Thus, the responses (e.g. from 'never' through to 'sometimes' to 'always') are divided numerically into a series of ordered responses (such as 1, 2, 3, 4, 5) which denote gradation in the possible range of responses.

In relation to the development of scales with this method, the researcher presents respondents with a large preliminary pool of items expressing favourable or unfavourable beliefs about the 'attitude object' (e.g. 'I feel pain all the time', 'I have severe pain', 'I have pain but it does not bother me', 'I am restricted in my activities because of the pain'), to which respondents reply in one of five ways:

strongly agree	agree	undecided	disagree	strongly disagree
5	4	3	2	1

It is convention for high numbers to signify favourable evaluation, so scoring is reversed where necessary. If an item is to be included on a Likert scale, respondents' responses to items must be compared, and only items that are highly correlated with other scale items are included in the final questionnaire (for internal consistency). The items selected are then tested on a new group of respondents, using the same five-point scale. The total attitude score is the sum of the responses. There is no assumption of equal intervals on the scale. Thus, the difference between 'agree' and 'strongly agree' may be perceived by the respondent to be greater than that between 'agree' and 'undecided'. The Likert scale can indicate the ordering of different people's attitudes, but not precisely how far apart or close these attitudes are. Likert scales provide ordinal level data.

The disadvantage of Likert scales, when used within a measurement scale which is totalled to produce a total scale score, is that while a set of responses will always add up to the same score, the same total may arise from many different combinations of responses, which leads to a loss of information about the components of the scale score (see Edelmann 1996).

Other forms of Likert scaling: visual analogue and numeric scales

A wide range of other formats have also been used (e.g. respondents may be asked to circle a number between 1 and 10, or to place a mark on a 10 cm line labelled – 'anchored' – at one end 'strongly agree' and at the other 'strongly disagree'). Sometimes respondents are asked to select a face to depict how they feel, with expressions on the faces ranging from 'delighted' to 'terrible' (Andrews and Withey 1976). Whatever the format, it is still basically a Likert scale and the task is the same: to indicate the extent to which the person accepts or rejects various statements relating to an attitude object (see Edelmann 1996).

The visual analogue scale (VAS) is a scale in the Likert style. A VAS is a line of a defined length (10 cm), usually horizontal, anchored at each end by a descriptive word or phrase representing the extremes (e.g. of a health state: 'worst', 'best'). The respondent places a mark on the line to indicate the point at which his or her response best answers the question being asked. A number of items which aim to assess pain, symptoms and quality of life use VASs, whereby the respondent makes a judgement of how much of the scale is equivalent to the intensity of the domain (e.g. severity of pain). One end of the line represents, in this example, 'no pain', and the other end represents, for example, 'pain as bad as you can imagine'.

A variation on the simple VAS, which is still a version of a Likert scale, is the numeric scale in which the horizontal (or vertical) VAS lines are bounded by numbers *and* adjectives at either end. The line may also have numerical values displayed at regular intervals (from 0–5, 0–10 or 0–100) in order to help respondents intuitively to understand the scale.

The Guttman scale

The Guttman method is a hierarchical scaling technique (Guttman 1944, 1950). Therefore, the items appropriate for a Guttman scale have to have the hierarchical property that individuals who agree with any item also agree with the items which have a lower rank on the scale. Thus, statements range from those that are easy for most people to accept to those which few people would endorse. An individual's attitude score is the rank of the most extreme item he or she endorses, since it is assumed that items of lower rank on the scale would also be endorsed.

In the scale construction, people are presented with a pool of statements and their response patterns to them are recorded. These response patterns ('scale types') follow a step-like order: the person may accept none of the statements in the set (so the score is 0), he or she may accept the first statement only (score = 1), the first and second statement only (score = 2), and so on. If the person accepts the third statement but not the first and second statement a response error is recorded, poor statements (high error rate) are discarded and the remaining items are retested.

This technique has been adopted in some scales of physical functioning. It is assumed that biological functions decrease in order, for example, that inability to perform particular functions implies inability to perform other functions of daily living, such as if one cannot bathe oneself, it is assumed that one also cannot dress oneself. One example is the Katz Index of Activities of Daily Living (Katz *et al.* 1963). These assumptions in scales of physical functioning are based on the untested belief that biological functions decrease in order, and are often questionable.

The problem with this method is that it is difficult to achieve a perfect unidimensional scale because attitudes and behaviours are often too complex and inconsistent. Thus, the claim of the scale to provide interval level data is questionable (the grouped categories aim to provide equal intervals).

Semantic-differential scale

The Thurstone, Likert and Guttman scaling methods all measure attitudes by assessing the extent to which people agree or disagree with various opinion statements. The semantic-differential scale (Osgood *et al.* 1957) differs from this approach by focusing on the meaning people attach to a word or concept. The scale title refers to the measurement of several different semantic dimensions, or different types of meaning reflected by the adjective descriptors.

The scale consists of an 'attitude object', situation or event and people are asked to rate it on scales anchored by a series of bipolar adjectives – for example, 'good–bad', 'fast–slow', 'active–passive', 'hot–cold', 'easy–hard'. Respondents' ratings express their beliefs about the 'attitude object'. Research by Osgood *et al.* (1957) indicated that most 'adjective dimensions' can be usefully grouped into three distinct categories: the largest number of adjectives ('good–bad' and 'happy–sad') reflect *evaluation*; 'strong–weak' and 'easy–hard' reflect *perceived potency*; and 'fast–slow', 'young–old' reflect *activity*.

As most attitude researchers are concerned solely with the evaluative dimension of the semantic differential, most scales express evaluative meaning only. Respondents rate an attitude object on a set of such 'adjective dimensions' and each person's rating (e.g. on a seven-point scale) is summed across the various dimensions, creating a simple measure of attitudes.

Research has established which adjectives express evaluative meaning, and therefore semantic-differential attitude scales are easy to construct, though the task of completing the scale may seem unusual to respondents. For example, we do not usually rate objects, situations or events on scales such as 'hard–soft' (Edelmann 1996). Semantic-differential scales do not conform to linear-scaling methodology.

Rasch scoring

The Rasch modelling approach to scaling has been less often used. It has been argued that the use of Rasch scaling results in greater accuracy and therefore improved measurement, for example, of health outcomes (Hays *et al.* 2000). With this method, scale items are ordered with the aim of creating a unidimensional construct (i.e. it taps one trait or ability), with additive items, and an interval level of measurement (Wright and Masters 1982; Wright and Linacre 1989). Using this method, for example, with a measurement scale of physical functioning, scale items would need to be ordered in relation to the degree of physical difficulty with each activity asked about. The assumption is that this would enable items with similar levels of difficulty to be identified and eliminated, and items then selected to measure the full spectrum of the construct (Granger *et al.* 1998).

Fitzpatrick *et al.* (2004) compared the relative precision of Rasch scoring versus conventional Likert scoring in discriminating level of satisfaction among patients undergoing hip replacement surgery. They used the Rasch scaling model based on the use of logits (e.g. the log-odds of the level of difficulty of an item relative to the difficulty of the total set of items analysed). Logits of greater magnitude represented increasing item difficulty or ability (Ludlow and Haley 1995; Fitzpatrick *et al.* 2004). They reported that considerable gains in precision were achieved with the Rasch scoring methods. However, the evidence base to support this method is still inconclusive.

Other methods

Oppenheim (1992) and Edelmann (1996) describe other methods of assessing attitudes. Most commonly used scales focus on the evaluative component, but psychologists are becoming more interested in the cognitive component of attitudes. One technique of assessing these is 'thought listing' (Petty and Cacioppo 1981). For example, after listening to or seeing a message, people are asked to write down in a specified time all their thoughts which are relevant to it. These thoughts are then rated and categorised: for example, according to whether they agree or disagree with the issue. This leads to the development of understanding about the beliefs and knowledge underlying attitudes. Similar information can be obtained by carrying out content analyses of material or group discussions, and analyses of body reactions (language) as people listen to (and react to) the messages presented to them. Other variations of projective techniques include sentence completion exercises, uncaptioned cartoon completion and picture interpretation (such as the Rorschach blots which stimulate people to identify ambiguous images).

Repertory grid techniques can be useful in providing information about people's individual constructs, inter-relationships and changes in attitudes over time (see Beail 1985). With this technique, the investigator presents three stimuli (a triad), such as photographs, to the respondent and asks him or her to say which two are the most alike and in what ways, and how they differ from the third. The constructs which underlie the distinctions are dimensions of the opinion. Respondents then relate the constructs to each other to form a grid. The constructs are listed in a grid down the left-hand side. Across the top are the stimuli, to each of which the construct is to be applied. The investigator takes the respondent through the grid step by step, ticking underneath each object said to possess the construct. The value of this method is that the constructs come from the respondent – not from the investigator. If the procedure is repeated over time, then changes can be measured. It is often used as pilot research for the development of semantic-differential scales.

Another method of measuring attitudes and desired behaviour is by use of vignettes (which simply means illustration). Short descriptions of the topic of interest, or case histories of patients, are presented to people along with pertinent questions. For example, doctors may be asked about what actions they would take if the patient was theirs. Investigators usually structure the method by giving people a list of response choices, such as possible actions. This provision of cues may result in bias and, for example, over-estimations of competence in the case of doctors. The validity of the method remains uncertain (see Sandvik 1995, for review). Many of these techniques have been restricted to clinical psychology, where they are used to gain insights into individual patients, as they are complex and time-consuming to administer and to analyse. Further, it is difficult to establish the reliability and validity of these methods.

Commonly used response scales

The most commonly used scale for measuring responses is the categorical scale, in the Likert format of a five- to seven-point scale, in which a respondent is asked to pick a category, such as 'none', 'very mild', 'mild', 'moderate', 'severe', 'very severe', which best describes their condition (e.g. severity of pain). It is commonly used because it is easily understood and analysed, though constructing them takes time.

The Likert method is the most commonly used response choice format in health status and HRQoL scales, apart from dichotomous 'yes/no' formats. Some health status questionnaires use a combination of dichotomous 'yes/no' response formats, Likert scales and VASs. While this variation may appear visually confusing, there is no evidence that any one scaling method produces superior results to the others. Categorical scales using words as descriptors (e.g. original Likert scale) and the VAS show similar responsiveness. The evidence on whether respondents find categorical scales easier to understand than VASs is contradictory. Researchers select scales primarily on the basis of the ease of constructing, administering and analysing the scale. Categorical scales (e.g. in the form of five- or seven-point Likert scales) are generally preferred because of their ease of administration, analysis and interpretation (Jaesche *et al.* 1990).

Scale values

It should be noted that many respondents will opt for a middle response category and prefer to avoid a decision at either end of response scales (e.g. positive or negative). A decision has to be made about removing middle points and instead forcing people to make a decision one way or the other (e.g. using a six-point rather than a seven-point scale). Too many scales can be boring for people, words may be conceptually easier for people to understand than numbers, though there is no consistent evidence for this, and alternative answers and statements on response scales should be balanced (e.g. 'very happy' should be balanced at the other end of the scale with 'very unhappy', and so on).

Rules for order and wording

Apart from the form of the questions and response type, the order and wording of questions can affect response and bias results. (See Box 13.8.) Detailed rules governing the design of questionnaires are found in texts by Sudman and Bradburn (1983) and Oppenheim (1992).

Question order

Funnelling

Most questionnaires adopt a 'funnel' approach to question order. With this technique, the module starts with a broad question and progressively narrows down to specific issues; this process necessarily involves the use of filter questions to 'filter out' respondents to whom the specific questions do not apply and direct them or the interviewer to the next question which applies to them. Unless computer-assisted interviewing is used, where applicable filters can be programmed, complex re-routing and manual skips of several pages in length should always be avoided as these create real potential for error.

Box 13.8 Types of questions to be asked first

The rules that apply to the ordering of questions can be found in most textbooks on methods (e.g. Bourque and Fielder 1995). The main rules are:

- Ask easy and basic (not sensitive or threatening) questions first in order to retain rapport and goodwill.
- Avoid asking for the respondents' socio-demographic characteristics at the beginning unless this is essential for the funnelling of the questionnaire – if a respondent objects to the personal nature of any of the details (e.g. ethnic status, income group), then rapport has been lost at the outset, with repercussions for completion.
- Ask the most important questions first, where no other rules apply (to ensure that important data is not entirely lost if the questionnaire is not fully completed, i.e. if the respondent tires and terminates the exercise before the end).
- Questions about behaviour should be asked before questions about attitudes to enhance reporting of socially undesirable behaviour (e.g. ask 'Have you ever smoked cigarettes?' before 'Do you think that smoking should be (a) permitted in public parks or (b) banned in public parks?'). If people express negative attitudes to smoking beforehand, they are then less likely to admit that they smoke.
- Ask about past behaviour before current behaviour on sensitive topics or undesirable behaviour in order to enhance reporting (e.g. 'Have you ever smoked cigarettes?', 'Do you smoke cigarettes now?').
- Ask general questions before specific questions on the same topic. Specific questions can influence response to more general questions, for example:
  How satisfied are you with your health? (*specific*)
  How satisfied are you with your life in general? (*general*)

The above will produce different responses from:

  How satisfied are you with your life in general? (*general*)
  How satisfied are you with your health? (*specific*)

With the first alternative ordering, respondents will generally exclude consideration of their health from their assessment of their satisfaction with their life in general – because they have already answered that question. Thus, minimalise order effects by placing general questions before specific questions.

There has been little research on the effects of question ordering and the order of batteries of measurement scales in relation to research on health. The issue is of importance because it is increasingly common for investigators to ask respondents to complete both generic (general) health status scales and disease-specific scales, or batteries of scales which more comprehensively cover pertinent domains of HRQoL. It could be hypothesised that if a disease-specific scale or battery is asked before a general health status scale, then the ratings of general health status would be more favourable because the disease-specific health status had already been considered and therefore excluded in replies to the general ratings. Thus, Keller and Ware (1996) recommended that the generic Short Form-36 Health Survey Questionnaire (SF-36) and the shorter Short Form-12 version should be presented to respondents before more specific questionnaires about health and disease, and that there should be a clear break between batteries of scales (making clear to respondents that they are starting a new module on the questionnaire) (Ware *et al.* 1993, 1995). However, the evidence from disease-specific studies and generic population health surveys suggests either that question order makes little difference to results (Barry *et al.* 1996), or that, in fact, worse scores are obtained by asking disease-specific questions before the generic SF-36 rather than the other way round (Bowling *et al.* 1999). Further research is needed on order effects in the context of health and disease. The investigator can only control order effects in interviewer-administered questionnaires (with self-administered instruments respondents can read through the questionnaire or battery of scales and start anywhere they choose to, even if asked not to). It should be pointed out that surveys can also have context effects on response. There is evidence that people report more ill health in the context of surveys on health topics than in general surveys which also include questions on health (Bowling *et al.* 1999). This is probably because they become more sensitised to their health in surveys which focus exclusively on it.

Question wording

Question wording can easily affect response. The use of leading questions, questions which do not reflect balance, complex questions and questions containing double negatives can all lead to biased replies. Loading questions (as when assuming behaviour) is a technique which must be carefully used and only in certain situations, such as threatening topics. These issues are outlined next.

Simplicity

It cannot be assumed that all people share the same frame of reference, values or understandings and interpret words in the same way. For example, different social groups will interpret 'dinner' differently, as manual workers regard it as a midday meal (traditionally, nourishment has been needed in the middle of the day by these groups because of the physical exertion demanded by their work), and professional workers (who have more sedentary occupations) regard it as an evening meal. There is also evidence that people distinguish ethnic group from ethnic origin, and their self-categorisation, in response to open-ended questions on ethnicity, is not consistent with traditional questionnaire (e.g. census) categories of ethnicity (Mortimer and White 1996; Pringle and Rothera 1996). Even the ever popular health status item 'Do you have any long-standing illness, disability or infirmity?' (Charlton *et al.* 1994; Charlton and Murphy 1997) apparently captures mostly medically diagnosed, chronic, physical diseases rather than people's experiences of ill health or non-diagnosed chronic conditions (Manderbacka 1998). Despite its questionable reliability and validity, variants of this question are used in government-sponsored health surveys worldwide (see Manderbacka 1998).

Therefore, it is important to use short, simple and familiar words and phrases that virtually all respondents will understand and conceptualise in the same way. It is also important to ensure that any translated questionnaires have been fully assessed and tested by panels of experts and lay people for meaning and cultural equivalence. The importance of these rules of questionnaire design are emphasised by cognitive research results which indicate that many people will respond to survey questions even when they do not understand the question (Clarke and Schober 1992).

Questions should avoid ambiguity (e.g. does 'doctor' refer to hospital doctor or GP, or both?), avoid negatives and certainly never use double negatives in questions (they are confusing and ambiguous – what does a 'no' reply actually mean?). They should be short (people will not remember long questions and only answer the last part) and jargon should be avoided (e.g. ask about brothers and sisters, not siblings; ask about where the respondent lives and not about place of residence). Gowers (1954) lists many simple alternatives for words. Questions should never include two questions in one ('double-barrelled') as this will lead to confusion; questions should each be asked separately.

Readability and cognitive checking

The Flesch scale, a readability yardstick, can be used in scale construction (Flesch 1948), and computerised versions are available. *Grammatik 5* (1992) will provide a report, comprising readability indexes (standard values that give the grade level required to read the document), sentence statistics and word count.

A number of interview techniques have also been developed to explore the way in which people interpret questionnaire items and to analyse their cognitive processes. 'Think-aloud' protocols can be used when testing new questionnaires. With these, people are asked to describe their thoughts while they are listening to each question, and also their interpretation of the question's intentions (Suchman and Jordan 1992). In-depth probing techniques are also used to check whether people interpret questions as intended. The process aims to mimic the process of natural conversation in which people routinely correct misapprehensions in order to facilitate meaningful communication.

Leading questions

It is important to avoid using leading questions and to train interviewers not to slip into them. Typical leading questions are: 'Don't you agree that . . . ?', 'You don't have difficulty with X, do you?', 'You don't have a problem with X, do you?', 'You haven't got pain, have you?' The provision of examples in brackets in questions can also be leading, and hence biasing. Some respondents may be uncertain about their reply and simply respond in relation to the examples. Leading questions bias respondents' replies: they are reluctant to contradict the interviewer, who appears to know what answer he or she is looking for, and will agree in order to proceed quickly to the next question (see Chapter 14). (See Box 13.9.)

Box 13.9 Leading questions bias respondents' replies

These questions will be deceptively casual and non-leading. You don't ask a prospective (dog) owner, 'Will you let your dog sleep on the bed if she wants to?' because he'll say, 'Why, of course!' just to shut you up. No, you ask, 'Where will the dog sleep?' If the prospective says, 'Out in the yard or maybe in the garage if she's lucky,' instead of, 'Wherever she wants,' this is a person who has no interest in the comfort or feelings of a longtime companion. This person does not get a dog.

(Heimel 1995)

Loaded questions

Loaded questions are questions which bias the respondent in a particular direction, hence leading to biased answers. Campbell and Garcia (1997) have provided 'spoof questions' to illustrate loaded questions on women's feelings on place of birth and maternity care, for example:

> Q: How important is it to you to give birth in the safety of a hospital labour ward with specialist doctors on the spot?
> A: Very important   Fairly important   Not important

> Q: How important is it to you to avoid the risks of infection and unnecessary intervention in a hospital labour ward?
> A: Very important   Fairly important   Not important.

It is important to avoid any element of bias in questions. Questionnaires are often open to the criticism that surveys can demonstrate whatever the investigator wants.

Balance

The failure to specify alternatives clearly in the question is also a form of leading question. For example, respondents should be asked 'Do you prefer to see the specialist in the hospital clinic or in your GP's surgery, or do you have no preference?' (and not just 'Do you prefer to see the specialist in the hospital clinic?'). The range of response options must be read to respondents in closed questions. (See Box 13.10.)

Box 13.10 Balanced questions

Cartwright and Anderson's (1981) work provides many examples of carefully worded and *balanced* questions:

Do you think the time it takes before you can get an appointment is reasonable or unreasonable?

Framing effects

The way in which the question is framed can also influence responses – the 'half-empty or half-full' effect. Framing is the expression of logically equivalent information (numerical or verbal) in different ways (Wilson *et al.* 1988).

Framing is problematic in research on people's preferences. Respondents will respond differently to questions about their preferences for treatment alternatives, depending on whether the treatments are presented positively, in terms of chances of survival, or negatively, in terms of mortality risk. Positive framing appears to be more effective than negative framing in leading people to select risky choices (Kühberger 1998; Edwards *et al.* 2001; Gigerenzer and Edwards 2003). Gigerenzer and Edwards (2003) suggested that doctors should use pictorial illustrations of risk as visual representations improved patients' comprehension.

Classic research by McNeil *et al.* (1982) involved presenting study participants with a hypothetical choice between two types of treatment for lung cancer (radiation therapy or surgery) and provided information on outcomes (immediate, at one year and at five years). Surgery was presented as offering greater life expectancy, but a higher risk of immediate death. However, this information on surgery was framed either in terms of mortality (i.e. negatively – 10 per cent mortality at one year) or in terms of survival (i.e. positively – one year survival rate of 90 per cent). While just 18 per cent of respondents favoured radiation therapy in the positive surgery survival frame, 44 per cent favoured it in the negative surgery mortality frame. All respondents, including clinicians, expressed a consistent preference for 90 per cent survival rather than 10 per cent mortality.

Similar biases occur when presented with quantities in other areas. Apparently, a well-known rule in marketing is that most people are not numerically sophisticated, and large quantities of small units sound much bigger than small quantities of large units. Hence CompuServe offered 650 hours of free internet access rather than one month's free trial (the small print stated that the 650 hours had to be used within one month, meaning that one would have to be online 21 hours per day) (*Statistics Watch* 1998). This is a common ploy in this sector. Evidence of consumers taking the bait was demonstrated by a court case brought by trading standards officers against a pie manufacturer in relation to trade misdescription, described in Box 13.11.

Box 13.11 Real-life example of effects of framing

The hostess of a luncheon party suffered a second embarrassment after finding that the chicken pies she had planned to serve contained less meat than she had expected . . . On Tuesday, however, as the pie makers pleaded guilty to misdescription, Lady N— J— also suffered the indignity of being criticised in court for trying to scrimp on the cost of the party . . . [She] had thought she was getting a bargain when she bought the pies . . . for less than 30p each . . . She was particularly pleased because a sign across the packaging claimed that the pies 'had 30 per cent more chicken pieces'. In fact they contained the same amount of chicken as other pies. The meat had simply been cut into smaller, and more pieces.

(Reported in *The Times*, 17 June 1999)

Appropriate response choices

A common problem is the design of questions which have inappropriate response choices: for example, as in 'Are you in favour or not in favour of private health care? Yes/No.' With this example, the 'yes/no' response choices are inappropriate: which alternative (in favour or not in favour) does the 'yes' response relate to? It does not offer a middle category and some people's responses will be forced into inappropriate categories. It could also be criticised as a leading question by asking about 'in favour' before 'not in favour' (see Oppenheim 1992). Such general questions are fairly crude, and relatively little information is obtained from them (e.g. what aspect of private health care is it that people are in favour or not in favour of?). Specific questions in relation to the topic of interest are preferable (see below).

Specific questions

Questions should be worded as specifically as possible. For example, do not ask 'Do you have a car?' Ask the more meaningful question: 'Is there a car/van available for private use by you or a member of your household?' And instead of asking simply for current age, ask for date of birth: age can be calculated from date of birth on the computer and it is more exact.

It is also important to use specific rather than general question wording when assessing satisfaction, for example. The question 'Are you satisfied or dissatisfied with your doctor?' is inadequate, as it does not provide the respondent with a frame of reference, and it will not provide any information on the components of satisfaction or dissatisfaction. It is also ambiguous: which doctor (hospital doctor or GP)? It is preferable to ask about the specific, such as 'Are you satisfied or dissatisfied with the personal manner of your GP?'

Complex questions

If complex questions are to be asked within a structured format, then they should be broken up into a series of shorter, simpler, questions which are more easily understood, even though this lengthens the questionnaire.

Rules for questions by type of topic

There are rules for asking questions about topics which are threatening, sensitive or embarrassing to respondents, about attitudes, knowledge, facts, frequency of behaviours, and questions which rely on the respondent's memory. These are outlined next, and further details can be found in Bradburn and Sudman (1974) and Oppenheim (1992).

Questions on threatening, embarrassing and sensitive topics

Some questions may lead the respondent to feel embarrassed or threatened by them. This makes the questions difficult to answer and to an under-reporting of the attitude or behaviour in question (i.e. biased response). These questions need careful construction to minimise bias (see Bradburn and Sudman 1974). They are best asked towards the end of a questionnaire. If the questionnaire is administered by an interviewer, it will have allowed time for good rapport to be established, and in a self-administered questionnaire if the easy and non-sensitive questions are asked first, the interest of the respondent will have been engaged. Further, if the sensitive questions are not completed, if they are asked towards the end, then this does not threaten the completion of the rest of the questionnaire (though the problem with self-administered questionnaires is that respondents can read through them before completing them and may not complete the entire questionnaire if they object to any of the questions).

In the case of threatening questions, or questions asking about undesirable attitudes or behaviour, loading the question can be appropriate. Assume the behaviour ('everyone does it'): 'Even the calmest parents smack their children sometimes. Did your child(ren) do anything in the past seven days to make you smack them?' In relation to cigarette smoking, where under-reporting is expected, it is preferable to ask 'How many cigarettes do you smoke each day?' rather than prefixing this with the lead-in 'Do you smoke?' (similarly with alcohol intake). These are the only circumstances in which presuming questions are permitted. Otherwise the question should be prefixed with a question to ascertain the behaviour, before asking only those who admit to it for further details (of frequency, etc.). There is also the danger of encouraging a positive bias in the results with this technique.

In the case of embarrassing questions, one technique is to prefix a personal question with an opinion question on the topic, but opinions and behaviour are not necessarily consistent. Open questions, as well as self-completed questionnaires and alternatives to question–response frames (e.g. card sorting, sealed envelopes, diaries, sentence completion exercises), are best for eliciting sensitive, embarrassing or undesirable behaviour.

Attitude (opinion) questions

These questions can be difficult to interpret, partly because of social desirability bias and partly because respondents may not have thought of the topic before being presented with it on the questionnaire, or by the interviewer – and thus may not have a considered opinion. Opinions are also multifaceted: for example, a person may feel that abortion is cruel but also feel that a woman has the right to choose. Thus, questions asked in different ways (i.e. with different wording) will obtain different replies – they are, in effect, different questions.

With attitude questions it is important to present both sides of a case, as offering no alternative can increase support for the argument offered (see earlier on leading questions and balance). Avoid tagging 'or not' onto the end of opinion questions – the inadequate statement of the alternative opinion can be confusing. As some people are automatic 'yes' sayers, avoid attitude questions that are all worded positively (see above on form and response sets). Moser and Kalton (1971) suggest asking 'Do you think . . . ?' rather than 'In your opinion ...?', and 'What is your attitude ... ?' rather than 'What is your attitude with regard to ... ?', as it is more natural and reflects everyday speech.

Interviewers, where used, are not permitted to vary the question wording with opinion questions (e.g. to facilitate the respondents' understanding) because changes in wording or emphasis can affect responses. While checks on the validity of the response can be made by, for example, checking behaviour against attitudes, these are not necessarily consistent in real life (see Wicker 1969; Stroebe and Stroebe 1995). The best method of ensuring the optimal validity of the replies is to use an attitude scale (e.g. a number of opinion statements). This is the most common method of dealing with inconsistency and maximising validity in social and psychological research, and distinguishes research on attitudes from opinion surveys by market researchers who simply analyse 'snap answers' to particular questions.

Questions about knowledge

Questions measuring respondents' level of knowledge about a topic should only be asked where respondents are likely to possess, or have access to, the information required, and are able to give meaningful replies. No one enjoys admitting ignorance, and respondents will guess the answer rather than do so.

Knowledge questions can also appear threatening to respondents if they do not know the answer. There are techniques for reducing the level of threat, for example using phrases such as 'Do you happen to know ...?' or (offhand) 'Can you recall ...?', and using opinion question wording in order to disguise knowledge questions: 'Do you think . . . ?' 'Don't know' categories should also be used in order to minimise guessing and to reduce feelings of threat. This reassures respondents that it is acceptable not to know the answer – no one likes feeling foolish or uninformed.

Factual questions

Factual questions, particularly those enquiring about personal details, should be introduced with an explanation about why the investigator is asking about them (e.g. in the case of socio-demographic details such as date of birth, ethnic status, occupation, and so on, to enable the investigator to analyse the views expressed by respondents by the types of people who have been interviewed). It should also be re-emphasised that no names will be included in the report about the study, the information is confidential and only the research team have access to it (see Atkinson 1967; Moser and Kalton 1971).

Questions asking for factual information should only be asked where respondents are likely to possess, or have access to, the information required, or respondents will be tempted to guess. Even in relation to factual information about the respondent's characteristics, there is potential for error. People might under- or over-state their age (e.g. if they round years up or down). Systematic reporting errors can occur in surveys of height and weight, as people have been shown to over-estimate their height and under-estimate their weight in postal questionnaires (Gunnell *et al.* 2000), especially obese individuals (Lawlor *et al.* 2002).

There is also potential for social desirability bias to influence replies (on alcohol intake, smoking behaviour, level of education, and so on). To describe a question as factual does not imply that the answers are correct. Recall of size, for example, varies with age. Rohde (2000) pointed out that it is a common experience that when an adult revisits a place known in childhood, it is smaller than expected; he cited the following example from Charles Dickens ([1861] 1958) in illustration: '... of course the town had shrunk fearfully since I was a child there. I had entertained the impression that the High Street was at least as wide as Regent Street, London or the Italian Boulevard at Paris. I found it little better than a lane.' Recall in relation to time frames is discussed later.

However, there are checks that can be made, such as comparing age with date of birth, checking information provided about use of health services with medical records (bearing in mind that the latter can contain errors or be incomplete) or asking people themselves to check. For example, in a study of prescribed medication that they are currently taking, people should be asked by interviewers to get the bottles and record the name, dose and frequency from the label.

Factual questions about the respondent's characteristics (date of birth, age, income, occupational status, ethnic status, marital status, etc.) are often known as *classification questions* (see Atkinson 1967, for examples) and are usually asked at the end of a questionnaire in order to avoid cluttering the flow of the questionnaire at the beginning, and also to avoid beginning the questionnaire with questions which might seem sensitive to some individuals (e.g. age, income, ethnic status) and adversely affect the successful completion of the interview/questionnaire. The exception is with quota sampling, where questions about personal characteristics have to be asked at the outset in order to select the sample with the correct quotas of people in different categories.

Frequencies of behaviour

It was stated earlier that when asking questions about frequency of behaviour on sensitive topics, it is appropriate to load the question and assume the behaviour in order to minimise social desirability bias in responses (e.g. smoking, alcohol intake). Whatever initial approach is made, quantification of the behaviour is the next step. In relation to alcohol intake, for example, both the frequency of the behaviour (drinking) and the amount drunk will need to be measured. For research purposes, the preference is to measure exact numbers, rather than vague categorisations, in order that averages can be calculated and more powerful statistical techniques employed.

There are several methods of quantification:

- Option 1 is to ask the respondent to state the amount drunk (e.g. on the last occasion or on a typical occasion) (with no pre-coded responses). The problem with Option 1 is that the respondent may be biased towards under-reporting the amount (if drinking is perceived as undesirable behaviour).
- Option 2 is to have narrow frequency response frames (e.g. 1 drink, 2–3 drinks, 4–5 drinks, 6+ drinks). This option is unappealing to respondents who drink more than four or five drinks. People may perceive the final code of 6+ drinks as indicating heavy drinking and be less inclined to tick it if this actually applies to them. Most people also dislike ticking the extreme anchors, especially when they have a negative implication.
- Option 3 is to have a wider response range (e.g. 1–3 drinks, 4–6 drinks, 7–8 drinks, 9–10 drinks, 11–12 drinks, 12+ drinks). This is more appealing to heavier drinkers and is the most likely to obtain the most accurate responses – people who drink more than four drinks can tick the second category without feeling that they are indicating they are heavy drinkers (as there are three further responses). It should be noted that it is more common research practice to start with the highest quantity and work downwards (e.g. 12+, 10–12, 7–9, 4–6, 1–3) in an attempt to encourage more accurate reporting (on the basis of the assumption that items at the top–middle are perceived by people as representing more 'normal' behaviour).

There are other challenges to designing questions about frequencies, particularly in relation to alcohol. Rehm et al. (1999) used a within-subject design in four surveys of alcohol consumption in order to compare a quantity frequency response, a graduated frequency response and a weekly drinking recall measure (i.e. all three measures of frequency were assessed in each respondent).

- The quantity frequency method starts with a question about the frequency of drinking episodes, and then asks about the usual or average number of drinks per occasion or during a reference time period. Usual quantity is difficult to report for many people as the amount consumed may vary considerably between drinking episodes and time periods. Also, usual drinking is, statistically, the mode, and is not equivalent to a mean, making it less useful for analysis. Less frequent, heavy drinking episodes may be disregarded by respondents (Rehm 1998) – but these may be of greatest research interest in relation to health effects.

- The *graduated frequency measure* starts by asking about the highest number of drinks consumed on any occasion during a time reference period (e.g. past 12 months). Filter questions then ask about the number of occasions on which specific quantities were consumed. This does not require so much averaging by respondents and captures more information on variability of alcohol intake.
- The *weekly drinking recall measure* asks for actual alcohol intake over the last seven days. This question type wrongly categorises less frequent drinkers as abstainers.

Rehm *et al.* (1999) reported that the graduated frequency measure consistently yielded higher estimates of the prevalence of high risk drinking and harm (as defined by consuming an average of >60g pure alcohol per day for males and >40g per day for females). Prevalence estimates of harmful drinking were almost five times higher for graduated frequency versus weekly drinking estimates, and almost three times higher for graduated frequency versus quantity frequency measures.

The World Health Organization (1996) has published the range of questions used in selected national health interview surveys across the world, though it did not recommend any particular approach (apart from quantification rather than vague response data) because of the methodological challenges and relative lack of methodological research on the best (least biasing) approach.

Another area which poses difficulties for valid measurement is food intake, and frequency of consumption of selected foods (e.g. fried foods, sugars, wholegrains, vegetables and fruit). While weighted food intake diaries over one week or more are more reliable than seven-day, or general frequency dietary questionnaires, these can be burdensome to respondents (and it is likely that they will guess weights, rather than actually weigh foods, and become more conscious of their diets and thus eat healthier diets during the study period). Even different diet questionnaires yield different rates of, for example, fruit and vegetable consumption (Michels *et al.* 2005).

Questions about time periods involving memory: time frames

Recall (memory) bias is always possible in questions asking about the past. The most reliable information will be obtained by using shorter time frames and asking respondents about more recent time periods. Asking about events beyond the past six months should be avoided, except on topics of high saliency to respondents (e.g. death, childbirth), where memory is better. The validity of the time period selected may also vary by age of respondent. Crawley and Pring (2000) carried out psychological experiments with people in three different age groups, asking them to date various groups of major events in society (e.g. the fire at Windsor Castle). They found that people aged 18–21 were more likely to believe that events occurred more recently than they had, and people aged 35–50 and 50 plus increasingly believed that more time had passed since the events had occurred than was the case.

Respondents can be aided in their recall by asking them to check any documents they have (e.g. payslips, pension books, bank statements), though some misreporting is still likely. Berney and Blane (1997) reported good recall of social circumstances over 50 years with the use of a life grid method, checked against available historical records.

There are also interviewer techniques to help respondents who seem to have difficulties with precise dates or periods: 'Was it more or less than three months ago?' Wide response codes can also assist here (e.g. 'In the past week/more than a week but less than two weeks ago/two weeks or more ago but less than a month ago', etc.). Respondents can also be given lists of likely responses to aid their memory. For example, if the question asks about which health professionals they have consulted in the past six months, then provide them with a comprehensive list on a showcard (as a memory jogger) from which to select their responses.

More reliable information is also obtained if behaviour within an exact time period is asked about, rather than usual behaviour. The time period of the question should be related to the saliency of the topic, as well as to reasonable recall periods in order to minimise recall (memory) bias.

Health status and quality of life scales usually ask respondents to rate themselves in relation to the past week (acute conditions), four weeks or three months (chronic conditions). Some scales have acute and chronic versions with different time frames (e.g. the SF-36; Ware *et al*. 1993). Time frames of between three and seven days are the most valid and reliable periods to use, though investigators will often want to find out about longer time periods (perhaps the past three months) – especially in the case of chronic, less common or less frequent health episodes. In the case of non-fatal injuries, one to three months is the longest recall time frame period advised, in order to avoid recall bias (Mock *et al*. 1999). If time frames are too short (e.g. 'today') then responses are less stable and reproducible, and also subject to regression to the mean in future follow-up studies. If the topic is salient to the respondent (e.g. pregnancy and childbirth, terminal care, more severe injuries), then longer time frames (such as 12 months) can be used, as they are less prone to recall bias (see Mock *et al*. 1999, for example). Otherwise it is unwise to ask respondents to recall periods of more than six months ago.

There is always the problem of the representativeness of the time period asked about. If seasonal variations are suspected, then the data collection period should be spread over a year to allow for this. Other difficulties arise if respondents have been asked about their 'usual behaviour'. Respondents' time references are unknown and people may under- or over-report the behaviour in question. Where usual behaviour is difficult to elicit, then respondents could be asked to keep a diary for a short time period to record the behaviour of interest, though only the most motivated will complete it.

Checking the accuracy of responses

Most researchers who attempt to check the reliability of the information given to them by respondents will check any factual data against records, where they exist and are accessible, and test the level of agreement between the data from the two sources (e.g. using the kappa statistic of concordance if the data is dichotomous). For example, in health care research, records may be available (with the patient's consent) with which to check prescribed medication, services received and medical consultations, tests, procedures or surgery performed and diagnosis. Research has indicated that people tend to over-report screening procedures, and that 'memory telescoping' occurs with screening (patients report the latest event to be more recent than the date in their records); however, the more major the procedure (e.g. major surgery), the higher the level of agreement between sources. Research also shows that between 36 and 70 per cent of self-reported diagnoses are confirmed by medical records, and between 30 and 53 per cent of diagnoses in records are confirmed by patients (Harlow and Linet 1989).

Other research on patients with prostate cancer has reported good agreement between self-reports and medical records for prior medical history but poor concordance for prior genitourinary diseases which had less explicit diagnostic criteria (Zhu *et al*. 1999). The agreement between self-reported data and medical records data will obviously vary by type of variable. The extent of concordance also varies by type of diagnosis (see review by Sandvik 1995). In relation to health data, it appears that overall, patients are reliable sources in relation to major events and conditions.

However, discrepancies do not necessarily imply that the patient was 'wrong'. While some patients will forget, some patients are not given full information and do not know their diagnosis or the names of any procedures carried out; in some cases the records may be in error, not the patient, which questions their use as a gold standard. For example, research, while limited, has reported only a weak correlation between the reported performance of procedures and their recording in notes, and the worst correlations were in relation to follow-up, guidance and advice (Norman *et al*. 1985; Rethans 1994).

Translating an instrument and cultural equivalence

Measurement instruments (e.g. health status scales) generally reflect the cultural norms of the society in which they were developed. Some items may not translate well, or at all, and items that were seemingly important in the original study population may appear trivial to members of a different culture (Guyatt 1993). Most instruments have been developed initially in English or American English languages. For an instrument to be used in international studies, and for consistent and valid analysis and comparison of results, the instruments must be conceptually equivalent to the original instrument, culturally relevant and acceptable to the target population within each target country, as well as being psychometrically comparable. Thus translation of a research instrument into another language does not consist simply of translation and back-translation before assessing its suitability for use. It is essential that the research team ensures congruency between words and their true meaning in the translated language, given the principle of linguistic relativism that the structure of language influences the manner in which it is understood. Sensitivity to culture and the selection of appropriate words are important. White and Elander (1992) have drawn attention to the most important principles of translation, including testing for its cultural equivalence, congruent values and careful use of colloquialisms. They suggested the following practice: secure competent translators who are familiar with the topic; use two bilingual translators (one to translate and one to translate back to the original language, without having seen the original); assemble a review panel, composed of bilinguists, experts in the field of study and members of the population of interest, who should refine the translations and assess equivalence, congruence and any colloquialisms used.

Apart from rigorous methods of translation and assessment for cultural equivalence, the psychometric properties of the instrument should be reassessed in each culture/ country that the instrument is to be used in, including item–scale correlations, comparisons of missing responses, scale correlation with any existing gold standards or other similar instruments and analysis of the psychometric properties of the instrument in relation to sub-groups within the population of interest (Reese and Joseph 1995). Meadows *et al*. (1997) described the principles of adapting measures for cross-cultural use, the problems associated with the forward-and-backward translation method and the types of equivalence in evaluating the appropriateness of the measure when administered in different cultures: content (each item of the questionnaire must describe a phenomenon relevant in each culture); experiental (situations and/or experiences included in the measure must be applicable in each culture); semantic (retention of the meaning of each item after translation); and conceptual equivalence (the validity of the concept in each culture).

Summary of main points

- Planning and piloting are essential at the outset of constructing a questionnaire.
- The format of the questionnaire can affect the answer obtained.
- With structured, pre-coded questions, the information obtained is limited by the questions asked and the response choices offered.
- Open-ended questions, without pre-coded responses, are essential where the topic is complex, or replies are unknown or too numerous to pre-code.
- Closed questions, with pre-coded responses, are preferable for topics about which much is known. Their advantage is that they are quicker and cheaper to analyse than responses to open questions.
- Closed questions carry the risk that replies may be forced into inappropriate categories.
- Closed questions give respondents clues about the answers expected, which they might not have thought of themselves.
- Respondents will more frequently endorse a statement than disagree with its opposite, and more frequently endorse the right-hand side statements. The direction of question wording and the response formats should be varied.
- The four main scaling methods are the Thurstone, Likert, Guttman and semantic-differential methods.
- The most common response scale is the Likert (rating scale). VAS and numeric scales are forms of Likert scales.
- The order and wording of the question can affect response.
- Easy and basic, non-threatening questions should be asked first; the most important questions should be asked first if no other rules apply.
- Questions about behaviour should be asked before questions about attitudes; general questions should be placed before specific questions.
- Leading questions, questions which do not reflect balance, complex questions and questions containing double negatives can lead to bias and should be avoided.
- Questions should contain simple and familiar words that everyone will understand.

Key questions

1 In what research situations are open and closed questions best suited?
2 What are the main effects of question wording, form and order on type of response?
3 Describe the main types of attitude scales.
4 What is the most commonly used attitude response scale?
5 What are the main techniques for asking questions on threatening, sensitive and embarrassing topics?
6 What types of questions should be asked first in a questionnaire?

Key terms

acquiescence response set
batteries of questions
closed questions
cultural equivalence
filter question
framing
funnelling
Guttman scale
leading questions
Likert scale
open questions
pilot study
pre-coded questions
prompts

question form
question order
question wording
rating scales
response set
scales of questions
scales (response formats)
scoring
semantic-differential scale
single item questions
stereotyped response set
Thurstone scale
visual analogue scale (VAS)
weighting item scores

Recommended reading

Bradburn, N.M. and Sudman, S. (1974) *Improving Interview Method and Questionnaire Design*. San Francisco, CA: Jossey-Bass.

Czaja, R. and Blair, J. (2005). *Designing Surveys*. Thousand Oaks, CA: Sage.

Oppenheim, A.N. (1992) *Questionnaire Design, Interviewing and Attitude Measurement*. London: Pinter.

Streiner, G.L. and Norman, D.R. (2003) *Health Measurement Scales: A Practical Guide to Their Development and Use*, 3rd edn. Oxford: Oxford University Press.

Sudman, S. and Bradburn, N.M. (1983) *Asking Questions*. New York: Jossey-Bass.

CHAPTER 14

Techniques of survey interviewing

Introduction

It has been pointed out that structured surveys try to measure facts, attitudes, knowledge and behaviour in such a way that if they were repeated at another time or in another area the results would be comparable. The qualities and training of interviewers are essential for the reliability and validity of the survey results. Interviewers must understand the nature of the study and exactly what is expected of them, from the importance of sampling and response rates to the way they ask and record the questions. Interviewers must also appreciate that no substitutes can be taken for sampled persons and that every effort must be made to interview those persons who are difficult to contact. This chapter describes techniques of structured interviewing. It is partly based on the training given by Professor Ann Cartwright to her research staff (I was once one of these) and on the detailed handbook for interviewers which is published by the Survey Research Center in Michigan (1976).

Types of interview

Face-to-face (personal) interview surveys involve interviewing people in their own homes or other sites. The interviews can be short and factual, lasting for a few minutes, or they can last for an hour or more. Structured interviews often include a combination of standardised questions, which are 'closed' (whereby the appropriate pre-coded response choices are checked, i.e. ticked or circled) or 'open-ended' (whereby the respondents' answers are written verbatim in the respondents' own words on the questionnaire). The third type of questioning is 'in-depth', whereby the interviewer uses unbiased probes as a stimulus to obtaining more detailed (in-depth) information about the topics in the interview schedule. With these, the interviewer writes down the respondent's responses, which may also be tape-recorded; after the interview a full report is written up. The latter is only used when the interviewer is highly trained and aware of the research issues.

Most of the rules which are described in this chapter also apply to telephone interviews. However, in telephone interviews there may be long pauses while the interviewer is recording the respondent's reply. The techniques for dealing with this are similar, for example, repeat the respondent's reply to fill the silence while recording it.

The interviewer

Essential qualifications for a good interviewer are sensitivity, and the ability to establish good rapport with a wide range of people, to be motivating, friendly and positive, trustworthy, sensitive, a good listener and not to interrupt respondents before they have finished speaking. Interviewers need to be committed and persevering, to adopt a neutral manner (showing neither approval nor disapproval), to have a clear voice, to be accurate in recording responses and to have legible handwriting. They must also be adept at leaving the respondent happy.

The characteristics of the interviewer can be biasing. People may respond differently to interviewers with different characteristics. Cosper (1972) reported that interviewers who adopted a 'business-like' approach, who wore dark suits rather than sportier suits, and those who were less educated found fewer drinkers of alcohol than interviewers who were 'friendly' and tried to gain the respondents' trust. The results of studies on interviewer bias are often inconsistent, but early studies also reported that young interviewers obtained less full and reliable results than older interviewers, and male interviewers obtained less full responses than females, particularly from males; female interviewers achieved their highest responses from males, except in cases of young female interviewers with young males (see Hyman *et al.* 1954; Webb *et al.* 1966, for reviews of classic studies).

Matching respondents up with interviewers least likely to produce bias by their characteristics would be practically difficult. Most researchers accept that these biases are inevitable and simply check for their presence and extent in the analyses (e.g. examining responses by age and sex of interviewer).

Preparation of interviewers

Interviewers must be prepared for their interviews with maps, name and address lists, time sheets, identity cards, visiting/appointment cards, letters of introduction and leaflets about the study to leave with respondents, non-response sheets (for recording details of each person who did not respond, such as refused, with reason, moved and address traced/untraced, and so on) and any relevant details about the sampling procedure. Interviewers should scan their name and address lists before leaving the office – if they know any of the individuals on the list they must return these and another interviewer will be allocated these respondents in order to ensure confidentiality and anonymity. They also need to plan their routes economically, so that they can call on people living near each other on the same day, and plan call-backs en route to other interviews.

Pencil or pen and computer-assisted interviewing

Some organisations request interviewers to use a soft, sharp pencil and others request them to use a blue or black pen (never red or green as these are generally used by editors, coders and the investigator back in the office). Some organisations prefer pen in order to enable them to monitor tightly errors and corrections made in the field. Pencil is easier to erase in case of error; errors in pen have to be clearly crossed through (such as two diagonal lines through the error). This is personal preference and there are no set rules across organisations.

Large organisations equip interviewers with laptop computers for face-to-face interviews which display the questionnaire and enable the interviewer to input the respondents' replies directly. Computer-assisted interviewing (known as CAI) is commonplace for telephone surveys. While the programming at the outset is time-consuming, the time saved at the coding and data entry stages can be enormous (the entered data by the interviewer are automatically coded and can be downloaded onto a main computer ready for analysis).

Interviewer handbooks

A typical handbook, or manual, for interviewers should be designed that is specific to the study they are working on. It will explain the aims of the organisation, the aims and sponsorship of the survey and techniques of interviewing. It will include a description of the study aims and design, including sampling techniques; the organisation and the timetable for the fieldwork; details of address lists, pay claims, documents about the study, the method of recording non-response and reasons; and then general and specific points about the questionnaire. It should emphasise the importance of accurate recording of the serial number on the questionnaire so that the respondent can be identified in the office for reasons of response checks, tagging for follow-up, and so on.

Specific information about the questionnaire usually given in interviewers' handbooks includes instructions on how to read out response categories. Sometimes the responses will be on showcards to be handed to respondents to aid recall, in which case there will be an instruction on the questionnaire ('Give showcard 1'). Sometimes the interviewer will be instructed to read out the response categories to respondents. In such circumstances the question may end with a colon (a colon can act as a prompt to interviewers to read out the response categories). Such information can be highlighted in the handbook. Information on skips and recording open-ended questions with verbatim quotations can also be reinforced in handbooks in relation to the relevant questions. Any signs and symbols used in the questionnaire should be explained in the handbook (e.g. < and > must be defined as less than and more than signs, as in <1 week, etc.). The handbook should also provide advice, where relevant, on tape recording, on using interpreters, on questions where the interviewer will need to be prepared to listen sympathetically (e.g. in the case of a death), on tracing respondents who have moved and on 'difficult to find' addresses. Definitions and examples can also be included. For example, in relation to the classification of occupations using the Registrar General's classification system in Britain, it is important that the interviewer records full details of occupation. The handbook can emphasise that it is important to record full and accurate information about occupation and that general descriptions are inadequate (e.g. 'secretary' is inadequate, as this description ranges from typist to company secretary). The handbook can encourage interviewers to probe, and remind them of the techniques for doing this, for example, 'What sort of secretary are you?', 'Can you describe what you actually do?'

The handbook can also give interviewers advice about what to do if respondents are tired or if they are worried about their well-being. It is never a good idea to break off the interview and continue on another day, as respondents may later refuse to continue. If the interview has to be stopped in the middle because the respondent is tired, for example, then break at an appropriate point (and not at upsetting or negative points). If interviewers are seriously worried about a respondent (e.g. a housebound person without any help, or an elderly person who is depressed or suicidal), they should first suggest professionals whom the respondent can contact; only in emergencies should the interviewer contact a professional on the respondent's behalf, and then signed consent should be obtained. The interviewer should be reminded that this is research interviewing and respondents should only exceptionally be referred to, or put in contact with, organisations or service providers; otherwise the representativeness of the sample, should any follow-up interviews be planned, will be affected.

The handbook can emphasise the correct order of asking any questions which are displayed in column format across the page. For example, in the case of the example in Box 14.1, the flow and speed are better if the symptoms are asked about first in column one, and then, after completing the whole of column one, the interviewer goes to the second column to ask about whether any of the symptoms that were reported have been consulted over. It is important that all interviewers use the same format in such cases.

Box 14.1 Correct order of asking questions

Sequence of questioning: go down the first column before the second column

In the past 4 weeks have you had any of these symptoms?			If yes to any: have you told your doctor about them?	
Symptoms:	Yes	No	Yes	No
Headache	—	—	—	—
Back ache	—	—	—	—
Stomach ache	—	—	—	—
Difficulty sleeping	—	—	—	—
Trouble with feet	—	—	—	—

Advice on safety can also be given in the handbook. If home interviews are being conducted in areas (e.g. certain inner-city areas) of high crime, researchers should also inform the police that they are carrying out the study, in case any potential respondents are suspicious and prefer to check for reassurance. In such areas, it is also important to ensure the safety of the interviewer. Some organisations, where calls out of daylight hours are involved, equip interviewers with mobile telephones in order to summon help quickly if necessary (though in the author's experience this has led to an increased chance of being assaulted, as the target becomes the mobile phone). If an interviewer feels uncertain about a respondent, then he or she should be encouraged to arrange to return with a second interviewer as companion. The office should ensure that it keeps up-to-date copies of interviewers' work schedules (this will also enable progress to be monitored). Interviewers should also ensure that they inform someone about their daily schedules for personal security purposes.

Interviewers' handbooks are no substitute for thorough training and briefing of interviewers; they are a complement to it.

Sampling by interviewers

Random sampling

Interviewers must be trained to use formulae for any additional sampling they have to do in the field. For example, if households have been sampled randomly using the postcode address file, but only one adult in each is required to be interviewed, the interviewer will have to be trained to sample the adult for interview on the doorstep. The interviewer will then need to use a random numbers table to select one adult per household for inclusion in the sample (weighting procedures are used in the analysis to correct for adults in households with fewer adults having a greater chance of inclusion in the sample). An example of the use of this method by the Office of National Statistics is outlined in Box 14.2. The approach is relevant to countries with central address files.

Box 14.2 Sampling procedure by interviewer

As the PAF [postcode address file] does not give the names of occupants of addresses, it is not possible to use the number of different surnames at an address as an indicator of the number of households living there . . . A rough guide to the number of households at an address is provided on the PAF by the multi-occupancy (MO) count. The MO count is a fairly accurate indicator in Scotland but is less accurate in England and Wales, so is used only when sampling addresses in Scotland. Addresses with an MO count of three or more, where the probability that there is more than one household is fairly high, are given as many chances of selection as the value of the MO count.

When the interviewer arrives at such an address, he or she checks the actual number of households and interviews a proportion of them according to instructions. The proportion is set originally by the MO count and adjusted according to the number of households actually found. A maximum of three households can be interviewed at any address. The interviewer selects the households for interview by listing all households at the address systematically then making a random choice by referring to a household selection table.

Addresses in Scotland with an MO count of two or less and all addresses in England and Wales are given only one chance of selection for the sample. At such addresses, interviewers interview all the households they find up to a maximum of three. If there are more than three households at the address, they are listed systematically and three of them are chosen randomly, as above, by means of a table. No addresses are deleted from the sample to compensate for these extra interviews but a maximum of four extra interviews per quota of addresses is allowed.

(Foster *et al.* 1995)

Sampling by interviewers can also be used to obtain booster samples of 'hard-to-reach groups'. For example, Bowling and Stenner's national population survey included mainly White British respondents, which reflected the national profile but produced insufficient numbers of people in ethnic minority groups for their group analysis. Thus they also worked with a survey organisation who used focused enumeration to sample main ethnic minority groups (known as an Ethnibus survey). Once the addresses had been sampled, interviewers were asked to visit each address to find out whether any members of the targeted groups lived there, and to invite them to participate in the study. In addition, residents were asked whether members of the targeted groups lived at that address, or in neighbouring homes:

> The Ethnibus was based on focused enumeration and stratified random sampling to ensure that samples were representative of the population. For sampling, Ethnibus used Census information on ethnicity across postal sectors, and listed the postal sectors according to concentration. Standard indicators of ethnic status were used, reflecting ethnic identity in the UK, and which reveal close connections between New Commonwealth countries and ethnic minority groups in the UK. Systematic random sampling was then used to ensure an even spread of postal sectors with differing concentrations. The number of addresses which were selected within the sector was proportional to the size

of the ethnic concentration, e.g. high concentration sector would yield high number of interviews. These addresses formed the starting point of the focused enumeration procedure. Ethnibus targeted: Indian, Pakistani, Black Caribbean, Chinese people. Sample boosting on the doorstep by interviewers was used to include greater numbers of people aged 65 and over. Interviews were obtained until target was achieved.

(Bowling and Stenner 2011, supplementary web file Appendix 1)

With focused enumeration (FE), there are strict interviewer protocols and formula that interviewers are required to follow during recruitment of respondents (RR), to prevent it being haphazard. Examples of the formula used in European wide surveys are illustrated in the technical report of the European Union Minorities and Discrimination Survey (European Union Agency for Fundamental Rights 2009, pp. 14–17), which was a survey of 27 European states:

FE relies on interviewers 'screening' addresses adjacent to the core issued address, e.g. the one that is identified via the RR procedure. During FE, any contact person at the RR address is asked to 'map' the immediate neighbours to find additional households where target minority persons might live. This is a method that keeps a random rule for respondent selection, but through proxy information, it provides better access to rare populations. Focused enumeration may cover any of the following dwelling units: any flats/houses one and two doors to the right and one and two doors to the left of the source RR address, and (if in a multi-story building) those DIRECTLY above and DIRECTLY under the flat where the interview took place. The aim was that interviewers could elicit information to screen out . . .

The FE approach is, in effect, a minority 'booster sample'. Because the focused enumeration booster sample was drawn from all sample PSUs – and because a fixed number of addresses is 'sampled' around each core sample address – the sample of addresses issued for screening by focused enumeration was representative of the coverage area (this assumes that the rules used by interviewers to identify the focused enumeration booster sample addresses were unbiased – which is a reasonable assumption for practical purposes).

With such methods, sample weights need to be applied in the analysis. For example, to compensate if some types of people had higher probability of being included in the sample than others (this is in addition to any sample weights used to compensate for known non-response by socio-demographic group).

Quota sampling

Other types of sampling conducted by interviewers include quota sampling. This is a technique common in market research and opinion polling. The geographical areas of the study are usually sampled randomly, after stratification (e.g. by type of region, parliamentary constituencies, socio-demographic characteristics of the area), and the quotas of people for interview are calculated from available population data (numbers (quota) of males, females, people in different age bands, and so on) in order to sample – and represent – these groups in the correct proportion according to their distribution in the population. The choice of the sample members is left to the interviewers. Interviewers are allocated an assignment of interviews, with instructions on how many interviews are to be in each group (men, women, etc.). They then usually stand in the street(s) allocated to them and approach passers-by, or call at random addresses in their allocated patches, until they have reached their quota of people willing to answer their questions. There is great potential for interviewer bias in the unconscious preferences operating in the selection of respondents.

Interviewer training

Interviewers require training so that they always ask the questions using the exact words printed on the questionnaire, and in the exact order they are in on the questionnaire, to minimise interviewer bias. Interviewers also need careful training and briefing, as well as experience, to enable them to find their way through complicated questionnaires while simultaneously maintaining rapport – to build up and maintain a sympathetic relationship, as well as trust – with respondents. They also need the skill to maintain the respondent's interest and motivation throughout. They should be able to communicate what is required of a respondent in terms of the interview and the information that is required. They need to be familiar with the form of the questions (i.e. pre-coded and open), and able to handle filter questions skilfully. The training must ensure that they are skilled at reading questions out carefully, at a reasonable volume and speed, paying attention to whether the respondent has heard and understood the questions. They must be accurate, and ring, tick or write in responses correctly.

Increasing interviewer training to periods of more than one day, writing questions so that the need for probing is minimised, tape recording interviews so that they can be checked in the office and reducing interviewers' workload can all lead to reductions in interviewer effects (bias) (Fowler and Mangione 1986). Interviewers must be trained (or briefed if they have already been trained) before they are given their lists of names and addresses to contact. The training and briefing consist of the research team and the interviewers going through the questionnaire question by question, together with any explanatory notes or instructions which have been prepared for interviewers about the questions. This is important in order to ensure that the interviewers understand why each question is being asked and what each means, and to clarify any final ambiguities. It is essential for the interviewers to know why questions are being asked, to enable them to probe adequately if respondents are not forthcoming or appear to misinterpret a question.

The interviewer training informs interviewers how to encourage respondents to participate (in a non-pushy manner), for example, by offering to return at a more convenient time, by offering to start the questionnaire to see how things go; and on how long it takes if respondents are slightly hesitant, and so on.

Interviewer bias

Interviewers must be trained to appear and speak in a neutral, non-judgemental manner. They must never appear surprised or disapproving in relation to a response. They are trained to display a uniform manner, expressing only polite interest. They must learn never to be embarrassed by questions or replies, and never to apologise for asking personal or embarrassing questions. If the interviewer thinks that a question is too personal (e.g. salary and total savings; frequency and adequacy of sex life), then the respondent will be influenced – he or she will detect this and decline to answer or give an inaccurate answer.

Interviewers must ask questions in a non-biasing and non-leading way. With interview surveys there is always the possibility of interviewer bias, whether owing to interviewers unconsciously asking a leading question, or respondents' deliberate social desirability bias (wanting to be seen in the best light and/or giving the answers they feel are expected of them). Interviewers' training teaches them not to ask leading questions which make assumptions about respondents or their replies (e.g. 'You haven't got chest pain, have you?' (leading); 'Have you got chest pain?' (non-leading)), to stick to the format of the questionnaire (question order and wording), to appear neutral, not to guess or make assumptions about respondents' likely answers, how to probe in a non-leading manner (e.g. 'Can you tell me more about that?', 'In what way?', 'Why do you say that?'), and to check for any obvious inconsistencies without making the respondent appear foolish or wrong (e.g. 'Can I check, have I got this down correctly?'). Interviewers should then have a minimum of one week's training whereby they role play for two or three days and then practise on a group of willing respondents from the population of interest (not actual sampled members for the main study). Where respondents agree, a tape recorder should be used for this and the investigator should listen to the recording while checking the questionnaire of the interview (this can detect any bias in the way the interviewer has asked the question and any ticking of wrong response codes, to facilitate subsequent retraining). Interviewers need to be instructed on how to fill in their time sheets and response/non-response forms (e.g. giving time and date of calls and reasons for any non-response). They need to be asked to return all completed forms and questionnaires to the office weekly so that their progress, accuracy, in relation to correct skips and lack of missing data, and response rates can be checked and any further training can be given if required. The main types of interviewer bias and error are summarised in Box 14.3.

Box 14.3 Potential biases and error in personal interviews

- Interviewer's characteristics, expectations and attitudes.
- Interviewer's behaviour:
    - not reading the questions or response choices out as worded;
    - directive, non-neutral probing;
    - inaccurate recording of responses.

Persistence in contacting respondents

Interviewers need to be committed and persistent – if no one is at home they have to call back at different times and days, and even at weekends or during the evening. They should use their initiative and ask neighbours when the person is likely to be in, while showing identity so as not to arouse suspicion or be mistaken for a potential burglar. Interviewers should always call in at the police station before commencing a study to explain that they will be in the area and leave identification. This is important in case respondents phone the police to check the identity of the interviewer and the authenticity of the investigation. It is reassuring to suspicious respondents to be informed that they can check the interviewer's authenticity with the police.

If there is difficulty in tracing an address, the interviewer should make enquiries locally, by contacting local people and shopkeepers, local post offices, the police station and the council office. If respondents are out when appointments have been made, a good interviewer will call again unannounced when next in the neighbourhood. Interviewers should be considerate and avoid disturbing people at inconvenient times (e.g. too early in the mornings, typical meal times).

Journeys also have to be planned with economy in mind. Interviewers have to be good planners: they should plan their routes economically to get through the greatest possible number of interviews per day, and always be aware of addresses requiring a call-back en route. Addresses near each other should be visited on the same day where possible, and call-backs planned when the interviewer is in the area anyway. Interviewers should be issued with visiting cards that can be left when respondents are out (e.g. 'Sorry I missed you, I will be in the area again on . . . My telephone number is . . . if you could call to arrange a convenient time'). Telephone contacts to arrange an interview are not advised: it is too easy for respondents to refuse.

Approaching respondents

Interviewers should dress neutrally, suitable for any kind of home, in order to minimise any bias (similarly the interviewer should not reveal personal details to the respondent – not even address, as this can be biasing). Before an interviewer approaches a respondent, the latter has usually been informed about the study, either by letter or by the investigator in person (e.g. while consulting a doctor), and asked if he or she would be willing to participate. If the information about the study has been sent by letter, the interviewer will not know in advance whether the person will agree to participate – and even those who have consented in advance can change their minds. The interviewer must approach potential respondents in a positive manner in order to encourage them to want to participate. The critical moment is when the interviewer introduces himself or herself. Response is likely to be increased if the interviewer looks happy, and appears positive and confident; it is likely to be decreased if the interviewer looks tense. Whether or not the person has been informed about the study beforehand, interviewers must always first show their identity photo-card, and inform the respondent about who they are and why they are calling ('Hello, I am . . . from the Department of . . . [show identity card]. We are carrying out a study about . . .'). At this point the interviewer should establish whom he or she wants to interview and ensure that he or she has approached the right person (interviews with the wrong person cannot be accepted).

Having located the respondent, the interviewer should give him or her a leaflet about the study, while explaining in a lively manner the purpose of the study, how the results will be used, its sponsorship, confidentiality, how the person's name was obtained and why it is important for him or her to respond. Investigators usually give interviewers the information in a standard format to read out (in a lively, not a dull, memorised patter). Leaving respondents with a letter and/or leaflet about the study is essential, especially in relation to frail and/or elderly people, in case anyone wants to check on the identity of callers. In relation to very ill respondents, it may be necessary to ask if someone can be interviewed on their behalf (a 'proxy' respondent).

Motivating people to respond

Interviewers must make respondents feel valued, interested in the topic, motivated to take part and important to the study (see Box 14.4). A good interviewer will have good intuition, know how to make positive doorstep introductions and have the ability to know when to retreat and when to reapproach reluctant respondents. However, there is little point in persuading reluctant respondents if the result is to increase survey bias in the responses obtained. Interviewers must be honest about the study and tell people how long the interview will take. In order to introduce the survey well, and encourage people to respond, interviewers must be familiar with the study and its aims. Interviewers should next state the desired course of action clearly. For example, instead of asking 'Are you busy now?' or 'Could we do the interview now?' (which may provoke a 'no' answer), interviewers should say 'I would like to come in and talk with you about this' (Survey Research Center 1976).

If interviewers appear hesitant, reluctant, unconfident, embarrassed or negative, they will encourage a negative response. Interviewers should assume that the respondent is not too busy for an interview there and then, and that he or she will be willing to take part – being confident but not pushy or aggressive. If the respondent really is too busy, then an arrangement should be made to return at a more convenient time. Similarly, as pointed out earlier, interview appointments should not be made by telephone – it is easier to say no by telephone than when faced with a friendly, positive interviewer on the doorstep.

Ultimately, if respondents adamantly refuse to take part, their wishes must be respected and the interviewer must apologise for bothering them and take leave. However, with the general decline in survey response rates, most interviewers will achieve about 65 per cent of the interviews they attempt, although lower response rates can be anticipated in certain types of area. All addresses should be visited in the first half of the fieldwork period, so that call-backs can be planned, particularly for anyone known to be away temporarily.

Often a respondent will change his or her mind after initially refusing, particularly if the refusal was owing to being busy. Interviewers could first try calling again a few days later if people initially refuse ('I was just passing and wondered if you might have time to take part now'). It is also worth considering whether a follow-up letter from the investigator on the organisation's notepaper can reverse a refusal. These letters can convince respondents that we genuinely would like to talk to them and that the topic is important. Follow-up letters are essential if the respondent did not speak the same language as the interviewer – the investigator can arrange for a translated letter about the study to be sent, and an interpreter offered. However, participation is voluntary and categorical refusals should be respected.

Box 14.4 Motivating people to respond

Typical questions asked by respondents when approached for an interview, and possible replies by interviewers, have been given by the Survey Research Center (1976) and include the following.

R: Why me?

I: We cannot talk to everyone but we try to talk to men and women of different ages in all walks of life. So we took a cross-section of people from the list of [voters] and you were one of them. This is what we mean by 'cross-section'. It is important to ensure that the study represents the population, so once we have chosen the names nobody else will do instead – otherwise we won't have a proper cross-section of people.

R: I don't know anything about this [research topic]; I'm not typical so there's no point in me taking part.

I: We are interested in your opinions and experiences even if you feel you do not know about this. Everyone's opinions are important. The results would not be valid if we only included those who were experts. It is important that we make sure that we represent everyone by interviewing a complete cross-section of people.

R: What good will it do me?

I: The study will not directly benefit the people we talk to, but it may help people in the future if we have information about what people need for planning purposes.

R: How will the results be used?

I: All replies are treated in strict confidence and no individuals can be identified in the report of the study as information is presented in figures in table form, and no names are used. The information is used for research purposes only and will not be passed on to anyone else. The results will be used for [e.g. planning health services for people in this area]. It is only by carrying out surveys like this that information can be obtained to do this.

R: I'm not sure about this!

I: Can we give it a try? Let me tell you the first question. I will stop at any time you wish and destroy the questionnaire.

R: I haven't got time.

I: I can call back at a more convenient time, how about . . . is that more convenient?

[Interviewer note: fill in appointment card and hand it to respondent to decrease chances of appointment being broken; if relevant, mention the long distance you have to travel for the interview.]

Interviewers must never break appointments.

Third parties and distractions

Another problem to be encountered is that, with home interviews, the person who answers the door may not be the person required for interview. The interviewer should establish a good rapport with the person who answers the door and quickly establish who the required informant is. Some marital partners, or children of older people, may be protective of the person one requires to interview and refuse on his or her behalf. Interviewers should always affirm that they would like to ask the person concerned themselves, except in circumstances where the person is ill, in which case the interviewer may have been instructed by the investigator to ask a carer ('proxy') to be interviewed instead (a proxy interview). The code of ethics is important with proxy interviews. Carers can be asked directly to give a proxy interview if the required respondent is unable to respond – for example, unconscious, mentally confused or severely mentally ill (e.g. psychotic) – otherwise the required respondent must give his or her consent to a proxy interview. Being blind, partially sighted or deaf is not a valid reason for conducting a proxy interview, as questions can be read out (for people with difficulty in seeing) or written down (for people with difficulty in hearing).

Caution should also be exercised when other people want to sit in on an interview between the interviewer and the respondent – whether or not the respondent is ill or frail. The presence of a third party (e.g. a spouse) can influence the respondent and lead to biased (wrong) answers. The interviewer should minimise any influences where possible. If there is only one room, then the interviewer should suggest that the respondent and interviewer sit in a corner of it to be quieter and more private. If this is not possible, and the other person interrupts at all, the interviewer should explain tactfully that it is only the views of the respondent that are wanted for the questionnaire and that the third person can give his or her views afterwards. The interviewer may have to explain further that he or she has been instructed only to obtain the views of the respondent so that the survey is representative.

The exception is where factual information is required (e.g. date of hospital attendance), and then there is no harm in another person helping to provide accurate information. If interpretation is required, another member of the household may offer to help. The offer of help should normally be accepted, but the interviewer should try to ascertain that it is the respondent's views, not the interpreter's, that are being obtained.

It is possible that a respondent does not want a friend or relative to know how he or she really feels or thinks about an issue. If a third party is present, the interviewer should try to encourage the respondent to show him or her to the door at the end of the interview – sometimes respondents say, 'That's not true what I told you . . . I'm really depressed but I didn't want him to know.'

There may be other distractions, such as loud televisions. If the interviewer lowers his or her voice the respondent will generally turn the television down. There may also be young children or babies present during the interview, and the interviewer will need to exercise patience if they are noisy or need frequent attention from the respondent, and continue to conduct the interview as smoothly as possible.

Beginning the interview

At the start of the interview it is important that the interviewer finds a place to sit where he or she can write comfortably. In case a table is not available, interviewers should carry a hard clipboard or pad with them. If the respondent has not invited the interviewer indoors, the interviewer should say, 'Do you mind if I come in as I have to write all this down?' Only short interviews (less than five minutes) can be successfully carried out on the doorstep.

Blank paper should also be taken, in case there is not sufficient room on the questionnaire for all the respondent's comments (though this is rare). Interviewers should sit facing the respondent, in a position where the respondent cannot look at what is being written.

Audio recording

If a tape recorder is to be used, the respondent's prior permission must be sought. Respondents are typically informed that its use helps the interviewer to check that he or she has recorded their views correctly and that most people agree to its use. If there is any anxiety about it, respondents can be informed that they will soon forget it is there, but refusals must be respected. In order to check for any reactive effects, one technique is to turn the recorder off at the end of the interview and 'chat' to respondents informally as a check on whether the respondent has anything else to add. Any new or inconsistent material that is raised should be noted later, along with separate interviewer notes about how the interview went.

It is important that the interviewer is familiar with the tape recorder, and regularly checks the play-back sound quality and the batteries. Longer tapes should be used to prevent the need for frequent turning over/changing during an interview.

Rapport

The reliability of the information collected is partly dependent on a satisfactory relationship being established between interviewer and respondent. If a respondent feels anxious or uneasy in any way, then he or she may not feel able or willing to express feelings or attitudes fully, or report behaviour. Interviewers need to be positive and encouraging without expressing their own views on the topic of the interview. They will need to exercise tact when bringing respondents who ramble back to the topic of the interview. They will need to be skilled at creating expectant silences to encourage responses, without letting silences drag or become embarrassing.

Interviewers should be sensitive to the needs of the respondent: he or she may need reading glasses to see showcards; people with difficulty hearing may be able to lip read or questions can be shown to them; all items, even showcards, can be read out to people who have great difficulty seeing. Interviewers must take care not to exhaust ill or frail people. Any of these difficulties should be noted on the front of the questionnaire.

Rules for structured interviewing

Questions asked by interviewers can cover a wide range of areas, including attitudes, knowledge, behaviour and descriptive data (from socio-demographic data to health status). Careful and precise interviewing techniques are essential in order to ensure the collection of complete, standardised and accurate data.

Pre-coded (closed) questions

With structured interviewing methods, each person in the sample is asked the same series of questions in the same order and worded in exactly the same way. Most questions will be pre-coded. A pre-coded question is one which is followed by a list of possible answers (response choices), with a code number opposite each, and respondents' replies are usually recorded by ticking or circling a pre-coded response category and writing in any verbatim open response answers (to any questions without pre-codes or without a suitable pre-coded response category, or to questions with pre-codes containing an 'other, please specify' category). The response choices are read out (or shown on a showcard) to respondents when they are required to reply in a certain way, in order to make specific comparisons among respondents. For example:

Q: Is your health:

Excellent	1
Very good	2
Good	3
Fair	4
Poor	5

When all the alternative responses are read out (or shown on a showcard), this is known as a *running prompt*. The response categories of 'don't know' and 'other' are never read out (unless there is a reason for this in the aims of the question). Some interviewers' schedules use a colon after the question to indicate that the response choices should be read out (e.g. Is your health: . . .). Other schedules print the instruction 'Read out' by the response categories. Interviewers are instructed never to ring a category that comes *nearest* to a respondent's reply (thus 'forcing' it into an inappropriate code); if in doubt they should repeat the question/response choices for the respondent to select one. If none of the categories apply, the respondent's reply must be recorded verbatim, in the respondent's own words. Some questions list 'other' response codes to allow for this, and the reply should still be written out. There is no need to read out the response choices for questions which can only be answered in one way: for example, 'How many children aged 16 and over do you have?'

Questions can involve the checking (ticking or circling) of just one response category (single code questions) or several responses may be checked (multicoded questions). Interviewers are usually taught to check one answer per question unless otherwise instructed on the questionnaire. With multicoded questions the instruction 'Code all that apply' usually appears on the questionnaire.

Open-ended questions

Some questions – for example, in relation to more complex issues – can be open-ended. With these, the respondent's answers are written in verbatim (in the respondent's own words). The following is an example of an open-ended question: 'What areas of your life have been most affected by your illness/condition?'

The interviewer must record everything that the respondent says, and probe to ensure the respondent's answer is complete. These replies are analysed in the office, and a coding frame is developed for them to be coded later. If there is not enough space under the question for the response to be recorded, then the interviewer should continue on a blank sheet and cross-reference it to the question number.

Filter questions

Some questions are called *filter questions* (also known as *funnelling* – see Chapter 13). This means that they are skipped for respondents to whom they do not apply. For example, males are not asked questions about cervical screening. Organisations vary in their layout of skip instructions for interviewers. Some put instructions to skip to a specific question in the right-hand margin of the filter question, some put the instruction immediately before the filter question. The format does not matter as long as it is clearly signposted (e.g. on inapplicable questions to be skipped) to ensure that interviewers do not make erroneous skips. Complex rerouting of questions should be minimised as it does make extra demands on the interviewer (as well as on the layout of the questionnaire). Computer-assisted interviewing (CAI) is invaluable for skips as they are automatic and do not depend on the skill and memory of the interviewer.

Interviewers should never decide themselves that a question is inappropriate. Unless there is a skip for specific groups of people marked in the questionnaire, *the questions must be asked* – only the respondent can decide if the question really is inappropriate, and then his or her reasons must be recorded.

Interviewing techniques

Interviewers are instructed to read each question slowly, and not to mumble, in order to enable the respondent to understand the question in full and to prepare a reply; to ask the questions in exactly the way they are worded and the order in which they appear on the questionnaire; to ensure that interviews are standardised and comparable; and to ask every question. Interviewers should look at the respondent after asking a question in order to pick up any embarrassment or lack of understanding and try to deal with this immediately.

Wording and order

It was pointed out in Chapter 13 that question wording affects response, and questions have to be carefully worded in order to obtain the most accurate and unambiguous response. It is important to avoid influencing respondents, and interviewers must avoid adding their own words and thereby changing the meaning of the question or leading respondents to respond in certain ways. Interviewers must never assume respondents' replies from previous answers or lead respondents to feel that they are expected to give a particular reply. Similarly, interviewers must never fill in respondents' answers from memory later. Interviewers must understand that changing the question wording and order can introduce serious bias.

The only question with which there is an exception to the rule is the question on gender:

Sex
Male   1
Female   2

With sex, the interviewer can check the appropriate code and does not need to ask the respondent, 'Are you male or female?'

Answering questions before they have been asked

It is common for respondents to appear to be answering later questions in their response to a current question. However, their answers must never be assumed and questions must never be skipped on the basis of a false belief that the respondent has already answered later questions. In order to avoid respondents becoming irritable in such circumstances, and to avoid the interviewer appearing to ignore what they have said, the interviewer can let respondents know that they are aware of their earlier response, and ask them for their cooperation again, by prefixing the question with, 'I know you have already mentioned this area, but can I just check . . . [read out the question as worded]?' or, 'Now you've already said something about this, but I'd like to ask you this question . . . [read out the question as worded].'

Where a respondent appears to have readdressed a question later, or given a reply to a later question early in the questionnaire, the interviewer should record the comments and cross-reference by asterisking and noting question numbers by the respondent's comments – as well as always asking the question when it is reached.

Question order also affects response, so it is important for interviewers to regain control of the order. The interviewer can tell the respondent that he or she cannot keep up with them and ask them to let the interviewer ask the questions in the order they appear on the questionnaire, so that he or she will not have to give the information more than once and can record the responses more accurately.

Inconsistency

People may be inconsistent about their attitudes and feelings. Interviewers should not try to make people consistent in relation to these. However, inconsistencies of fact should be detected and sorted out with the respondent: for example, by saying, 'Can I check? I don't seem to have got this down right.'

Need for reassurance

If the respondent appears to need reassurance, the interviewer should affirm that 'There are no right or wrong answers on this, we are just trying to obtain your ideas.'

Sometimes respondents ask interviewers what they think, but interviewers must never succumb because they can bias respondents into giving a similar reply. Interviewers must simply explain that it is the respondents' opinions that matter. Respondents will soon learn that it is the role of the interviewer to read out questions as they are written, and not give opinions, and it is their role to reply as best as they can.

Misunderstandings

Questions which have been misunderstood can be repeated just as they are worded in the questionnaire. If the respondent just needs time to think, then do not hurry him or her, and create a comfortable atmosphere if a silence occurs in these circumstances.

If the respondent really does not understand the word used in a question the interviewer can say 'whatever it means to you'. If he or she gives a correct definition, then the interviewer can say so and repeat the question. If the lack of understanding is genuine, then the interviewer must simply make a note of this by the question and move on to the next question. In some cases, investigators will give the interviewer a handbook of notes about the questionnaire and include alternative definitions of words for interviewers to use, so that if the respondent's definition is wrong, the interviewer can guide him or her to the right meaning without changing the wording of the question.

In some cases, the handbook can also give suggestions for prompting (suggestions of answers). On the whole, however, these techniques are often avoided because they can lead to bias as well as a different response from the one intended (question wording affects response). Although questionnaires should use simple and short words that most people understand, there will occasionally be someone who really does not understand particular questions (though this should be rare, except in cases where the first language spoken by the respondent is not that which the questionnaire is written in).

Wherever the interviewer has offered an alternative definition, or reworded a question, or probed further for a response, this must be recorded next to the question to facilitate its interpretation by the investigator.

Reluctance to respond to items

If a respondent does not want to reveal particular information – for example, personal details such as income or evaluation of his or her sex life – then the interviewer should first confirm that the information is confidential, and that replies will be presented in tables of figures and no person can be identified. If respondents remain reluctant, then their wishes should be respected and the interviewer should move on to the next question. If interviewers appear embarrassed at such questions, respondents are more likely to refuse to respond. If interviewers appear 'matter of fact' in manner, the information is usually forthcoming, and is less difficult to obtain than imagined, though the extent of response bias (underestimates of income, alcohol intake, etc.) is unknown.

Uncertainty, don't know and vague replies

Some respondents will be unable to make up their minds about which response category applies to them, but interviewers must never suggest likely responses. Instead, they should say neutrally, 'Which code do you think might be closest to the way you feel?'

A 'don't know' reply can have several interpretations: the respondent may not understand the question and does not want to admit it; the phrase 'don't know' may simply be giving him or her time to think; the respondent may be using the phrase evasively because he or she is reluctant to answer the question; or he or she may genuinely not know the answer. The last is important survey information, and the interviewer has the responsibility of ascertaining that a 'don't know' response reflects this and none of the former reasons. The most effective technique is to repeat the question. Probing can be used next: 'Which of these comes closest to your . . . ?' The same techniques are used for dealing with vague replies.

It is important that interviewers always record a don't know or any inadequate responses in order to inform the coder that the question has not been omitted in error.

Probing

A probe is a stimulus which is used to obtain more extensive or explicit responses from people. Some respondents have difficulty verbalising their responses, have not thought about the topic before, have difficulty forming a reply or may not wish to reveal their true feelings. Others may give unclear or incomplete replies. In such cases, probing is required. The Survey Research Center (1976) has described the function of probing as to motivate – without bias – the respondent to clarify and enlarge upon what he or she has said and to help the respondent to focus on the content of the question. The Center has published an entire chapter on probing, which contains techniques for encouraging respondents to clarify or enlarge upon their answers, or even to return to the point of the question (see Box 14.5).

Box 14.5 Examples of non-directive probes

- Repeating the question just as it is written.
- An expectant pause, accompanied, for example, by a nod of the head (if used sensitively).
- A verbal 'mm' or 'yes' followed by an expectant pause.
- A quizzical glance followed by an expectant pause.
- Repeating the respondent's reply as the interviewer is writing it down can stimulate the respondent to further thought.
- Neutral comments or questions, such as: 'Anything else?' 'Any other reason?' 'How do you mean?' 'What do you mean by . . . ?' 'Could you tell me more about your thinking on that?' 'Why do you feel that way?'

(Survey Research Center 1976)

These probes must be used gently, and not in a demanding tone of voice, which will discourage respondents. It is important that interviewers understand the aim of the questions in order to probe effectively. Finally, longer sentences, which give respondents time to think, are likely to elicit more information than short ones, for example, 'Are there any other reasons why you feel that way?' is more effective than a curt 'Any other?' The latter is more likely to elicit a 'no' in response (Survey Research Center 1976). Similarly, negative probes should never be used, as they will encourage negative responses (e.g. 'Nothing else?', 'Is that all?').

Directive probing techniques are permissible when one is eliciting factual information. For example, if respondents are asked about their social network *size* (e.g. number of relatives, friends and neighbours he or she has had contact with in a specific time period), and respondents appear to have omitted the partner they live with (which is common as they tend to be taken for granted), it is acceptable to use directive probes to focus the question by asking 'Does that include your wife/husband/partner?' If a respondent has difficulty remembering the date of an event, the interviewer can assist by asking 'Was it more or less than a year ago?' and so on.

Redirecting

It is common for respondents to go off the topic and talk about other issues not relevant to the questionnaire. The interviewer has to be skilled at bringing respondents tactfully back to the point. If this is done firmly from the outset, then the problem is less likely to recur throughout the interview. In some sensitive areas (e.g. if a respondent has been bereaved, or is terminally ill), the interviewer will need to be prepared to be a sympathetic listener to some extent, before bringing the respondent gently back to the questionnaire using neutral techniques. Techniques for dealing with going off the point include, 'Perhaps we can talk about that later. What I'm really interested in here is [repeat the question].'

When respondents digress at any length, interviewers should note this on the questionnaire (e.g. R talked about the state of the economy). All comments, explanations and probes made by the interviewer should also be recorded on the questionnaire. For example, probes can be recorded simply by the letter P, followed by any responses the respondent makes. When the question has been repeated the interviewer can simply record RQ.

The end of the interview

Interviewers must leave the respondent in a positive frame of mind. This can be difficult if the topic of the interview is stressful or distressing (e.g. about bereavement). After the interview has been completed, the interviewer should be prepared to spend time, if appropriate, listening to the respondent in order to leave him or her in a positive frame of mind. If requested, at the end of the interview the interviewer should also be prepared to spend time explaining the study further and answering the respondent's questions. This is only polite after respondents have given up their time for the study.

At the end of the interview, the interviewer should check through the schedule to ensure no questions have been omitted, thank respondents for taking part, ask them if they have any questions they would like to ask about the study and leave them feeling positive and willing to take part in surveys again.

Recording responses

Information must be recorded or entered onto computer (if computer-aided interviewing is used) accurately, and legibly if by hand. Apart from always recording the response, interviewers should also record the tone in which replies are given where it appears relevant (e.g. a reply in a sceptical, cynical or hurried tone which appears to contradict the response or response category chosen).

Interviewers should record any necessary information, or verbatim quotes, during the interview – they will be forgotten afterwards and information will be lost. With practice, interviewers become accomplished at recording responses while respondents are talking – interviewers cannot afford to spoil the rapport gained with the respondent by having respondents sitting waiting for them to finish writing. One technique of maintaining respondents' interest while the interviewer is recording their response is to repeat their response while writing it down. This also tends to prompt further comments.

Any answers by the respondent that are written out (rather than simply a response category checked) by the interviewer must be recorded verbatim (i.e. written out in full in the respondent's own words). This is essential in order to ensure that meaning is not lost or distorted, and enables these quotations to be used in reports as illustrative material and/or coded later in the office when they have been analysed and a suitable coding frame has been developed. Notes, summarising, paraphrasing or paraphrasing in the interviewer's words (e.g. 'She said that she did not feel happy') where full recording is requested are not acceptable. For example, the difference is illustrated by comparing the following.

Verbatim:
'I feel unhappy because I can't get outdoors and I've lost my independence and control. I can't go shopping or go and see my family or anything. To keep your independence is what's so important.'

Summarised:
'Unhappy, can't get out for shopping, visiting.'

The summarised version lacks the depth of the full reply, and is less revealing about what is really important to the respondent (independence).

Interview notes

Some investigators ask interviewers to write a short description at the end of the questionnaire about the respondent, any other people present and how the interview went. This can be invaluable for the coders. However, abusive or critical personal remarks about respondents are not appropriate.

Debriefing

Debriefing sessions between the investigator and the interviewers are important. These should take place after any piloting (interviewers know when questions were misunderstood or too difficult for respondents and need to be changed), and periodically throughout the study, as well as at the end. Important information for the investigator is obtained from these feedback sessions, and they also help the interviewers to feel valued and part of a team, and to feel there is a cathartic opportunity to talk about how the interviews went. Investigators should always be prepared to be sympathetic listeners to an interviewer (in the same way that psychotherapists need to be counselled after client work).

Quality control

Fabricated interviews are rare, but have been known to occur. If an interviewer has been detected fabricating an interview or falsifying the data collected, then the entire batch of interviews from that interviewer should be treated as suspect and discarded. It is possible to check for faked data (e.g. over-consistent responses). The office can send thank-you letters to respondents, and invite them to provide feedback on self-completion cards about how they felt the interview went. Some organisations send field supervisors to recall or telephone samples of respondents to check that they were interviewed. If interviewers are informed that these checks are routine, then they are less likely to be tempted to fake interviews and risk detection.

High interviewing standards should also be maintained by quality control in the office – as questionnaires are returned they should be checked for obvious errors, missed data, legible writing, and so on. In the case of missed data, interviewers can be requested to recall on the respondent and obtain the data. Interviewers with high error rates should be retrained.

Large survey organisations maintain the interviewing standards of their interviewers by organising basic and advanced training sessions and refresher courses.

Summary of main points

- People may respond differently to interviewers with different characteristics.
- Interviewers should speak in a neutral, non-judgemental manner, and never appear surprised or disapproving.
- Interviewers should ensure the collection of complete, standardised and accurate data.
- Computer-aided interviewing with laptop computers increases accuracy; entered responses can be automatically coded and stored.
- If respondents do not understand the question, it should be repeated slowly; if this fails, the interviewer should ask respondents what they think it means.
- Some questions are called filter questions (also known as funnelling). This means that they are skipped for respondents to whom they do not apply.
- Interviewers must never assume respondents' replies from previous answers or lead respondents to feel they are expected to give a particular reply.
- Techniques for dealing with respondents who go off the point include 'Perhaps we can talk about that later. What I'm really interested in here is [repeat the question].'
- It is essential to check returned interviews for faked data (e.g. over-consistent responses), missing data, legible writing and obvious errors.

Key questions

1 What are the methods interviewers can use for increasing response rates to a study?
2 What types of sampling can interviewers carry out?
3 What qualities and skills do interviewers need?
4 Why is it important that interviewers ask questions in the same way and in the same order?
5 What is a running prompt?
6 Explain the term 'leading question'.
7 In what circumstances are directive and non-directive probing appropriate?
8 How can potential interviewer biases be checked?

Key terms

closed questions
direct probes
filter questions
funnelling
indirect probes
interviewer bias
interviewer effects
open-ended questions

pre-codes
quota sampling
rapport
redirecting
response
running prompt
skips
verbatim recordings

Recommended reading

Fowler, F.J. (2009) *Survey Research Methods*. Thousand Oaks, CA: Sage.

Fowler, F. and Mangione, T. (1989) *Standardized Survey Interviewing: Minimizing Interviewer-related Error.* Thousand Oaks, CA: Sage.

Survey Research Center (1976) *Interviewer's Manual*, revised edn. Ann Arbor, MI: University of Michigan, Survey Research Center, Institute for Social Research.

CHAPTER 15

Preparation of quantitative data for coding and analysis

Introduction

Once the research data have been collected, the process of preparing them for analysis begins. Coded data allow the researcher to reduce large quantities of information into a form than can be more easily managed, usually by computer programs. Quantitative data will need to be sorted and coded, and even qualitative data will need to be indexed or categorised by some rigorous method, in preparation for analysis. The aim is to develop a system for the assignment of numbers to observations (the data). This chapter describes the process of coding quantitative data. Because qualitative data are often based on grounded theory and the categorisation process is developed throughout the research process, the description of the coding of qualitative data is integrated in the relevant chapters on qualitative methods, rather than here.

Coding

Coding is a method of conceptualising research data and classifying them into meaningful and relevant categories for the participants in the study (the unit(s) of analysis). Regardless of the mode of administering the questionnaire, a number is assigned to a category, which is called the code (e.g. with the variable sex, code 1 is assigned to females and code 2 to males). Coding formats need to be included on or within the questionnaire, whether it is a paper, electronic (e.g. via a laptop), internet-based or telephone direct data entry questionnaire survey. It is developed after the data have been collected in cases where categories for answers are not all known beforehand, and where respondents' replies do not fall into pre-coded response categories: e.g. for open-ended questions and pre-coded questions which have an 'other, please specify' code. The latter coding of quantitative data is carried out at the end of the data collection period, once all the codes have been finalised (especially as some codes may require extension).

If previous knowledge or theory was used to construct response categories (pre-coded questions) before the instrument was administered to respondents, then this is called *deductive* coding. When a study is exploratory, or when there is little previous knowledge or theory to inform the development of codes at the outset of the study, then the coding is designed after analysing a representative sample of answers to questions, and it is called *inductive* coding. The advantages of this approach are flexibility, richness of the codes and opportunity to develop new categories that might not otherwise have been thought of (they are derived from the data, rather than the data being constrained by being forced to fit pre-codes). The disadvantage is the time-consuming nature of the task (see Box 15.1).

Box 15.1 Steps in developing a coding frame

- Write down a list of replies from a sample of the questionnaires (e.g. 30, depending on the questionnaire and size of the study).
- Identify the main categories of these replies.
- Include final 'other, please specify' codes to include replies not thought of.
- Try to include code items for all the main themes which occur in order to minimise the 'other' code obtaining a frequency value higher than any of the main codes, which is never informative. A sense of balance also needs to be maintained here to prevent the list of code items becoming overlong, which is difficult for coding and leads to tiny frequency distributions for rarely occurring codes.
- If people have given a reply which fits more than one category (e.g. more than one reason for dissatisfaction with health care given), then each reply will need to be coded separately and they should all be allowed for in the coding up to a

pre-defined level (e.g. code up to six replies; if more than six replies, code the first six given). It is important to specify the number of replies that will be coded because the corresponding number of coding boxes for each reply has to be designed and printed onto the coding sheet.
- Finalise the codes to be used, and design the coding frame for the question with the code items in order of the most commonly occurring listed first.
- Assign a numerical value to each coded item.
- Test the coding frame on another batch of questionnaires (e.g. 30, depending on the study).

The basic rules for the development of the coding scheme (known as the *coding frame*) for quantitative data are that the codes must be mutually exclusive (a response must fit into one category (code) only), coding formats for each item must be comprehensive and the codes must be applied consistently (see J. Fielding 1993). In contrast, the coding rules for qualitative data permit the allocation of responses to more than one category in order to facilitate conceptual and theoretical development.

Direct data entry and electronic questionnaires

Most large research organisations train their interviewers to use electronic versions of the questionnaire via personal computers in computer-assisted telephone interviews, or laptop computers in computer-assisted face-to-face interviews. The advantage is that data can be entered, automatically coded and transmitted nightly via the telephone to a central computer which processes the data. In addition, programs can be designed to minimise errors and assist interviewers with question skips; they also prevent interviewers from moving to the next question unless a response at each question has been entered.

Manual coding and data entry

Otherwise, for example if the questionnaires are self-completed manually (e.g. postal), then they will need coding entirely in the office. Interview data can also be hand-coded by the interviewer during or after the interview ('field coding') directly onto the paper questionnaire. However, it usually requires coding, or the coding to be completed, back in the office by a coder, or team of independent coders. The latter method is generally preferred, because it takes place in a less rushed routine setting and is usually less prone to coding errors.

Some simple self-completion questionnaires do not require further coding if the respondent has ticked the numerical code corresponding to his or her reply. It is rare, however, to be able to dispense with office coding completely, as most questionnaires allow for the later coding of 'other' response categories, or any open-ended questions that have been included in the questionnaire. The codes may be entered by the coder onto the questionnaire in the boxes designed for this (usually in a right-hand margin) or in clearly labelled coding boxes on a separate coding transfer sheet. The use of the latter increases the costs of the study (design, paper and printing) but has the advantage that the questionnaire is less visually cluttered (by the omission of the coding boxes).

Coding boxes

Coding boxes are allocated for each question. Each box must contain only one number. Thus, for answers which have been allocated a two-digit code (e.g. number of miles: 40), two coding boxes will be provided – one for each number. If more boxes are provided than there are numbers in the answer recorded on the questionnaire, then noughts should be written into the boxes preceding the first number of the response (e.g. 040).

Coding transfer sheets

The paper or electronic coding sheets used for data input will either be the completed, pre-coded questionnaires, or coding transfer sheets for each questionnaire which contain the transferred codes from each question. The latter are used if the investigator does not wish to clutter the questionnaire with numerical codes and coding boxes, though this then doubles the administrative effort and paper costs. (See Box 15.2.) Both methods must indicate exactly where in the individual's computer record each item of data is to be placed. This is usually done by allocating variable names to each question, which are stored in the computer's data entry program (in a predefined sequence) as well as on the coding frame (the variable name is usually a summary of the question in eight or less digits and/or the question number).

Box 15.2 Example of coding transfer sheet

Question:	Coding boxes:	Variable name:
Serial no.	☐ ☐ ☐ ☐	SERIALNO
1 Where saw specialist	☐	Q1SPEC
2 Given a choice	☐	Q2CHOICE

The code book

For quantitative data, a code book of the data should be prepared. (See Box 15.3.) This is simply a master copy of the questionnaire, with the question number, the question, the full range of valid codes written in, including missing and 'do not apply' values (known as *value labels* by computer packages), the number of columns available for each response (code boxes for transfer to the computer columns) and the variable label, which will be required for its identification on the computer (usually a maximum of eight digits). Either the question number can be used for the variable label or a short word (e.g. the word 'class' could be used to identify the social class code).

Some investigators write these details by hand onto a copy of the questionnaire; others will retype the entire code book. If all the codes are already known and typed onto the questionnaire before it was printed, and if the coding boxes are already known and printed in the right-hand margin, then a few hand additions of extra codes and the variable names are all that is needed. The code book is needed for coding and reference.

Box 15.3 Example of code book

Questionnaire for patients

Master copy code book

	Code boxes	Variable name
Serial no.:	☐ ☐ ☐ ☐	SERIALNO

1 Where did you see the specialist this time?

At GP's surgery	1	
At hospital outpatient clinic	2	☐ Q1SPEC
Missing response	9	

2 Did your GP offer you the choice of seeing a specialist in the GP's surgery or at the hospital?

Yes	1	
No	0	☐ Q2CHOICE
Missing response	9	

Numerical values for codes

Quantitative analysis requires the information gathered to be coded either quantitatively (in the form of a measurement such as weight in kilogrammes or age in years) or 'qualitatively' (e.g. in the form of a homogeneous category so that the numbers in each group can be counted). Thus, for sex, the groups are male and female; for marital status, the groups are married, cohabiting, single, widowed, divorced, separated. As was pointed out earlier, each of these coded groups will require a numeric value before it can be entered onto the computer, counted and analysed. For example, each of the following dichotomous response choices could be scored 0 and 1 respectively: true, false; died, survived; been an inpatient in past 12 months, not been an inpatient in past 12 months. Items with more than two response categories must be given a value for each point: for example, the categories of strongly agree, agree, disagree, strongly disagree could be allocated 4, 3, 2, 1 respectively.

The basis for defining groups for coding may be natural (e.g. sex, blood group), agreed by convention (e.g. *International Classification of Diseases*; World Health Organization 1992; Registrar General's Classification of Occupations (Britain) for social class and socio-economic grouping; Office of Population Censuses and Surveys 1980) or defined by the investigator for the purposes of the study. For standard socio-demographic data, the codes used for national datasets should be used, or be compatible with them, in order that the data can be compared with national data (in Britain, the codes should aim to be compatible with the codes used by the Office for National Statistics, which conducts the annual General Household Survey; see Foster *et al.* 1995). The advantage of conventional classifications (where they exist) over ad hoc coding schemes is that they enable the results of different studies to be compared.

It is wise to collect and code precise information where possible, as data can always be collapsed and recoded once on the computer if the range of codes used is too wide, resulting in some codes having few responses. For example, the investigator should collect exact age of first pregnancy rather than age group, such as under 25, 25–34, 35+. Wrong decisions based on the collection of grouped data at the data collection stage cannot be reversed at the analysis stage.

It helps to avoid coding errors if the numerical codes for commonly occurring items are consistent (e.g. for a single column code: yes = 1 and no = 0; don't know = 7; inadequate = 9; does not apply = 8). Although some coding frames do alternate 'no' replies between code 2 and code 0, this only serves to increase coding errors (coders like to learn the codes where possible and avoid consulting the code book for every question as they become familiar with the coding, so the investigator needs to aid their memory and hence accuracy). This explains why some health status questionnaires (e.g. the Short Form-36; Ware *et al.* 1993) carry the instruction to reverse/change some codes later on the computer – not at the hand-coding stage – in order to facilitate consistency with coding and avoid coder confusion and error.

Coding open questions

Open questions allow respondents to use their own words and form their own response categories. Responses must then be listed by the investigator after the data have been collected, then grouped by theme for the development of an appropriate coding frame (this can often be done on the basis of analysing a random sample of 30–50 questionnaires, and then testing the coding frame on further batches). Only then can coding take place.

Even with a largely structured questionnaire, with pre-coded response choices there is likely to be a need to list and develop a coding frame for the various 'other, please specify' or 'please state why . . .' ('safety net') response choices that were offered to respondents whose replies did not fit the codes given (see Box 15.1).

Examples of data obtained from open-ended questions in patients' self-administered questionnaires about their visit to specialists' clinics in general practice (Bowling *et al.* 1995b) are given in Box 15.4.

The expectations given by most of the patients in this study (about 400) were fairly similar, and a multiple response coding frame with numerical codes attached was easily developed for them (e.g. a diagnosis/labelling of problem = 1, cure = 2, treatment/surgery as cure = 3, procedure/surgery for investigation = 4, and so on).

Not all comments are as concise as these, and they often require more than one code ('multicodes') to ensure that all items mentioned have been accounted for. For example, at the end of the same questionnaire the patients were asked if they would like to make any other comments about their visit to the specialist's clinic, and many wrote a quarter to half a page of comments.

It can be seen in Box 15.5 that a range of issues emerged, each of which will require coding (e.g. patient's travelling time saved = 1, patient's travelling expenses reduced = 2, patient's travelling time increased = 3, patient's travelling expenses increased = 4, prefers familiar surroundings of GP's surgery = 5, GP's premises unsatisfactory = 6, and so on). The alternative to giving each possible response its own code is to code yes (mentioned) = 1 or no (not mentioned) = 0 in relation to each item for each respondent (allowing for an 'other' code for anything which does not fit the codes, though these should be few in number). In this case a coding box will need to be allocated for each item. In the former coding example, a smaller number of boxes could have been allowed because the (unique) codes could have been coded into any of the allotted boxes which would be labelled, for example, first comment, second comment, third comment, and so on. The investigator would need to ensure that enough boxes were included to allow for the maximum number of comments made per respondent (or make a rule: up to a maximum of six comments allowed for, although this results in loss of information). The decision is the investigator's, depending on how he or she wishes to analyse the data. One problem with the multiple response coding boxes is that the application of statistics is limited (the computer package can be instructed to add responses up across X categories (boxes) and produce a frequency listing by type of comment, for example, the MULT-response facility in SPSS – Statistical Package for the Social Sciences – but tests of differences cannot be applied to such tables), whereas, if each item is given the 'yes/no' code, and its own box, all types of non-parametric statistical manipulations are possible.

Box 15.4 Examples of responses to open-ended questions

What did you expect to happen as a result of seeing the specialist?

    'A diagnosis.'

    'Complete cure.'

    'A solution to my problems.'

    'I expected to be told exactly what the problem was.'

    'I thought he would put his finger on the root of the problem and advise treatment.'

    'I expected to be given an operation to find out what was wrong with me.'

    'I wanted the cyst removed which was causing a lot of pain.'

Box 15.5 Examples of 'other comments'

As I have no car and am on a low income I am very pleased with the new facility which suits my needs. It also means my daughter has less time off school when these visits are necessary. Previously we visited [hospital] which meant a 45-minute bus trip each way incurring an expensive fare and waiting a long time in a very hot hospital. I also feel it is good for a child to see the specialist in fairly well known surroundings.

The clinic was held in the basement of a GP's surgery and the waiting area was a small dark poky corridor. This was very unsuitable for young children and it would have proved very tedious with a 3-year-old if the wait had been longer than 20 minutes. It was not any more convenient to attend this surgery than to attend the local outpatient department. We were seen, however, by a consultant who works from [different district] and not our local X hospital, and our son will be operated on in [next district] which is at least 25 miles away from our home.

In some cases, investigators may simply choose to code the nature of the comments raised (e.g. positive = 1, negative = 2, mixed = 3) and use the quotations in illustration. This decision is entirely dependent on the importance of the question, the quality and importance of the information contained in the answers and personal preference.

Even if the coding is comprehensive, a human element is always added to research reports if people's comments can be included in illustration.

Coding closed questions

Closed questions require that any groupings should be defined before the data are collected. The response is then allocated to the pre-defined category, with a number assigned. The response is then itself an item of data ready for transfer to coding boxes, data entry and analysis (e.g. yes = 1 and no = 2). It is important at the design stage of the questionnaire to ensure that a recorded response is always requested. For example, if the questionnaire simply asks respondents to tick items that apply to them (as in the Sickness Impact Profile; Bergner *et al.* 1981), it will be unknown whether unticked items imply a 'no' response or whether the respondent forgot or declined to answer them.

It was pointed out earlier that some survey organisations give interviewers laptop computers and respondents' replies to closed questions are entered and automatically coded, ready for data processing back in the office. This requires the prior construction of the coding schedule (frame), and is possible only with highly structured surveys, where the subject is well known, as are the likely responses. It is more common for coding to be transferred or carried out in the office by hand. An instruction sheet for coders is usually designed (which may be on a coding frame) which clarifies any likely ambiguities and specifies how the coding is to be carried out.

Computers will generally be used to code data that are already in numerical form (e.g. age from date of birth, and coding into age groups after initial analyses of relevant cut-off points).

Checking returned questionnaires

As the questionnaires or other data collection forms are returned to the office, the investigator should check for missing data (interviewers can be asked to return to respondents to collect them, or they may need retraining if consistent errors are found) and ineligible writing. Fabricated data, while rare, should always be checked for at the coding and analysis stages. They may be revealed by checking for data sets that are too 'clean' or consistent.

Verification

Preferably two coders should be used to code the entire data set independently; the investigator should appoint an independent checker to check any discrepancies between the two sets of coding, correct any errors and reach agreement over any genuine differences in interpretation.

Human data entry and direct data entry systems

Programmed electronic *optical scanners* may be used to read the codes directly into the computer data entry program, and automatically produce the data files, though some require the data to be on optical scanning sheets (like the ones used in computer-graded multiple choice examinations in universities, which candidates complete directly with their responses). However, there is evidence that scanning methods in research have unacceptably high error rates. For example, survey staff at the Office of Population Censuses and Surveys (now ONS) found that 6 in 14 postal questionnaires had been incorrectly scanned (NHS Health Survey Advice Centre 1996).

As with the coding, the process of verification of office data entry involves two data entry persons independently entering the data, and the use of a computer program which can check for any differences in the two datasets, which then have to be resolved and corrected by a member of the research team.

Human coding (verified) and data entry, or direct data entry (e.g. with electronic versions of the questionnaire used with telephone interviews or face-to-face interviews with a laptop computer), are usually preferred. With the latter, the computer displays each question on the screen and prompts the interviewer to input the response directly, whereupon it is programmed to store it under the correct code. Computer-assisted direct data entry systems are programmable to prevent out-of-range codes being entered, and ensure consistency with data formats. Coded data ultimately form a data matrix stored in a computer file. Statistical software packages contain facilities for entering the data which can be read directly by that package, though many packages can translate data typed into other programs (e.g. word processing packages).

Creation of the system file

The computer package chosen for analysis will have a facility for the creation of a system file before the data can be entered. For example, the SPSS system file will require the labelling of all the variables and their response choices, the number of columns to be assigned to each and determination of which codes are to be assigned as missing in the analyses (e.g. 9s or blanks for inadequate responses and 8s for 'does not apply'). This should be done before the coding has been completed so that it is ready before the data entry is due to commence.

Cleaning the data

Once the data have been stored in computer-readable form (e.g. on disk), the next task is to eliminate the more obvious errors that will have occurred during the data collection, coding and input stages. An *edit* program will need to be specified. This should look at missing values, skips, range checks and checks for inconsistency. This will require a set of instructions for the computer package used that will automatically examine, and draw attention to, any record that appears to have an error in it (the package will require the investigator to specify the values that are acceptable for each variable). The 'dirty' item can then be checked against the original data sheet and corrected. In some cases it may be worth returning to the original data source (respondent, record, etc.) to check responses.

Range checks

For data fields containing information about a continuous variable (e.g. height), observations should fall within a specified range. Thus, if the height of an adult male falls outside the normal range it should be checked. For data fields containing information about a categorical variable (e.g. sex), observations should consist of valid code numbers. Thus, if the codes for sex are 1 = male, 2 = female and 9 = unknown, then code 3 would be invalid, and the data sheet or source should be re-examined. Most data entry packages automatically prevent out-of-range codes being entered – for example, if the computer package has been told that the only codes to a question are 1 (for 'yes') and 2 (for 'no'), then it will not permit any other digits (0, 3+) to be entered.

Consistency checks

Often certain combinations of within-range values of different variables are either logically impossible or very unlikely (e.g. height by weight is an obvious variable to check). Other obvious methods of checking for errors include checking ages of respondents by, for example, type of medical specialty treated (then any children treated in geriatric wards, elderly people in paediatric wards, men in gynaecology wards, etc. can be checked and corrected).

These checks will not eliminate all the errors introduced during the data collection, coding and data input (entry on to computer) phases. Mistakes may be made that do not result in out-of-range values or inconsistencies. There is no substitute for careful recording of data, coding, data entry and verification (e.g. standard professional practice is double coding and double data entry, and then the investigator checks any inconsistencies).

Checking for bias in the analyses

Response bias

As much information as possible should be collected about non-responders to research (e.g. age, sex, diagnosis, socio-economic group) in order that the differences between responders and non-responders to a research study can be analysed, and the extent of any resulting bias assessed. Two questions should be asked in order to check for response bias:

1 Are there any groups of people that have tended not to respond (e.g. males, younger people)?
2 If so, has this biased the results and affected their representativeness (e.g. are the non-responders likely to be different from the responders in relation to the variables under investigation)? This may be speculative, but there may be indications of differences in the results or in the existing literature.

In order to check for age bias, for example, the investigator should compare the age structure of the respondents with that of the non-responders, or that of the study population as a whole. Tests for statistically significant differences between the numbers and means obtained should be carried out.

Interviewer bias

Where more than one enumerator, interviewer or observer has been used, comparisons can be made between the data collected by each one. Where each data-gatherer covers a different set of people, differences in totals and distributions for each variable should be tabulated by each of them, and examined for bias.

Missing values and data checks

There are two types of missing values: first, where a question is deliberately blank because it did not apply to the individual respondent (the respondent legitimately skipped it and was 'routed' round it); second, where a reply was expected but not given, which is known as an 'inadequate' response.

It is customary to use default system missing values in statistical data packages where data are inadequate or missing (e.g. respondent did not reply or interviewer forgot to ask the question). An example is the 'SYSMIS' dots in SPSS (. or .. or .... depending on the column width of the variable), or the code 9 (or 99, 999 for double or triple column variables, and so on). In the case of the 9s being a legitimate coding value, for example, in the case of the variable age and a respondent who is aged 99, then a triple coding box should be used and the inadequate value is increased to 999 – a value that will not be a legitimate code (no one will be aged 999). Some investigators use 8 (or 88, 888, and so on) for questions which do not apply to the respondent (DNAs); for example, skips in the questionnaire will be employed so that men will not be asked about breast screening or cervical cytology. The inadequate (9s) and do not apply (8s) response codes are then set to missing on the computer (identified as missing values), so they are not routinely included in the analyses (but can be pulled back in if required for any reason). If these are not coded, any blank columns can simply be set to 'missing values' using the 'SYSMIS' procedure.

With SPSS the frequency counts show the missing values (and provide a set of percentages with them counted in and a second set of percentages with them counted out), though none of the other statistical analyses show them (they just give a total missing values count at the end of each table, which enables the researcher to check that the correct number of cases have been entered into the analysis). The investigator should always check the numbers of cases assigned as missing (8s and 9s) for each question and double check that question X was not asked to X cases to which it did not apply (which should equal the number of 8s). This is an essential part of the initial data cleaning exercise.

Missing values, whether due to office error or respondent item non-response, can lead to biased estimates (e.g. people who are anxious might be less inclined to respond to a question about their quality of life), are always problematic in analyses, and in estimates of the sample's representativeness. There are various techniques for addressing missing values in the analyses, to enables the data to be analysed (see Barladi and Enders 2010). Weighting adjustments are often used to compensate for incomplete coverage of populations and total non-response. Imputation methods that assign values for missing responses are used to compensate for item non-responses. Some investigators create dummy variables to code for missing observations, though there is the danger of bias.

The most common method for dealing with missing data, if it is minimal, is to exclude cases with missing data from analyses, using only complete data; assuming that data are missing at random, it leads to unbiased parameter estimates. However, this can considerably reduce the sample size. Some investigators substitute a mean for the missing data (e.g. if the respondents' quality of life item scores are missing, one could substitute the mean for the sample). While not influencing the sample mean, the increase in sample size does increase the denominator for calculating the standard error, thus reducing the standard error.

Other researchers use linear regression to model or predict what the missing score should be on the basis of other completed variables, with the advantage of using some data from the missing cases to make the estimate, rather than making full assumptions. However, the problem of error variance is still present and this method increases the sample size and reduces the standard error. In order to deal with the problem of increased noise due to imputation, Rubin (1987) developed a method for averaging the outcomes across multiple imputed data sets to account for this. Each imputed data set is analysed separately and the results are averaged except for the standard error (SE). The SE is constructed by the within variance of each data set as well as the variance between imputed items on each data set. These two variances are added together and the square root of them determines the SE, thus the noise due to the imputation, as well as the residual variance, are introduced to the regression model (Rubin 1987). This does not totally eliminate the problem, but it does reduce it. Advanced methods of multiple imputation have been developed (Azur et al. 2011). One example is known as multivariate imputation by chained equations (for an example, see Dale et al. 2013), though these methods have the disadvantages of being time-consuming to learn and to conduct, and one has to be very careful in assessing the validity of the results. See Box 15.6 in which Katz (1999) summarises various methods for various data.

Box 15.6 Katz on methods for estimating missing data

Katz (1999) summarised the various methods of estimating missing data:

- for cross-sectional data:
  - Assign the sample mean.
  - Assign the subgroup mean (conditional mean).
  - Model the value of the missing data by using other covariates in the analysis (simple imputation).
  - Model the value of the missing data by using the other covariates in the analysis and include a random component (multiple imputation).
- for longitudinal data with repeated measurements of the respondent:
  - Carry the last measured observation forward.
  - Model the missing observation based on serial values.
- in multivariable analysis:
  - Delete cases with any missing data.
  - Create dichotomous variables to represent missing data.
  - Try harder to obtain the missing data.
  - Decrease the number of independent variables in the analysis.
  - Estimate the values of missing data.

Computer packages for the analysis of quantitative data

The investigator must decide which computer package to use for the analyses. This is dependent on the type of data obtained and the analyses required (see Andrews *et al.* 1981). For straightforward analyses in health and social sciences, SPSS is probably the most popular (Norusis 1993). Epi Info is sometimes used in public health research (Dean *et al.* 1995). Hierarchical (multilevel or multilayered) data sets – data collected at different levels of society (e.g. patient, doctor, clinic, hospital; or individual within household, household) – are easier to analyse using multilevel analysis (Goldstein 1995; Rasbash and Woodhouse 1995). Packages which are appropriate for analysing complex longitudinal data, including survival analyses (analysis of time to event data), include STATA, BMDP, SAS and S-Plus (Hosmer and Lemeshow 1999); of these, STATA is increasingly used. A statistician should be consulted over the appropriate package for the data and planned analyses.

The analysis

Statistical tests for the analysis

The investigator should be clear from the outset of the research what the unit of measurement is, for example, numbers of patients or numbers of doctors' clinics. This information would have been needed for the initial power calculation and design of the study, as well as at the analysis stage. Also required at the outset is the level of the data collected (nominal, ordinal, interval, ratio), as this determines the type of statistical tests that are appropriate in the analysis of the data.

The investigator may wish to use univariate statistics (descriptive statistics for the analysis or description of one variable, e.g. frequency distributions, statistics of central tendency, dispersion, e.g. range), bivariate statistics (descriptive statistics for the analysis of the association between two variables, e.g. contingency tables, correlations, tests of differences between group means or proportions), or multivariable analyses (techniques which allow for the measurement of the effects of one variable on an outcome to be measured, while controlling for the effects of other variables, thus removing their effects, e.g. multiple regression, logistic regression). There are now several readable statistical textbooks which describe the range of tests available, the assumptions underlying their use and their appropriateness (e.g. Bland 1995; Katz 1999).

Stages in the analysis

Once the data have been cleaned, the investigator should produce descriptive statistics first, in order to be able to describe the findings and look at any skewness. The distributions will inform any required recoding of the data (e.g. age into age groups) and the variables which have a sufficient spread of responses for them to be analysed with bivariate statistics (e.g. contingency tables). The results of the bivariate analyses will inform the investigator whether multivariable analyses should be performed with any of the variables (e.g. multiple or logistic regression), depending on the type of data and the aims of the study. It is important to go through these initial stages in order to obtain a feel for the data and the findings. A surprisingly large amount of insight can often be obtained from analysing simple two-by-two contingency tables. It is increasingly common for investigators to launch straight into multivariate analysis and statistical modelling, and even more common for research publications to present only these, leaving both the investigator and the reader relatively ignorant about the basic characteristics of the data. It is also common to present the results of multivariate analysis inadequately (see Bender 1996). A statistician should always be consulted.

The data should be examined for patterns in the numbers: what is the trend in the data – does the trend go up, down, or is there no trend, is it reversed or is there no clear pattern?; what is the extent of any trends, changes or differences – e.g. proportional differences in disease incidence between groups, geographical areas, time periods? The nature of trends should be noted (are they steady, sharp rises or falls, erratic?), and absolute and relative differences. Ways of looking for patterns in tables, graphs, scatter plots, pie charts and histograms (bar charts) have been clearly described by McConway (1994b).

It should be restated that statisticians often argue that there is an over-emphasis on hypothesis testing and the use of P values in experimental and descriptive research, at the expense of focusing on the magnitude of differences and changes. Some statisticians even argue that significance tests should not be used at all in descriptive research. There is also heated controversy about the validity and appropriateness of one-tailed significance tests and of statistics for small samples (e.g. Fisher's exact test, Yates's continuity corrections for contingency tables using chi-square tests). As was emphasised earlier, investigators should consult a statistician about the appropriate approach to their analyses, ideally when the study is designed.

Critical analysis

The analysis will need to focus on what aspects of the data support or refute or cast doubt upon the original hypotheses of the study. The data should be analysed and presented critically, drawing attention to any weaknesses in the study design, the instruments of data collection and the sample (e.g. high sample non-response or item non-response). Alternative explanations for any associations reported should be considered, along with any potential extraneous variables which might have intervened and confounded the results.

Summary of main points

- Coding is a method of conceptualising research data and classifying them into meaningful and relevant categories. The number assigned to an observation is called the code.
- Data consist of observations of values for variables.
- Coding errors can be minimised by ensuring that the numerical codes for commonly occurring items are consistent.
- As questionnaires are returned to the office, routine checks should be made for missing data so that they can be obtained and entered where possible.
- Analyses of the characteristics of responders and non-responders, where basic data on the latter have been obtained, provide information on response bias.
- Analyses of the data by each interviewer used provide information on interviewer bias.

- The coding and data entry should be verified by another person.
- Checks in the analyses should be made for out-of-range values, consistency and missing values (data cleaning).
- After the data have been cleaned, investigators should produce descriptive statistics first, in order to become familiar with the data, and then decide what recoding is required and which cross-tabulations are worth carrying out.
- Decisions about multivariable analysis can be made after analysis of the bivariate data for trends and patterns.

Key questions

1 Distinguish between inductive and deductive coding.
2 What are the rules for coding quantitative data?
3 What are the steps in developing a coding frame?
4 Explain range and consistency checks.
5 How can fabricated data be detected at the coding and analysis stages?
6 How can response bias and interviewer bias be checked for in the analyses?

Key terms

bivariate
closed questions
codebook
coding
coding boxes
coding frame
coding transfer sheet
consistency checks
critical analysis
data cleaning
data entry
deductive coding
direct (electronic) data-entry
edit

electronic questionnaire
inductive coding
missing values
multicodes
multivariable
open questions
optical scanning
range checks
response bias
response errors
system file
unit of measurement
univariate
verification

Recommended reading

Fielding, J. (1993) Coding and managing data, in N. Gilbert (ed.) *Researching Social Life*. London: Sage.

Fowler, F.J. (2009) *Survey Research Methods*. Thousand Oaks, CA: Sage.

McConway, K. (1994) Analysing numerical data, in K. McConway (ed.) *Studying Health* *and Disease*. Buckingham: Open University Press.

Pallant, J. (2007) *SPSS Survival Manual: A Step by Step Guide to Data Analysis Using SPSS*, 3rd edn. Maidenhead: Open University Press.

Qualitative and mixed research methods

Introduction

The chapters in this section describe the main qualitative research methods, and also those which combine qualitative and quantitative approaches in a research study. Unstructured interviewing and focus group techniques are qualitative methods of data collection. Some methods, such as observational studies, can be carried out in either an unstructured or structured way, and may be combined in a single study. Other methods, such as case studies, consensus methods and action research, often use triangulated qualitative and quantitative approaches to data collection. Document research can involve the qualitative extraction of data from records (as in the analysis and presentation of narratives as evidence) or a highly structured and quantitative approach.

The distinction between qualitative and quantitative research can also be blurred at the analysis stage, as some investigators employ a variety of methods to interpret qualitative data (from highly structured content analyses using a computer software package to unstructured narrative analyses).

In social science, there is often an interplay between qualitative research observations and the development and refinement of the hypotheses, and consequently the categories to be used in the analysis. The categories for coding the data are often developed during and after the data collection phases, and this is therefore an inductive approach. It was pointed out earlier (see Chapter 6) that this is known as *grounded theory* (Glaser and Strauss 1967). One strength of qualitative methods is that the investigator is free to shift their focus as the data collection progresses – as long as the process does not become disorganised and lose its rigour. The preference for hypothesis generation rather than hypothesis testing should not be assigned too rigorously, as otherwise qualitative research will be restricted to speculation, and at some stage hypotheses will require testing (see Silverman 1993). Because of the interplay between the stages of qualitative research, and the tendency towards grounded theory, the design, methods and analysis of each qualitative method will be considered together in this section.

Qualitative research

Qualitative research is a method of naturalistic enquiry which is usually less obtrusive than quantitative investigations and does not manipulate a research setting. It aims to study people in their natural social settings and to collect naturally occurring data. It aims to understand the individual's view without making any value judgements during the data collection (an 'emic' perspective) (Carter and Henderson 2005). The focus is on the meanings that the participants in the study setting attach to their social world. Its strength is the ability to study people in the 'field', i.e. in their natural settings. Qualitative researchers acknowledge that there can be multiple interpretations of a situation or social realities. They aim to avoid the assumption that their own view is the predominant reality, and to interpret how people conceptualise the world in order to understand their actions. As social and health problems can have multiple causes, research investigating these utilises a wide range of methodological approaches, though frequently in isolation rather than embracing combined methods in a single research study. (See later sections on mixed methods and realistic evaluation.)

Qualitative research describes in words rather than numbers the qualities of social phenomena through observation (direct and unobtrusive or participative and reactive), unstructured interviews (or 'exploratory', 'in-depth', 'free-style' interviews, usually tape-recorded and then transcribed before analysis), diary methods, life histories (biography), group interviews and focus group techniques, analysis of historical and contemporary records, documents and cultural products (e.g. media, literature). Demonstrable advantages of qualitative research over quantitative methods have been shown in situations in which there is little pre-existing knowledge, the issues are sensitive or complex and the maximum opportunity for exploration and inductive hypothesis generation is desired.

The use of qualitative research methods in social sciences was relatively commonplace prior to the 1920s, after which survey research and statistical techniques of analysis began to advance. Critics attempted to counterbalance positivist approaches, rejecting the idea that knowledge is based on measurable observations of an objective reality, and developed frameworks of research rigour in qualitative research (Glaser and Strauss 1967; Denzin 1970). Qualitative methods are now popular in health (e.g. nursing) and social care research. There is also greater use of both qualitative and quantitative approaches within the same research study in order to collect more comprehensive data and wider understanding of the research problem. (See section on mixed and combined research methods/approaches later.) This has led to a blurring of the incompatibilities between the paradigms of qualitative and quantitative research approaches, and the development of a more pragmatic middle ground, seeking to avoid the earlier clashes between quantitative versus qualitative paradigms (Morgan 2007; Cresswell 2009; Moriarty 2010).

Moriarty (2010) summarised the theoretical and philosophical approaches that have influenced qualitative research, both of which emphasise the importance of language and interpretation, including:

- Interpretivism, emphasising people's interpretations of phenomena and situations, rather than 'reality'.
- Constructivism, based on the belief that human phenomena are socially constructed rather than objectively 'real'.
- Critical theory, as in critical discourse analysis, emerged from critical linguistics, which views language socially, and focuses on the ways social and political domination are reproduced in text and talk. Critical discourse analysts want to understand, expose and resist social inequalities.

■ Activism, which criticises the traditional division between researcher and research participants and aims to empower the latter in the research process.

Qualitative research methods have their theoretical origins in social, psychological and anthropological sciences, and philosophy. Moriarty (2010), following Snape and Spencer (2003), summarised the main, core characteristics of qualitative research, emphasising:

■ in-depth and interpretive approaches to understanding the participants' worlds;
■ small samples, possibly sampled using salient criteria;
■ data collection involving close, interactive and developmental research contacts between researcher and participants, enabling exploration of emerging themes;
■ production of rich, detailed, extensive and informative data;
■ analysis which is open to emerging concepts and ideas, producing detailed descriptions and classifications, leading to identification of patterns of association, or typologies and explanations;
■ outputs which focus on interpretations of social meaning through mapping and re-presentations of participants' worlds.

Qualitative research is the main method used by anthropologists in participant observations and/or qualitative interviewing of members of a culture (ethnography), and by social scientists whose approach is rooted in a phenomenological perspective. The latter argue that structured measurement scales and questionnaires are unsatisfactory, because it is unknown whether all the important domains are included and this method does not capture the subjectivity of human beings. Qualitative techniques have a wide range of applications in health care research. Qualitative research methods have been commonly used in research documenting the experience of chronic illness (Abel *et al.* 1993), and in the functioning of organisations, though they have been less frequently used in the assessment of outcomes of treatment. This is because the testing of causal hypotheses takes place in a context that subscribes to the traditional, positivist view of science, which requires adherence to the scientific method and uses experimental research designs and structured, standardised methods. While qualitative methods were not designed to test causal hypotheses, it is appropriate for the investigator to exercise curiosity and devise qualified hypotheses about cause-and-effect relationships in relation to the phenomenon observed (e.g. 'It is possible that . . .'). The qualitative investigator has the advantage of getting close to the research material, and can obtain a great deal of in-depth information that can be tested in subsequent quantitative studies if necessary and appropriate. Qualitative research can also enhance quantitative research by placing quantitative data in meaningful social contexts.

Rigour in qualitative research

Kirk and Miller (1986) distinguished between three types of reliability in relation to qualitative research: quixotic reliability, in which a single method yields consistent results (the authors used the term 'unvarying', which is not necessarily useful; see Silverman 1993); diachronic reliability, which is the stability of the observation over different time periods; and synchronic reliability, which is the similarity of the observations within the same period (e.g. using triangulated methods or more than one observer/interviewer per situation/case). In quantitative research these forms of reliability are tested by scales measuring internal consistency, test–retest and inter-rater reliability exercises (see Chapter 7). Not all qualitative researchers accept that they need to establish the credibility of their research results by using such methods. It is argued that if the existence of criteria against which knowledge can be measured is accepted, then the qualitative researcher's essential challenge to 'universal truth' must be rejected, and the epistemological underpinnings of qualitative methods are contradicted (Weaver and Atkinson 1994; Kelle and Laurie 1995; see Murphy et al. 1998).

There needs to be more recognition of the value of using triangulated research methods in order to enhance the validity of quantitative, as well as qualitative, research (Webb et al. 1966). (Also see Chapter 9, the section on triangulated methods, and Chapter 19 on mixed research methods.) Different methods should, in theory, yield comparable results in relation to the same topic and the same research setting. On the other hand, it is possible that inconsistencies may be found between the observed setting and people's accounts of the setting when interviewed. In this case, the methods should be used in a complementary fashion (i.e. to find out about people's differing perceptions of events that occurred in settings that were observed). The different perspectives of qualitative researchers towards the issue of validating their findings have been described in some detail by Murphy et al. (1998).

Reactive effects and research processes for research rigour

While the value of qualitative research is that it studies people in their natural settings and is arguably less reactive than quantitative methods, there is still a great deal of scope for reactive effects. For example, in observational studies, or in unstructured interviews where the investigator returns more than once to the respondents, there is potential for a Hawthorne effect as well as bias on the part of the investigator (leading to the recording of impressions and perceptions).

There are several other processes for ensuring that qualitative research is conducted in a rigorous manner. The researcher should be honest about his or her theoretical perspective and/or values at the outset, the research should be conducted in an explicit and systematic way in relation to the design, data collection, analysis and interpretation, and the investigator must aim to reduce sources of error and bias. Ideally, more than one investigator takes part and the independent reports of each can be analysed for their consistency (reliability). Meticulous records need to be kept about the research process and the investigator should keep a *separate* diary of his or her feelings and interpretations. In order to ensure rigour in research, the careful recording of the data throughout is essential. This refers not just to the field notes but also to other sources of data used (e.g. documents, tape recordings). If audiotapes or videotapes are used, then another member of the research team can independently categorise items as a check against bias and the intervention of perception. The aim is that another investigator should be able to analyse the data in the same way and reach the same conclusions. The categorisation of the data, as in coding quantitative data, is simply a method of assigning units of meaning to the material. It is important that the concepts and themes should be searched for and categorised in a systematic way. It is also important to avoid writing the research report based on the investigator's impressions.

Mays and Pope (1996) compiled a checklist for the assessment of rigour in qualitative research studies, which is included in Box V.1.

> ## Box V.1 Assessing rigour in qualitative research
>
> - Were the theoretical framework of the study and the methods used always explicit?
> - Was the context of the research clearly described?
> - Was the sampling strategy clearly described and justified?
> - Did the sampling include a diverse range of individuals and settings, if appropriate, in order to enhance the generalisability of the analysis?
> - Was the fieldwork clearly described in detail?
> - Were the procedures for analysis clearly described and justified?
> - Can the research material and the procedure for its analysis be inspected by an independent investigator?
> - Were triangulated methods used to test the validity of the data and analysis?
> - Were the analyses repeated by another researcher to test the reliability of the data and analysis?
> - Was enough of the raw data (e.g. transcripts of interviews) presented in a systematic fashion to convince the reader that the interpretation of the investigator was based on the evidence and is not impressionistic?
>
> (After Mays and Pope 1996)

Section contents

CHAPTER 16

Unstructured and structured observational studies

Chapter contents

Introduction

The casualty patients are attended in a new building, situated in Smithfield, at the north-east corner of the hospital property. It consists of a large, well-ventilated room, capable of seating about 600 persons. The males sit at one end, and the females at the other . . .

Four porters act under the curator of the surgery in maintaining order. The room has frequently been overcrowded. There is no exact record of the total daily attendances, the new cases only being entered in the registers . . .

It is estimated that not less than a thousand patients frequently attend on a Monday or Tuesday morning, of whom at least two thirds are medical . . . The medical consulting rooms are too small, they are very insufficiently ventilated and in summer the heat and unpleasant atmosphere are much complained of. There is scarcely sufficient room for the physician and one patient, and yet several are admitted at the same time . . . Should the physician of the former week desire to see any of the patients for whom he had prescribed, he is compelled to examine them in the public waiting-room; in fact, to a considerable extent, the work is done in public . . .

On the morning in question, 120 patients were seen and dismissed in an hour and ten minutes, or at the rate of 35 seconds each . . . The patients are entitled at least to decent examination and reasonable care. But they are dismissed with a doubtful dose of physic, ordered almost at random, and poured out of a huge brown jug, as if the main object were to get rid of a set of troublesome customers . . .

The social position of the out-patients . . . is for the most part that of the labouring and pauper classes . . . Now and then patients present themselves who appear to be unfit objects of charity . . . but . . . the discomfort of waiting in close association with a set of dirty people is, or ought to be, sufficiently deterrent to those who can afford to pay . . .

Whilst manifest improvements have been introduced elsewhere, Bartholomew's comparatively stands still . . .

(The *Lancet* investigation into the outpatient department of the London hospitals, *Lancet*, 1863)

Methods of careful observation, coupled with investigation, have long been used in western medicine, dating back to its foundations with Hippocrates of Cos (*c.*450–*c.*370 BC). As the above extract from the *Lancet* in 1863 illustrates, this was not confined to biological and clinical experiments. Indeed, systematic *observation* is the classic method of enquiry in natural science. It is also a mainstream method within the social sciences, particularly in organisational analysis (e.g. in the study of functioning of organisations (e.g. hospitals), and in the evaluation of new management and business processes). Social psychologists frequently include observation with their experimental designs. For example, multiple methods were used in Milgram's (1963) classic experiment of obedience, in which blinded research subjects (volunteers) were ordered to administer electric shocks to a victim with electrodes attached to his wrist (unblind research 'confederate'), increasing in intensity with each incorrect answer given by the victim during a word-pair learning exercise. The shocks were hoax shocks, unknown to the subjects. The duration and latency of the shocks were recorded by timing devices. The unblinded observers of the experiment watched the process through a two-way mirror, made recordings of the experiment, took photographs, made notes, and interviewed the subjects afterwards. Although the study would be ethically unacceptable today, it was a powerful method of illustrating the strength of the obedience tendencies shown (and the acceptance of the reality of the situation by subjects), despite subjects' distress at the pain they thought they were causing to the victim learner (the latter had been instructed to protest (e.g. by pounding on the wall) when 300 volts had been reached).

Observation is also a classic tool in its own right in both sociology and psychology. Goffman's (1961) classic work on institutions developed from his research as a participant observer (hospital porter) in a psychiatric institution. The study is rich in its description of routines in traditional, 'total' institutions and how they lead to individuals' depersonalisation, humiliation, loss of identity and autonomy, and could ultimately be psychologically destructive. He described how 'stripping' of self-identity was used to facilitate the uniform management of 'inmates'. Stripping included not only the loss of personal possessions and clothing, but also intrusions of privacy and submission to demeaning practices, for example, force feeding, being forced to eat with a spoon or a cup, having to ask for things like a drink of water or to go to the toilet; 'Often he is considered to be of insufficient ritual status to be given even minor greetings, let alone listened to.' Evidence that these practices still persist in long-stay institutions for older people was provided in the observational study by Clark and Bowling (1989, 1990). Observational studies on children's wards have also shown how a high wall of status separated the children from even the lowest grades of staff, resulting in degradation of the child patient (Holm and Smidt 1997). Such studies need to be carried out continually in order to increase awareness and maintain alertness about what it is like to be a patient and/or dependent on others for help.

Given their powerful influence when well conducted and analysed, it is surprising that observational methods are not used more frequently by contemporary social scientists who are surrounded by their subject matter (Moser and Kalton 1971). Their increasing rarity, particularly in the health field, is partly due to research funding priorities (towards quantitative research methods) and the increasing role and concerns of local district ethics committees. Moreover, the observations need to be systematic and the subject matter must be appropriate, which is not always possible in relation to social life.

While sociologists use mainly qualitative, unstructured observational techniques in natural settings, psychologists tend to use quantitative observational approaches, with structured coding schemes to record verbal and non-verbal communications and behaviours, in either natural or laboratory settings. However, there is often an overlap between the two approaches, with many investigators developing structured coding forms for recording routine data, along with unstructured, qualitative field notes and narratives. Even when the approach to data collection has been qualitative, many sociologists code their qualitative data and use content analysis for a more structured analysis, as well as presenting narrative accounts. Because of such overlap, each technique is included in this chapter.

Observation

Observation of behaviours, actions, activities and interactions is a tool for understanding *more* than what people say about (complex) situations, and can help to comprehend these complex situations more fully. It can be participative or non-participative, structured and quantitative (with a checklist, categories to check, rating scales) or unstructured and qualitative (direct recording of events and stories as they occur). It can be acknowledged and overt or concealed. As the setting for the observations is usually deliberately chosen by the investigator, the sampling technique is purposive. The settings are usually natural, but they can be laboratory settings, as in psychological research.

Qualitative observations are frequently referred to as ethnography. Ethnography is derived from anthropology and adheres to the philosophy of phenomenology. It is based on the need of the investigator to understand the 'symbolic world' of the group of interest (the meanings people develop about their experiences) and the study of behaviour in natural, as opposed to the experimental, laboratory settings of, for example, psychologists (N. Fielding 1993). It involves a triangulated approach to research: for example, using a combination of unstructured interviews and record research to supplement and validate the observations.

In social science, the definition of observation is not limited to 'watching' but extended to the *direct* gathering of information by the investigator using the senses, generally both sight and hearing. Observation is a research method in which the investigator systematically watches, listens to and records the phenomenon of interest. Observation does not depend on people being willing to be interviewed or the existence of accurate and complete documents. It does not depend on the memory or knowledge of interviewees, or their reporting of attitudes and behaviour – all of which can be the subject of bias. Observation has other limitations, however, such as observer bias, the reactive effects of the observer's presence and the impossibility of observing a large random sample of people, organisations or other units of study.

Participant observation

Participant observation is a qualitative observational technique which involves the observer (researcher) in the activities of the group being observed. Events are observed and recorded, together with the interpretation and explanation of them by the other 'actors' (participants). It is the best method for understanding the experiences of people, and the meanings they attach to them, though the types of observations are also limited by the social role undertaken by the observer. The method was developed first by anthropologists, but became a popular technique of social research in the early part of the twentieth century, in particular with the study of social deviance by social interactionists. Its history has been briefly described by May (1993).

Classic studies showing the valuable insights that can be obtained using participant observation include Goffman's (1961) study of the total institution, Becker *et al.*'s (1961) study of medical students, and Glaser and Strauss's (1965, 1968) research on dying. With careful attention to ethical safeguards, it has also been found to be a valuable tool when studying children and families, especially enabling observation of children exhibiting their affections, pleasures and dislikes to family members, and parents' normalisation of events – all findings which were missing in interview transcripts (Carnevale *et al.* 2008).

Concealed participant observation

The participant observer may be honest about his or her role in the group, or may conceal the investigation and pretend to be a normal member of the group (e.g. obtaining employment as a porter in a hospital and observing the social setting in which he or she is participating). Different approaches have been described by Patton (1990). Concealment does raise ethical questions in relation to the lack of informed consent. On the other hand, concealment is sometimes the only way to increase knowledge about society. (See Box 16.1.) For example, access to a maximum security prison will necessarily be as an employee (Fleisher 1989).

Box 16.1 Concealment in Rosenhan's study

One of the best-known examples is Rosenhan's (1973) participant observation study in the USA, in which the members of his research team feigned the characteristics and behaviour of people with a diagnosis of schizophrenia (e.g. 'hearing voices'). They acted as 'pseudo-patients' in order to gain entry to a psychiatric hospital for their observations. All but one of them were admitted with a diagnosis of schizophrenia. Once admitted, they stopped pretending they had any symptoms, but their diagnoses were not changed. One researcher's medical case notes contained the recording 'engages in writing behaviour'. Only the other patients appeared suspicious about the genuine status of the researchers as patients. Such research when concealed can also carry dangers: the research team has to find a way out of the situation (discharge in this case). Their study, although covert, was widely reported and highly regarded. It was used as evidence about the unreliability of psychiatric diagnoses and the consequences of labelling (see Chapter 3).

Concealment can also lead to a great deal of emotional stress on the part of the observer: the stress of not 'fitting in', of knowingly creating deception, of discovery, and even stress owing to the desire to abandon the research and properly join the group under study. Lofland and Lofland's (1995) answer to dealing with stress is to keep in contact with fellow researchers, with whom problems can be discussed and placed in context, and to keep a diary, which is essential to the research process as well as therapeutic.

Gaining access

Gaining access in overt observational studies

Observation and participant observation may be overt. Gaining access to the desired setting in overt observational studies is potentially a problematic area, but this is not necessarily so, especially if the observer's presence is legitimised by sponsorship of a credible organisation or by an introduction by someone within the setting or organisation (Pope 2005).

However, there may be suspicions about academics and their motives among local communities, as well as feelings of personal and professional threat. Time must be spent forging links with the community of interest before access can be expected, and explanations should be offered about how the study can be mutually advantageous (Hornsby-Smith 1993).

In overt observation, access is usually obtained through negotiations with a 'gatekeeper' (e.g. the head of an organisation). The first step is writing to the heads of organisations on official headed paper about the aims, nature and confidentiality of the study, and its potential value. The 'gatekeeper' may also be interested in the research data, and the investigator has to be honest about the raw data on individuals being confidential, while undertaking to provide the organisation with the research report. This permission is often given without consulting the members being studied, and the investigator needs to be aware of this, because the observations then become covert.

Gaining access in covert observational studies

If the study is to be covert (e.g. one of informal group behaviour), then the investigator has to become an accepted member of the group before the research can be undertaken. It has its own induction processes, as was discovered in one study of British Steel Corporation directors:

> The observer . . . has to enter the symbolic world of those he is to observe: he must learn their language, their customs, their work patterns, the way they eat and dress and make himself respectable. There is an initial period when he must understand what expectations are held of him and when he is taught how he can behave. But he also has to teach respondents so that he can carry out his observer role effectively.
>
> (Brannen 1987)

Lofland and Lofland (1995) emphasised the importance of trade-offs, or reciprocating favours, in gaining access and trust. They cited examples such as offering lifts, offering to make the tea or coffee, and so on. This is illustrated by Whyte's (1943) study, also cited by the former authors. (See Box 16.2.)

Box 16.2 Whyte and gaining acceptance in order to be an observer

Whyte's (1943) classic study of 'street corner society', also cited by the former authors, provides examples of the difficulties of gaining access; he eventually accepted help from a contact in a local settlement house. He recorded the following conversation between himself and his contact.

Observer: I want to see all that I can. I want to get as complete a picture of this community as possible.

Contact: Well, any nights you want to see anything, I'll take you around. I can take you to the joints – gambling joints – I can take you around to the street corners. Just remember that you're my friend. That's all they need to know. I know these places, and if you tell them you're my friend, nobody will bother you. You just tell me what you want to see and we'll arrange it.

Hardware: video- and audiotapes

Human observation has potential for being erratic, as the observer becomes familiar with, and responds to, the research setting. Selective auditory perception also operates to lead listeners to be most likely to 'hear' sounds that correspond to the sounds of their own language (Osgood 1953) or the language system of the observer. Neither random assignment of observers nor random time sampling for observations can reduce this type of selectivity and bias: hence the popularity in social science of using audio recordings in interview studies, which contain more material and are uncontaminated. The video recorder provides another dimension. There is a mass of available TV and radio material which has largely been ignored as a source of historical data worthy of analysis.

Research in the social sciences involving this hardware has tended to use hidden audio- and videotapes, as well as two-way mirrors, whereby people could be observed unnoticed (e.g. new students at freshers' parties were observed by the staff using two-way mirrors on my own degree course, in order to study the methods of social interaction of new students). Such unobtrusive methods would now be regarded as highly intrusive and unethical unless the people's prior consent has been obtained or they are set in highly public places (e.g. high streets, along with all the other security video cameras on which there are no legal constraints). Videotaping, as well as the use of two-way mirrors, has traditionally been of particular value in psychology research: for example, to study body language and eye movements (see Webb *et al.* 1966, for a review).

It is common for research involving in-depth interviews to audiotape interviews, with respondents' permission, and later transcribe and code the content, as well as extract narratives for their qualitative and rich insights. This is an expensive and time-consuming process, but it works well with complex subjects, and on subjects about which little is known. Respondents quickly forget the recorder is turned on and the reactive effects are believed to be minimal. However, many investigators believe in the technique of turning the recorder off at the end of the interview and continuing to 'chat' to respondents as a check on whether the respondent has anything else to add. These investigators are likely to be familiar with the request from respondents during interviews: 'Don't write this down, but . . . '.

One problem of using video cameras to study social phenomena is the high 'dross' rate (collection of a large amount of irrelevant data). To avoid this, some investigators step in and manipulate a situation, in order to record the reaction. The best-known public example of this was the classic television programme *Candid Camera*, in which the production team gave up simple observation and turned to introducing confederates who would behave in such a way as to direct attention to the topic of study and more quickly produce usable material. This is now a common method employed by the media (see Webb *et al.* 1966, for a review). These methods do have potential reactive effects (awareness of being studied). If a video camera is conspicuously sited it can potentially change behaviour. The ethics of this method, given that the person's prior consent is not obtained, has been largely unaddressed.

Video material is less commonly used for research material (except in media studies), partly because of potential reactive effects and partly on ethical grounds: used in public places, there may be ethical objections if people have not had the opportunity to consent; used in personal situations, video cameras would probably be seen as intrusive. However, they have been successfully used in documentary analysis and people tend to get used to the camera (as they do to audiotapes and observers) and behave as normal. Videotape recordings can be transcribed and categorised, using content analysis of behaviour, interactions, and so on, although this is more complex than with audiotapes.

Establishing validity and reliability

Reducing observer bias

The *rigour* required of qualitative research means that attempts must be made to reduce bias and errors throughout the research process. Observer bias is a systematic difference between a true situation and that observed owing to observer variation in perceptions (i.e. interpretation). Observation requires accuracy in perception of detail, and careful training and rehearsal in order to reduce the tendency to report interpreted (perceived and inferred) events, rather than the events themselves. Participant observers need to be careful that their involvement in the research setting does not restrict their perception or understanding of it.

Methods to test for observer bias involve inter-observer comparisons. There are always problems with the potential for bias and the recordings of perceptions rather than events, though ideally the use of two observers per situation, where possible, can help to overcome this. Training in recording observations as objectively as possible is essential (making repeated comparisons of observations between pairs of observers until their accounts are similar). The results of the comparisons will not be in the form of statistical coefficients of concordance but of discussion of the observations made. Ideally, the investigator should observe unfamiliar social settings and interactions, as he or she is then less likely to ignore or take activities for granted.

Reducing reactive effects

The other real potential for bias in observation studies is owing to the reactive effect of the research arrangements – the Hawthorne effect, where people change in some way simply as a result of being studied (Roethlisberger and Dickson 1939). The effect of the observer appears to erode over time (Clark and Bowling 1990); thus it is arguable that the analysis of observation data should commence after a time period when the reactive effect of the observer has worn off. However well integrated the observer becomes within the setting, there is always potential for a reactive effect and therefore bias. It is important that the observer maintains an awareness of this.

One source of ethical concern owing to the need to minimise reactive effects is responding to urgent needs. For example, if one is observing a hospital ward and a patient falls over, should one go and assist the patient, or reduce reactive effects and simply record the whole process? The latter could be regarded as unethical in human terms but it is the correct procedure in research terms. It poses a dilemma for the observer that is not always easily resolved.

Representativeness of the observations

It is important for the observer to spend as much time as possible in natural observational settings, and to include different days and times to ensure that the data are comprehensive and to enhance their validity and reliability. It is essential to know how typical the events and interactions observed are. As pointed out above, it is also important to spend enough time in the research setting to overcome the reactive effects of the observer's presence and his or her biases and assumptions.

Observation and triangulated methods

Ideally, observational methods should be part of a triangulated research methodology (use of three or more methods), so that observed events, behaviours and attitudes can be verified by independent sources (e.g. records or interviews). Objective observations are impossible to achieve, but the observer is still required to convince others that his or her accounts are credible and not mere subjective perception. If more than one observer is used, their accounts can be compared, but this still does not indicate the extent to which the recorded observations are accurate from the point of view of those being observed. It is possible that the investigator can use independent, multiple research methods (e.g. validate observations using interview methods), and checks against these can establish some evidence of congruence and internal consistency. Naturalistic investigators believe that contamination of the results through the presence of the observer in the setting being observed and subjectivity of interpretation is inevitable. Thus, they focus on the 'confirmability' of the data from different sources.

Social interactionists would argue that this positivist approach to validity and reliability misses the point of their method. They would argue that validity is confirmed when the observer learns the social norms and rules of the group being observed, and can successfully relate these to others who could also 'pass' in the same setting (Hughes 1976). These perspectives have been discussed more fully by N. Fielding (1993).

Structured observations: what to record

The prior definition of phenomena to observe, the preparation of structured observation schedules and the use of techniques such as time sampling operate within a quantitative, deductive approach to research. The researcher has begun with a conceptual definition, specified what is to be observed and standardised with a validated measuring instrument, and then proceeds to make the observations in order to test the theory.

Observation is a difficult technique, given that observational schedules are rarely transferable across studies and settings. Unlike in survey research where existing questionnaires can often be used, in observational research the investigator usually has to start from the beginning and assess the situation, carrying out extensive piloting in an attempt to discover which aspects of observation are countable and codeable and which aspects demand narrative descriptions.

The first decision with observational research is to decide what to observe and the clear definition of all variables of interest. The decision should be based on theory, and the observation schedule should be restricted to the phenomena of interest or the task will become unmanageable. The observer should keep separate notes (memos or a diary) about additional information, rather than rely on retrospective memory later on at the analysis stage.

Erlandson *et al.* (1993) pointed out that much is to be gained by looking, listening, feeling and smelling, rather than simply talking. They emphasised the value of recording any critical incidents (specific events in the social context being studied that reflect 'critically' on the operation of that context) on index cards (each on a separate card). The incident should identify the people, location and time; it should be verifiable by more than

---

Box 16.3 Structuring observations

- The setting. What is the physical environment like? What is the context? What kinds of behaviour are promoted or prevented?
- The participants. Describe who is in the setting, how many people and their roles. What brings them together and who is allowed there?
- Activities and interactions. What is going on? Is there a definable sequence of activities? How do people relate to the activity and relate to, and interact with, each other?
- Frequency and duration. When did the situation being observed begin? How long does it last? Is it recurring and, if so, how often, or is it unique? How typical of such situations is it?
- Subtle factors. Informal and unplanned activities; symbolic and connotative meanings of words; non-verbal communication (e.g. dress, space); unreactive indicators such as physical clues; what does not happen but should?

(Merriam 1988)

---

one source; it should help to define the operation of the organisation being observed. Erlandson *et al.* used this technique themselves in observational studies, together with a log which forms a record of what is happening to the observer. They also cited Merriam's (1988) observational checklist as a guide on how to structure observations, which is presented in Box 16.3.

Other items that should be recorded are objects (buildings, furniture, equipment, and so on), the purposes of the activities and events observed, and feelings displayed in relation to people, events and activities (Stringer 1996).

Fennell *et al.* (1994) give several examples of Lipman's (1967) non-participation observational study of residential care homes. This is illuminating as he included detailed sketches of seating, and logbooks of who was in the room and chair occupancy. With his system, a figure of 100 per cent by a chair in the lounge indicated that it was always occupied by the same person – as opposed to low frequency values by a chair, indicating that it did not 'belong' to anyone. It is an insightful study of the symbolic attachment to, and possession of, chairs in such settings, in contrast to the philosophy of residential care of 'free seating', for example:

> Once Mrs M, a small and frail woman of 90, found the contentious chair No. 25 occupied by Mrs. A . . . Mrs M demanded . . . that the chair be vacated. Mrs A refused, claiming the chair was hers. After some argument, Mrs M lifted her walking stick and began beating Mrs A about the head and shoulders . . . .
> (1967, p. 566)

The observer should develop a *system* for recording observations. The field notes in observational studies need to include descriptions and accounts of people, tasks, events, behaviour and conversation. They should be restricted to what is being observed. The field notes are the log of the phenomenon being observed; they form the continuous description of the setting and its people, relationships, hierarchies, interactions, roles, rules, actions, events, conversations, and so on. It is usually helpful to draw maps of the setting, indicating layout, people present and their movements. The recordings should be organised by time and kept in chronological order. Raw behaviour should be recorded, not just the observer's interpretation of the meaning of the behaviour. The observer also needs to use a system of shorthand codes for recording routine phenomena (e.g. double quotation marks are used to denote verbatim quotes; single quotation marks are used for paraphrases; parentheses are for contextual information or the investigator's interpretations; a solid line is used to partition time periods) (Kirk and Miller 1986; Silverman 1993).

At the end of each observational session, the observer should write the field notes up in full (and not permit a gap of more than a day or memory bias will begin to take effect and distort or delete any events the observer did not have time to record, the meaning of additional shorthand, and so on). Both the actual field notes and the full transcription made afterwards should be kept and made available for inspection by others in order to satisfy queries about the reliability of the material. The observer should also record separately in a diary – either manually or dictated on to an audiotape – his or her feelings (e.g. anxiety, embarrassment, excitement) and impressions about the situation, and any points about how the observational period went (this is where ideas and interpretations can be recorded, not with the field data). This requires discipline and time. During the observations and writing up of field notes, ideas for analysis will begin to occur. They should all be recorded in the diary that should be maintained for each day's fieldwork.

Lofland and Lofland (1995, pp. 89–96) described in detail the types of field notes to take. They emphasised that the process of observation for most naturalistic researchers involves a sequence of making mental notes, jotted notes, then full field notes. These are private documents, and they require one to be disciplined and to allow enough time:

- *Mental notes:* The aim of mental notes is to orientate oneself, and aid memory. Loffland and Lofland described it as 'directing your mind to remember things at a later point . . . preparing yourself to be able later to put down on paper what you are now seeing' (1995, p. 90). It is useful to carry small (paper format) notebooks for this purpose, as jotting down handwritten notes is likely to be quicker than typing into portable electronic notebooks.
- *Jotted notes:* These include, for example, phrases, quotations, and key words that are noted inconspicuously during observations. Their function is to jog memory when field notes are written up. These can include jogged memories as current observations bring back a memory of events on past observational sessions that were omitted in error from the field notes.
- *Full field notes:* At the end of each observation day or period, all mental notes and jotted notes need to be converted promptly (i.e. within hours) into a log of observations, before memory starts to fail and recall bias comes into play. Memory will start to fade by waiting even a day. Some investigators talk into digital audio recorders instead of jotting down mental notes, sometimes coupled with obtrusive video recordings. All notes, whatever the format, still have to be transcribed, which is a time-consuming process, especially in the case of the latter. Lofland and Lofland (1995, pp. 93–5) described the main contents of field notes as running descriptions of events, people, overheard conversations, interactions; changes in settings or people; drawn maps of layout and people. Jogged memories can also be included. These all need to be organised chronologically, with dates and times noted. At this stage, analytical ideas should begin to emerge – all should be written down (e.g.

in brackets), even if they seem trivial. Field notes are also used for recording one's impressions and feelings of the people, interactions and settings under observation, and possible influences on these feelings (e.g. one's personal emotional state, including feelings of embarrassment and why). The latter can help to identify any personal biases later on.

Time sampling

An observational schedule based on time sampling can be helpful – it involves the selection of observational units at different points in time. This helps the researcher to structure the observations over time to ensure representation of time and day of the week, and can be helpful in the analyses. For example, one could make random 15-minute observations at different times of day on each day of the week. Or one could select a different person to observe every hour, and so on. A structured observational schedule, perhaps organised by day and time period, with spaces for ticking off pre-coded activities and behaviours, will help to structure the observations and also be easier to analyse. It does not prevent the use of freehand observational notes on separate sheets. (See Box 16.4.)

Box 16.4 A study using time sampling of GP consultations

Observation methods were used in early studies of GPs' workloads. For example, Buchan and Richardson (1973) observed 23 doctors conducting over 2000 consultations. They recorded face-to-face consultation times by patients' condition and social class of patient, length of time doctors took to perform examinations of the patient by type, and the proportion of the consultation time spent on medical history-taking, examination, reading and writing by type (e.g. sickness certificates).

Recording observed (non-verbal) body language

There is a wide range of quantitative and obtrusive laboratory techniques for recording and coding non-verbal behaviour physiologically (e.g. changes in electrical skin conductance, as in sweating, the electrical activity of the brain, heart rate, blood pressure, pupil size and changes, and so on) (see Rozensky and Honor 1982; Scherer and Ekman 1982; Siegman and Feldstein 1987). In addition, a number of standard notation and coding systems have been developed by psychologists for coding observational data. The recording of non-verbal (e.g. eye contact, gestures, use of hands, body posture, blushing) and spatial behaviour (movements towards and away from others, movements to maintain distance or closeness) also needs to be decided on, and the aspects of this carefully defined. There have been many studies of these behaviours by social psychologists, increasingly with the use of video recorders, though traditionally two-way mirrors were used to observe unsuspecting people.

Recording systems have been developed for body motion in research settings (Birdwhistell 1970), and anthropology has a system of notation for recording posture, touching behaviours, voice volume and other characteristics (Hall 1965). Some medical specialties (e.g. neurology) and specialists in physical education have borrowed methods of notating movement from dance notation (Causley 1967). Non-verbal facial behaviour can be categorised and analysed with a coding scheme called the Facial Action Coding System (FACS), which can identify and code over 7000 different combinations of facial actions (Ekman and Friesen 1978).

Unstructured observations

In contrast to the deductive method, a qualitative and inductive approach will begin with the observations, and postpone definitions and structures until a pattern has been observed. Much qualitative research, particularly observational research, adopts a *grounded theory* approach (Glaser and Strauss 1967). The researcher develops the conceptual categories *from* the data and then continues with the fieldwork in order to elaborate these, while the data are still available for access. The researcher works to fit the theory to the data by checking in the field as the research proceeds. This process has been described by Erlandson *et al.* (1993). While a deductive approach carries the risk of losing the richness of observational research and the spontaneity of the research situation which should lead to insights, an inductive approach carries the risk of ending up with masses of unstructured notes which are difficult to organise and analyse. Often, a combination of approaches will be helpful, beginning with just observing the social setting of interest until the setting reveals which aspects are of interest, what is appropriate for coding and ticking on a structured schedule and what is best left to observational notes.

Recording the research data in the field can be problematic in participant, as well as some non-participant observation, with observers often resorting to discreet, hastily scribbled notes at inconspicuous times, or a facility for making mental notes and transcribing these to paper during frequent trips to the toilet. Note-taking is easier in covert observation, though there can still be an element of disruption if group members being observed see the observer sitting in the corner making copious notes about them. These can all lead to reactive effects, which, along with memory bias and recordings which appear incomplete or confused, can impair the reliability and validity of the research data. Pope (2005) described the practicalities of making field notes in hospital settings:

> It is not always appropriate to take notes contemporaneously – conversations over lunch, or when walking to a meeting, may have to be remembered and written down later. Sometimes it is necessary to focus on the action without writing. Like others before me, I found that toilet breaks provided an excellent opportunity to quickly write notes, especially if privacy was required. My jottings, which run to many notebooks, are embarrassingly scruffy, consisting of fairly untidy writing, hasty sketches, and idiosyncratic abbreviations and shorthand . . . I aim to write up these notes – even if only in neat longhand – on the same day and to type them as soon as possible as field notes . . . Field notes . . . provide the raw material for the analysis. My own notes can be characterised . . . as realist. I try to document the minutiae of life in the setting and offer a single reading or version of events.

As with structured observations, the observer should also develop a system of shorthand codes for recording routine phenomena, and record his or her feelings about the situation at the end of each observational period.

Combining structured and unstructured recordings

Observational data can be collected and analysed using a combination of methods: for example, coded events and illustrative narratives. An example of this combined method is the observational study of the quality of life in nursing homes and hospital wards for elderly people by Clark and Bowling (1989, 1990). They developed an observational schedule that recorded codeable events and made qualitative recordings of observations. Two observers recorded situations until their accounts were consistent during the piloting. The observers simply recorded everything they saw and then analysed the accounts in order to develop the codeable section of the observation schedule. This consisted of objective events such as contacts between patients, between patients and visitors and between patients and staff (by type of staff), staff responses to requests from patients to be given a drink of water and to be taken to the toilet (these responses were also timed), number of falls and types of activities. Interactions were also recorded, such as whether communications between staff and patients consisted of requests, comments only or conversations of more than one sentence, and whether the content was positive, negative or neutral. The last inevitably required more subjective assessment on the part of the observer, as did a further category of observations: whether the patient looked happy, unhappy or neutral, and whether he or she looked engaged, disengaged or neutral. The investigators defined each of these descriptions carefully. Comparisons of the observations of the two observers at the outset revealed that while 'positive' and 'negative' categorisations coincided, discrepancies arose over the categories 'neutral' and 'other'. These more subjective observations require the presence of at least two observers in order that reliability checks can be carried out.

The schedule was eventually divided into 15-minute intervals for recording (in order to provide a time reference for observations), with the structured codes across the top and a space at the side for free descriptive recordings of what was happening. There was also a space for diagrammatic representation of where labelled patients were sitting in relation to each other, and a space for recording every 15 minutes the number of patients, staff and visitors present. Such a complex observational exercise is only possible if several observers are used or the setting under observation is relatively inactive (as was the case in institutions caring for elderly people).

This method led to the collection of valuable data on the processes of care, which were not collectable by any other method, and to rich descriptive data on quality of life. The wider evaluation study, which was based on a randomised controlled trial (RCT), had found no significant differences between patients in geriatric wards and small, purpose-built nursing homes in relation to life satisfaction and satisfaction with care (partly owing to elderly people's reluctance to be critical of health care). However, the observational data revealed clear differences between settings, and the structured observational data (e.g. content analysis counting negative and positive interactions, choice offered at mealtimes, disengagement, professionals' responses to requests for help and number of minutes taken to respond, existence and type of entertainment and activities) were clearly supported by the narratives (see Box 16.5), which showed the quality of life to be poorer in the hospital setting.

Box 16.5 Examples of narrative recordings

The narrative recordings from Clark and Bowling (1989, 1990) clearly illustrate the value of narrative recordings of observations in illustration of categorised analyses.

> The domestic comes in and hands tea out . . . Clara does not want her tea so the nurse forces her to drink it. Clara is fighting against this. The nurse then holds her hands and forces her head up threatening 'I'll throw you out of the window if you don't drink it' . . . . The nurse goes out and returns with milk in a beaker and tells her she has brought her a cold drink as she doesn't want tea. Clara, who is always reluctant to eat or drink and used to be fed with a syringe, does not look happy about this. She is forced to drink it while the nurse holds her hands down. The main problem was that she did not appear to be able to breathe. The feeding took 9 min. and in that time she was given only three breaks for breath. (Hospital ward)

> [At lunch time] Mary is watching one of the patients who does not like being force fed with a beaker of Complan. She says angrily to Jane, 'It's no good them force feeding them because it doesn't do them any good. It gives them indigestion and makes them unhappy. It's no good at all.' [Thirty min. later] The domestic is in a hurry to clear up the dishes; she says, 'I'm on my own.' She removes Daisy's and Jane's sweets before they have finished. She actually removed the spoon from Daisy's hand, and Jane had not even started on her sweet. (Hospital ward)

> A nurse helps Sara into the room and says, 'Coffee is over, you've missed it. Would you like a cup of coffee?' Sara says, 'Yes.' The nurse goes to the kitchen and returns with a cup of coffee for her . . . Sara smiles and says, 'Thank you' . . . Harriet is reading. The nurse notices and asks, 'Would you like the light on? It's a bit dark because of the bad weather.' Harriet says, 'Yes' and the nurse turns on the light . . . Another nurse helps in Maud. Edith and Amy say, 'Hello' to her. Edith asks her if she has had her breakfast. Maud says, 'Yes.' Catherine sees me and says, 'Good morning. I've just had a bath. I like having a bath.' She has a broad smile on her face . . . (Nursing home)

(Clark and Bowling 1989, 1990)

Theoretical analysis of observational data

The concepts and themes selected for analysis will depend on the aim of the study and the theoretical perspective of the observer, as well as the material collected. Feldman (1995) described four techniques of analysis used by social scientists, which are based on theories of ethnomethodology, semiotics, dramaturgy and deconstruction. They are summarised below.

Conversation analysis focuses on talk in social interactions, and discourse analysis analyses all types of verbal and textual material. Conversation analysis, which is associated with ethnomethodology, treats all talk as social action, basing analyses on naturally occurring situations and conversational interactions. It aims to study responses, including silences and speech fillers ('ums and errs') in order to understand the situation. (Also see the section on conversation sampling.) Ethnomethodologists search for the *processes* by which people make sense of interactions, events and society. They believe that the meanings and symbols ascribed to these phenomena form the basis for their future behaviour and interpretations. The focus is on *how* sense is made of situations, rather than *what* sense is made. The approach is based on the assumption that actions and interactions have social meanings for participants and that people assume that others share the same meanings, and will actively seek to maintain this shared knowledge. Garfinkel (1967) undertook research demonstrating these shared meanings and documented how people became upset when understandings were not shared (see Garfinkel 1967, pp. 38–44, 75):

(S) 'How are you?'

(E) 'How am I in regard to what? My health, my finances, my school work, my peace of mind, my . . . ?'

(S) (Red in the face and suddenly out of control) 'Look! I was just trying to be polite. Frankly, I don't give a damn how you are.'

Garfinkel rejected the positivist theory that people are governed by rules, and argued that interpretation and behaviour are specific to the context and its meaning. A weakness of the method is that the introduction of audio- and or video-recordings into the social setting is 'unnatural' and has the potential to change it, as well as being time-consuming to analyse.

Ethnographic research, while always open to criticisms of potential observer bias, has also offered insights into health and social care settings. For example, Scourfield and Pithouse (2006) examined the use of lay and professional knowledge in child protection services, and showed that social workers' knowledge about the topic was influenced by gendered lay ideas as well as professional knowledge.

Semiotics, dramaturgy and deconstructionism are highly specialised techniques for analysing observational data, and are outlined briefly. A semiotician focuses on the rules for combining elements of speech and attempts to understand the processes by which meaning is attached to language. For example, the term 'buildings' can have several adjectives (competing meanings) attached to it (physical structure, residence, community), several connotative meanings (institutions, homes, neighbourhoods) and several institutional concerns (e.g. from legitimation of organisational role to location of power and control). The textual context is considered as a whole, as the elements of speech derive their meanings from their relationship with other elements (see analyses of documents in Chapter 19).

A dramaturgist focuses on the roles people are in and their strategies for producing desired effects; he or she is looking for a performance, and the categories include scenes, actions, roles, actors, meanings and motives. The technique is usually used in studies of organisational rituals, but can also be used to analyse individual roles (e.g. parent).

A deconstructionist is searching for the multiple meanings implicit in texts, speeches, conversations or events. He or she looks for the dominant ideology and the alternatives that could be used to interpret the material. For example, disruptions (e.g. a joke) reveal the possibility of other meanings being ascribed to a situation. These investigators look for what is *not* said, silences and gaps, as the written or verbal exchange is seen as a partial representation of what is actually happening.

These theories and processes are too complex to be described in a general text, and interested readers are referred to Feldman (1995).

Categorisation of observational data

More generally, observers also have to balance the need for their analysis to be coherent and to revolve around identified themes against the selective (biased) use of materials, so that the observations do not appear to fit too neatly into the analytical framework selected. The rule is to work from the data and not from a theory, with a sift through the data to find fragments that appear to fit it.

The categorisation of the data may be basic for profiles (e.g. number of people, groups, meetings observed) or analytic. The analysis of the data is dependent on the themes identified during the fieldwork. For example, Becker and Geer (1982), in their observational study of a medical school, prepared their data for analysis by coding them into separate incidents, and summarised medical students' actions for each incident. They tentatively identified major themes and categories during their fieldwork stage and marked these with a classification number which represented the code number of the theme or category to be used in the analysis. Whyte (1943), in his classic observational study of street-corner society, began to consider the analysis during the data collection period, and attempted to facilitate the process at first by storing all his observational field notes in strict chronological order. He later decided that this was unhelpful, as he needed to sub-divide his notes into themes and categories. He then set about physically sorting his notes into separate piles representing the different social groups studied, rejecting the alternative sorting system of classifying the material by topic (politics, family, church, and so on). He recounted the difficulties of doing this without knowing, at that time, what the relevant topics for analysis would be. His honesty is insightful and demonstrates the need to have a coding system in the margins of field notes in order to be able to cross-reference with notes classified differently: observations can fit into more than one category and thus flexibility must be inherent in the classification system used. This process is now facilitated by computer programs for qualitative data (see below).

It was pointed out earlier that the process of analysis with observational data is to transcribe fully the field notes after each observational period (in order to minimise recall bias) if it was not possible during the observational period, to search for common themes and to categorise them. It is important to ensure that the categorisation and resulting analysis are conducted rigorously, and do not appear anecdotal; they should address coherent themes. The categorisation should also be carried out in a standard way so that an independent investigator would be able to categorise the data in the same way.

If a systematic and rigorous approach to the analysis of the data is undertaken, the data should be read in order to select key themes that emerge from them, and then the entire dataset should be categorised (i.e. indexed) in relation to these themes. It can also be categorised in relation to theoretical ideas. If categorisation is decided upon, computer software is available which allows the entry of transcripts from observational or in-depth interview material, and its indexing by theme and subsequent analysis (for advice, see Weitzman and Miles 1995). Pfaffenberger (1988) and J. Fielding (1993) have described the coding process for qualitative data and suggest various steps to be taken in the process (see Chapter 17 for examples of computer software and the analysis of in-depth interviews).

The traditional rule of mutual exclusivity for coding applies only to quantitative data. With qualitative data, the multiple coding of single items is permissible, as well as often being necessary, for *analytic* coding (Lofland and Lofland 1995). Analytic coding requires multiple coding which can be cross-referenced for conceptual and theoretical development.

With qualitative data, the development of categories is experimental at first. Becker (1971) suggested that *sequential analysis* should be carried out with the data, in which the data are continually checked against the interpretation until the investigator is satisfied that the meaning is correct. The investigator should review the frequency with which categories have been applied to the data, reject those that are rarely applied (unless this is important for the analysis) and focus on the more frequent categories. It may be necessary to elaborate on the last and to collapse codes. Some observational studies will involve frequency counts of very basic data (number of people at social gatherings, number of times social groups meet, and so on). Others will involve more sophisticated counts (number of utterances, conversations, and so on).

Some social scientists argue that the categorised data then lose their dynamic and spontaneous quality. Interactionists would also argue that this process distorts the nature of the social situation. The data are no longer purely qualitative. Given that observations cannot be 100 per cent complete, it could be argued that this categorisation process confers a false scientific respectability on the data and that only the raw qualitative data should be presented, analysed and interpreted. Content analysis is described further in the next two chapters in relation to in-depth interviewing and document analyses.

Narratives

The practice of rigour does not prevent the data from also being presented qualitatively in narrative format (i.e. in full transcript in illustration). Transcripts should be used to illustrate situations, and also be subjected to content analyses and used to support theoretical interpretations. Clark and Bowling's (1989, 1990) observational narratives (see Box 16.5) were used in illustration of life in institutional settings, and in illustration of the structured observational data collected. For example, the unit of analysis in the structured observations was the number of observational sessions (analysed in sub-units of 15 minutes each), and totals were calculated in relation to the number (and proportion) of sessions in which patients were involved in recreation, drinking, verbal and non-verbal interaction with others, sitting doing nothing, and so on. The structured and unstructured data were interpreted in relation to Goffman's (1961) theory of institutions, which emphasised the dehumanising and demeaning nature of institutional routines.

For example, many interactions could be interpreted as demeaning practices (e.g. stripping of self-identity, which Goffman (1961) described as a mechanism to facilitate the uniform management of people in institutions). These included staff forgetting patients' names, ignoring needs to help, restraining patients, force feeding, supplying all patients with plastic cups and beakers with spouts, and spoons rather than cutlery at meal times, regardless of need, and removal of cutlery and food from patients before they had finished their meals. Observed summaries of these practices, to illustrate this, included the examples in Box 16.6.

Box 16.6 Further examples of narrative recordings

> Two nurses are feeding the patients. Sweet is served . . . Everything has been served by the nurses in relative silence . . . (15 minutes later) Rose tries to get up from her wheelchair. The nurses see her and persuade her to walk over to the armchairs to sit down – this is her restraining chair (a chair with a tray fastened to the front). She goes over and sits, but when she realises they are going to fasten her in she starts screaming and becomes hysterical. She fights and kicks the nurses. (30 min. later) . . . Rose is still crying and banging on her table which is restraining her . . . Rose's banging is getting on the other patients' nerves. They shout, 'Pack it in'. She bangs with more force . . . (Hospital ward)

This observational study showed the value of using both structured logs and narrative recordings, and which consistently supported and illustrated the findings of each. Analysis of the structured logs showed that there were no positive patient–nurse interactions in the ward setting, and that most of the comments between patients on the ward were negative. The logs also showed that a third of lucid patients' requests for help (e.g. to go to the toilet or for a drink of water) in the ward were ignored by the nurses. The narratives illustrated this clearly, for example:

> X is shivering badly and muttering that she is cold. The nurses have begun to wheel patients away and put them to bed (1.45 p.m.), [30 minutes later] – X is shivering badly. Her dress is up to her waist and she is completely naked from the waist down. Z begins to call for a nurse and bangs her hand on the arm of her chair. The nurse in the room ignores her. A district nurse comes in and talks to the patients. She notices X shivering and felt her skin. She went to get her a cardigan. Z is calling 'Can I have a drop of water please?' She calls again and again, and although there are nurses in the room they ignore her. Z becomes agitated and taps her hand vigorously to attract attention. She becomes distressed and still the nurses ignore her . . . X is still shivering badly, she occasionally calls for help . . . [30 minutes later] – X is now shivering quite violently, even though she is now wearing a cardigan that the district nurse put on her and the room is very warm. She calls for the nurse again and again, but no-one pays her any attention . . . [30 minutes later] . . . X is still shivering uncontrollably. I feel her hands and they are frozen. Two nurses have seen her but have done nothing . . . (Hospital ward)
>
> (Clarke and Bowling 1989)

The study also illustrated the need for clear guidance on the ethics of observing social settings, including the circumstances in which observers should intervene and assist (e.g. in situations where people are at risk of harm), debriefing observers, and feedback to managers of settings (in anonymous form).

Audio-observation: conversation sampling

Conversation sampling is a method of analysing societal attitudes by listening techniques (rather than visual observing). For example, an investigator might attempt to study attitudes to current wars or conflicts by conversation sampling. Conversations can be sampled in a range of situations (e.g. in public places, on public transport or from radio phone-in programmes).

The disadvantage of this method is the amount of irrelevant conversation one has to include. The validity of the method is also questionable. If conversations on buses are sampled and recorded, the problem is that the population travelling by bus is not stable or representative, and can be affected by the season, the weather and the type of area. Audible conversations are likely to be different in content from inaudible conversations. All these can explain changes in the topic and content of the conversation.

However, conversation sampling has proved to be a valuable source of data, bearing in mind these limitations. For example, there have been studies showing differences between men and women in the way they converse and phrase instructions, the content of their conversation, and so on. The first published study of conversations was by Moore (1922), who slowly walked up Broadway from 33rd to 55th Street each evening for several weeks and wrote down every overheard audible conversation, collecting 174 fragments for analysis. While this is hardly representative of the population, the method can provide insightful data for developing hypotheses for further testing. The design can also be improved by sampling conversations in a wider variety of settings and time periods. Within settings, the sampling process is usually well defined (e.g. random samples of short or long conversations, complete or sections of conversations in defined situations). For example, one could decide to sample consecutive telephone calls to an ambulance station over a period of time in relation to the first five seconds of conversation. This approach was adopted by Schegloff and Sacks (1974) in relation to calls to a police station in the USA. The rules, processes and consequences of telephone conversation were mapped out by them (the answerer of the telephone speaks first, and the caller provides the topic, the orderly sequence – turn taking – of the conversation, understandings, and so on). Their research was cited by Silverman (1993) as an example of conversational analysis. He drew attention to the significant implications of this work for 'a distribution rule for first utterances' – which is that the answerer speaks first – by reference to an anecdote cited by one of these authors. In this, a woman adopted a strategy of silence after receiving a series of obscene telephone calls. Her friends became irritated by this practice because she broke the rule that the answerer speaks first, but the tactic was successful as the obscene caller would not speak until she had said 'hello' first in accordance with the distribution rule for first utterances.

Not all the early research on conversations would be regarded as ethical or possible today. Webb et al. (1966) gave several examples of early research designs, including the following by Henle and Hubble (1938): 'The investigators took special precautions to keep subjects ignorant of the fact that their remarks were being recorded. To this end, they concealed themselves under beds in students' rooms where tea parties were being held, eavesdropped in dormitory smoking rooms and washrooms, and listened to telephone conversations.'

Recording and analysing verbal communication

Linguistic and extra-linguistic behaviour (e.g. volume and pitch of voice, speed of speech) will need to be taken account of, in either manual or audio recordings of events. Communication can be studied quantitatively in units of sentences or phrases, and can be categorised in relation to form rather than topic. Verbal communication also contains elements of *paralanguage:* voice quality, pauses, and so on. The study of verbal form and paralanguage is known as *process analysis*. This is in contrast to schemes for coding and analysing words: for example, the classification of sentences or phrases by topic (as in content analyses of documents). Process coding schemes require the definition of the unit of analysis (e.g. the sentence, the phrase) and the sampling process (e.g. random samples of short or long, complete or sections of conversations in defined situations). At its most basic, the technique permits the counting and timing of behaviours such as silence, interruptions, pauses, speed of speech and utterances (as in studies of personality traits) (Chapple 1949).

Although conversations are usually analysed in units (e.g. sentences, phrases), the analysis needs to take account of the wider context of the conversation and each unit (e.g. by analysing the narrative and not units in isolation). There are various methods for analysing conversations, from content to process and linguistic analyses. The latter two techniques are highly specialised and complex, and focus on the use of language and type of speech behaviour (see above). The analyses in ethnomethodological research in relation to social meanings are also specialised (Boden and Zimmerman 1991). Silverman (1993) provided examples of the analysis of conversations by type of content (e.g. charge–rebuttal sequences), though he pointed out that this type of analysis is open to the criticism (e.g. by ethnomethodologists) that it is based on taken-for-granted assumptions about the structure of the conversation and its interpretation by the parties involved.

Summary of main points

- Qualitative research data should be collected rigorously and systematically, using more than one investigator in order that checks on reliability can be made.
- Meticulous records should be kept, and a separate fieldwork diary.
- The categorisation of the data should be carried out systematically and impressionistic material avoided in the report.
- Observation can be participative (overt or concealed) or unobtrusive (direct and open), structured (with a checklist, categories to check, rating scales) or unstructured (direct recording of events and stories as they occur).
- Conversation sampling is a method of analysing societal attitudes by listening techniques.
- Objective observations are impossible to achieve, but observers are still required to convince others that their accounts are credible and not mere subjective perception.
- Observational methods should be part of a triangulated research methodology (use of three or more methods), so that observed events, behaviours and attitudes can be verified by independent sources (e.g. records or interviews).
- Recording and coding systems have been developed for non-verbal body language and motion in research settings.
- In contrast to the deductive method, an inductive approach begins with the observations, and postpones definitions and structures until a pattern has been observed.
- With qualitative data, the multiple coding of single items is permissible, in order to facilitate cross-referencing for conceptual and theoretical development.

Key questions

1 Explain the concept of rigour in relation to qualitative research.
2 What type of research questions are qualitative methods appropriate for?
3 How can the reliability of observational research be enhanced?
4 Discuss the ethical implications of undisclosed participant observation.
5 How can the observer attempt to gain access to the social situations of interest?
6 Distinguish between structured and unstructured observation.
7 What research issues are appropriate for audio-observational research?

Key terms

audio-observation
body language
classification
concealed observation
conversation sampling
deconstruction
dramaturgy
ethnomethodology
grounded theory
induction
naturalistic enquiry
non-verbal behaviour
observation

observer bias
overt observation
participant observation
reactive effects
rigour
semiotics
sequential analysis
structured observation
time sampling
triangulated methods
unstructured observation
verbal communication

Recommended reading

Adamson, J. (2005) Combined qualitative and quantitative designs, in A. Bowling and S. Ebrahim (eds) *Handbook of Health Research Methods: Investigation, Measurement and Analysis.* Maidenhead: Open University Press.

Carter, S. and Henderson, L. (2005) Approaches to qualitative data collection in social science, in A. Bowling and S. Ebrahim (eds) *Handbook of Health Research Methods: Investigation, Measurement and Analysis.* Maidenhead: Open University Press.

Donovan, J. and Sanders, C. (2005) Key issues in the analysis of qualitative data in health services research, in A. Bowling and S. Ebrahim (eds) *Handbook of Health Research Methods: Investigation, Measurement and Analysis.* Maidenhead: Open University Press.

Glaser, B.G. and Strauss, A.L. (1967) *The Discovery of Grounded Theory: Strategies for Qualitative Research.* New York: Aldine Publishing.

Lofland, J. and Lofland, L.H. (1995) *Analyzing Social Settings*, 3rd edn. Belmont, CA: Wadsworth Publishing Company.

May, T. (1993) *Social Research: Issues, Methods and Process.* Buckingham: Open University Press.

Mays, N. and Pope, C. (1996) Rigour and qualitative research, in N. Mays and C. Pope (eds) *Qualitative Research in Health Care.* London: British Medical Journal Publishing Group.

CHAPTER 17

Unstructured inter

Chapter contents

Introduction

An 'unstructured interview' simply means a face-to-face interview using an interview schedule with the topics listed but with few specific questions and no fixed questions; these interviews aim to be carried out 'in-depth'. When investigators require more specific information a semi-structured format is used. With this method the interviewer guides the interview on the topic of interest by asking specific, open-ended questions. The interview is still carried out in-depth. Individual unstructured interviews are expensive and time-consuming. Unstructured interviews follow an *interpretive approach*, where the aim is to analyse how people understand their social worlds and the meanings of events. These interviews will be described in this chapter.

⌐red interviews

⌐f unstructured, in-depth interview

⌐uctured, in-depth interviews aim to delve deep beneath the surface of superficial ⌐ponses to obtain true meanings that individuals assign to events, and the complexities ⌐f their attitudes, behaviours and experiences. This method allows the respondents to tell their own stories in their own words, with prompting from the interviewer. Graham (1984) emphasised the importance of documenting people's 'stories' and other personal accounts (diaries, letters) in leading to more enlightened research, in which people are the subjects and not the objects of the research, and in leading to 'a sociology which places a particular emphasis on experience and subjectivity as the route to theory'.

These interviews can be topic- or event-based, or they can be historical or cultural. Cultural interviews are between members of a shared culture and involve explorations of people's experiences and the knowledge and values they pass on to the next generation. The interviews are often repeated. As culture is often communicated through stories, the interviewer should listen at length in order to elicit these. The potential value of such an approach with new research topics, compared to structured interviews which carry the danger of forcing responses into inappropriate codes, is shown in Box 17.1.

Box 17.1 Example of the inappropriate use of structured questionnaires on little-known topics, illustrating the need for an unstructured, in-depth approach

It was still pitch-dark, and it was drizzling. Elio was coming home from the night shift, and he was tired and sleepy; he got off the streetcar and walked toward home, first by a street with an uneven roadbed, and then along a small alley that was not lit. In the darkness he heard a voice that asked him: 'Would you agree to an interview?' It was a slightly metallic voice, devoid of dialectal inflection; strangely, it seemed to him that it was coming from below, close to his feet. He stopped, a bit surprised, and answered yes, but that he was in a hurry to get home.

'I'm in a hurry too, don't worry,' the voice answered. 'It won't take two minutes. Tell me: how many inhabitants are there on the earth?'

'More or less, four billion. But why are you asking me, of all people?'

'Purely by chance, believe me. I did not have the opportunity to select. Listen, please: how do you digest?'

Elio was annoyed. 'What do you mean, how do you digest? Some digest well, some don't. Who are you anyway? I hope you're not trying to sell me some medicine at this hour, and here in the dark in the middle of the street?'

'No, I'm just collecting statistics,' the voice said, unperturbed. 'I come from a nearby star, we are supposed to compile an annual directory of the galaxies' inhabited planets, and we need some comparative data. Why do you spend so much time washing yourselves and washing the objects around you?'

Elio, with a certain embarrassment, explained that one washes only a few times each day, and that one washes so as not to be dirty, and that if one stays dirty there is the danger of catching some disease.

'Right, that was one of our hypotheses. You wash in order not to die. How do you die? At what age?' . . . he said there weren't any rules, both young and old die, very few got to be a hundred. 'I understand. Those who use white sheets and wash their floors live long.' Elio tried to rectify this, but the interviewer was in a hurry and continued, 'How do you reproduce?'

(Levi 1990)

Unstructured, in-depth interviews have been described as 'guided conversations' (Lofland and Lofland 1995), as 'testimony studies' when used within evaluations of services (St Leger *et al.* 1992) and as life or oral histories. Life history, or oral life history, research involves face-to-face unstructured interviews which aim to allow the respondent to talk in depth and at length about past events. It uses narrative research methods of collecting and analysing data based on the stories people tell during interviews about their lives (see Rubin and Rubin 1995, for types of interview). These approaches are usually combined with other data such as photographs, documents, and letters. Unlike other methods of qualitative research, where analyses are based on categorisations of data, true narrative approaches aim to preserve the integrity of the original data and contexts, and can be time-consuming. However, one limitation is that people's memories fade, and problems of recall bias are likely to increase over time.

Life story or oral history approaches are also an important source for enhancing historical research (Berridge 1996). Common features in all disciplines include: the generation and use of people's natural propensity for story-telling and using these to explore particular social and historical issues; the ideal of empowering and respecting the narrator; and enhancing the researcher's understanding of the individual, of social life and of social interactions (Atkinson 1998). According to theories of psycho-social development, reviewing life experiences into a cohesive story are developmental tasks associated with later life (Erikson and Erikson 1997). With these oral histories, the investigator chooses a period of time, or an event, and asks individuals involved to describe what happened (e.g. during the Second World War).

With the life history, the personal life events of the respondent are explored. The interviewer requires skill in order to ensure that the history is an account of the person's life, including themes in their life that they regard to be important. Opening questions include, for example, 'I'd like to find out about your life. Could you tell me about it, for example, as if you were telling me the story of your life?' Useful probes for detail during the interview are 'What happened next?', 'What did you do?', or 'How did that make you feel?'. A checklist of open probes should cover the interviewee's childhood, education/life, occupation/work life, marriage/cohabiting/living arrangements, key relatives and friends/personalities, stresses, ethnic and religious background. Reflection techniques, by simply repeating the person's words, also encourage people to talk more about something.

These interviews can carry much memory bias and the danger of the reinterpretation of events, and require cross-checking with other sources of information (see Thompson 1988). Concern about accuracy of life histories has led to use of probing and prompting about dates, key life transitions, or reference points to enhance recall (Humphrey 1993; Walter *et al.* 1987). A life grid approach has also been developed to facilitate more accurate collection of recall data. While it has been used in quantitative research, Parry *et al.* (1999) described its application in qualitative interviews on smoking in older age, and life changes throughout the life course. They used an A3 grid divided into five columns for each respondent, covering key external events, age, family, work/leisure, housing, health and smoking. An adapted example of their prepared grid is shown in Box 17.2. Direct events under each column heading were entered (e.g. family, work/leisure, housing, health, smoking/start and quitting dates) and events under each heading were entered during the interview chronologically (e.g. marriages, divorces, redundancies, etc.). The interviewer was able to cross-reference direct and indirect indicators with smoking behaviour and probe around these associations. The completion of the life grid was described as a mutual endeavour between interviewer and respondent, and shifts some control to the latter. They also reported that respondents found the challenge of solving discrepancies in their life grid accounts as rewarding, for example:

Interviewer: I see from the grid that you stopped smoking when you were living in Leeds, was that right? You said it was between 64 and 68? So it would be the same time you were living in Leeds.

R19: Ah no, here it's a good job you pointed that . . . actually em, no, I stopped smoking before I went to Leeds, it must have been between 62, 64 then this happened. Sorry about that.

Interviewer: That's fine.

R19: It's just that you bring, I should have had my diary, well that wouldn't be in my diary anyway because I wouldn't show that one.

Interviewer: No, that's fine, this is the very reason why we use the grids. They are clever.

R19: No, you're quite right, I didn't smoke while I was in Leeds. Quite right, yes.

Interviewer: You stopped before then?

R19: Yes, I stopped before then.

Box 17.2 Example of prepared life grid

Key external events	Age	Family	Work/ Leisure	Housing	Health	Smoking
1915						
1960	45					
Physician's report on nation's health						
US Surgeon Gen. Report when health warnings appeared on cigarette packets were introduced						
1965	50					

England won World Cup
Football

Apollo Moon landing
1970   55

(Parry *et al.* 1999)

The *advantages* of unstructured interviews in general are that more complex issues can be probed, answers can be clarified and a more relaxed research atmosphere may obtain more in-depth as well as sensitive information. The *disadvantages* are that the data are time-consuming and difficult to collect and analyse (e.g. with content analyses and narratives), there are greater opportunities for interviewer bias to intervene and, because it is a time-consuming method, it is expensive and only feasible with small samples, which then leads to the questionable representativeness of the data.

Research in sociology is often based on qualitative techniques, and clearly illustrates the importance of conducting unstructured interviews in order to understand how patients define their medical conditions and treatment. For example, Morgan's (1996) data from in-depth interviews with people with hypertension demonstrate how much information we lose in standard, pre-coded questions asking people to rate their health as excellent, good, fair or poor. For example, one of her respondents with hypertension described herself as: 'Delicate – no, not delicate – I can't think of the word for it. I wouldn't say I'm an ill person, but I wouldn't like to say I'm healthy. I don't know whether that makes sense really. You feel as though it's always there, but it doesn't affect you.'

While there is inevitably potential for interviewer bias in qualitative interviews, the greater involvement and participation of the interviewer in the interaction aim to prompt greater depth, and it is assumed that once the level of communication has reached this 'depth', then respondents will reveal their 'true' inner feelings, attitudes and behaviour. (See Box 17.3.)

Box 17.3 Cornwell's study and the value of repeating interviews

Cornwell's (1984) research on people's attitudes to health, illness and medical care was based on repeated in-depth interviews with respondents over several months. However, she found that at the outset of the study, even using qualitative interviewing techniques, people only revealed their 'public accounts', and it was not until they were interviewed several times, and began to regard the research as part of their lives, that they revealed their true feelings and beliefs to the interviewer – their 'private accounts'. This study demonstrates how important the rapport and familiarity between investigator and respondent in qualitative research are.

In-depth interviewing: sample selection and size

Qualitative interviewing is usually based on small sample sizes, and the sampling techniques preferred include convenience sampling, purposive sampling, snowballing and theoretical sampling. These methods of sampling, which are used in qualitative research, were described in Chapter 8, along with other sampling methods, and will be more briefly described here. *Convenience sampling* refers to the sampling of subjects for reasons of convenience, for example, easy to recruit, near at hand, likely to respond. *Purposive sampling* is a deliberate non-random method of sampling, which aims to sample a group of people, or settings, with a particular characteristic. *Snowballing* is a technique used where no sampling frame exists and it cannot be created. Initial respondents are asked to suggest others whom they know are in the target group and who could be invited to take part, and so on. Its disadvantage is that it is limited to members of a specific network. *Theoretical sampling* involves the generation of conceptual or theoretical categories during the research process. The principle of this method is that the sampling aims to locate data to develop and challenge emerging hypotheses (Glaser and Strauss 1967). The sampling stops when no new analytical insights are forthcoming (i.e. theoretical saturation). This method necessitates the coding and analysis of data during the ongoing sampling process owing to the interplay between the collection of the data and reflection on them. No attempt is made to undertake random sampling.

The data obtained from qualitative interviews are used to increase our insight into social phenomena rather than assume representativeness. Nonetheless, the issue of non-representativeness of people, and hence the limitations upon generalisability of results, is a criticism that is frequently encountered. The sample to be interviewed could, in theory, be randomly selected to satisfy generalisability, though given the small numbers usually required, the chances of the sample being representative of a wider population of interest are usually slim. Moreover, there might not be a suitable sampling frame of the population group of interest. For example, Oakley's (1974) study of housework was based on a sample of 40 married working-class and middle-class women with at least one child under 5 years of age. The sample was taken from two GPs' lists of patients in London: one in a working-class and the other in a middle-class area. Thus, though an attempt was made to obtain a representative sample of the population of interest, the samples were not probability samples from which precise population estimates can be made. Probability sampling is not practical in small-scale qualitative research, especially when no sampling frame of the group of interest is obtainable.

A common problem facing the researcher undertaking qualitative, in-depth interviewing is the question of sample size. Sample sizes are necessarily small because of the complexity of the data, which are expensive and time-consuming to analyse, and because the data aim to provide rich insights in order to understand social phenomena rather than statistical information. A sample size of 'one', however, obviously cannot give rise to any generalisations, but there is no clear guideline about what constitutes an appropriate cut-off point. The 'rule of thumb' applied most frequently is that when the same stories, themes, issues and topics are emerging from the study subjects, then a sufficient sample size has been reached.

The process of the interview

As with structured interviewing, respondents should be informed of the aims of the study, its sponsorship, where their names were obtained and confidentiality. A covering letter containing this information should be given to them to keep.

Although the interviews are unstructured, there will usually be
questions about the respondent's socio-demographic characteri
as structured interviews (e.g. sex, date of birth, occupation, e⌐
date and place of interview). A post-interview comment shee⌐
the interviewer to record information about his or her feelings
rapport, insights, disruptions, and so on.

Unstructured, or in-depth, interviewing uses a simple checklist of topi⌐
than fixed questions, and there are no pre-codes. The interviews should be au⌐
recorded (with respondents' permission) in order that they can be analysed in deta⌐.
later. This also enables the interviewer to attend to the informant, rather than manually
recording all the responses, and communicate that the respondent is being listened to.
Tape recorders are rarely intrusive as people forget about the recorder once the interview
gets under way. It was pointed out in Chapter 16 that, in order to check for any reactive
effects, one technique is to turn the recorder off at the end of the interview and 'chat' to
respondents informally as a check on whether they have anything else to add.

A good quality recorder, as well as tapes, should be used in order to enhance the
sound quality of the playback and minimise research material lost due to inaudibility.
The interviewer should still take some notes – for example, key words and phrases – in
order to keep account of the topics that have been covered, as well as a back-up to failed
recordings (and batteries should be regularly checked).

If the interviews are based on grounded theory, the process is iterative. The data
are collected and theories and potential concepts and categories are developed during
the process, more data are collected and the theories, concepts and categories tested,
and so on until an understanding of the phenomenon is achieved. The questioning is
redesigned during the process as new themes emerge which need to be explored. This
continuous process stops when theoretical saturation has been reached and additional
interviews add nothing more to the topic of interest (Glaser and Strauss 1967; Bryant and
Charmaz 2010).

Transcription and coding should be undertaken during the interviewing period. The
investigator should code the content by theme (computer packages are available for this).

Various annotation guides for transcribing are available, which suggest standard
shorthand symbols (notation) for the transcriber (Potter and Wetherell 1987). Each
transcribed script should be read by two independent coders, and a thematic coding
frame developed. Thematic categorisation should then be undertaken by two independent
coders, and codes for any discepancies agreed with a third independent coder, in order
to ensure methodological rigour. Categories and themes for coding will be derived
directly from analysing the interview material, as well as from the conceptual ideas the
investigator has while conducting and listening to the interviews.

Techniques of in-depth interviewing

Interviewer skills

In-depth interviewing requires highly skilled interviewers, who are fully aware of the aims
of the study. The aim is to encourage respondents to talk freely and spontaneously about
their feelings, experiences, attitudes and behaviour.

interviewer must learn to explore any symbols and meanings of the respondent, recognise that his or her own perspective is only one way of looking at the world. s important that the interviewer does not ask questions that indicate lack of cultural omprehension, but is skilled at encouraging the respondent to talk, and listens in order to find out about events, attitudes, experiences, motives and reactions. The interviewer must be trained to cope with alternating phases of openness, withdrawal, trust, distress and embarrassment. It is important for the interviewer to be skilled at bringing the respondent back to a positive frame of mind and certainly to leave him or her feeling calm (Rubin and Rubin 1995). For example, at the end of the interview, topics with no emotional or threatening content can be raised, and respondents should always be told what valuable information they have given as the interview is being closed.

Need for neutrality

The neutral introduction of the study's aims, and an emphasis on confidentiality, are required in the same way as for structured interviewing. Ice-breaking questions are important at the beginning, in order to relax the respondent and set the agenda (e.g. 'Can you tell me what you like about your job?').

While unstructured interviewing allows for greater social interaction between interviewer and interviewee, with few constraints on the interview schedule, interviewers should still aim to minimise their own, potentially biasing, role, limiting their interactions to encouraging nods and expressions, and non-directive, neutral probes. They must resist the urge to agree or disagree with respondents and they need to perfect the art of creating expectant, not embarrassing, silences.

Some interpretive sociologists will disagree with the need for strict neutrality, and encourage interviewers to interact with respondents and conduct 'normal' conversations. This interaction is then treated as research data and analysed as such. Such an approach should only be attempted when the investigator is highly skilled, and it has to be carefully analysed because of the increased potential for interviewer bias. Examples of this approach are presented later in the section on narrative format.

Generally, however, the 'unstructured, in-depth' interviewer should avoid leading questions, biasing questions, double negatives, two questions in one, and so on. The interviewer should also follow the same rules as in structured interviewing in relation to the use of neutral probes and prompts (e.g. 'Can you tell me more about that?', 'Did anything else happen?'). However, there are circumstances in which leading questions are useful: for example, with behaviour and attitudes that are likely to be under-reported (see Chapter 14 on structured survey interviewing techniques).

Oppenheim (1992) offers advice on wording for unstructured, in-depth interviews (e.g. when neutral acknowledgement is needed: if respondents become distressed because of painful memories, the interviewer could say 'I appreciate that talking about things like this is not easy' or 'Knowing something about your personal experience of X will be very valuable in guiding our research'). With structured interviews, conducted within a framework of positivism, the interview–respondent interaction is of interest only in relation to interviewer bias and error, response bias and whether the interviewer has departed from the interview protocol (Brenner 1981). In contrast, unstructured interviews are regarded by qualitative researchers as a social encounter and the social context of the interview is taken into account in interpretation of the data (see Silverman 1993).

Checklists

There are several techniques available for in-depth interviewing. At a basic level, the researcher conducts the interview with only a simple checklist of topics to cover. The checklist should include the issues the investigator wishes to probe and salient points about them – for example, 'Can you tell me about your illness? How did it affect you at first?' (Probe emotional, physical, behaviour.) 'How does it affect you now?' (Obtain current perspective. Obtain any instances when it led to stress.) 'How did others react towards you?' The checklist should be used flexibly and is simply a guide to the topics to raise when talking to the respondent.

Critical incidents techniques

In other situations, various techniques may be used. These include critical incidents techniques. For example, the interviewer asks respondents about key events (e.g. illnesses) in their past in order to discover how they are likely to react to, act upon (e.g. consultations with doctors) and cope with future situations; or GPs are asked what they did in identified recent clinical situations.

Other techniques include sequential, or chronological, interviewing (e.g. respondents are asked to tell their 'story' to the interviewer in their own way, they are asked further about events as they are thus reported and they may be asked to reflect back on previously stated beliefs in relation to any new material). Information about people's life histories (biographies) can be collected with this technique.

Preparing questions

Erlandson *et al.* (1993) emphasised that the key to obtaining rich data is asking good questions that have been prepared beforehand to reflect the basic research questions, and careful listening and recording. The questions must not be overly structured, however, or they will constrain the respondent. They cited Patton's (1990) list of six basic kinds of questions that can be used to obtain different types of data, which is displayed in Box 17.4.

Box 17.4 Basic types of question

- Questions to elicit descriptions of experiences, behaviour, actions and activities (e.g. 'What are the most memorable experiences you have had as an administrator?').
- Opinion or value questions to inform about people's goals, intentions, desires and values (e.g. 'Why are you a teacher?').
- Questions about feelings in order to obtain an understanding of emotional responses (e.g. 'How did you feel when the administration moved you to a different grade?').
- Questions about knowledge and factual information (e.g. 'How many teachers are there in this school?').
- Questions which determine what sensory stimuli – sight, sound, touch, taste or smell – respondents are sensitive to (e.g. 'Why do you like plants in your room?').
- Background questions that aim to understand the respondent's previous experiences (e.g. 'Will you briefly explain your educational background?').

(Patton 1990)

Obtaining more depth

Rubin and Rubin (1995) point out that there are three basic types of qualitative interview questions: (1) main questions with which to begin and guide the conversation; (2) probes to clarify answers and to request further information; and (3) follow-up questions which pursue the implications of replies to main questions.

Main questions

In preparing the list of main questions or topics, the investigator works out the main questions which act as devices for covering the events or processes of interest. These can be global questions which enable the respondent to describe the situation of interest in his or her terms (e.g. 'How does X usually work?'; 'Describe a typical day . . .'; 'Describe what happened last time . . .').

Probing questions

Probing questions can simply be requests for extension, such as 'Can you tell me more about . . . ?' 'Is there anything else . . . ?' 'What happened then?', or simply be an expectant repeat of the respondent's sentence in a way that suggests that more information is desired. They can be encouragement or *prompting* questions, such as 'Uh huh?', 'Yes?', 'Go on'. They can be example questions, such as 'Can you give me an example of . . . ?' (Rubin and Rubin 1995; Stringer 1996). Probes need to be well timed and neutral. Care also needs to be taken not to act like an inquisitor (Rubin and Rubin 1995), nor to try and control the discussion so that the interview follows the researcher's agenda and not what is important to the respondent. Follow-up questions should focus on issues that are important to the subject of study, and can simply be 'Would you talk a bit more about . . . ?' Rubin and Rubin (1995) provide examples of each type of question in relation to cultural interviews and topic-based interviews.

Referring back as follow-up questions

More depth can be obtained by asking respondents to describe events backwards in time, or by asking them to go over points already covered later on in the interview or during a second interview, explaining the need for clarification of some points. Detail can always be directly solicited, but it is important to establish a pattern for requiring detail early on in the interview, and the respondent will soon learn to respond to this and provide it automatically. Types of neutral follow-up questions which can obtain more depth include: 'What do you mean by [repeat the respondent's statement]?'; 'Are the problems you mentioned getting any better or worse?'; 'Could I ask you a few more questions about . . . ?'; 'How are you dealing with . . . ?' (Rubin and Rubin 1995).

Analysis and presentation of in-depth interview data

In order to analyse and present qualitative data, the investigator must be thoroughly familiar with the field notes, the tape recordings and their transcriptions and any other data collected. Making sense of these data in order to analyse and present them is challenging, time-consuming and expensive. At the transcription stage it is worth adopting certain transcription symbols. Silverman (1993) gives instances of these. For example, left brackets indicate the point at which a current speaker's talk is overlapped by another's talk; numbers in parentheses indicate elapsed time in silence in tenths of a second; underscoring text indicates some form of stress (via pitch or amplitude); empty parentheses indicate the inability of the transcriber to hear what was said; double parentheses contain the author's descriptions rather than the actual transcriptions.

Once transcribed, data can be organised by topic, and themes coded into categories (and some may fit more than one) as the research is in progress, in order to make the final task more manageable. Ongoing analysis while collecting data can also inform and improve the research process (see Glaser and Strauss 1967). The analysis of qualitative research data requires considerable interpretation by the investigators. It is this feature which is both a strength and a weakness of the method. The two most common approaches are to analyse and present the data in either a categorised or a narrative format.

Several authors have summarised the main approaches to analysing qualitative interview data (Donovan and Saunders 2005; Green 2005). These include grounded theory approaches, in which theory should emerge from, and is grounded in, data, and adaptations of this method (Bryant and Charmaz 2010; and see section on grounded theory in Chapter 6). Essential to the approach are methods of constant comparison, in which the data collection and analysis are cyclical processes of comparing segments of data in order to inform subsequent data collection, to generate theory inductively from the emerging themes and to develop conceptual categories to understand relationships in the data. Methods of analysis also include narrative approaches, which emphasise story telling, usually using unstructured, in-depth interviewing. Structural elements of the story are identified, as well as the role of the interviewer in its production. Instead of categorisation, the context is preserved, and longer sections of talk are presented in illustrations and examples of meanings. Content analysis is the simplest, and sometimes superficial, approach to the analysis of qualitative data, involving the identification of codes with which to categorise the data. A popular method of analysis in applied health and social research is the framework approach. This involves identification of a thematic framework which reflects the aims of the study as well as inductively reflecting the key or recurring themes emerging from the data; this framework is developed into an index which lists the categories for analysis. (See section later on the framework approach.)

Categorising qualitative data: content analysis

Coding

Glaser and Strauss (1967) argued that coding is essential for the invariable analysis of qualitative data. Coding means relating sections of the data to the categories which the researcher has either previously developed or is developing on an ongoing basis as the data are being collected. To facilitate this process, it is important for the investigator to note constantly the categories, or potential categories, in the margins of the raw material. Ultimately, a 'storage and retrieval' system will need to be developed that permits the storage of the data under the relevant categories, re-labelling as required, and the easy retrieval of these for analysis.

Framework approach

One approach to sorting, categorising and interpreting qualitative data is the framework approach. This involves familiarisation by reading the interview transcripts to obtain an overview of the material; the identification of a thematic framework (e.g. drawing on any themes identified in the interview (topic) guide, themes emerging from respondents, and analytic themes emerging from repeated analyses); applying the thematic framework systematically by coding (indexing) each fragment or section of the transcript; charting by rearranging the data according to the identified themes; mapping and interpretation (aggregating patterns, searching for structure, synthesising the findings) (Ritchie and Spencer 1994).

Framework analysis was developed for applied, policy relevant research, using a more structured topic guide than used by most qualitative studies. The process of analysis is similar to thematic analysis, but is more informed by *a priori* reasoning. Ritchie and Spencer (1994) described five stages in framework analysis, which are summarised in Box 17.5.

Box 17.5 Stages of framework analysis

1. Familiarisation with the range and diversity of the data often by selection of a representative sample for full analysis.
2. Identification of a thematic framework which reflects, *a priori*, the aims of the study, as well as inductively reflecting themes emerging from the data; this framework is developed into an index which labels categories for analysis.
3. Indexing, in which the thematic framework is applied systematically to the data set. The text is annotated with numerical codes from the index, supported with text descriptors to elaborate the index heading.
4. Charting, in which the data are rearranged according to the appropriate thematic references, in order to facilitate comparison of themes across cases.
5. Mapping and interpretation, in which the charts are reviewed in order to identify patterns and typologies, and associations across the data.

(Ritchie and Spencer 1994)

Content analysis

When presenting qualitative data in a categorised manner, the investigator carries out a content analysis. The procedure is basically as follows: data are collected, coded by theme or category and finally the coded data are analysed and presented. One method of analysing the data is known as the *grounded hermeneutic method*. It enables themes to emerge from the respondents' own stories, and the use of methods of *constant comparison* (Strauss and Corbin 1990; and see Donovan and Sanders 2005). With this method, after a small number of interviews have been completed, their themes and categories are developed, comparisons are made with subsequent interviews, and similarities and differences between them are examined. This then influences the subsequent sampling, interviews, refinement of themes and categorisation, and analysis.

In order to satisfy criteria of reliability, the field data (e.g. audio- and videotape recordings, written field notes and/or text) should be listened to, viewed and/or read by a team of investigators to agree the categories used. The categorisation exercise should be carried out by the investigator and also by an independent investigator. Their categorisations should be compared and any discrepancies discussed and final categorisation agreed.

The time-consuming nature of this method of research should not be underestimated. Audio-taped interviews, for example, have to be transcribed from the recording before they can be analysed. For one hour of tape recording one should allow between two and four hours transcribing, depending on the skill and speed of the transcriber and the clarity and complexity of the interview material.

Traditionally, qualitative data have been hand-sorted and categorised by theme, which has had the advantage of the researcher maintaining a close relationship with and awareness of the original data. Analyses of qualitative data involved a massive 'cut and paste' process, whereby relevant themes were highlighted in transcripts and then cut out and pasted onto index cards, which were then organised into theme order. The index cards also permitted space for cross-referencing, with that unit's themes coded onto different cards, as well as cross-references to the original source to enable the investigator to trace it back to its original context. Matrices or spreadsheets could also be constructed, with concepts and themes displayed along the top row, and the variables of interest listed in the left-hand margin so that they could be cross-referenced with the concepts.

An example of manual categorisation is Scambler and Hopkins's (1988) research on epilepsy, which included interviews with 94 people with the condition. The authors stated:

> Excepting some demographic and other precoded material, data from the taped interviews were transcribed on to sets of 'topic cards'. These corresponded to a series of topics generated during the pilot investigations and explored during the interviews; a set of fifty or more was produced for each person, the precise number depending on his or her age and marital status at onset. The problem of overlap of data relevant to more than one topic, and hence to more than one topic card, was resolved by a system of cross-referencing. The cards brought together and afforded easy access to all statements made during the interviews pertinent to any selected topic. The data on the cards were then of course available for both qualitative and quantitative analysis.

Manual categorisation is still widely practised for small studies, but is time-consuming for large databases. Computer packages are now commonly used for categorisation of data, and have advantages over manual categorisation (see later).

Another example of content analysis, which was used in quantitative as well as qualitative analyses, can be found in Calnan and Williams (1996). They present data from an earlier study by one of the authors on women's perceptions of medicine, based on in-depth, tape-recorded interview techniques. Each respondent was asked to assess her GP in relation to whether she considered him or her to be 'good' or 'bad', and asked about why she made that assessment. The data were analysed and the women's reasons were listed and coded into categories such as: good doctor, sympathetic, knows her personally, immediately refers to specialist, examines thoroughly, gives a lot of time, treats children well, listens; bad doctor, routinely gives prescriptions, treats everything as a waste of time, will not make house calls at night, does not listen, abrupt/rude manner, uncaring. Using these codes they could analyse the data by, for example, social class, and they demonstrated that women in higher social class groupings used different criteria to make their assessments than women in lower groupings.

Scambler and Hopkins (1988) carried out a content analysis of the information they collected in relation to the social effects of epilepsy. This showed that the principal cause of the distress experienced by four out of five of their respondents at the onset of their condition (e.g. first seizure) was the reaction of other people (often their families) to them. The authors' data yielded three typical features of family responses, and used the verbatim descriptions of respondents to illustrate the content analysis (see Box 17.6).

Box 17.6 The use of verbatim descriptions in illustration of content analyses

It was possible, however, to discern three typical features of family responses (to first onset of epilepsy): concern, bewilderment and helplessness. All are reflected in the following account of onset by a troubled and shaken spouse:

> I just didn't know what the hell was happening: it was as simple as that! I had never seen anybody have a – whatever it was! I didn't know what to do quite frankly. And it was, if I remember rightly, about 2.30 a.m., or something like that, and it was – it was just frightening, that's all I can say. I didn't know what to do. I think that's what frightened me more than anything: I just didn't know what to do, how to cope. I didn't know what I should be doing – whether I should be trying to stop it, or do something; I just didn't know.

(Scambler and Hopkins 1988)

Rules for coding

With *quantitative* analysis, the coding rule is generally that codes should be mutually exclusive so that a single unit of data can only be coded in one category. Quantitative coding does permit the use of multiple codes for replies to single questions in questionnaires to fit instances where respondents have mentioned several things in one reply. For example, in reply to a question about what the good qualities of their GPs are, people might say that their doctor is good at examining them, a sympathetic listener, good at explaining things, and so on; each thing mentioned would need to be coded (the question is multicoded). In contrast, in *qualitative* coding, a single item is permitted to be coded in more than one category in order to permit cross-referencing and the generation of several hypotheses.

The first stage is to develop the categories (themes) into which the data will be coded. J. Fielding (1993) stated that if the research stems from a theory, then the codes should be chosen to represent the theory and the data coded to fit the categories (which she terms 'coding down'). If the aim is to describe the data in order to generate theory, then the opposite rule applies and the categories can be developed from the data ('coding up'). In practice, it is preferable to code up in all cases, but to ensure that additional theoretical codes are included and to apply them to all relevant instances.

Pfaffenberger (1988) and J. Fielding (1993) have made suggestions for the coding of qualitative data, including those shown in Box 17.7.

Box 17.7 Steps in the coding process

1. Take the first batch of 20 or so sets of data (e.g. questionnaires or the field notes or transcripts).
2. Mark off and note down the responses (or significant features or quotes) on filing cards, using a new card for each new response or concept.
3. With questionnaires, code the same question for the batch before moving on to coding new questions to enhance consistency.
4. For interviews or transcripts, code short segments (e.g. paragraphs) at a time. Some researchers have collected the data in time periods (e.g. 15-minute intervals) or other meaningful units (sentences in conversation, line breaks in accounts) to facilitate coding and analysis, but this is not always possible. The decision about where to make line breaks is determined by the investigator and transcriber.
5. Develop codes that can interlink different units of data.
6. Change and refine the categories as understanding increases and improves.
7. Sort the file cards into related categories.
8. Repeat the process on another 20 questionnaires or other datasets and then again until no new categories are generated.
9. Develop the instructions for coding.
10. Develop a framework that links the codes together typologically.

(Pfaffenberger 1988; J. Fielding 1993)

Criticisms and potential weaknesses of this approach are that the very process of categorising and coding the data disembodies it from the person who produced it and from the interactive nature of the interview. The value of qualitative data is in the richness of its insights and the analysis of narratives and individuals' stories. Care is required in order not to lose the qualitative nature, and richness, of the data.

Electronic computer programs for analysing qualitative data

It was mentioned earlier that until the development of computer packages to analyse qualitative data in the 1980s, 'cut and paste' techniques (e.g. cutting sections of data and pasting them on to index cards that could be filed under the appropriate category) were the most widely used for organising (categorising), storing and retrieving qualitative data. While this method is still commonly used, as many investigators feel that they are closer to their data by using manual procedures, it is also increasingly common to use a computer package to store and categorise the data by theme. The themes are not allocated numerical values by the computer program; instead they are categorised and stored by their contextual theme, using labels of up to ten characters. The themes also maintain their contextual position in the raw transcripts which have been entered into an associated word processing program. There are various computer programs available for qualitative categorisation and analysis (e.g. ETHNOGRAPH (Seidel and Clark 1984; www.qualisresearch.com; accessed September 2013), QSR NUD.IST (Richards and Richards 1990) and the updated QSR NVIVO (www.qsrinternational.com/products_nvivo. aspx; accessed September 2013) and Atlas (Scientific Software Development 1997;

updated version: www.atlasti.com/qualitative-software.html; accessed September 2013). Some are particularly valuable for theory-building, having the facility to code the text into several different categories and to link between codes, as well as between memos and text, memos and codes, and different segments of text (Prein and Kelle 1995). The programs will retrieve segments of marked text by single codes or combinations of codes, and these can be easily compared. There can be multiple linkages between segments of text. This is essential for grounded theory approaches as they concentrate on extracting the meanings that emerge from the data and the type of coding used. The use of computers with grounded theory has been explored by Lonkila (1995). Advice on the selection of appropriate computer packages is given in Weitzman and Miles (1995).

While programmed coding of words and phrases, with 'look up' tables and dictionaries stored in the machine, can be carried out by qualitative analysis packages, concept-matching inevitably remains a problem and there is no match for the trained human brain. However, hypotheses can be tested and theories can be built by employing the networks of categories generated on the computer. The investigators' field 'memos' can also be stored and retrieved if required. Less well developed is the storage, linkage and retrieval of diagrams and maps drawn of the field setting or phenomenon of interest.

Computerised categorisation and analysis are becoming increasingly popular, and arguably make the process more systematic and hence rigorous. While some investigators object to the distance computers impose between them and their data, it is the only practical method of organising and analysing larger qualitative studies. For example, Dingwall et al.'s (1983) research on child abuse resulted in more than 7000 pages of observational and interview data and the authors described how the use of a computer retrieval system was the only realistic method of organising them.

It is important to emphasise that simply counting the number of times an item or concept has been mentioned during unstructured interviews is not necessarily meaningful. Frequency does not necessarily equate with social significance of the topic. This type of content analysis may be useful in document analyses, depending on the aim of the document and the aim of the research, but should be used with caution in other types of research. The theoretical and methodological issues involved in the use of computers in qualitative research have been explored by several authors in an edited volume by Kelle (1995).

Narrative format

By contrast, the narrative approach stresses the importance of the story the respondent has to tell, focusing on presentations of the actual transcripts. All qualitative reports, even those which include a content analysis, will also include sections of the transcripts alongside the investigator's interpretations of them. Data need to be presented so that their richness is not lost.

The emphasis in narrative format is placed on analysing the content or structure of the narrative in its original and intact form. This is also known as discourse analysis. Data are sometimes, but not always, coded by theme or category, and these coded data are used to develop an analysis of the situation. Gerhardt (1996) has used narratives to present and analyse her data collected from interviews with patients with endstage renal failure in relation to their experiences with dialysis and transplantation. She obtained

234 tape-recorded in-depth interviews with patients in South-east England, and these comprised over 600 hours of tape-recorded material. She presented the transcripts of the interview in short 'blocks' she called 'meaning units' (Box 17.8).

Box 17.8 Example from Gerhardt's (1996) analyses

113 P: well my mother

114 she was willing

115 to give me a kidney

116 but I didn't want it

117 because

118 well

119 if she gives me a kidney

120 that's to say

121 if the kidney

122 doesn't work on me

123 then I will still be disabled

124 and probably

125 my mother starts feeling bad . . .

The narratives were then analysed in relation to their content and the investigator's analysis can refer to the line numbers as evidence of the validity of the approach, for example:

The second step in his action story is his decision not to accept his mother's offer of a live-donor organ (115–33). He again tells an argumentative narrative rather than a full-fledged story, stating the fact(s) and then giving reason(s). The facts were: 'My mother was willing to give me a kidney but I didn't want it' (113–16). The reason is: If this live donor transplant would fail, the situation would be worse than now, that is, he would be still 'disabled' (123), and she could 'start feeling bad' (125). From this it follows that he rejected the offer . . .

Others report the full interaction between interviewer and patient in their narratives and use them to illustrate their interpretations. The extract from Radley (1996) in Box 17.9 demonstrates not only how the researcher uses the dialogue for analysis, but also how the interview can be a spontaneous and dynamic interaction, with the spontaneity of the interviewer rewarded with further meaningful information from the respondent.

Semiotics is described elsewhere in relation to the analysis of observational studies and document research. It should also be briefly referred to here, as some investigators analyse interview narratives in relation to semiotics. With semiotics, the textual context is considered as a whole, as the elements of speech derive their meanings from their relationship with other elements. Barrett (1996) gives examples of the importance and social relevance of this method of analysis in relation to understanding elderly people's use of the term 'managing' in the context of assessments of their need for social care. He showed how for 'non-economically fragile' older people 'managing' seems to mean acting within a longer-term view, with a positive outlook in relation to the future (e.g. 'Oh yes, I do manage on my money'; 'I couldn't manage if there wasn't a bit in the bank'; 'You've got to manage'). In relation to the 'economically fragile', 'managing' seems to mean a shorter-term view and 'getting by' (e.g. 'We manage week by week but there's nothing to spare'; 'We're managing at the moment'; 'We get by, we manage'). He explored this use of language in terms of how it affected people's lives and its symbolism of other features of their lives.

Box 17.9 Example of the interview as interaction

Interviewer: What have you been told about the operation by the hospital?

Patient: That I'm not very pleased with. I went Tuesday and they told me and my wife it could be touch and go if I even come through it because I've got heart disease.

Interviewer: You knew that before?

Patient: I didn't know, no. It puts you off a bit.

Interviewer: Has that made you think twice about whether you want it doing?

Patient: No, I still want it doing, but I wish they hadn't told me. My doctor he played hell about it. He said they [the doctors at the hospital] shouldn't have told you at all.

The man's wife was also confused and angry. She said: 'Our doctor, he don't know nothing about it . . . He says as far as he's concerned all he knows he's got to have that bypass. We know that. What is this bloody diseased heart?'

These comments show the uncertainty engendered in the patient (and family) by a diagnosis that was not accepted, perhaps because it was at variance with what they had previously understood.

(Radley 1996)

Summary of main points

- Unstructured interviews aim to delve beneath the surface of superficial responses to obtain true meanings that individuals assign to events, and to understand the complexities of their attitudes, behaviours and experiences.
- There are three basic types of questions which are used in unstructured approaches: main questions which guide the interview, probes, and follow-up questions.
- Transcription and coding should be undertaken during the interviewing period.
- Once transcribed, data can be organised by topic, and themes coded into categories (and some may fit more than one) as the research is in progress, in order to make the final task more manageable.
- With *qualitative* coding, a single item is permitted to be coded in more than one category in order to permit cross-referencing and the generation of several hypotheses.

- Individual unstructured interviews are expensive and time-consuming.
- The advantages of unstructured approaches are that more complex issues can be probed, answers can be clarified, and in-depth, as well as sensitive, information elicited.
- The disadvantages of unstructured approaches are that the data are time-consuming and difficult to collect and analyse.

Key questions

1 Describe the main sampling methods for qualitative interviews.
2 What interviewer skills are needed for unstructured interviewing?
3 What types of questions are asked in unstructured interviewing?
4 Outline the advantages and disadvantages of unstructured interviewing.
5 Explain the principles of content analysis.

Key terms

content analysis
convenience sampling
cultural interviews
framework approach
in-depth interviews
interpretive sociology
interviewer bias
life grid
life history
narrative format
naturalistic enquiry

oral history
process analysis
purposive sampling
reactive effects
semiotics
snowballing
spatial behaviour
testimony studies
theoretical sampling
unstructured interviews

Recommended reading

Bryant, A. and Charmaz, K.C. (2010) Grounded theory in historical perspective: an epistemological account, in K.C. Charmaz and A. Bryant (eds) *The SAGE Handbook of Grounded Theory*. London: Sage, pp. 31–57.

Carter, S. and Henderson, L. (2005) Approaches to qualitative data collection in social science, in A. Bowling and S. Ebrahim (eds) *Handbook of Health Research Methods: Investigation, Measurement and Analysis*. Maidenhead: Open University Press.

Erlandson, D.A., Harris, E.L., Skipper, B.L. and Allen, S.D. (1993) *Doing Naturalistic Inquiry: A Guide to Methods*. Newbury Park, CA: Sage.

Fielding, J. (1993) Coding and managing data, in N. Gilbert (ed.) *Researching Social Life*. London: Sage.

Kitzinger, J. (1995) Introducing focus groups, *British Medical Journal*, 311: 299–302.

Minichiello, V., Aroni, R. and Hays, T.N. (2008) *In-depth Interviewing*. Melbourne, VIC: Pearson Education Australia.

Rubin, H.J. and Rubin, I.S. (1995) *Qualitative Interviewing: The Art of Hearing Data*. Thousand Oaks, CA: Sage.

Silverman, D. (1993) *Interpreting Qualitative Data: Methods for Analysing Talk, Text and Interaction*. London: Sage.

Focus groups

Chapter contents

Introduction

A focus group is a group of people, brought together, to discuss, or focus on, a specific research issue, or issues, to enhance understanding, using open-ended questions. They are 'focused' because the process involves a collective activity (Kitzinger and Barbour 1999). Group discussions are frequently mislabelled as focus groups. It should be noted that the essence of a focus group is the interaction between the participants to generate the data. Earl-Slater (2004) described good practice for focus groups as having:

- a clear objective;
- clear and consistent principles;
- a predefined time scale;
- good management;
- accurate recordings of progress, events, decisions;
- a safe environment in which to share thoughts, feelings and impressions; and being non-threatening;
- a clearly defined end-point;
- knowledge from the outset about what will be done with the information obtained.

Focus group interviews

Focus group interviews are held with small groups of people in the target group of interest. They are encouraged to interact with each other and the group leader in addressing (focusing on) the issues of interest. Focus group interviews follow an *interpretive approach*, where the aim is to analyse how people understand their social worlds and the meanings of events.

They aim to explore specific issues. They have the advantage of making use of group dynamics to stimulate discussion, gain insights and generate ideas in order to pursue a topic in greater depth. They can be used to provide a 'safe' discussion in which to explore sensitive subjects which might be perceived as embarrassing or difficult to discuss during personal interviews (e.g. sexual relationships), and to provide a context in which groups can generate and explore their own questions, discuss and 'make sense' of their attitudes and ideas. They can be used to examine not only what people think, but how they think and why they think in that way, their understandings and priorities (see Kitzinger 1995). It is a useful technique for exploring cultural values, and beliefs about health and disease. The group processes can help people to explore their views and generate questions in ways that they would find more difficult in face-to-face interviews (Kitzinger 1996). These methods are popular in communications and media studies, market research, health promotion research among different cultural groups (e.g. explorations of concepts of illness causation, prevention, and health knowledge) and action research. In the case of the latter, investigators are keen to make participants feel that they are an active part of the research process (Kitzinger 1996).

Group composition

Confidentiality is not obtained in group settings, and the presence of others can be inhibiting to some respondents. Groups have to be carefully balanced in relation to the age, sex and ethnic status of respondents: for example, if young people, women, or people in ethnic minority groups are in disproportionately fewer numbers in the group they may feel socially constrained and not contribute freely to the discussion. It may sometimes be necessary to have single-sex groups in similar age ranges in order for the atmosphere to be permissive and relaxed. Market researchers aim for members who do not know each other, though in social and health research in local communities group anonymity is not necessarily aimed for (depending on the topic).

There are no guidelines about the number of focus groups to aim for. Many investigators aim for between 6 and 20, but this is dependent on the complexity of the topic. A focus group will typically contain between about 6 and 12 participants, and a group leader (e.g. the investigator) who uses an unstructured guide (topic/question list) to stimulate and guide discussion. The leader needs to be skilled at creating a relaxed atmosphere, leading group discussions and handling conflict, as well as drawing out passive participants. Groups usually last between about one and two hours, and a comfortable environment is provided with refreshments. Some investigators ask participants to participate in games: card sorting exercises (e.g. with statements printed on them), specially designed board games, 'cake cutting' or coloured disc games, for example, in groups about health priorities and allocation of resources. The groups are tape-recorded, and some are video-recorded. The investigator also makes observational notes during the meetings.

Appropriate topics for focus groups

Market and media researchers are the most skilled in this technique, and they generally produce the richest and most insightful reports. However, they do not always provide the rich data hoped for. For example, Mulholland (1985) explored the following hypothesis using focus group techniques on the topic of advertisements promoting smoking: 'the use of . . . surreal imagery can be a very powerful way of attracting consumers' attention but it should be used with great care. The images are often very emotionally charged and can sometimes harm rather than help the advertiser's cause.' Two focus groups were used, comprising six and five members, for group discussions lasting for two to three hours each. One group was composed of men aged 18–24 and the other of women aged 18–24. Comfortable chairs, alcohol and snacks were provided in order to create a pleasant and relaxed atmosphere. The members were shown a series of advertisements and were encouraged to talk freely and give their emotional and instinctive responses to them. It was reported that the women were less inhibited in their responses than the men, who were more limited to 'surface rationalisations' and did not want to appear foolish in front of their peers. It was concluded that the groups were not totally successful at probing beneath rational consciousness, and consequently the investigator decided to conduct supplementary in-depth one-to-one interviews with a small sample ($n = 5$). The investigator concluded that this was the most fruitful method, as it was easier to overcome inhibitions and obtain deeper meanings on a one-to-one basis. Some of the examples cited are shown in Box 18.1.

Box 18.1 Benson & Hedges poster 'Venus Fly Trap'

This poster is visually very striking. It shows what appear to be flesh-eating plants in an abandoned greenhouse, with one of them grasping a packet of B & H. The picture had a grotesque appeal, but even superficial analysis revealed disquieting associations.

'It's weird. They live on live food, don't they . . . insects and things like that. If you think about it, that's quite morbid, because you could say the same about a packet of cigarettes – they live on human beings and it will eventually kill them' (woman, 18–24, smoker).

They were likened to Triffids which survive even when human life is extinct. 'Everything else is dead and disregarded and abandoned and these plants still live on' (woman, 18–24, smoker).

'It's a peculiar plant. It could be after the nuclear war . . . man has disappeared but you still get the packet of cigarettes' (man, 18–24, smoker).

The authors reported that the committed smokers, who did not wish to question their reasons for smoking and the health issues involved, did not associate these images of death and destruction with the cigarettes. The less committed smokers who wanted to shake off their addiction did relate the imagery to the harmful effects of cigarettes and were disturbed by it. These differences which were perceived between committed and non-committed smokers were repeatedly demonstrated in relation to other smokers' advertisements, and the authors reported that the value of the qualitative one-to-one techniques in eliciting these was apparent.

The success of the method will depend on the topic. Bowling (1993b) found that focus group methods worked well and provided the richest data in relation to the public's views of priorities for health services, and, in contrast to the above example, were less inhibiting for respondents than one-to-one interviews. This was because respondents in the latter situation often appeared to feel embarrassed in front of the interviewer if they found the exercise difficult. In a group situation members could see that everyone found the exercise difficult and that this was more apparently 'expected' and 'allowed'. Long silences while thinking the issues through were easier in a group situation, but could turn into awkward silences in front of an interviewer in a one-to-one situation. See Box 18.2 for another example of the use of focus groups with older people and their carers.

Box 18.2 Example of focus group methods: older people and their carers

Bagshaw and Unell (1997) used a series of focus group methods with older people and their carers in order to inform their programme on the research and development of outcomes for community care. Their report is informative in relation to the range of approaches used with the focus groups, and the rich data that resulted. The objectives of the focus groups included determination of how easy or difficult it is for people to think about the concept of outcomes; identification of the concepts and words that are meaningful and acceptable to people when talking about outcomes; exploration of people's understandings of common words and phrases used in community care documents; to find out what service users and carers expect community services to achieve for themselves as individuals; and to obtain views about the priorities that users and carers attach to particular outcomes. They conducted nine focus groups in three stages (levels) in different locations, each one including a group for carers, a group for older people, and a group for people with physical impairment (average attendance 8.4 people). The different levels allowed for a rural–urban spread and also permitted the researchers to reflect on each stage and refine their methods. The first-level groups were asked to reflect on the subject of outcomes in response to direct questions (e.g. 'What do support and services enable you to do that you could not otherwise do?'), and asked to dream about an ideal world and the ideal help or support they would get, and finally to prioritise the help and support. The second and third levels used a more indirect approach with the use of cameos (short case studies of an imaginary person in the situation of a carer/older person/person with a physical impairment). The participants in the second level were asked to identify good and not so good aspects of the situation and to suggest improvements, and to imagine what the person's life might be like in six months' time if improvements had been made. This was followed by brainstorming techniques based on the meanings and significance (to them) of words used in official documents about community care. The third level also used the cameos to identify the good and not so good aspects of the circumstances and then worked in small groups with a list of words and phrases with the aim of choosing the most important in relation to the person in the cameo. This was followed by a discussion about whether the choice would have been the same or different if they had applied their own circumstances, and about the most important two concepts (Bagshaw and Unell 1997).

QOL-S domain	Focus group members' suggestions
Relations with other people	
Relationships with parents, siblings and other relatives – communicating, visiting and helping. Close relationships with spouse or significant others. Close friends.	The different items in this domain were regarded as overlapping with each other. For example, 'Close friends' could also be relatives and other siblings. Satisfaction with sexual life was not explicit in this instrument.
Social; community and civic activities	
Helping and encouraging others, participating in organisations and volunteering.	Social activities were regarded as the same as cultural ones, such as visiting museums and exhibitions, because society offers these activities. One of the items described two very different areas: helping or encouraging others and participating in organisations. Volunteering was not a familiar activity for Swedish people.

Source: Leidberg et al. (2012).

Table 18.1 Selection of focus group participants' suggestions for alterations to the quality of life questionnaire-Swedish version (QOL-S)

Focus group methods have also been used to develop measurement scales and to test their content validity. Leidberg et al. (2012) used five focus group interviews with women to examine the validity of the Swedish version of the Quality of Life (QoL) scale. Eighteen out of 25 who were invited agreed to take part. The opening question was 'What does quality of life mean to you?', and later the participants were asked about specific domains in the measure. Their analysis of the transcripts showed that participants' perceptions of QoL were congruent with the measurement scale, though further attention to translated items and overlapping items was needed. Some of the emerging suggestions reported are shown in Table 18.1.

Weaknesses of focus groups

Weaknesses of focus groups include possible unrepresentativeness of the target group, members' fear of expressing certain views, and dominance of views by certain group members. These issues need to be managed by a skilled, trained facilitator (or moderator). Earl-Slater (2004) summarised the potential pitfalls of focus group methods, including:

- bad management;
- use of amateur moderators, or moderators who have vested interests in the topic (can bias the group);
- no particular focus;
- failure to brief moderator of true purpose of the group;
- too small or large a group;

- too much is attempted in a single session;
- insufficient flexibility to cope with all issues emerging in the group.

Methods of analysis

The methods of analysis are the same as for in-depth interviews. The methods include category analysis (e.g. content analyses), narrative format and paralinguistic behaviour analyses, depending on the aims and scope of the study (see Pfaffenberger 1988; J. Fielding 1993) and the earlier discussion on analysis of unstructured, in-depth interviews).

Content analysis

With a content analysis, the key themes and concepts are identified in the transcripts (or on the computer), and these are categorised. The process is the same as with content analyses of unstructured interviews, except that discussions within groups are compared.

A frequency count of the number of issues and views expressed by type can be undertaken, taking into account tone and non-verbal behaviour (bearing in mind that frequency does not necessarily equate with social significance). Kitzinger (1995) recommended that the content analysis should make full use of focus group data, and use special categories for certain types of narrative (e.g. questions, jokes, anecdotes, censorship, changes of mind, deferring to the opinions of others). She also recommended the use of contextual illustrations of the conversations, rather than isolated quotations.

In the example of the exploration of community care outcomes given earlier, content analysis was applied to the transcripts of the audio-recordings of the meetings, and the authors provided interpretations of the emerging themes alongside their presentation of verbatim examples, for example:

> Being in control was a concept that triggered lively debate among the people with physical impairment, most of which concerned positive assertions about the need to control your life. This was in marked contrast to the older people. One older person at level 2 said that control was a horrible word, especially when talking about warden-controlled accommodation. Being in control of people doing the housework was important to the people with physical impairment at level 1: 'She does what I want her to do and not what I don't want. You know, I mean I am in control'; 'I am in charge. That's all what matters is that I am in charge' . . .
>
> (Bagshaw and Unell 1997)

Exploration of meanings and concepts in narratives

Sometimes focus group transcripts can be presented to illustrate quantitative data. For example, Bowling (1993b) undertook both quantitative questionnaire surveys and qualitative focus group discussion in order to measure the public's priorities for health services. The rich qualitative data were used to shed light on why people made the priority ratings they did. For example, people ranked life-saving treatment, particularly for children, as high. The group discussions among community groups in the same area as the study led to an understanding of why people made these ratings (see Box 18.3). Reviews of the use of focus groups have been conducted, though generally concluding that studies are weak (see Box 18.4).

Box 18.3 Focus group on priority setting in health services

Group A

Respondent 2 (R2): If there is a hundred to one chance that they may survive, they should be given that chance.

R3: You give them that chance.

R4: Whilst there's a life . . .

R3: That mental patient is still alive. Him being mental is not going to kill him. That unit for that baby will help it.

R5: But it says here they are unlikely to survive.

R3: Yes, but without it, it's not going to, you've made the decision . . . If the person is still alive and not in pain, then they've still got a good quality of life, whereas if you've got a person who could die without treatment, you've got to give that person a chance to live. You haven't got the right, there's only one person who's got the right to say 'No, you don't live' and He's up there.

R5: If a child is really unlikely to survive it really does seem a bit naive to plough a lot of money into it.

Box 18.4 Reviews of use of focus groups in research

Webb and Kevern (2001) searched nursing databases on the reported use of focus groups in research. They found that the greatest use was with service development projects, and that most reports were relatively unsophisticated in their use of the method. In particular, the stated use of content analysis and grounded theory was not rigorous; there were incompatibilities between stated adoption of phenomenological perspectives and approaches to focus group research and analysis; and participants' interaction, while stated to be a benefit of the method, was rarely reported or discussed. They reported that some authors referred to using grounded theory as a method for data analysis, though there was no indication of using concurrent data collection and analysis, as the method requires. With grounded theory, themes arise from the data, rather than being predetermined by a research question. Data should be subjected to constant comparative analysis, as data collection, using theoretical sampling, is ongoing. Theoretical sampling is used to collect further data to corroborate or otherwise the analyses, and elaborate on the categories developed. Strauss and Corbin (1990, p. 23) stated that a grounded theory is one that is 'discovered, developed, and provisionally verified through systematic data collection and analysis of data pertaining to that phenomenon'. They regarded data collection, its analysis and emerging theories as having a reciprocal relationship. Kitzinger (1994) also, in a review of over 40 reports of use of focus groups, stated that none concentrated on the conversations between participants, and few cited quotations from more than one participant at a time. In sum, the focus group method is only useful if applied appropriately, conducted and analysed rigorously.

Summary of main points

- Focus groups are interviews with small groups of people who are encouraged to interact with the group leader and talk to each other in addressing (focusing on) the issues of interest.
- Focus groups have to be carefully composed and balanced in relation to the characteristics of respondents to prevent people from feeling socially constrained.
- Focus group interviews follow an interpretive approach where the aim is to analyse how people understand their social worlds and the meanings of events.
- The advantages of such approaches are that complex issues can be probed.
- The disadvantages are that the data are time-consuming and difficult to collect and analyse, and there are greater opportunities for interviewer/facilitator bias to intervene.

Key terms

content analysis
convenience sampling

focus groups

Recommended reading

Bloor, M., Frankland, J., Thomas, M. and Robson, K. (2001) *Focus Groups in Social Research.* London: Sage.

Kitzinger, J. (1995) Introducing focus groups, *British Medical Journal*, 311: 299–302.

CHAPTER 19

Mixed research approaches

Chapter contents

Introduction

The complementary use of combined (mixed) qualitative and quantitative research designs in a study was relatively common before the development and increasing use of statistics; it is again increasing in popularity. Creswell and Plano Clark (2007) defined mixed methods as the combination of quantitative and qualitative approaches in order to provide a better understanding of research problems than either approach alone. Such research provides strengths that offset the weaknesses of quantitative and qualitative research when used alone; more comprehensive evidence about the research issue; and more comprehensive answers, and also encourages the use of multiple paradigms. They classified mixed methods into four main types: triangulated, embedded, explanatory and exploratory research (see Box 19.1). Mixed methods address issues of what works, and with what effect, as well as questions relating to magnitude of effect.

Box 19.1 Main types of mixed methods

Triangulation: to obtain different but complementary data on the same topic to best understand the research problem.

Embedded: one data set plays a supportive, secondary role in research based primarily on the other data type.

Explanatory: a two-stage mixed methods design where qualitative data helps to explain or build upon initial quantitative results.

Exploratory: the results of the first method (qualitative) help to develop or form the basis of the second method (quantitative).

(Creswell and Plano Clark 2007)

As well as using different methods to complement each other (drawing on the strengths of each method, on the basis that each has different weaknesses and strengths), there have long been advocates of the use of what has generally been termed 'triangulated methods' (in order to minimise research bias and enhance the validity of the results by testing the consistency of findings obtained by different methods). The investigation of complex or sensitive issues in health care can benefit from a more flexible, mixed methods approach. For example, Bowling and colleagues (Bowling *et al.* 1991; Clark and Bowling 1989, 1990) used structured survey, randomised controlled trial (RCT) and non-participant observation methods to measure quality of life for older people in nursing homes versus long-stay hospital wards. While the structured measures were found to be insensitive to differences between the institutionalised older people in each setting, the observations supported marked differences between the two settings. Moreover, while experimental designs may provide information on whether interventions work, they do not always shed light on *why* they work. Mixed methods research offers the potential to obtain deeper understandings of people and events. At RAND, in the USA, Gonzalez Morganti *et al.* (2013) used mixed qualitative and quantitative research methods in order to develop a more complete picture of how emergency departments contributed to the US health care system, and their use for non-emergency conditions. Their approach was primarily quantitative analysis (using routine hospital data, health insurance data, patient and clinician surveys), supplemented by qualitative interviews and focus groups with emergency department and other clinicians. Their use of several methods provided context and explanations for the main observations, particularly the way the departments served a wide range of societal roles.

There is a debate about the validity of the process of mixing qualitative and quantitative methods given that each methodology is derived from opposing philosophical backgrounds. There are some social scientists who adhere more rigidly to either deductive or inductive philosophies, and who regard the combined use of qualitative and quantitative techniques as 'invalid', or 'contradictory'. There may also be a danger that qualitative research, when conducted in quantitative research environments, becomes little better than 'research with quotes'. However, as Adamson (2005) argued, in her description of the philosophical perspectives of combined designs, while each approach emerged from different epistemological positions, they have achieved some independence from their roots. The common distinctions between qualitative and quantitative designs, and their polar philosophical assumptions include inductive versus deductive research, individualism versus collectivism, constructivism versus positivism, researcher control versus participatory, and natural versus artificial research settings. For further details of these, the range of typologies of mixed methods, and examples of the use of mixed methods, readers are referred to Adamson (2005).

This chapter describes *realistic evaluation*, which uses a mixed methods research design. It also describes specific approaches which generally involve the use of a combination of qualitative and quantitative approaches to data gathering ('mixed methods research'). For example, case studies may use triangulated methods comprising observation, unstructured interviews, document research and structured questionnaires. Consensus methods involve a combined semi-structured and structured approach in relation to questionnaires, semi-structured and structured meetings of experts, and quantitative summaries. Action research also combines unstructured group meetings, focus groups, unstructured interviews, document research and structured questionnaires. Finally, document research can be quantitative, as in the analysis of vital population statistics by demographers, and/or qualitative, as in some historical research (e.g. oral histories), or a combination of both approaches, as in media analyses, diary analysis and historical research more generally. The different methods are described in Parts 19.1–19.4.

19.1 Realistic evaluation and blurring of boundaries

Realistic evaluation is an interpretive orientation, based on critical realism towards research methods, situated between positivism and relativism. It aims to unpick the mechanisms whereby interventions or programmes work. The effectiveness of these is not dependent on simple outcomes. The framework aims to understand the mechanisms through which interventions produce change; the social context which triggers these mechanisms; and to develop predictions about the patterns of outcomes, according to the context and mechanisms triggered (Pawson and Tilley 2007). It uses a *mixed methods approach,* which holds that using more than one method within a research project produces a more complete picture of the research phenomena. Thus, it is a good example of the *blurring* of boundaries between qualitative and quantitative methods. Realistic evaluation is based on the philosophy of realism, which acknowledges that social or health interventions are embedded in complex, multiple social systems, within which social structures, and its layers, interact to form social contexts. In effect,

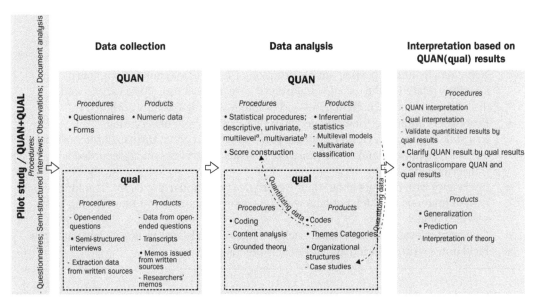

Figure 19.1: Summary of realistic evaluation, with embedded quantitative methods (QUAN) and supportive qualitative (qual) mixed methods design

Source: Pommier *et al.* (2010).

relationships between variables are not fixed, or necessarily replicable, but influenced by context. This approach holds that, as particular interventions may work differently in different situations, the investigator needs to find out what mechanisms work, in what conditions, and why, in order to lead to specific outcomes (Pawson and Tilley 1997). Pawson and Tilley argued that realistic evaluators should not simply be pluralists, but that methods should be chosen to test the hypotheses/propositions (i.e. rather than the investigator's personally preferred methods applied regardless). It is theory-driven, as it aims to understand and make explicit underlying assumptions about how interventions work. The mixed methods research design within a realistic evaluation approach, is one in which qualitative approaches have a supportive, secondary role to quantitative methods, and the approaches are combined throughout the research process and writing up. Pommier *et al.* (2010) used realistic evaluation, with a mixed methods embedded design whereby qualitative methods supported quantitative methods –'QUAN(qual)', to evaluate a health promotion programme in schools. Their summary of their embedded design is shown in Figure 19.1.

Realistic evaluation is an increasingly popular concept in social, educational and health promotion research, though neglected in health services research, yet its principles would fit well with the evaluation of complex clinical interventions in health care. (See section on complex interventions in Chapter 10.) Few published examples exist of its use in practice, though methodological rules are emerging. Rycroft-Malone *et al.* (2010) applied a realistic evaluation approach to the study of clinical protocol-based care, and report several examples of 'what works for whom, how and in what circumstances'. They used a combination of methods, including those derived from ethnography. These are summarised in Box 19.2.

Box 19.2 Summary of combination of methods used in realistic evaluation by Rycroft-Malone *et al.* (2010)

- Non-participant and participant observation of nursing and multi-disciplinary activities related to the use of standardised care approaches. Observations and discussions recorded in field notes and/or audio-recorded as appropriate.
- Post-observation interviews guided by issues arising from observations.
- Key stakeholder interviews exploring views in general about the use, influences on use, and impact of standardised care approaches. Interviews audio-recorded and transcribed in full.
- Interviews with patients about their experiences of standardised care. Tracking of patient journeys in which patients were interviewed a number of times during their service contact.
- Review of relevant documentation, such as copies of guidelines, protocols, and pathways.
- Field notes written during and after each site visit.

19.2 Case studies

The study of single or small series of cases

A case is a single unit in a study (e.g. a person or setting, such as a clinic or hospital). A case study is a research method which focuses on the circumstances, dynamics and complexity of a single case, or a small number of cases. The numbers are necessarily small as the cases are intensively explored in-depth, retrospectively, currently and sometimes over time, through, for example, detailed observations, interviews and information from records. Multiple research methods are usually employed in order to investigate fully complex situations and to validate the findings (e.g. Sidell's 1995 case study of elderly people's understanding of health and illness combined qualitative interview methods, analysis of official statistics and policy analysis).

It is a valuable method for the study of complex social settings and is useful in the exploratory, early stages of research, and for generating hypotheses. It is also used as a biographical research method (i.e. unstructured interviews to obtain a narrative of a respondent's life), as well as by investigators with a phenomenological perspective (Stake 1995). Case study approaches have long been used by clinicians in relation to the understanding of disease.

Case studies on a small scale carry little financial cost, although larger case studies (e.g. of an organisation) over a period of time can be costly and time-consuming. They are often undertaken with a view to the single case(s) contributing to an understanding of wider situations, though the material they generate is not generalisable. The aim of the case study is to understand the case selected for study. Quantitative survey methods can be used subsequently to assess how typical the situations and/or organisations studied are. The case study, as with other qualitative approaches, is reliant on the skills of the investigator to interpret the data in a rigorous manner, rather than reporting selective perceptions. The approach to focus groups research also varies with the perspective of the investigator (Box 19.3).

Box 19.3 Yin's approach to case study research

Yin's (2003) approach to case study was based on a constructivist paradigm – that truth is relative and dependent on one's perspective. This paradigm 'recognizes the importance of the subjective individual meaning, but does not reject some notion of objectivity'. One of the advantages of this constructivist approach is the close collaboration between the researcher and the participant, while enabling participants to tell their stories, and describe their views of reality. This enables the researcher to better understand their actions. According to Yin (2003), a case study design should be considered when:

- the focus of the study is to answer 'how' and 'why' questions;
- the researcher cannot manipulate the behaviour of those involved in the study;
- the researcher wants to cover contextual conditions because of a belief they are relevant to the phenomenon under study; or
- the boundaries are not clear between the phenomenon and context.

Examples of case studies

Korman and Glennerster (1990) conducted a case study describing the administrative, financial and political activities leading to the closure of a large mental handicap hospital. This research was pursued for seven and a half years and involved the investigators undertaking observations (of meetings) and analysis of minutes, records of committee meetings and documents. The results of their analyses were fed back in interviews with key figures. The feedback process allowed the participants to correct and enlarge upon the investigators' accounts and for an agreed 'collaborative' version to be produced, which was based on 'a collaborative understanding of events'. Their report is a mixture of quantitative data (e.g. descriptive information about patients, staffing levels, ward closures and financial cost data) and qualitative descriptions.

Bury (1988) used a case study approach to present material from his study of 30 people with arthritis, all of whom were interviewed at least twice. His unstructured interview schedule covered the experience of the onset of the condition and development of the illness, its impact on work and home life, and the process of seeking medical help. He used the case study approach to illustrate some of the processes involved, and also the collective data for the analysis (e.g. to analyse the impact of the illness on social relationships). Some sections from the opening of one of his case studies are shown in Box 19.4 in illustration of the case approach adopted.

Box 19.4 Legitimisation and chronic illness – the case of Mrs M

Mrs M lived in a Manchester suburb with her husband and two children, both of whom were in their late teens. She was 46 years of age at the time of the first interview and had worked for some years as a telephone operator. During the previous five years, she told me, she had been to her GP from time to time with various problems, indicating some form of rheumatism. But these had not been interpreted by her doctor or herself as meaning that she had a specific or serious arthritic complaint. On one occasion she had experienced pain in her big toe, and had thought she might be suffering from bunions. This was dismissed by her GP although no alternative explanation was offered. Subsequently she reported pains in her knees and had been prescribed four aspirins a day on the general understanding that she might have a touch of rheumatism . . . Her early visits to the GP gave her no grounds for further thought about the problem.

But the symptoms did not entirely disappear. As time went on, she noticed that her body was beginning to fail her. She said:

> I'd say it started properly about 18 months ago. I noticed that it was awkward to carry bags, shopping bags. I think the very first thing was my knees. I felt as though they were going to give way when I was going up and down stairs. There are three flights at work. Well, I'm on the third floor, so if the lift wasn't working I had to walk up and this is how I noticed it. And also I never used to wait for the lift coming down, I used to always run down. I had to stop because I felt as though I was going to fall.

Even so, Mrs M kept trying to minimise the problem in her mind. When I asked her what she thought was happening she said, 'I didn't think anything really, I just never thought anything.' Then her elbows and one of her shoulders began to ache. She found she was knocking herself painfully and couldn't bear carrying a shoulder bag. And this made her think that it was something more than just her previous 'rheumatic' symptoms. Their severity and persistence began to be worrying. Still, she hung on to a view of herself as basically healthy (as most people with chronic illness do). She did not want to see herself crossing the dividing line, even though her healthy self-image was becoming difficult to sustain.

She stated that she consulted her GP again. This time he began to consider that she might have a specific rheumatic condition and indeed the word 'rheumatoid' seems to have been introduced at this point . . . Mrs M said she was dismayed to hear him use this term, but because it was couched in such a vague context she hoped its use signified less than she feared.

(Bury 1988)

A case study approach was also used to examine types of decision-making among 12 nursing students, and the factors influencing their decision-making (Baxter and Rideout 2006). The researchers chose a case study design because the case was the decision-making of nursing students, but the case could not be considered without the context of the nursing school, and its clinical and classroom settings in which decision-making skills were developed and used. Inductive analysis revealed three key encounters that demonstrated students' decision-making: encounters with the patients, nursing staff, and clinical tutor, and each showed emotion- and also knowledge-based responses to situations. This information had potential implications for curriculum development.

The analysis

The case study approach is usually based on unstructured interviews and, where appropriate, observations and document analyses. The methods for these are described below and in Chapters 16 and 17. The methods of analysis are those belonging to the particular methods used. What does differ is the presentation of the results. The traditional style of the research report (statement of the problem, literature review, research design, data-gathering, analysis, conclusions) does not suit the case study. Stake (1995) suggested that the report of a case study should follow three stages: (1) a chronological or biographical description of the case; (2) the investigator's approach to understanding and investigating the case; and (3) a description of each, in turn, of the major components of the case. Vignettes, which describe particular episodes, should be included in the report.

19.3 Consensus methods

Methods for establishing and developing consensus

Methods are increasingly being used to establish the extent of consensus, and in some cases to develop it, in areas of uncertainty in clinical medicine and health policy, when there is a lack of definitive evidence about the effectiveness and appropriateness of health care interventions.

There are three main methods of establishing consensus views: (1) the Delphi method; (2) consensus development panels; and (3) nominal group processes. These methods are often used in combination and aim to produce quantified estimates of consensus through the use of a mixture of quantitative and qualitative techniques. There can be problems of selection bias with these techniques. For example, those experts willing to participate may not be representative of the total population targeted. This is a potential problem because the type of participants affects the results. The methods have been described by Fink *et al.* (1984), Jones and Hunter (1996) and Murphy *et al.* (1998).

There is debate about the validity and reliability of consensus methods, and no agreement about which method is the most appropriate (Jones and Hunter 1996; Murphy *et al.* 1998). Current opinion appears to be that the results of consensus development methods should be interpreted cautiously, and tested for their validity against observations.

Delphi technique

The Delphi technique is described as a qualitative method (Earl-Slater 2004), using open-ended questions, to obtain the ideas or attitudes of a number of people anonymously. With Delphi methods participants do not meet others to discuss the topic, or know what each other's responses are. A large number of individuals across diverse locations and areas of expertise can be included anonymously, thus avoiding bias from group interactions and domination by one or a few experts. It preserves individuals' identities and is an economical method of contacting large numbers of people.

The method includes cycles of feedback by post or internet/email, rather than face-to-face discussion. It is a structured process using a series of questionnaires rounds to collect information. Rounds are continued where there is still potential for obtaining further information, and until group consensus is reached. For example, experts may be sent a questionnaire containing several open-ended questions about their ideas

Points to consider	Recommendations for planning and using the Delphi procedure	Recommendations for reporting the Delphi procedure
Questionnaire for the first round	Define the study objective and what you expect of participants. Are the selection criteria appropriate for the study objective? If the objective is to develop a new QI and to evaluate whether an indicator has the appropriate characteristics for the concept being assessed, use validity as the selection criterion. If the objective is to evaluate the availability in medical records of information relevant to a QI, use feasibility as the selection criterion. Use a 1–9 Likert rating scale and define the steps on the scale clearly (e.g. indicate what the lowest and highest ratings mean). Allow the panel to comment and to add QIs. Define consensus and criteria for stopping the Delphi procedure.	Study objective, method for QI selection, number of QIs in the first questionnaire, criteria for QI selection, how questions were formulated, and definition of consensus.
Experts	Create a heterogeneous group of experts (healthcare professionals, informal caregivers, patients). Ask the potential panel participants about their willingness to participate; send an information letter explaining the Delphi procedure and benefits from participation; include an agreement form with the letter. Invite a very large number of experts, if possible from different countries.	Composition and characteristics of the panel, number of participants (diagram of participant flow), response rate for each round, whether special techniques were used to invite participants, and geographic scope of the Delphi procedure.
Sending questionnaires	Use two methods (Internet and mail) to target as many people as possible and to increase the response rate.	Report the method(s) used to send the questionnaires.
Next rounds	Construct the next questionnaires based on the results of the preceding rounds. Exclude QIs for which there was no consensus. Send each participant a personalized questionnaire with: • Quantitative group results (median, minimal, and maximum ratings) • Qualitative feedback: abstract of panel members' comments • The participant's own response to illustrate position versus the group	Flow of QIs with the QIs eliminated and added at each round. Method used to inform the participants of the results of previous rounds.

(continued)

| Final round | If agreement is reached among panel members: End the Delphi procedure. When reaching a consensus is difficult or consensus is unclear, a physical meeting is recommended. | Report the number of rounds whether a meeting was held (and if there was a meeting, what the participants did and who attended), duration of the Delphi procedure, results for each QI score and list of selected QIs. If possible, include a copy of the questionnaires in an appendix. |

Source: Boulkedid *et al.* (2011).

Table 19.1 Guidance for using and reporting Delphi procedures performed to select health care quality indicators (QIs)

and experiences of the topic in question. Their responses would be compiled into a questionnaire under a limited number of topic headings or statements that is then recycled back to the experts, asking them to rank their level of agreement with them. The rankings are then summarised in another questionnaire and fed back to the participants, who are asked again to rank their level of agreement. These re-rankings are analysed to assess the degree of consensus. If a substantial amount of disagreement remains, then a further cycle of feedback and re-rankings may ensue. An example is Moscovice *et al.*'s (1988) use of the method to establish health priorities. The Delphi procedure is valuable for achieving a consensus about issues where none existed previously.

Earl-Slater (2004) summarised the questions that arise with Delphi methods as:

- Who to include and how to include them.
- How to keep participants distant from any group pressures.
- The topic.
- How to collate responses.
- How to manage and moderate the process.
- The time scales involved.
- Internal rewards for participation.
- External rewards beyond the participants.
- How many waves to conduct.
- Whether additional questions emerge as a result of the Delphi exercise (rather than the primary question being changed).
- What to do with the information obtained.

Findings of a systematic review of use of the Delphi method for selecting health care quality indicators suggested the need to improve the use and reporting of this technique (Boulkedid *et al.* 2011). Table 19.1 summarises the authors' resulting guidance for using and reporting Delphi procedures performed to select health care quality indicators (QIs).

Consensus development panels

This is sometimes called the consensus development conference. The method involves organising a meeting with panels of experts in a particular field, or panels of lay people, or mixed, brought together to discuss specific topics, usually with the aim of improving understanding of an area or developing a consensus. For example, it is a process whereby experts in a specific area meet to determine whether or not a consensus exists about criteria of good practice. A facilitator is required who is either an expert on the topic or a non-expert who has credibility with the participants. The process can be expensive and requires a high level of organisation. The method is usually used to assess health care technologies by large health care organisations, government organisations and bodies representing medical doctors (Perry and Kalberer 1980; Stocking et al. 1991).

Nominal group process

Formal consensus methods such as the nominal group technique are often used as part of guideline development. This method is also known as the 'expert panel'. With this method, the experts who are participating in the process are asked to decide on their individual views on the topic before meeting. For example, they rank the appropriateness of a health care intervention on a numerical Likert scale (e.g. from 0 ('never indicated') to 9 ('always indicated')). The results are summarised and presented to participants at the subsequent meeting, sometimes along with a review of the relevant literature. At this meeting they discuss the rankings and their differences. They are asked to re-rank the issues in the light of the group's discussion. The final analyses of the re-rankings are fed back to the participants. A facilitator is also required for this (see Box 19.5). Examples of its use in clinical medicine include the consensus panel approach to establishing appropriateness criteria for cholecystectomy and for prostatectomy (Hunter et al. 1994).

Box 19.5 Example of a combined Delphi and nominal group process method for establishing appropriateness criteria: the Rand method of developing appropriateness criteria and its use in utilisation review

Investigators at Rand in the USA developed a systematic method for generating criteria of appropriateness that could be applied equally to health care interventions carried out in different institutions (Brook et al. 1986; Kahn et al. 1988). It has been clearly summarised by Hicks (1994).

Method

The method involves a review of the literature on effectiveness and current practice in relation to the intervention in question. This leads to the generation of a catalogue of indications for the intervention. Then a small panel of nine expert clinicians is appointed, each of whom is sent a copy of the review and the catalogue of indications. They are asked to rate the appropriateness of performing the procedure for each potential indication on a nine-point scale (1 = extremely inappropriate, 9 = extremely appropriate). Next the panel meets. They are each reminded of their own ratings and given an anonymous breakdown of the other panellists' ratings, followed by discussion of areas of disagreement, and then panellists anonymously re-rate the complete set of indications.

Analysis

In relation to each indication, the mean score and a measure of the panel's agreement are calculated. Where the mean score is between 1 and 3, and there is general agreement, then the indication is classified as inappropriate. Similarly, where the mean score is between 7 and 9 and there is general agreement, then the indication is classified as appropriate. Where the mean is between 4 and 6, or where there is disagreement among the members of the panel, then the indication is classified as equivocal.

Outcome

This method has been successfully applied in the USA, and has been used by many US health insurance companies in pre-intervention or pre-hospital admission reviews (e.g. as a condition for paying a medical fee, the companies require that doctors obtain prior approval before intervening on any patients insured with them), and its provider organisations also use it as a means of assessing the appropriateness of individual doctors' practices (Hicks 1994).

Criticisms

The method has been criticised for ignoring patients' and carers' preferences, over-estimating rates of inappropriateness, ignoring intuitive clinical assessments, relying on criteria of appropriateness that have been finalised by consensus rather than by scientific evidence, for applying a limited definition of appropriateness which does not take into account resources and the individuality of the patient, for not making the intended outcomes of care explicit in the definition of appropriateness, and for not making explicit which risks and benefits panellists took into account or ignored when making their judgements (see Hicks 1994, for a review). The latter omission makes it difficult for users of the appropriateness ratings to understand their meaning, and therefore impossible to judge whether the criteria are appropriate for use in their own practice. This has restricted its international adoption, despite the foundations of the criteria being based on scientific reviews of the research literature, and not just clinical practice. As Hicks (1994) concluded, '. . . although measures of appropriateness may seem to be objective, the process by which they are produced, although systematic, remains highly subjective'. An example of cultural differences has been provided by Brook *et al.* (1988). They pointed out that, for a patient with angina on mild exertion (class III), coronary artery bypass surgery was rated by a US panel to be appropriate, with a median rating of 7 on the nine-point scale of appropriateness. However, a panel of physicians and cardiologists in the UK rated the procedure as clearly inappropriate (median rating of 2/9). Similar cross-cultural differences have been found in neurology (Hopkins *et al.* 1989).

The analysis

The results from these consensus methods are not always straightforward to analyse, and the level of agreement obtained may depend on whether or not the views of outliers were included or excluded (e.g. see Scott and Black 1991). Jones and Hunter (1996) and Murphy *et al.* (1998) have described the methods used to analyse and feed back the results of consensus methods. They point out that agreement with statements is usually summarised by using the median and measures of dispersion or spread of judgements (interquartile ranges), which are fed back to participants at each stage. The median is preferred to the mean as it is more robust to the effect of outliers. Jones and Hunter (1996) also described the rules that have been developed for the analysis of scaled data. For example, with a nine-point scale, scores 1–3 represent the region where participants feel intervention is not indicated; 4–6 represent the region of equivocality; and 7–9 represent the region where it is felt that intervention is indicated. Strict agreement is obtained if all rankings fall within *one* of these regions; a broad definition of agreement is obtained if ranks fall within *any* three-point region. Tests for whether extreme rankings lead to the misrepresentation of the final results involve the analysis of the rankings with the exclusion of one extreme high and one extreme low ranking per statement.

Hutchings *et al.* (2005) assessed the effect of design features and clinical and social cues in formal consensus development processes. They used a factorial design to examine the appropriateness ratings of groups of GPs and mental health professionals in relation to four mental health interventions for three conditions. The groups differed in the provision or not of a systematic literature review, group composition, and realistic or idealistic assumptions about the health service resources available. Their analyses found the technique to be robust. Raine *et al.* (2004) also examined influences on group judgements in general practitioners and specialists, in relation to clinical appropriateness of mental health therapies in three medical conditions. They reported agreement with the research evidence for 51 per cent of 192 scenarios used. Agreement was more likely to be achieved if the group comprised only GPs, if a literature review was provided, or if the evidence was consistent with doctors' beliefs. Murphy *et al.* (1998), on the basis of an early review of the literature, presented the issues which require consideration, such as group composition, the influence of the way the information is presented on decision-making, the structuring of interactions, and the analysis.

19.4 Action research and rapid appraisal techniques

Action research

Action research is undertaken by participants in social situations to improve their practices and their understanding of them. The method was designed to study social systems with an aim of changing them (i.e. to achieve certain goals). It is a community-based method. Community-based action research has frequently been employed in a wide range of settings, from hospitals and health clinics to clubs, factories and schools. The method is used by teachers, social workers, doctors, nurses, community workers, and so on in their local working environments in order to define needs and problems, devise methods to deal with the problems and improve services. Examples include the investigations of people's health problems and behaviours by health professionals in an area, with the aim of developing appropriate treatment and preventive programmes (e.g. in relation to community health issues or health promotion projects).

Hart and Bond (1995) have described the history of action research, which, they point out, was a term coined by Lewin (1946), its founder, to describe a method of generating knowledge about a social system while simultaneously trying to change it. The stress of action research today has shifted from its early emphasis on rational social engineering to a method of community or organisational development by awareness-raising, empowerment (an ability to influence decision-making) and collaborative investigation between trained researchers, professionals (e.g. nurses and doctors) and lay people, with the help of designated mediators (facilitators). The revival of interest in action research stems from some disillusionment with the use of positivist methods of evaluation. Action researchers do not treat participants as subjects but empower them to act on their own behalf as active participants in making changes (Hart and Bond 1995).

Hart and Bond selected seven criteria which distinguish different types of action research, and which together distinguish action research from other methods. Action research:

1 is educative;
2 deals with individuals as members of social groups;
3 is problem-focused, context-specific and future-oriented;
4 involves a change intervention;
5 aims at improvement and involvement;
6 involves a cyclic process in which research, action and evaluation are interlinked;
7 is founded on a research relationship in which those involved are participants in the change process.

Action research is a popular technique for attempting to achieve improvements by auditing processes and critically analysing events. It is a critical, self-reflective, bottom-up and collaborative approach to enquiry that enables people to take action to resolve identified problems. Action research involves a participatory and consensual approach towards investigating problems and developing plans to deal with them. Although it uses the methods of social science, it does not treat people as 'subjects' of study: the research process is presented to lay people and professionals in an accessible way, and undertakes the research in a way that is user-friendly. This has the potential to lead to solutions that are appropriate for local communities, and to a local commitment to them.

Action research uses multiple research methods, most of which are qualitative, though some quantitative surveys may also form part of the process. It involves research in the field and close involvement with the key players in order to identify problems, implement reforms and audit or evaluate the consequences (e.g. in educational research and audit by managers in the health services). Action researchers often use focus group and in-depth interview methods, as they want participants to feel part of the decision-making, as well as standardised questionnaires. The information is usually gathered quickly and the overall approach to data-gathering is known as *rapid appraisal techniques*. These are described later, under 'Rapid appraisal'.

The phrase 'Look, think, act' has been coined to describe action research (Stringer 1996). By 'look', Stringer means that participants should define and describe the problem to be investigated and its context; by 'think', he means they should analyse and interpret the situation in order to develop their understanding of the problem; by 'act' he means that they should formulate solutions to the problem. He defines community-based action research in terms of a search for meaning:

> It provides a process or a context through which people can collectively clarify their problems and formulate new ways of envisioning their situations. In doing so, each participant's taken-for-granted cultural viewpoint is challenged and modified so that new systems of meaning emerge that can be incorporated in the texts – rules, regulations, practices, procedures, and policies – that govern our

professional and community experience. We come closer to the reality of other people's experience and, in the process, increase the potential for creating truly effective services and programs that will enhance the lives of the people we serve.

Stages of action research

Stringer (1996) proposed the following steps for 'setting the stage', 'looking', 'thinking' and 'acting'.

Setting the stage

Because action research attempts to engage local people in formulating solutions to identified problems, the investigator's role is that of facilitator in the process of investigating people's interpretations of the situation and problem, in developing negotiation and consensus, and in handling conflict. At the beginning of the project it is essential to identify the stakeholders, ensure they all know who else is involved in the project, its aims and events, and establish a positive climate of interaction and activity that all are involved in (e.g. doctors, nurses, managers, patients, the public, other key community figures and leaders). It is important to arrange meetings with people and to maintain regular contact, in order that they feel continuously involved and feel some ownership of the project. Facilitation and networking skills are essential. It is also important to find out from each person involved who else he or she thinks should be contacted and included in discussions. The groups, for example, can be encouraged to develop their own profiles, or lists, of the history of the setting or community; who are involved (e.g. nurses, doctors, community leaders, community workers, the local public) and relationships between them; what type of groups are involved (e.g. socio-economic groups, ethnic groups); and what resources are available and from whom. The investigator, in the role of the facilitator, must appear legitimate but neutral and non-threatening to all groups involved, and thus his or her role has to be carefully negotiated with each of the relevant social groups. The facilitator must not be seen to be closely associated with any particular group; members must be able to feel that they can talk to the facilitator freely and in the knowledge that their comments will not be passed on to other groups.

Looking

The facilitator must next enable participants jointly to describe the situation and the problem. Stringer (1996) suggests the following steps which the facilitator must take in this process: gathering information (e.g. by interviewing participants in each 'stakeholder group' about the group, events, the setting, and so on, using the techniques of unstructured interviewing; participating in the setting and observing activities and events, using the techniques of observation, and analysing documents); helping each 'stakeholding group' to develop a descriptive account of the problem and its context; working with the groups to develop a joint descriptive account. Stringer advised against the common practice in action research of calling public meetings on the issue of interest, because these are usually held on alien territories (e.g. schools, agency offices) and there is usually a poor turnout for them. Instead, he recommended that public meetings should only be organised once the stakeholder groups have met on neutral terms to clarify their positions. He pointed out that while larger projects will involve informal meetings, public meetings and the organisation of committee meetings to structure the implementation of plans and proposals (e.g. working parties, steering groups, agency, inter-agency and community committees), most smaller projects will require only inter-group meetings. These include: focus group meetings, where people with similar interests or agendas discuss specific issues; in-group forums, which are meetings of single interest or stakeholder groups to discuss specific issues; responsive informal meetings as needed; agency-specific meetings to enable employees to discuss common interests or agendas; community group meetings where members of the community meet for these discussions. There is usually a need to conduct these processes with relative speed, and this technique is called *rapid appraisal* (see below.)

Thinking

The facilitator next needs to organise meetings to enable participants to understand and interpret the situation. This may involve sending participants copies in advance of descriptive accounts developed during the previous stage. These are summarised at the meeting, and participants are organised into small groups (e.g. of six different stakeholders) to discuss the issues and negotiate their perspectives, which they summarise on charts, and present to other groups in a common session at the end. Follow-up activities are arranged, for example, to plan the next phase.

Acting

The solutions to the problem should be planned by all the 'stakeholder groups'. This involves the groups reviewing the issues and agreeing on their priorities. They can do this in small group meetings and then come together for common sessions. The next stage is the setting of goals, objectives and tasks on the basis of the priorities of members of each group, who then again come together for a plenary meeting. At the implementation stage there will be a need for support and assistance from the facilitator and continual reviewing of progress by the participants; at some stage, an evaluation of the project by the stakeholder groups may be required. These processes, together with the supportive role of the facilitator during these and the implementation stages, have again been described in detail by Stringer (1996). A useful toolkit for action research was compiled by Hart and Bond (1995), and includes: a self-assessment questionnaire designed to assist with thinking about the research problem and the proposed research; groupwork guidelines, factors the facilitator should consider, advice on starting programmes, ice-breaking games; ethical guidelines; advice on diary keeping for facilitators as a form of field notes, self-reflection and evaluating performance and progress; advice on evaluation (e.g. using basic records, local information, surveys and so on); and the use of structured attitude scales.

Action research usually aims to conduct the stages of the research fairly quickly, and then uses the techniques of rapid appraisal.

Rapid appraisal

Action researchers often use rapid appraisal techniques for the swift assessment of local views and perceptions of problems and needs. This is based on a combination of interviews with key people and group meetings (Ong *et al.* 1991). Rapid appraisal is a qualitative technique for community assessment. The aim is to gain insight quickly into the population of interest and into the community's own perspectives of its needs. It is usually undertaken within an action research programme which aims to translate the findings into areas for action (e.g. by health service managers or primary health care teams). It can be used to establish the foundations for an ongoing relationship between service purchasers, providers and the public (Pickin and St Leger 1993). The advantage of rapid appraisal is its greater *speed* in comparison with other methods. Interest in the use of the technique in relation to health needs in Britain has increased as a result of the NHS Management Executive's (1991) statement that purchasers of health care will need to discover and respond to the views of local people about the pattern and delivery of health services.

The scientific rigour and validity of the approach involve the use of triangulated research methods. The method involves working in the field with mainly qualitative approaches, in order to learn from local people, and includes an initial series of multidisciplinary meetings to examine the research questions and determine the methods; demographic profiles; semi-structured interviews with selected respondents; sometimes a postal survey; social and geographical mapping; concluding with workshops to summarise the findings (e.g. identified community needs in relation to health or social services) and agree priority areas for action (the action research programme). Thus data can be diverse and include existing written records, interviews with a range of local informants and observations in the neighbourhood.

Using rapid appraisal techniques to assess health needs of residents

Murray and Graham (1995) used rapid appraisal techniques to assess the health needs of residents living on a council estate (670 homes) in Edinburgh. They used rapid participatory appraisal techniques, which involved the collection of local data by a team consisting of a GP, a health visitor, two social workers and a community education worker. This team collected data from existing documents about the neighbourhood, made direct observations of the neighbourhood and conducted interviews and focus groups with key informants (community leaders, local residents selected to represent different age and social groups and with different health problems, and people with professional knowledge about the community because of their work). In addition, information held in the local general practice was collated (e.g. number of consultations, incidence of acute illnesses, hospital referrals, details of repeat prescribing), small area statistics were analysed (on hospital-based morbidity, births and deaths) and a postal survey on the health of 435 residents was carried out. As is often found in these exercises, the rapid appraisal exercises showed that the most important 'health needs' identified by people were outside the remit of the health service (e.g. a bus route into the estate, play areas for small children, a local supermarket). An example of the use of rapid appraisal methods in Latin America was to assess local needs, design the intervention and evaluate a food security programme. The exercise was described in detail, along with the processes of identifying and defining local concepts, and clarifying these (Bergeron 1999). The monitoring of progress of activities in relation to stated goals, and evaluation of overall impact was described, and is summarised below as:

- *Informants*: Beneficiaries of project activities.
- *Format*: Focus group session including 8–10 informants, held in a quiet, private area.
- *Materials*: Large chart prepared in advance, listing activities in rows, and whether each had an impact on income, food access, and food availability in columns. The last column is left for explaining reasons of impact or lack thereof.

The method of carrying out this exercise is:

- List the activities undertaken by the project in that community (e.g. obtained from community project officers, later validated with local informants in the village, to ensure that the activities noted in project paperwork indeed correspond to those deployed in the community).
- Considering each activity in turn, ask villagers whether this activity had the effect of increasing income, food access, or food availability in the community (taking care with definitions).
- Informants are asked about the reasons for the success (or failure) of the activity.
- The activities considered to be the most successful (in terms of villagers' priorities) are listed, followed by the less successful ones, and so on, until all the activities have been listed and ranked in relation to one another.
- This exercise is also undertaken with the technical staff in charge of the programme.
- Comparing assessments between project managers and beneficiaries validates the findings and provides a more complete and balanced evaluation of activities.
- Prior steps: Identify activities realised in this community with project staff.
- Validation: Compare beneficiary and project staff evaluations. Discuss discrepancies in joint discussions.

Examples of rapid appraisal carried out by health authorities and general practice teams within action research programmes are given by Ong and Humphris (1994). They also provided a guide to the steps in conducting rapid appraisal. They stated that the first step is preparation and the selection of the team to undertake the rapid appraisal. The second step is to hold a workshop (e.g. two days) with the aim of choosing a target area, to identify key questions based on information profiles and to choose respondents for study. Next is the fieldwork stage (e.g. interviews and analysis of the data), followed by a further workshop (e.g. a half-day) with the aim of deriving a list of needs. This is followed by a further fieldwork stage in which respondents are returned to and are asked to rank in priority the needs/issues compiled. Next is the analysis of this exercise and a workshop (e.g. a half-day) to discuss the results, prepare a feedback meeting and develop proposals. This is followed by an open meeting to formulate concrete plans for action, and then a final meeting to develop plans and assess actions.

Although the advantages of rapid appraisal include the potential to collect information quickly from local populations, and the involvement of local populations in planning and evaluation, there are inevitable limitations of the method. Apart from the intense and time-consuming nature of the fieldwork, analysis and ensuring public participation at each key stage, there is potential for bias and lack of generalisability where different groups of people and professionals are not adequately represented in interviews, and susceptibility to manipulation by informants; there may be researcher bias unless findings are analysed by independent individuals; lack of clear procedures for validation of findings; the data are limited due to the brief time frame of the research, and limited resources used. The training and skills of the research team are key to the quality of the information obtained and analysed.

Public involvement

Public involvement is increasingly regarded as a key element of the research process, and many grant bodies require details to be included in the grant application about how the public/service users, as well as key stakeholders, will be involved in the research from the outset. Active public involvement in research includes helping to identify and design the research questions, to ensure the study has lay/user relevance. In some cases it can include active participation in the data collection, and in reflecting on the findings (Park 1999). Appropriate methods of public involvement, of course, depend on the research task. A guide to public involvement and types of participation has been described by Earl-Slater (2004). In the social sciences, true participatory research emphasises the joint ownership of the research. It involves inclusion of interested groups – for example, health professionals, lay carers, patients and other members of the public – on an advisory committee to oversee the research, which necessitates careful management to enhance trust and to reduce the effect of power differentials on effective participation. The advantages of this method include enhancing the social significance (e.g. lay relevance) of the research, and empowering lay groups.

A systematic search of the literature on consumer involvement, which found 286 documents explicitly mentioning consumer involvement in identifying and prioritising the research topic, reported that the barriers to consumer involvement include: poor representation of consumers; consumers' unfamiliarity with research and research programmes' unfamiliarity with consumers; negative attitudes and poor working relationships; and difficulties in communication and time constraints (Oliver *et al.* 2004).

Methods of ensuring equitable access and inclusion (e.g. by age, sex and ethnic group) are important, and this means accessible venues. In order that people can feel involved they also need resources – thus the investigator needs to provide lay summaries of the study and study materials in user-friendly, plain language formats, translated where needed. Participants also need to feel respected and supported. Where appropriate, training may need to be provided (Macaulay *et al.* 1999).

Honorariums need to be costed into the grant proposal for lay members in recognition of the value of their time; these and reimbursement of their travel expenses need prompt payment (www.involve.org.uk).

19.5 Document research

Documents as sources of, or for, research

A document is a written, audio or visual image record. It can be a source *of* or *for* research (May 1993), depending on the theoretical perspective of the investigator. For example, investigators holding a positivist perspective might access and use official government statistics (e.g. on crime or suicide rates) *for* their research, but will reject most unofficial documents (e.g. diaries, literature) as subjective and unscientific. They acknowledge that the reliability and validity of such documents are rarely perfect, but strive to find ways to improve them. In contrast, investigators holding a phenomenological perspective will view all types of documents as a source *of* but not *for* research because they are all viewed as social constructions and it is the process of construction which merits research attention. For example, Sudnow (1968), who is a social interactionist, showed how crime statistics in the USA reflected the process of 'plea bargaining' through which defendants were encouraged to plead guilty. Similarly, Prior (1987) described how coroners used their 'common sense' in their decisions about whether an autopsy should be undertaken, and treated sudden and violent deaths as more suspicious among people in the manual classes and among the unmarried. They were therefore more likely to perform an autopsy on them than on middle-class or married people. Thus, official statistics on cause of death reflect decision-making processes which themselves require investigation.

While positivist investigators had always recognised the problems within the secondary data (i.e. records and statistics) they analysed, the upsurge of interest in phenomenological perspectives (e.g. social interactionist, symbolic interactionist and labelling theories) during the 1960s meant that the actual study of the construction of records was seen as a separate and legitimate field of investigation. As Silverman (1993) put it, records are a 'potential goldmine for sociological investigation'.

Whichever theoretical stance is taken, no document can be regarded as a completely accurate representation of the phenomenon of interest, but, within limitations and taking their social context and process of construction into account, they can be valuable sources of data about society.

Types of documents

Documents are socially produced material and include public archival records such as public actuarial records (demographic characteristics of the population, such as births, deaths and marriages), political and judicial archival records (such as court decisions, budget decisions, and so on), government department documents (such as crime statistics on numbers of arrests and convictions by type), ongoing archival records of other public and private institutions in society, and mass media records. Some public records are derived from census data. Other documents include personal papers, diaries, literature, art, cartoons and photographs. Historians and biographers make extensive use of archives of policy papers and other documents, as well as personal letters, in their reconstruction of events (e.g. Berridge 2007). Epidemiologists rely on data on mortality, incidence, prevalence and exposure rates to diseases for ecological studies (Rothman 1986). Video and audio recordings and photographs are also social documents and are often underused as research sources. Visual arts can be an important source of information about society and its values. Cultural constructions, or media analyses, are another form of document analysis. It is possible to analyse societal values and practices from analyses of past and current popular media, for example, all national newspapers (broadsheet and tabloid), women's magazines, television and radio programmes. Thomas (2010) searched district archives, sanitary reports, newspaper articles and letters, hospital and medical reports, as well as other archived documents in order to describe the Lambeth cholera outbreak of 1848–49 and its aftermath. These revealed rich data on various treatments used by doctors and also lay people (e.g. alcohol).

Thus, it can be seen that documents can be classified in many different ways: for example, public or private, official or unofficial, individual or corporate (Pickin and St Leger 1993). The methods of extracting data from documents, and their analysis, can be either qualitative (as in narrative analyses of, for example, diaries) or highly structured and quantitative (as in the demographic analyses of population trends over time from public records of births, deaths and marriages, and so on).

Advantages and disadvantages of documents as sources

The advantages of document research include their relative non-reactivity with the investigator, convenience and low cost in comparison with other research methods. Higher costs are involved if extensive national or international searching, or any restoration or translation, is required. Many archives also have the advantage of covering entire populations for long time periods.

Comprehensive and systematically collected databases, maintained over time, for large populations can provide valuable information which can form a basis for designing descriptive and analytic research studies. St Leger *et al.* (1992), for example, state that, in relation to large, clinical databases, it can be possible to explore how patients' outcomes alter according to differences in their characteristics and clinical management.

Investigators from both positivist and phenomenological perspectives have criticised document research, the former because documents (apart from official statistics) are seen as too subjective and impressionistic, and the latter because documents reflect society's biases and are simply social constructions of reality. Thus the process of their construction should be investigated, rather than the content of the documents themselves. In sociology, for example, one of the most frequently cited misuses of official statistics in relation to theory was Durkheim's (1951) analysis of suicide rates, referred to earlier. He argued that the suicide rate can be explained sociologically by analysing suicide levels in relation to religion, season of the year, time of day, race, sex, education and marital status. He performed these analyses across several countries, obtaining the data from available archives. The work has been held up as flawed because of the biases in official statistics on suicide. For example, in Catholic countries a low suicide rate was reported, not because it accurately reflects a low rate in socially cohesive societies, as was hypothesised, but because of the social taboo and unlawful nature of suicide leading to such deaths being categorised as 'death by misadventure' rather than suicide.

Authenticity, bias, error and interpretation

Document research requires careful investigation, first, to ensure that the required documents are available, accessible and authentic, and, second. to sift through often overwhelming amounts of data, but also to produce balanced accounts. It is important for the investigator to be aware of the authenticity, completeness and representativeness of documents and the meanings of words and classification schemes used in their compilation. The results stemming from the use of historical (past) sources and documents will be determined by the sources used, their completeness and who they were originally compiled or written by (in relation to bias). Each of these sources can be subject to editing, error, loss and falsification, which the investigator must be aware of.

Historical records may be imperfect: for example, demographic records prior to the nineteenth century are so imperfect that estimates cannot be reliably made from them. Errors in data analysis of records can also occur due to time sampling. Economic conditions, wars and environmental conditions can all influence record-keeping.

Official statistics may be subject to classification errors and, more importantly, changes in the definitions of classifications over time, making comparisons difficult or impossible (crime and unemployment statistics are well known for changing definitions and classifications). This requires investigators to be meticulous in detecting these in order to be able to interpret their documents accurately. For example, when one is analysing causes of mortality over time, it is likely that increases and decreases in many causes of death are simply due to changes in the definition of the medical condition, and even fashion (e.g. doctors in Britain are advised not to record 'old age' as a cause of death on death certificates, and thus the recorded number of deaths owing to 'old age' has fallen).

Accounts found in letters, diaries, etc. may be exaggerated, biased and unrepresentative. Works of art and literature are also used as sources of past life, and are subject to the same limitations. The main sources of bias in document research stem from the selective deposit and selective survival of recorded material, whether the material consists of letters, diaries, official or other documents. Some documents may have been removed or destroyed, which leads to bias – are they missing because their contents reflect negatively on an organisation or society? Some documents may also be subject to bias through subjective editing or variations in editing. The document analyst must be aware of bias from the person who authorised and compiled the document, the method of storage and its completeness.

There are many other problems in interpreting the past. For example, apart from changing terminology and classifications, the meaning attributed to words may also change over time and between places, thus creating difficulties in comparisons of rates (e.g. of disease, death, crime, employment) over time. There can also be bias owing to the perspective of the compiler or commissioner (the latter is relevant when analysing official statistics, e.g. crime or unemployment statistics). For examples of the methodological problems of relying on official statistics, see Kitsuse and Cicourel (1963), Doyal (1979), Government Statisticians' Collective (1979) and Miles and Irvine (1979).

It is important to attempt to ascertain the source and aims of any documents used in research, and any potential biases. Pickin and St Leger (1993) suggested using the following criteria when assessing documentary sources: authenticity, credibility and freedom from distortion, representativeness and clarity of meaning. The range of documents for research, and the pitfalls, have been described by Macdonald and Tipton (1993) and May (1993). Everything in document research has to be checked from more than one angle, and nothing can be taken for granted. This is where multiple, or triangulated, research methods become essential (Webb *et al.* 1966; Denzin 1970, 1978).

Types of document research

The approaches of sociologists, both positivists and phenomenologists, were outlined previously. Other prominent types of document analyses are historical, demographic and media analyses. These are briefly described next.

Historical research

Much historical research, and also policy analysis, is dependent on document analyses. Good policy analysis delves deeply into the material under study and is time-consuming – in effect, becoming historical and of historical interest. Historical and policy research and analysis are essential in order to provide insights into society and the interrelation of events. Like surveys, they are required for the documentation of social change. Historical research methods include qualitative narratives, such as careful compilation and interpretation of relevant information in order to chronicle events. This includes information from diaries, newspaper reports, minutes of meetings, official documents and oral histories. Historical research methods also include quantitative analysis of trends, using sources such as official statistics relating to births, deaths, marriages and diseases, and information from other records.

An example of historical research which used triangulated methods is Berridge's (1996) analysis of the construction and definition of AIDS over time as a policy problem in the UK. She used a range of unofficial and official documents, official statistics, publications, press material and popular literature (fiction), and carried out interviews (oral histories) with a wide range of key figures. The work is an illustration of how the author integrated the material from a wide range of sources to produce a coherent analysis of events, assumptions, activities, consequences, official and unofficial responses and interpretations which shaped UK health policy in this field. Berridge (1994) described the difficulties of conducting archive research in Britain, because access to the required official documents was officially inhibited owing to the operation of a 30-year rule, preventing access to government records for that period. However, she described how they could be partly accessed – but not cited – through contact with key people, complemented with reliance on oral histories (which she acknowledges can involve reinterpretations of the past, problems of memory bias over dates and events, and so on):

> What therefore happens is a phenomenon familiar to many contemporary historians: what I have called 'archives on the run' or 'ad hoc archives'. Archives are picked up, sometimes literally, where they present themselves. Here are some examples from the AIDS research. A member of a gay group had been on a government health-education committee about which there was much controversy. Some civil servants saw it as indicative of the hidden gay agenda for AIDS – that the threat to the general population should be stressed to avoid the danger of a public backlash against gays. Another gay member of the committee had, in the course of an interview, maintained that a senior civil servant had made astonishing, and indeed, quite hilarious, suggestions about how to contain the epidemic. 'Avoid male prostitutes' or 'don't come to London' were, he considered, the messages which should be stressed. My interviewee rifled through his filing cabinet and gave me the minutes of the committee as well as the early papers of his own organisation. I staggered back with brimming carrier bags full of material vital for assessing these competing stories, as well as for filling in the ad hoc nature of the initial organisational response. (I am well aware that minutes are only one form of constructed history data.)
>
> On another occasion an interview with a leading haemophilia consultant who had been involved from the earliest days in the issues round AIDS and haemophilia provided important oral testimony. But he also handed over evidence he had prepared for the haemophiliac compensation case. This was a file neatly detailing and referencing the history of the blood-supply issue in the UK together with information on the operation of the international plasma trade, and documentation of how his own views about AIDS and its impact on the blood supply and blood products had changed over time.

Demographic research

Demography is based on the analysis of population statistics relating to births, deaths, marriages, diseases, and so on. Historians often use demographic methods. James (1994) cites the demographic study of England from 1541 to 1871 by Wrigley and Schofield (1981) as an example of this overlap. They analysed national demographic patterns over several centuries, focusing primarily on church registers of baptisms, marriages and burials (parish registers). Although these were required to be kept since 1538, few survive and, among those that do, there are breaks in registration, and incomplete or defective registrations in most registers, particularly during periods of war, famine and plague as well as owing to human errors. The first task was to locate the registers and assess their reliability by working with local historians across England. Wrigley and Schofield developed a statistical method to identify and deal with short breaks and incomplete periods, though many registers still remained unusable. The other problem encountered was the accuracy of the records – some children might not have been baptised and couples might have lived out of wedlock. As the authors stated, this form of study can only be approximation. The statistical techniques used by demographers were described in Chapter 4.

Media analyses

Media analyses are a form of document research. The data extracted from media analyses can be categorised and analysed quantitatively and/or qualitatively in order to provide rich insights on societal attitudes and behaviour (see Aldridge 1993, for an example of media analyses to document society's attitude to suicide). Media analyses usually focus on written material (e.g. newspapers and magazines), though film, radio, television (e.g. advertisements, news broadcasts) and cyberspace also provide material for research. Newspapers have published indexes, usually available in large public libraries. Investigators can use keywords to search for relevant items. These inevitably provide limited perspectives, and are biased by editorial selectivity. More thorough analysis involves a search of the original sources and investigators should conduct their own independent content analyses.

Analysis of documents

Data extracted from documents and records can be analysed systematically either qualitatively or quantitatively. With qualitative techniques, the focus is on the social and cultural context of the document and its production.

Semiotics

Early linguistic research focused on the meaning of words and historical changes in meaning. This was abandoned in favour of a semiotic approach which analyses the rules of combining elements of speech (language) rather than simply utterances of speech. Semiotics is the systematic study of signs and symbols within society. These do not exist autonomously, but derive their meaning from the system in which they are used. The approach rejects the quantified method of content analysis and instead focuses on the codes in each text, which is considered as a whole. The text is analysed to extract the codes which reflect the message contained in it; it is, in effect, a method of structuring a text. Silverman (1993) presents a narrative analysis of fairy tales by Propp (1968) as an example of a semiotic approach. Propp argued that the fairy tales within different cultures share similar themes, which can be broken down into elements (dragon, king, daughter, kidnap), each of which can be replaced (witch, chief, wife, vanish) without altering the story's basic structure, because each element has a function (evil force, ruler, loved one, disappearance). Propp isolated 31 functions (e.g. prohibition, violation, disappearance) in 100 tales analysed. These functions were contained in seven 'spheres of action' (the villain, the provider, the helper, the princess and her father, the despatcher, the hero, the false hero). The plots took four forms: development through struggle and victory; development through the accomplishment of a difficult task; development through a combination of these two; and development through neither. While this has since been modified by other investigators, it serves here as a clear illustration of how semiotics can be used in the analysis of narratives (see Silverman 1993, for a more detailed description). It illustrates the principle that signs derive their meaning from their relationship with *other* signs. This approach does not provide an analysis of the text within the context of its social construction (Macdonald and Tipton 1993), but it is a method of analysing the text itself.

Content analysis

Alternatively, a quantitative content analysis, involving the systematic and objective identification, linking and counting of specified characteristics, can be carried out in order to compare categories and to make inferences from the data (see Holsti 1968; Frankfort-Nachmias and Nachmias 1992). The procedure is the same as the techniques for content analysis described in Chapter 17 on unstructured interviewing, and involves the investigator categorising the data to make comparisons and to produce counts of the frequency with which words, phrases, themes, and so on occur. The computer software available to facilitate this process was also described in Chapter 17. This method of analysis relates only to the content of the document and is not an analysis of the process by which the document was produced.

Objectivity in the analysis can be enhanced by ensuring that the coding (inclusion or exclusion of data items into the categories of interest) is carried out according to an explicit set of rules. The rules should clearly describe the category and inclusion and exclusion criteria. This will enable other researchers to obtain the same results from the data. This ensures that the investigator does not only extract data which are likely to support his or her hypotheses. For example, the rule could be that in the documents of interest, which should relate to a specified period, all key symbols will be extracted (the key symbols relate to the topic of interest, and might include countries, references to war, references to unemployment, and so on). When a specified key symbol is found it is scored as present, and the context is recorded (and can be coded into meaningful categories and/or quite simply into, for example, positive, negative or neutral text).

It is important, however, to remember that the frequency with which phrases occur in a text does not necessarily equate with their importance or meaning, and this is a relatively unsubtle approach to analysis. The context (context unit) has to be taken into account when one is recording and coding items (recording unit). The recording unit is the smallest body of content (e.g. a word, term, theme, person, paragraph, item) in which the appearance of a key symbol is counted. The context unit is the largest body of content (e.g. a book, speech, article) examined in characterising a recording unit. Themes are often used as recording units, particularly in the study of attitudes and values. The units are eventually classified and coded into comprehensive and relevant categories, which can be counted.

The enumeration systems used are usually based on: a time–space system (e.g. space, inches, columns) or units of time (minutes) to describe the relative emphases of the different categories in the document; an appearance system which searches for the appearance of the category; a frequency system which records and counts every occurrence of the category; and an intensity system (used with attitudes and values) which involves the construction of scales (such as the Thurstone scale) (Frankfort-Nachmias and Nachmias 1992).

Holsti (1968) has produced a very helpful checklist of the most commonly employed types of categories used in content analyses, which is also partly reproduced by Frankfort-Nachmias and Nachmias (1992). In Box 19.6 one of the categories ('What is said') is shown.

Box 19.6 Categories for content analysis

'What is said' categories

- Subject matter. What is the communication about?
- Direction. How is the subject matter treated (e.g. favourably or unfavourably)?
- Standard. What is the basis on which the classification by direction is made?
- Values. What values, goals, or desires are revealed?
- Methods. What methods are used to achieve goals?
- Traits. What are the characteristics used in describing people?
- Actor. Who is represented as undertaking certain acts?
- Authority. In whose name are statements made?
- Origin. Where does the communication originate?
- Location. Where does the action take place?
- Conflict. What are the sources and levels of conflict?
- Endings. Are conflicts resolved happily, ambiguously or tragically?
- Time. When does the action take place?

Examples of content analyses of media documents

Jacobson and Amos (1985) carried out a survey of women's magazines in the UK in order to elicit the magazines' coverage of smoking, and policy on advertising in general and cigarettes in particular. In this context, an earlier content analysis was carried out of the 1984 issues of the two top-selling youth magazines. The research included counts of the proportion of photographs published in the magazines which showed someone smoking, and which showed pop stars smoking or holding cigarettes, and the number of items and pages covering cigarette smoking in other named women's magazines.

Similarly, Manstead and McCulloch (1981) conducted a content analysis of 170 British television commercials in order to examine their portrayal of men and women (i.e. sex-role stereotyping). The investigators videoed all commercials transmitted by one television company between 6.00 and 11.30 p.m. during a seven-day period (totalling 493 commercials), excluding 309 repeat advertisements, and those showing only children or fantasy characters, from their final sample. This left 170 advertisements for coding by two independent coders. They made 2152 codings, of which discrepancies occurred between them in relation to 86 (96 per cent agreement achieved), mainly in relation to whether arguments were scientific and the type of reward involved. A maximum of two (the most prominent) central adults were coded for each commercial in relation to the characteristics shown in Box 19.7.

Box 19.7 Example of codes used in content analysis of commercials

Mode of presentation
- Voice (disembodied voiceovers)
- Visual

Credibility
- Users of the product
- Authority sources (of information)
- Other

Role
- Spouse
- Parent
- Homemaker
- Worker
- Professional
- Celebrity
- Interviewer/narrator
- Boyfriend/girlfriend
- Sex object
- Other

Location
- Home
- Store
- Occupational setting
- Other

Arguments
- Scientific (including factual evidence)
- Non-scientific (opinions or testimonials in favour of the product)
- No argument

Reward type
- Opposite sex approval
- Family approval
- Friends' approval
- Self-enhancement (in health or appearance)
- Practical
- Social/career enhancement
- Other
- None

Product type

- ■ Body
- ■ Home
- ■ Food
- ■ Auto (cars and accessories)
- ■ Sports
- ■ Other

(Manstead and McCulloch 1981)

While content analysis is popular and widely used, it does have limitations. For example, the coding process is subjective, which necessitates the use of two coders. However, it has been argued that once the coders have been trained, the investigator may simply be testing the ability to enforce his or her theoretical biases (Durkin 1985, 1986). The other problem is that content analysis concentrates on counting the frequencies at which a phenomenon occurs, and rarely analyses its contextual meaning and organisation, and by this process of reduction may thereby misrepresent the data. This emphasises the importance of replicating research in order to assess the consistency of findings between studies.

Diary methods

The diary method involves the respondent keeping a daily record of activities or events (e.g. symptoms). Diary methods, structured or unstructured, can be valuable when detailed information needs to be collected, and there is no other method. They are also a form of document research. Respondents are also less constrained by diaries (unless they are heavily structured) than by questionnaires with fixed choice responses. It is only practical to use this method with small, committed samples of people (and remembering that several sample members will discontinue the diary or not fully complete it over the study period). It is also unreasonable to expect people to complete diaries for long periods of time.

This method, because it is less affected by recall bias, can be a valuable check on the reliability of information collected retrospectively by questionnaire from a larger sample (the diary sample can be a motivated subset of the study population), though non-completion is often a problem. Diary assessment is not a substitute for questionnaire and interview methods, but it can contribute further information – it is complementary.

The diary method ranges from the collection of data about activities and events to symptom diaries. Diary methods can be unstructured – simply asking the patient to record the item when it occurs – or structured, whereby the diary is completed daily (or more than daily) according to instructions. For example, people might be asked to enter any symptoms they experience (and their nature and severity) on a daily basis over a month into a diary, or to enter any items (e.g. over-the-counter medication, medical appliances) purchased in relation to a medical condition. The diary instructions should clearly specify the need to fill it in at the requested intervals and for accuracy. Letters and telephone calls offering encouragement may motivate respondents to continue completing the diary.

Hyland and Crocker (1995) and Hyland (1996) have described the use of the diary method within a double-blind, controlled trial of asthma treatments. The study involved patients completing a quality of life diary for seven days out of a two-week baseline period, and during the first week of every month during a six-month treatment period. A questionnaire assessing quality of life was also administered at baseline, and at three and six months after treatment. The diaries were reported to have better longitudinal correlations with the physiology of the respondents in comparison with the questionnaires, while the questionnaires had better cross-sectional correlations with physiology. Thus the authors concluded that diaries are better longitudinal instruments, with patients' own recordings of problems over time being more sensitive to change, and that questionnaires are better cross-sectional instruments. Hyland reported the problem of floor and ceiling effects in diaries, and suggested that respondents showing their effects could be excluded from the analysis (i.e. people reporting no problems/ incidence throughout the study period, or people reporting daily problems throughout), or respondents with floor effects (non-zero problem incidence) at baseline could be excluded from entry into the rest of the study. A decision to exclude a group from analysis should be taken cautiously – they may be an important group, rather than idiosyncratic in their diary completion, worthy of study.

Logging

A variation of a diary method is logging, as in time sampling, where a bleep sounds at either random or fixed intervals to prompt respondents to record their feelings or behaviour at the time. Such logging methods were used in early studies of GPs' workload, whereby doctors would record their activities on specially designed sheets at specific intervals. For example, Floyd and Livesey (1975) used the bleep method of time (or activity) sampling to study the work of five doctors.

Non-completion

Respondents may fail to complete a diary, or fail to complete it on particular days, and even complete it retrospectively (e.g. hastily just before returning it to the researcher). Hyland (1996) suggested that it is wise to accept that non-completion on some days should be expected and allowed for in the design. He further suggested that the use of electronic diaries could overcome some problems, by not permitting retrospective completion, and by reducing the burden on the respondents and also on the investigator by electronic downloading of diary information. Perry *et al.* (2011) used diaries in the context of their RCT of the effects of home and class-based exercise programmes on activity, and reported problems in the correct completion of diaries to record falls in older people. They found associations between incorrect completion and low level of education and non-English as a main language. They also concluded that diaries may under-report the rate of falls as those at higher risk were less likely to return diaries, despite being more likely to report falls. Alternative strategies for analysing diaries and their structure have been described by Alaszewski (2007).

Analysis of diaries

Diaries can generate a large volume of data for analysis. They can also yield quantitative data (e.g. on expenditure, weighed food intake, symptoms experienced). Hyland (1996) suggested analysing problem incidence rates: the proportion of days when respondents reported a problem or the topic of interest out of all days when they recorded either a problem or no problem. This calculation is only possible when respondents have high completion rates. Low completion rates lead to statistical noise and the topic or problem count becomes unstable. Hyland further suggested deciding on a completion cut-off point at the outset of the study, below which respondents' data are considered invalid. Content analyses can also be performed on diaries, though the investigator needs to be confident that their level of completion merits this.

Summary of main points

- The case study is a research method which focuses on single or small series of cases, using triangulated research methods.
- There are three main methods for establishing consensus views: the Delphi method, consensus development panels and nominal group processes. These are often used in combination.
- Action research is problem-focused, educative, reflective, critical and 'bottom-up', aims to involve participants and is oriented towards improvement and change.
- The technique of gathering information quickly in action research is commonly referred to as 'rapid appraisal'.
- A document is a written, audio or visual image. Documents can be a source *of* or *for* research.
- The methods of extracting data from documents, and their analysis, can be either qualitative (as in narrative analyses of, e.g. diaries) or highly structured and quantitative (as in analyses of public records of births, deaths and marriages).
- Documents need to be checked for authenticity, completeness, representativeness and the meanings of words and classification schemes used.
- Diary methods, structured or unstructured, can be valuable when detailed information needs to be collected, and there is no other method.
- A variation of a diary method is logging, as in time sampling, where a bleep sounds at either random or fixed intervals to prompt the respondents to record their feelings or behaviour at the time.
- Mixed research methods can be used to complement each other, leading to a blurring of approaches (drawing on the strengths of each method, on the basis that each have different weaknesses and strengths) or for triangulation (in order to minimise research bias and enhance the validity of the results).

Key questions

1   What research issues are appropriate for case study methods?
2   What are consensus methods?
3   What are the principles of action research?
4   Explain the term 'participation' in action research.
5   What is rapid appraisal?
6   Distinguish between diary methods and logging.
7   What are the main types of documents used in research?
8   What are the main problems in document research?
9   Distinguish between qualitative and quantitative record research and analysis.

Key terms

action research
actuarial records
archives
authenticity
case studies
consensus development panels
consensus methods
content analyses
Delphi methods
demography
diary methods
document research
empowerment of participants
error
expert panel
focus group
historical records

history
logging
media analysis
mixed methods
nominal group process
questionnaires
rapid appraisal
realistic evaluation
recall bias
representativeness
semiotics
stakeholders
subjective editing
time sampling
triangulated research methods
unstructured interviews

Recommended reading

Adamson, J. (2005) Combined qualitative and quantitative designs, in A. Bowling and S. Ebrahim (eds) *Handbook of Health Research Methods: Investigation, Measurement and Analysis.* Maidenhead: Open University Press.

Creswell, J.W. and Plano Clark, V.L. (2011) *Designing and Conducting Mixed Methods Research.* Thousand Oaks, CA: Sage.

Hyland, M.E. and Crocker, G.R. (1995) Validation of an asthma quality of life diary in a clinical trial, *Thorax*, 50: 724–30.

Silverman, D. (1993) *Interpreting Qualitative Data: Methods for Analysing Talk, Text and Interaction.* London: Sage.

Stake, R.E. (1995) *The Art of Case Study Research.* London: Sage.

Stringer, E.T. (1996) *Action Research: A Handbook for Practitioners.* London: Sage.

Glossary

acquiescence response set ('yes-saying'): respondents will more frequently endorse a statement than disagree with its opposite.

actuarial records: public records about the demographic characteristics of the population served.

archives: ongoing records maintained by institutions within society.

attrition: loss of sample members over time in longitudinal and experimental research with post-tests.

average costs: the total costs divided by the total number of units of output.

bias: deviation in one direction of the observed value from the true value of the construct being measured, due to systematic errors in the research methods (as opposed to random error).

bivariate statistics: descriptive statistics for the analysis of the association between two variables (e.g. contingency tables, correlations).

blind: concealing the assignment of people to experimental or control group in experiments. Concealment can be from the people or from both the people and the person carrying out the intervention, for example, the treating doctor ('double blind').

capital costs: the costs of land, buildings and equipment.

case: a single unit in a study (e.g. a person or setting, such as a clinic, hospital).

case study: a research method which focuses on the circumstances, dynamics and complexity of a single case, or a small number of cases.

causal hypothesis: a statement that it is predicted that one phenomenon will be the result of one or more other phenomena that precede it in time.

causal relationships: observed changes (the 'effect') in one variable are owing to earlier changes in another.

central limit theorem: the sampling distribution approaches normality as the number of samples taken increases.

central tendency: (a) Mean: the arithmetic mean, or average, is a measure of central tendency in a population or sample. The mean is defined as the sum of the scores divided by the total number of cases involved. (b) Median: this is the middle value of the observations when listed in ascending order; it bisects the observations (i.e. the point below which 50 per cent of the observations fall). (c) Mode: a measure of central tendency based on the most common value in the distribution (i.e. the value of X with the highest frequency).

clinical trial: an experiment where the participants are patients.

closed question: the question is followed by predetermined response choices into which the respondent's reply is placed.

cluster: a sample unit which consists of a group of elements.

cluster sampling: probability sampling involving the selection of groupings (clusters) and selecting the sample units from the clusters.

coding: the assignation of (usually numerical) codes to each category of each variable.

cohort: the population has a common experience or characteristic which defines the sampling (e.g. all born in the same year).

concept: an abstraction representing an object or phenomenon.

confidence interval: a confidence interval calculated from a sample is interpreted as a range of values which contains the true population value with the probability specified.

confounding factors: an extraneous factor (a factor *other* than the variables under study), *not controlled for*, distorts the results. An extraneous factor only confounds when it is related to dependent variables and to the independent variables under investigation. It makes them appear connected when their association is, in fact, spurious.

content analysis: the systematic analysis of observations obtained from records, documents and field notes.

control group: the group in the experimental research that is not exposed to the independent variable (intervention).

control variable: a variable used to test the possibility that an empirically observed relationship between an independent and dependent variable is spurious.

coping: the cognitive and behavioural efforts to manage the internal and external demands of the stressful situation.

cost–benefit analysis: assignation of a monetary value to the benefits of a programme, and making comparisons with the monetary costs of the programme for an assessment of efficiency.

cost-effectiveness analysis: comparison of different programmes producing the same type of non-monetary benefit in relation to their monetary costs for an assessment of efficiency.

cost minimisation: compares the cost of achieving the same outcome.

cost–utility analysis: relates the cost of a scheme to a measure of its usefulness or outcome (utility).

crisis theory: the individual strives towards homeostasis and equilibrium, and therefore crises are self-limiting as people work towards achieving stability.

critical appraisal: the careful and systematic examination of research to assess its reliability, validity, value and relevance in a particular context.

cross-sectional study: collection of data at one point in time.

data cleaning: after the data have been entered on to the computer, they are checked to detect and correct errors and inconsistent codes.

deduction: a theoretical or mental process of reasoning by which the investigator starts off with an idea, and develops a theory and hypothesis from it; then phenomena are assessed in order to determine whether the theory is consistent with the observations.

dependent variable: the variable the investigator wishes to explain – the dependent variable is the expected outcome of the independent variable.

determinism: assumes that everything is caused by some factor in a predictable way; explanations that are based on a few narrowly defined factors to the exclusion of all others.

disability-free life expectancy: an indicator that aggregates mortality and morbidity data for a population into a single index; it represents the average number of years that a person of a given age may expect to live free of disability.

dispersion: a summary of a spread of cases in a figure (measures include quartiles, percentiles, deciles, standard deviations and the range).

ecological fallacy: relationships between variables are estimated at one level of analysis (e.g. the clinics) and then wrongly extrapolated to another (e.g. the individual patients).

ecological studies: research where the unit of observation is a group of people rather than an individual (e.g. schools, cities, nations).

effect size: a numerical index of the magnitude of an observed association.

empirical: based on observation.

empiricism: a philosophical approach that the only valid form of knowledge is that which is gathered by use of the senses; explanations should be based on actual observations, rather than theoretical statements.

ethnography: the study of people in their natural settings; a descriptive account of social life and culture in a defined social system, based on qualitative methods (e.g. detailed observations, unstructured interviews, analysis of documents). This method is used by anthropologists.

ethnomethodology: a method for the study of a cultural group (ethno), but more specifically the methods of the people; the study of how people use social interaction to make sense of situations (to create their 'reality') (*see also* phenomenology, interpretive approach, symbolic interactionist approach).

evaluation: application of research methods with the aim of critically evaluating the effectiveness of programmes.

evidence-based practice: the explicit, judicious use of best evidence, integrated with expertise, in decision-making about patient/client care.

experiment: a scientific method used to establish cause and effect relationships between the independent and dependent variables. At its most *basic*, the experiment is a situation in which the independent (experimental) variable is fixed by manipulation by the investigator or by natural occurrence. The *true* experimental method involves the random allocation of participants to experimental and control groups. Ideally, participants are assessed before and after the manipulation of the independent variable in order to measure its effects on the dependent variable.

experimental group: the group that is exposed to the independent variable (intervention) in experimental research.

field research: research which takes place in a natural setting.

focus groups: a research method of interviewing people while they are interacting in small groups.

frequency distribution: the number of observations of each of the values within a variable.

functionalism: theory based on the interrelationships within the social system as a whole; how they operate and change, and their social consequences for individuals, sub-systems and societies.

grounded theory: the investigator develops conceptual categories from the data and then makes new observations to develop these categories. Hypotheses are derived directly from the data.

health behaviour: an activity undertaken by a person for the purpose of preventing disease or detecting it at an asymptomatic stage.

health lifestyle: voluntary health behaviour based on making choices from the alternatives that are available in individual situations.

health need(s): need for health has been variously defined and measured in terms of need for health, expressed need (demand) for (effective) treatment, and ability to benefit from treatment.

health service needs: need for effective services.

hierarchical data: data on different levels or layers (e.g. household, individual member of household).

holistic: the phenomenon of interest is viewed in terms of the relationships between each level of the system. Holism identifies the whole of the social system as more than the simple sum of the individuals within it. Holism is at the centre of sociological theory.

hypothesis: a tentative solution to a research question, expressed in the form of a prediction about the relationship between the dependent and independent variables.

hypothetico-deductive method: beginning with a theory and, in a deductive way, deriving testable hypotheses from it, the hypotheses are then tested by gathering and analysing data and the theory is supported or refuted (*see* deduction).

idiographic: research which studies individuals, and which attempts to understand people or social situations in relation to their unique characteristics, without attempting to make generalisations.

illness behaviour: the perception and evaluation of symptoms of ill health, and subsequent action taken (or not).

incidence: cases (e.g. of disease) which first occur in a population in a defined period of time.

incremental analysis: examination of the incremental change in effectiveness and costs of moving from one type of care to another.

incremental costs: the extra costs of moving from one service to another.

independent variable(s): the explanatory or predictor variable – the variable hypothesised to explain the dependent variable(s).

individualistic or reductionist fallacy: inferences about groups are wrongly drawn from data about individuals.

induction: begins with the observation and measurement of phenomena and then develops ideas and general theories about the universe of interest.

inferential statistics: these enable the researcher to make inferences about the characteristics of the population of interest on the basis of observations made on a sample of that population.

information bias: misclassification of, for example, people's responses due to error or bias.

interaction: the direction and/or magnitude of the association between two variables depends on the value of one or more other variables.

interpretive approach: the theoretical perspective that social scientists must include the meaning that social actors give to events and behaviour; symbolic interactionists and ethnomethodologists hold interpretive perspectives and subscribe to the philosophy of phenomenology.

interval data: the data points (classes) are ordered and the size of the difference between the points is specified, but the zero point and unit of measurement are arbitrary (e.g. temperature – the zero point differs on the two scales commonly used).

intervening variable: the independent variable affects the dependent variable through the intervening variable. This is also referred to as indirect causation.

interview: a research method which involves a trained interviewer asking questions and recording respondents' replies. Interview questions can be structured (printed on a questionnaire with set question wording and pre-coded response categories), semi-structured (mostly open-ended questions, i.e. with no pre-coded response categories) or unstructured and in-depth (listed topics about which interviewers probe respondents for their views and experiences).

leading question: question phrased in a way which leads the respondent to believe that a certain reply is expected.

level of measurement: categorisation of measuring instruments, and their resulting data, into four types: nominal, ordinal, interval, ratio.

longitudinal: at more than one point in time.

marginal costs: the extra cost of producing one extra unit of output.

meta-analysis: quantitative synthesis of primary data from several studies to produce an overall summary statistic.

missing data: information that is not available for a particular case (e.g. person) for which other information is available (e.g. owing to item non-response).

moderating variable: the variable that determines the effect of one variable on another.

multivariable analysis: allows for the measurement of the effects of one variable on an outcome to be measured, while controlling for the effects of other variables (e.g. multiple and logistic regression analysis).

naturalistic research: descriptive research in natural, unmanipulated, social settings using less obtrusive, qualitative methods.

need: includes felt need (want), expressed need (demand), normative need (experts' definitions which can change over time in response to knowledge) and comparative need (comparisons with others and considerations of equity).

nominal data: the classes are mutually exclusive, but have no intrinsic order or value (e.g. classification of capitals: Berlin, London, Milan, Paris, Stockholm).

nomothetic: the science of general laws; a belief in general laws that influence behaviour or personality traits and therefore aims to generalise research findings.

normal distribution: a mathematically defined curve which is an ideal or a theoretical distribution that occurs frequently in real life, especially in sampling. The normal distribution is a symmetrical, bell-shaped curve, rising smoothly from a small number of cases at both extremes to a large number of cases in the middle; and the average (mean) corresponds to the peak of the distribution; it is enveloped by a curve and equation.

null hypothesis: a statement that there is no relationship between the dependent and independent variables.

number needed to treat: the number of people who need to receive the intervention (e.g. prescribed medication) for a given period in order that one more person will have the specified successful outcome, compared with the number who would have that outcome without the intervention.

observation: a research method in which the investigator systematically watches, listens to and records the phenomenon of interest.

odds: the ratio of the probability of an event occurring, to that of it not occurring.

operationalise: the development of proxy measures which enable phenomena to be observed empirically (i.e. measured).

opportunity cost: the value of the best alternative use of a programme's resources (i.e. the value forgone by the investment in the programme).

ordinal data: classes which can be placed in rank order (e.g. bigger than, preferred to) but in which the amount by which one class is bigger/preferred is not specified (e.g. behaviour and attitudes: much more, more, about the same, less, much less; strongly agree, agree, neither agree nor disagree, disagree, strongly disagree; social class: I professional, II semi-professional, IIInm non-manual, IIIm manual, IV semi-skilled, V unskilled).

P **value:** *P* is the symbol of the probability associated with the outcome of a test of a null hypothesis (i.e. the probability that an observed inferential statistic occurred by chance, as in $P < 0.05$); p (small p) is used for proportions. Statistical tests exist which, in appropriate study designs and samples, can test for the probability of observing the values obtained.

paradigm: a set of ideas (hypotheses) about the phenomena under inquiry.

paradigm shift: this occurs if, over time, evidence accumulates which refutes, or is incompatible with, the paradigm, and thus the old paradigm is replaced by the new one.

participant observation: a research method in which the investigator takes part in (i.e. has a 'role' in) the social phenomenon of interest.

patients' preferences: the weighing up, consideration and expression of a value for alternative choices of action (e.g. of type of health service delivery or treatment).

perspective: a way of interpreting empirical phenomena.

phenomenological sociology: based on the concept of the social construction of reality through the social interaction of people (social actors), who use symbols to interpret each other and assign meanings to perceptions and experiences (*see also* ethnomethodology, interpretive approach, symbolic interactionist approach).

phenomenology: the philosophical belief that, unlike matter, humans have a consciousness. They interpret and experience the world in terms of meanings and actively construct an individual social reality.

placebo: inert treatment given to controls in trials.

positivism: positivism aims to discover laws using quantitative methods and emphasises *positive facts*. It assumes that human behaviour is a reaction to (i.e. determined by) external stimuli and that it is possible to observe and measure social phenomena, using the principles of the natural scientist, and to establish a reliable and valid body of knowledge about its operation based on empiricism and the hypothetico-deductive method.

power calculation: a measure of how likely the study is to produce a statistically significant result for a difference between groups of a given magnitude (i.e. the ability to detect a true difference).

precision: the ability of a measure to detect small changes in an attribute.

prevalence: percentage of population affected (e.g. with a specific disease) at any given time.

prevalence ratio: the number of cases (e.g. of disease) in a population at one point in time, expressed as a ratio of the population's size.

prospective study: collection of data over the forward passage of time (future).

publication bias: bias stemming from the fact that positive findings are more likely than negative findings to be published.

qualitative research: social research which is carried out in the field (natural settings) and analysed largely in non-statistical ways.

quantitative research: the measurement and analysis of observations in a numerical way.

random error: the errors in the study (usually from the sampling) randomly vary and sum to zero over enough cases; random error results in an estimate being *equally* likely to be above or below the true value.

random sampling: this gives each of the units in the target population a calculable and non-zero probability of being selected.

randomisation: assignment at random of people to experimental and control groups in experiments.

range: a measure of dispersion which is based on the lowest and highest values observed.

ratio data: scores are assigned on a scale with equal intervals and a true zero point.

reactive (Hawthorne) effect: a guinea-pig effect (awareness of being studied). If people feel they are being tested, they may feel the need to create a good impression, or if the study stimulates new interest in the topic under investigation, then the results will be distorted.

reductionism: the view that the phenomenon of interest can be explained within the lowest level of investigation (e.g. in biology, the cellular or chemical level). In sociology, this is known as atomism, which argues that the social system is no more than a collection of individuals, and in order to understand the social system we simply need to understand individuals.

reductionist fallacy: inferences about groups are wrongly drawn from data about individuals.

regression to the mean: an extreme measurement on a variable of interest which contains a degree of random error; on subsequent measurements, this value will tend to return to normal. The implication is that if a group of patients with a severe disease rating at a particular point in time have been selected for study, they may improve in the short term independently of any intervention simply because of the random variation inherent in the disease.

relative risk: the incidence rate for the condition in the population exposed to a phenomenon divided by the incidence rate in the non-exposed population.

relativism: no single system of knowledge or beliefs (or 'social facts') exists; it is dependent on context (i.e. culture).

reliability: the extent to which the measure is consistent and minimises random error (its repeatability).

research design: this refers to the strategy of the research – how the sampling is conducted, whether a descriptive or experimental design is selected, whether control groups are needed, what variables need to be operationalised and measured, what analyses will be conducted.

research methods, or techniques: these are the methods of data collection – interview, telephone, postal surveys, diaries and analyses of documents, observational methods, and so on. They are also the instruments to be used.

response rate: the number and percentage of people who respond positively to the invitation to take part in the study.

responsiveness: a measure of the association between the *change* in the observed score and the change in the true value of the construct (*see also* sensitivity).

retrospective study: collection of data over past time (looking backwards).

reverse causation: the causal direction of the observed associaion is opposite to that hypothesised. Experiments deal with reverse causation by the manipulation of the experimental (independent) variable, measuring the dependent variable before and after this manipulation.

sample: a subset of a population.

sampling: techniques used to obtain a subset of a population without the expense of conducting a census (gathering of information from *all* members of a population).

sampling distribution: the distribution of means of all possible different samples of *n* observations that can be obtained from this population. It has a mean equal to the population mean. It is a normal distribution (assuming the sample size is large enough).

sampling error: any sample is just one of an almost infinite number that might have been selected, all of which can produce slightly different estimates. Sampling error is the probability that any one sample is not completely representative of the population from which it was drawn.

sampling frame: a list of the sampling units from which the sample can be drawn.

secondary data: existing sources of data that could be used for research purposes.

selection bias: bias in the sample obtained.

sensitivity: ability of the actual gradations in the scale's scores to reflect changes in condition adequately; probability of correctly identifying the affected person; proportion of people who have a condition/disease who score positive on tests for it.

sensitivity analysis: a method for making plausible assumptions about the margins of errors in the results, and assessing whether they affect the implications of the results. The margins of error can be calculated using the confidence intervals of the results or they can be guessed.

Sick Role: a social 'niche' where people who are ill are given the opportunity ('rights') to recover in exchange for obligations aimed at recovery and a return to normal social roles.

simple random sample: a probability sampling method that gives each sampling unit an equal chance of being selected in the sample.

skewed distribution: a distribution in which more observations fall on one side of the mean than the other.

social stratification: the structured inequalities that exist between social groups owing to the unequal and systematic distribution of rewards and resources.

specificity: a measure of the probability of correctly identifying a non-affected person (i.e. 'non-case') with a measure; the proportion of people without a condition/disease who score negative for it when tested.

spurious association: an observed association between the dependent and independent variables which is false (spurious) because the association is caused by a third extraneous variable which intervenes. If the latter is controlled, the observed association disappears (see confounding factors).

standard deviation: this is the most common measure of dispersion. It is based on the difference of values from the mean value (the spread of individual results round a mean value); it is the square root of the arithmetic mean of the squared deviations from the mean.

standard error: this is a measure of the uncertainty in a sample statistic; the standard deviation of the sampling distribution is called the standard error. It is related to the population variation. The standard error of a mean is the standard deviation of the population divided by the square root of the sample size. The formula is given in standard statistical texts.

standardised mortality rate: deaths, for example, per 1000 of the population standardised for age.

standardised mortality ratio: compares the standard mortality rate for the standard (whole) population with that of particular regions or groups (index population), and expresses this as a ratio.

statistical significance: significance at the 0.05 per cent level means that five times in 100 the results could have occurred by chance, i.e. if the test was performed 100 times, on five occasions significant results will occur by chance.

stigma: the social reaction which leads to a spoilt identity and application of the label of deviant in society.

survey: a method of collecting information from a sample of the population of interest (known as a sample survey).

survival analyses: analysis of time to event data (e.g. from date of first diagnosis of a specific disease to date of death).

symbolic interactionist approach: perspective concerned with the meanings of phenomena to individuals, and how these meanings are produced in social exchanges. It focuses on the details of interactions between individuals, rather than the wider social system, and in particular the use of symbols in communications and in the creation of a sense of self and a sense of social reality (*see also* phenomenology, ethnomethodology, interpretive approach).

systematic error: the errors in the study result in an estimate being more likely to be either above or below the true value, depending upon the nature of the systematic error in any particular case.

systematic random sampling: a sample in which every *k*th case is selected from the population (*n*) (with a random starting point).

systematic research: the process of research should be based on an agreed set of rules and processes which are rigorously adhered to, and against which the research can be evaluated.

systematic review of the literature: review prepared with a systematic approach, using predetermined criteria, to minimise biases and random errors, and including components on materials and methods.

theory: a set of logically interrelated propositions and their implications.

triangulation: the use of three or more different research methods (i.e. multiple methods) to investigate the phenomenon of interest.

type I error (or alpha error): the error of rejecting a true null hypothesis.

type II error (or beta error): the failure to reject (i.e. acceptance of) a null hypothesis when it is actually false.

unidimensional: the items comprising a measurement scale form a single dimension that reflects one concept.

univariate statistics: descriptive statistics for the analysis (description) of one variable (e.g. frequency distributions, statistics of central tendency and dispersion).

validity: the rigour of a study, with bias minimised, enhancing results and estimates.

validity, ecological: the realism of the research results in real-life settings, outside the artificial research setting.

validity, external: the extent to which the research findings can be generalised to the wider population of interest and applied to different settings.

validity, internal: the extent to which the instrument is really measuring what it purports to measure.

variable: an indicator assumed to represent the underlying construct or concept, produced by the operationalisation of the latter.

References

Abbey, A. and Andrews, F.M. (1985) Modelling the psychological determinants of life quality, *Social Indicators Research*, 16: 1–34.

Abel, T., Geyer, S., Gerhardt, U., Siegrist, J. and van den Heuvel, W. (eds) (1993) *Medical Sociology: Research on Chronic Illness*. Bonn: Informationszentrum Socialwissenschaften.

Acheson, D. (1988) *Public Health in England: The Report of the Committee of Inquiry into the Future Development of Public Health Function* (Chairman: Sir Donald Acheson). London: HMSO.

Acheson, R.M. (1978) The definition and identification of need for health care, *Journal of Epidemiology and Community Health*, 32: 1–6.

Acquadro, C. and Jambon, B. (2005) The quality of life newsletter becomes the patient-reported outcomes newsletter, *Patient Reported Outcomes*, 34: 1.

Adamson, J. (2005) Combining qualitative and quantitative designs, in A. Bowling and S. Ebrahim (eds) *Handbook of Health Research Methods: Investigation, Measurement and Analysis*. Maidenhead: Open University Press.

Adamson, J., Cockayne, S., Puffer, S. and Torgerson, D.J. (2006) Review of randomised trials using the post-randomised consent (Zelen's) design, *Contemporary Clinical Trials*, 27: 305–19.

Addington-Hall, J. and Kalra, L. (2001) Who should measure QoL? *British Medical Journal*, 322: 1417–20.

Ahmed, S., Addicott, C., Qureshi, M. *et al.* (1999) Opinions of elderly people on treatment for end-stage renal disease, *Gerontology*, 45: 156–9.

Ajzen, I. (1988) *Attitudes, Personality and Behavior*. Chicago: Dorsey Press.

Ajzen, I. (1991) The theory of planned behavior, *Organizational Behavior and Human Decision Processes*, 50: 179–211.

Alaszewski, A. (2007) *Using Diaries for Social Research*. London: Sage.

Albrecht, G.L. and Devlieger, P.J. (1999) The disability paradox: high quality of life against all odds, *Social Science and Medicine*, 48: 977–88.

Aldridge, D. (1993) Observational methods: a search for methods in an ecosystemic paradigm, in G.T. Lewith and D. Aldridge (eds) *Clinical Research Methodology for Complementary Therapies*. London: Hodder & Stoughton.

Allen, C. and Beecham, J. (1993) Costing services: ideals and reality, in A. Netten and J. Beecham (eds) *Costing Community Care: Theory and Practice*. Aldershot: Ashgate Publishing.

Altman, D.G. (1980) Statistics and ethics in medical research, III: how large a sample? *British Medical Journal*, 281: 1336–8.

Altman, D.G. (1991) *Practical Statistics for Medical Research*. London: Chapman & Hall.

Altman, D.G. (1996) Better reporting of randomised controlled trials: the CONSORT statement, *British Medical Journal*, 313: 570–1.

Anderson, R. (1989) Research on health behaviour: an overview, in *Proceedings of a Symposium on Health Behaviour Research: Its Application in Health Promotion*, Pitlochry, Scotland, 1986. Copenhagen: WHO.

Anderson, R. (2008) New MRC guidance on evaluating complex interventions, *British Medical Journal*, 337: a1937.

Anderson, R. and Bury, M. (eds) (1988) *Living with Chronic Illness: The Experience of Patients and their Families*. London: Unwin Hyman.

Anderson, R., Kravits, J. and Anderson, O.W. (eds) (1975) *Equity in Health Services: Empirical Analyses in Social Policy*. Cambridge, MA: Ballinger.

Anderson, T.F. and Mooney, G. (1990) *The Challenges of Medical Practice Variations*. Basingstoke: Macmillan.

Andresen, E.M., Rothenberg, B.M. and Kaplan, R.M. (1998) Performance of a self-administered mailed version of the Quality of Well-Being (QWB-SA) questionnaire among older adults, *Medical Care*, 36: 1349–60.

Andrews, F.M. (1984) Construct validity and error components of survey measures: a structural modelling approach, *Public Opinion Quarterly*, 48: 409–22.

Andrews, F.M. and Crandall, R. (1976) The validity of measures of self-reported well-being, *Social Indicators Research*, 3: 1–19.

Andrews, F.M., Klem, L., Davidson, T.N. *et al.* (1981) *A Guide for Selecting Statistical Techniques for Analysing Social Science Data*. Ann Arbor, MI: Survey Research Center, Institute for Social Research, University of Michigan.

Andrews, F.M. and Withey, S.B. (1976) *Social Indicators of Well Being: Americans' Perceptions of Life Quality*. New York: Plenum Press.

Antman, E.M., Lau, J., Kupelnick, B. *et al.* (1992) A comparison of results of meta-analyses of randomized controlled trials and recommendations of clinical experts: treatments for myocardial infarction, *Journal of the American Medical Association*, 268: 2408.

Antonovsky, A. (1984) The sense of coherence as a determinant of health, in J.P. Matarazzo (ed.) *Behavioral Health*. New York: Wiley.

Armitage, P. and Berry, G. (1987) *Statistical Methods in Medical Research*, 2nd edn. Oxford: Blackwell Scientific Publications.

Ashmore, M., Mulkay, M. and Pinch, T. (1989) *Health and Efficiency: A Sociology of Health Economics*. Milton Keynes: Open University Press.

Atkins, L. and Jarrett, D. (1979) The significance of 'significance tests', in J. Irvine, I. Miles and J. Evans (eds) *Demystifying Social Statistics*. London: Pluto Press.

Atkinson, J. (1967) *A Handbook for Interviewers: A Manual for Government Social Survey Interviewing Staff, Describing Practice and Procedures on Structured Interviewing*, Government Social Survey, No. M136. London: HMSO.

Atkinson, R. (1998) *The Life Story Interview*, Qualitative Research Methods Series 44. Thousand Oaks, CA: Sage.

Azur, M.J., Stuart, E.A., Frangakis, C. and Leaf, P.J. (2011) Multiple imputation by chained equations: what is it and how does it work? *International Journal of Methods in Psychiatric Research*, 20: 40–9.

Backett, K.C. and Davison, C. (1995) Lifecourse and lifestyle: the social and cultural locations of health behaviour. *Social Science and Medicine*, 40: 629–38.

Bagshaw, H. and Unell, J. (1997) *Examining Outcomes in Community Care: Report on Focus Groups*. York: Social Policy Research Unit, University of York.

Balas, E.A. and Boren, S.A. (2000) Managing clinical knowledge for healthcare improvements, in J. Bemmel and A.T. McCray (eds) *Yearbook of Medical Informatics*. Stuttgart: Schattauer, pp. 65–70.

Baltes, P.B. and Baltes, M.M. (1990) *Successful Aging: Perspectives from the Behavioral Sciences*. New York: Cambridge University Press.

Bandura, A. (1977) Self-efficacy: toward a unifying theory of behaviour change, *Psychological Review*, 84: 191–215.

Bandura, A. (1986) *Social Foundations of Thought and Action: A Cognitive Social Theory*. Englewood Cliffs, NJ: Prentice Hall.

Bandura, A. (1997) *Self-Efficacy: The Exercise of Control*. New York: Worth Publishers.

Barber, J.A. and Thompson, S.G. (1998) Analysis and interpretation of cost data in randomised controlled trials: review of published studies, *British Medical Journal*, 317, 1195–200.

Barendregt, J.J. and Bonneux, L. (1999) The trouble with health economics, *European Journal of Public Health*, 9: 309–12.

Barendregt, J.J., Bonneux, L. and van der Maas, P.J. (1994) Health expectancy: an indicator for change, *Journal of Epidemiology and Community Health*, 48: 482–7.

Barladi, A.N. and Enders, C.K. (2010) An introduction to modern missing data analyses, *Journal of School Psychology*, 48: 5–37

Barreto, S.M., Swerdlow, A.J., Smith, P.G. and Higgins, C.D. (1997) Risk of death from motor-vehicle injury in Brazilian steelworkers: a nested case control study, *International Journal of Epidemiology*, 26: 814–21.

Barrett, D. (1996) Research, theory and practice: misunderstanding verbal language during community care assessments, in J. Phillips and B. Penhale (eds) *Reviewing Care Management for Older People*. London: Jessica Kingsley.

Barry, M.J., Walker-Corkery, E., Chang, Y. *et al.* (1996) Measurement of overall and disease-specific health status: does the order of questionnaires make a difference? *Journal of Health Services Research and Policy*, 1: 20–7.

Bartley, M., Ferrie, J. and Montgomery, S.M. (1999) Living in a high unemployment economy: understanding the health consequences, in M. Marmot and R.G. Wilkinson (eds) *Social Determinants of Health*. Oxford: Oxford University Press.

Barton, J. (1996) Weighting for non-response: an overview, *Briefing*, 4: 14–16.

Battista, R. (1993) Practice guidelines for preventative care: the Canadian experience, *British Journal of General Practice*, 43: 301–4.

Baxter, P. and Rideout, L. (2006) Decision making of 2nd year baccalaureate nursing students, *Journal of Nursing Education*, 45: 121–8.

Beaglehole, R., Bonita, R. and Kjellström, T. (1993) *Basic Epidemiology*. Geneva: WHO.

Beail, N. (ed.) (1985) *Repertory Grid Technique and Personal Constructs: Applications in Clinical and Educational Settings*. Beckenham: Croom Helm.

Bech, P. (1995) Commentary on: 'A standardized psychiatric consultation lowered costs of care and improved physical functioning in somatising patients', *Evidence-Based Medicine*, 1: 32.

Becker, H. (1963) *Outsiders: Studies in the Sociology of Deviance*. New York: Free Press.

Becker, H. (1971) *Sociological Work*. London: Allen Lane.

Becker, H. and Geer, B. (1982) Participant observation: the analysis of qualitative field data, in R.G. Burgess (ed.) *Field Research: A Sourcebook and Field Manual*. London: Allen & Unwin.

Becker, H.S., Geer, B., Hughes, E.C. and Strauss, A.L. (1961) *Boys in White: Student Culture in Medical School*. Chicago: University of Chicago Press.

Becker, M.H. (1974) The health belief model and personal behaviour, *Health Education Monographs*, 2: 326–73.

Becker, M.H. and Rosenstock, I.M. (1987) Comparing social learning theory and the health belief model, in W.B. Ward (ed.) *Advances in Health Education and Promotion*. Greenwich, CT: JAI Press.

Begg, C., Cho, M., Eastwood, S. *et al.* (1996) Improving the quality of reporting of randomized controlled trials: the CONSORT statement, *Journal of the American Medical Association*, 276: 637–9.

Bekker, H., Thornton, J., Airey, C.M., Connelly, J.B. *et al.* (1999) Informed decision-making: an annotated bibliography and systematic review, *Health Technology Assessment*, 3 (1).

Bell, S.J., Airaksinen, M.S., Lyles, A. *et al.* (2007) Concordance is not synonymous with compliance or adherence, *British Journal of Clinical Pharmacology*, 64: 710–11.

Beller, E.M., Glasziou, P.P., Altman, D.G. *et al.* (2013) PRISMA for abstracts: reporting systematic reviews in journal and conference abstracts, *PLoS Medicine*, 10: e1001419.

Benbassat, J., Pilpel, D. and Tidhar, M. (1998) Patients' preferences for participation in clinical decision-making: a review of published surveys, *Behavioural Medicine*, 24: 81–8.

Bender, R. (1996) Logistic regression models used in medical research are poorly presented, *British Medical Journal*, 313: 628 (letter).

Ben-Shlomo, Y. and Kuh, D. (2002) A life course approach to chronic disease epidemiology: conceptual models, empirical challenges, and interdisciplinary perspectives, *International Journal of Epidemiology*, 31: 285–93.

Berger, P. and Luckman, T. (1967) *The Social Construction of Reality: A Treatise in the Sociology of Knowledge*. Harmondsworth: Penguin.

Bergeron, G. (1999) *Rapid Appraisal Methods for the Assessment, Design, and Evaluation of Food Security Programs*. Technical Guide No. 6. Washington, DC: International Food Policy Research Institute.

Bergner, M., Bobbitt, R.A., Carter, W.B. *et al.* (1981) The Sickness Impact Profile: development and revision of a health status measure, *Medical Care*, 19: 787–805.

Berkanovic, E. (1982) Who engages in health protective behaviours? *International Quarterly on Community Health Education*, 2: 225–37.

Berney, L. and Blane, D. (1997) Collecting retrospective: accuracy of recall after 50 years judged against historical records, *Social Science and Medicine*, 45: 1519–25.

Berridge, V. (1994) Researching contemporary history: AIDS, *History Workshop Journal*, 38: 228–34.

Berridge, V. (1996) *AIDS in the UK: The Making of Policy, 1981–1994*. Oxford: Oxford University Press.

Berridge, V. (2007) *Marketing Health: Smoking and the Discourse of Public Health in Britain, 1945–2000*. Oxford: Oxford University Press.

Berry, D.A. (1996) *Statistics: A Bayesian Perspective*. Belmont, CA: Duxbury Press.

Berry, R. (2011) *Older People and the Internet: Towards a 'System Map' of Digital Exclusion*. London: International Longevity Centre.

Biddulph, J. (2005) Mathematical models in health care, in A. Bowling and S. Ebrahim (eds) *Handbook of Health Research Methods: Investigation, Measurement and Analysis*. Maidenhead: Open University Press.

Billingham, L.J., Abrams, K.R. and Jones, D.R. (1999) Methods for the analysis of quality-of-life and survival data in health technology assessment, *Health Technology Assessment*, 3(10).

Bilotta, C., Bowling, A., Casè, A. *et al.* (2010) Dimensions and correlates of quality of life according to frailty status: a cross-sectional study on community-dwelling older adults referred to an outpatient geriatric service in Italy, *Health & Quality of Life Outcomes*, 8: 56.

Bilotta, C., Bowling, A., Nicolina, P. *et al.* (2011) Older People's Quality of Life (OPQOL) scores and adverse health outcomes at a one-year follow-up: a prospective cohort study on older outpatients living in the community in Italy, *Health and Quality of Life Outcomes*, 9: 72.

Bilotta, C., Bowling, A., Nicolina, P. *et al.* (2012) Quality of life in older out-patients living alone in the community in Italy, *Health and Social Care in the Community*, 20: 32–41.

Birdwhistell, R.L. (1970) *Kinesics and Context: Essays on Body Motion and Communication*. Philadelphia, PA: University of Pennsylvania Press.

Bisig, B., Michel, J.P., Minder, C.M. *et al.* (1992) Disability-free life expectancy: available data in Switzerland, in J.M. Robine, M. Blanchet and J.E. Dowd (eds) *Health Expectancy* (first workshop of the International Healthy Life Expectancy Network (REVES)). Studies on Medical and Population Subjects No. 54. London: HMSO.

Black, N. (1990) Quality assurance of medical care, *Journal of Public Health Medicine*, 12: 97–104.

Black, N. (1996) Why we need observational studies to evaluate the effectiveness of health care, *British Medical Journal*, 312: 1215–18.

Black, N. (2009) Health services research: the gradual encroachment of ideas, *Journal of Health Services Research and Policy*, 14: 120–3.

Black, N., Brazier, J., Fitzpatrick, R. and Reeve, B. (eds) (1998) *Health Services Research Methods: A Guide to Best Practice*. London: BMJ Publishing.

Blalock, H.M. (1972) *Social Statistics*, 2nd edn. London: McGraw-Hill.

Blalock, H.M. and Blalock, A.B. (1971) *Methodology in Social Research*. London: McGraw-Hill.

Bland, J.M. and Altman, D.G. (1986) Statistical methods for assessing agreement between two methods of clinical measurement, *Lancet*, 1: 307–10.

Bland, M. (1995) *An Introduction to Medical Statistics*. Oxford: Oxford University Press.

Blane, D., Davey Smith, G. and Bartley, M. (1993) Social selection: what does it contribute to social class differences in health? *Sociology of Health and Illness*, 15: 2–15.

Blane, D., Gopalakrishnan, N. and Montgomery, S.M. (2008) Quality of life, health and physiological status and change at older ages, *Social Science & Medicine*, 66, 1579–87.

Blane, D., Netuveli, G. and Stone, J. (2007) The development of life course epidemiology, *Revue d'Épidémiologie et de Santé Publique*, 55: 31–8.

Blaxter, M. (1983) The causes of disease, women talking, *Social Science and Medicine*, 17: 59–69.

Blaxter, M. (1990) *Health and Lifestyles*. London: Routledge.

Blaxter, M. and Patterson, L. (1982) *Mothers and Daughters: A Three Generational Study of Health, Attitudes and Behaviour*. London: Heinemann Educational.

Blazer, D. (2002) Self-efficacy and depression in late life: a primary prevention proposal, *Ageing and Mental Health*, 6: 315–24.

Bloom, A. (1968) *The Republic of Plato*, translated with notes and an interpretive essay. New York: Basic Books.

Bloombaum, M. (1983) The Hawthorne experiments: a critique and reanalysis of the first statistical interpretation by Franke and Kaul, *Sociological Perspectives*, 26: 71–88.

Bochner, S. (1983) Doctors, patients and their cultures, in D. Pendleton and J. Hasler (eds) *Doctor–Patient Communication*. London: Academic Press.

Boden, D. and Zimmerman, D.H. (eds) (1991) *Talk and Structure: Studies in Ethnomethodology and Conversation Analysis*. Berkeley, CA: University of California Press.

Bollen, K.A. and Curran, P.J. (2006) *Latent Curve Models: A Structural Equation Perspective*. Hoboken, NJ: John Wiley & Sons Inc.

Bond, M., Bowling, A., Abery, A. *et al.* (2000) Evaluation of outreach clinics held by specialists in general practice in England, *Journal of Epidemiology and Community Health*, 54: 149–56.

Bone, M.R. (1992) International efforts to measure health expectancy, *Journal of Epidemiology and Community Health*, 46: 555–8.

Boore, J. (1979) *Prescription for Recovery*. London: Royal College of Nursing.

Booth, C. (ed.) (1899–1902) *Labour and Life of the People of London*, 17 volumes. Basingstoke: Macmillan.

Bottomley, A., Jones, D. and Claassens L. (2009) Patient-reported outcomes: assessment and current perspectives of the guidelines of the Food and Drug Administration and the reflection paper of the European Medicines Agency, *European Journal of Cancer*, 45: 347–53.

Boulkedid, R., Abdoul, H., Loustau, M., Sibony, O., *et al.* (2011) Using and reporting the Delphi method for selecting healthcare quality indicators: a systematic review, *PLoS ONE*, 6: e20476.

Bourque, L.B. and Fielder, E.P. (1995) *How to Conduct Self-administered and Mail Surveys.* Thousand Oaks, CA: Sage.

Bowling, A. (1989) Implications of preventive health behaviour for cervical and breast cancer screening programmes: a review, *Family Practice*, 6: 224–31.

Bowling, A. (1993) *What People Say about Prioritising Health Services.* London: King's Fund.

Bowling, A. (1994) Social networks and social support among older people and implications for emotional well-being and psychiatric morbidity, *International Review of Psychiatry*, 6: 41–58.

Bowling, A. (1995) What things are important in people's lives? A survey of the public's judgements to inform scales of health-related quality of life, *Social Science and Medicine*, special issue on 'Quality of Life', 10: 1447–62.

Bowling, A. (1996a) Health care rationing: the public's debate, *British Medical Journal*, 312: 670–4.

Bowling, A. (1996b) The effects of illness on quality of life: findings from a survey of households in Great Britain, *Journal of Epidemiology and Community Health*, 50: 149–55.

Bowling, A. (1996c) The most important things in life: comparisons between older and younger population age groups by gender. Results from a national survey of the public's judgements, *International Journal of Health Sciences*, 6: 169–75.

Bowling, A. (1998) Variations in population health status, *British Medical Journal*, 317: 601 (letter).

Bowling, A. (1999) Ageism in cardiology, *British Medical Journal*, 319: 1353–5.

Bowling, A. (2001) *Measuring Disease: A Review of Disease-specific Quality of Life Measurement Scales*, 2nd edn. Buckingham: Open University Press.

Bowling, A. (2005a) *Measuring Health: A Review of Quality of Life Measurement Scales*, 3rd edn. Buckingham: Open University Press.

Bowling, A. (2005b) Mode of questionnaire administration can have serious effects on data quality, *Journal of Public Health Medicine*, 27: 281–91.

Bowling, A. (2005c) *Ageing Well: Quality of Life in Older Age.* Maidenhead: Open University Press.

Bowling, A. (2005d) Just one question: if one question works why ask several? *Journal of Epidemiology and Community Health*, 59: 342–5.

Bowling, A. (2007a) Aspirations for older age in the 21st century: what is successful ageing? *International Journal of Aging and Human Development*, 64: 263–97.

Bowling, A. (2007b) Health status assessment, in S. Ayers, A. Baum, C. McManus, S. Newman, K. Wallston, J. Weinman and R. West (eds) *Cambridge Handbook of Psychology, Health and Medicine*, 2nd edn. Cambridge: Cambridge University Press.

Bowling, A. (2007c) Quality of life assessment, in S. Ayers, A. Baum, C. McManus, S. Newman, K. Wallston, J. Weinman and R. West (eds) *Cambridge Handbook of Psychology, Health and Medicine*, 2nd edn. Cambridge: Cambridge University Press.

Bowling, A. (2009a) Psychometric properties of the Older People's Quality of Life Questionnaire Validity. *Current Gerontology and Geriatrics Research.* 2009; open access online journal: http://dx.doi.org/10.1155/2009/298950.

Bowling, A. (2009b) *Research Methods in Health: Investigating Health and Health Services.* 3rd edn. Maidenhead: McGraw-Hill.

Bowling, A., Bond, M., Jenkinson, C. and Lamping, D. (1999) Short-Form 36 (SF-36) health survey questionnaire: which normative data should be used? Comparison between the norms provided by the Omnibus Survey in Britain, the Health Survey for England and the Oxford Healthy Life Survey, *Journal of Public Health Medicine*, 21: 255–70.

Bowling, A., Culliford, L., Smith, D., Rowe, G. and Reeves, B. (2008) What do patients really want? Patients' preferences for treatment for angina, *Health Expectations*, 11: 137–47.

Bowling, A. and Ebrahim, S. (2001) Measuring patients' preferences for treatment and perceptions of risk, *Quality in Health Care*, 10: 12–18.

Bowling, A. and Ebrahim, S. (eds) (2005) *Handbook of Health Research Methods: Investigation, Measurement and Analysis.* Maidenhead: Open University Press.

Bowling, A., Farquhar, M. and Grundy, E. (1996) Outcome of anxiety and depression at two and a half years after baseline interview: associations with changes in psychiatric morbidity among three samples of elderly people living at home, *International Journal of Geriatric Psychiatry*, 11: 119–29.

Bowling, A., Formby, J., Grant, K. and Ebrahim, S. (1991) A randomised controlled trial of nursing home and long stay geriatric ward care for elderly people, *Age and Ageing*, 20: 316–24.

Bowling, A., Gabriel, Z., Dykes, J. et al. (2003) Let's ask them: a national survey of definitions of quality of life and its enhancement among people aged 65 and over, *International Journal of Aging and Human Development*, 56: 269–306.

Bowling, A., Grundy, E. and Farquhar, M. (1995) Changes in network composition among the very old living in inner London, *Journal of Cross-Cultural Gerontology*, 10: 331–47.

Bowling, A., Hankins, M., Windle, G., Bilotta, C. et al. (2013a) A short measure of quality of life in older age: the performance of the brief Older People's Quality of Life questionnaire (OPQOL-brief). *Archives of Geriatrics and Gerontology*, 56(1): 181–7.

Bowling, A., Hart, D. and Silman, A. (1989) Accuracy of electoral registers and family practitioner committee lists for population studies of the very elderly, *Journal of Epidemiology and Community Health*, 43: 391–4.

Bowling, A., Reeves, B. and Rowe, G. (2010) The Patients Preferences Questionnaire for Angina treatment: results and psychometrics from 383 patients in primary care in England, *Quality and Safety in Health Care*, 19: 1–7.

Bowling, A., Reeves, B. and Rowe, G. (2012b) Do treatment preferences for patients with angina change? An 18-month follow-up study, *Health Expectations*, 15: 351–9.

Bowling, A., Rowe, G., Lambert, N., et al. (2012a) The measurement of patients' expectations for health care: a review and psychometric testing of a measure of patients' expectations, *Health Technology Assessment*, 16(30).

Bowling, A., Rowe, G. and McKee, M. (2013b) Patients' experiences of their healthcare in relation to their expectations and satisfaction: a population survey, *Journal of the Royal Society of Medicine*, 10: 143–9.

Bowling, A., Seetai, S., Morris, R. and Ebrahim, S. (2007) Quality of life among older people with poor functioning: the influence of perceived control over life, *Age and Ageing*, 36: 310–15.

Bowling, A. and Stenner, P. (2011) Which measure of quality of life performs best in older age? A comparison of the OPQOL, CASP-19 and WHOQOL-OLD, *Journal of Epidemiology and Community Health*, 65: 273–80.

Bradburn, N.M. (1969) *The Structure of Psychological Well-being*. Chicago: Aldine.

Bradburn, N.M. and Sudman, S. (1974) *Improving Interview Method and Questionnaire Design*. San Francisco, CA: Jossey-Bass.

Bradshaw, J. (1972) A taxonomy of social need, in G. McLachlan (ed.) *Problems and Progress in Medical Care: Essays on Current Research,*

seventh series. Oxford: Oxford University Press for Nuffield Provincial Hospitals Trust.

Bradshaw, J. (1994) The conceptualisation and measurement of need: a social policy perspective, in J. Popay and G. Williams (eds) *Researching the People's Health*. London: Routledge.

Brannen, P. (1987) Working on directors: some methodological issues, in G. Moyser and M. Wagstaffe (eds) *Research Methods for Elite Studies*. London: Allen & Unwin.

Brazier, J., Deverill, M., Green, C. et al. (1999) A review of the use of health status measures in economic evaluation, *Health Technology Assessment*, 3: 1–158.

Brazier, J., Harper, R., Jones, N.M.B. et al. (1992) Validating the SF-36 health survey questionnaire: new outcomes measures for primary care, *British Medical Journal*, 305: 160–4.

Brazier, J., Harper, R., Waterhouse, J. et al. (1993a) Comparison of outcome measures for patients with chronic obstructive pulmonary disease, paper presented to the Fifth European Health Services Research Conference, Maastricht, December.

Brazier, J., Jones, N. and Kind, P. (1993b) Testing the validity of the EuroQol and comparing it with the SF-36 health survey questionnaire, *Quality of Life Research*, 2: 169–80.

Brennan, P. and Croft, P. (1994) Interpreting the results of observational research: chance is not such a fine thing, *British Medical Journal*, 309: 727–32.

Brenner, M. (ed.) (1981) *Social Method and Social Life*. London: Academic Press.

Brenner, M.H. (1987a) Economic change, alcohol consumption and disease mortality in nine industrialised countries, *Social Science and Medicine*, 25: 119–32.

Brenner, M.H. (1987b) Relation of economic change to Swedish health and social well-being, 1950–1980, *Social Science and Medicine*, 25: 183–96.

Brewin, C.R. and Bradley, C. (1989) Patient preferences in randomised controlled trials, *British Medical Journal*, 299: 313–15.

Briggs, S.R. and Cheek, J.M. (1986) The role of factor analysis in the development and evaluation of personality scales, *Journal of Personality*, 54: 106–48.

British Medical Association (1985) *Presenting a Paper: How to Do It, 1*, 2nd edn. London: BMA.

British Sociological Association (1991) *Statement of Ethical Practice*. London: BSA.

Britten, N., Campell, R., Pope, C. *et al.* (2002) Using meta ethnography to synthesise qualitative research: a worked example, *Journal of Health Services Research and Policy*, 7: 209–15.

Britton, A., McKee, M., Black, N., McPherson, K., Sanderson, C. and Bain, C. (1998) Choosing between randomised and non-randomised studies: a systematic review, *Health Technology Assessment*, 2: 1–119.

Brook, R. (1992) Improving clinical practice: the outcomes v. process controversy in the US. Conference on Healthy Outcomes, organised by *Health Services Journal*, London, 19–20 November.

Brook, R.H. (1994) Appropriateness: the next frontier, *British Medical Journal*, 308: 218–19.

Brook, R.H., Chassin, M.R., Fink, A. *et al.* (1986) A method for the detailed assessment of the appropriateness of medical technologies, *International Journal of Technology Assessment in Health Care*, 2: 53–63.

Brook, R.H., Kosecoff, J.B., Park, R.E. *et al.* (1988) Diagnosis and treatment of coronary disease: comparison of doctors' attitudes in the USA and UK, *Lancet*, 1: 750–3.

Brook, R.H., Ware, J.E., Rogers, W.H. *et al.* (1984) *The Effect of Coinsurance on the Health of Adults: Results from the Rand Health Insurance Experiment*. Report no. R-3055-HHS. Santa Monica, CA: Rand.

Brown, C.A. and Lilford, R. (2006) The stepped wedge trial design: a systematic review, *BMC Medical Research Methodology*, 6: 54.

Brown, H.I. (1977) *Perception, Theory and Commitment: The New Philosophy of Science*. Chicago: University of Chicago Press.

Brown, J. (2005) Economic evaluation, in A. Bowling and S. Ebrahim (eds) *Handbook of Health Research Methods: Investigation, Measurement and Analysis*. Maidenhead: Open University Press.

Brunner, E. and Marmot, M. (1999) Social organisation, stress and health, in M. Marmot and R.G. Wilkinson (eds) *Social Determinants of Health*. Oxford: Oxford University Press.

Bryant, A. and Charmaz, K.C. (2010) Grounded theory in historical perspective: an epistemological account, in K.C. Charmaz and A. Bryant (eds) *The SAGE Handbook of Grounded Theory*, London: Sage, pp. 31–57.

Buchan, H., Gray, M., Hill, A. and Coulter, A. (1990) Needs assessment made simple, *Health Service Journal*, 100: 240–1.

Buchan, I.C. and Richardson, I.M. (1973) *Time Study of Consultations in General Practice*, Scottish Health Service Studies No. 27. Edinburgh: Scottish Home and Health Department.

Bulmer, M. (1982) The merits and demerits of covert participant observation, in M. Bulmer (ed.) *Social Research Ethics*. London: Macmillan.

Burge, P., Devlin, N., Appleby, J. *et al.* (2004) Do patients always prefer quicker treatment? A discrete choice analysis of patients' stated preferences in the London Patient Choice Project, *Applied Health Economics and Health Policy*, 3: 183–94.

Bury, M. (1988) Meanings at risk: the experience of arthritis, in R. Anderson and M. Bury (eds) *Living with Chronic Illness: The Experience of Patients and their Families*. London: Unwin Hyman.

Bury, M. (1991) The sociology of chronic illness: a review of research and prospects, *Sociology of Health and Illness*, 13: 451–68.

Bush, J.W. (1984) General health policy model: quality of well-being (QWB) scale, in N.K. Wenger, M.E. Mattson, C.D. Furberg and J. Ellinson (eds) *Assessment of Quality of Life in Clinical Trials of Cardiovascular Therapies*. New York: Le Jacq.

Bush, T.L., Miller, S.R., Golden, A.L. and Hale, W.E. (1989) Self-report and medical record report agreement of selected medical conditions in the elderly, *American Journal of Public Health*, 79: 1554–6.

Butler, J. (1999) The modern doctor's dilemma: rationing and ethics in healthcare, *Journal of the Royal Society of Medicine*, 92: 416–21.

Byrne, R., Davies, L. and Morrison, A.P. (2010) Priorities and preferences for the outcomes of treatment of psychosis: a service user perspective, *Psychosis: Psychological, Social and Integrative Approaches*, 2: 210–17.

Calnan, M. (1987) *Health and Illness*. London: Tavistock.

Calnan, M. (1988) Towards a conceptual framework of lay evaluation of health care, *Social Science and Medicine*, 27: 927–33.

Calnan, M. and Williams, S.J. (1996) Lay evaluation of scientific medicine and medical care, in M. Calnan and S.J. Williams (eds) *Modern Medicine: Lay Perspectives and Experiences*. London: University College London Press.

Campanelli, P. (1995) Minimising non-response before it happens: what can be done, *Survey Methods Bulletin*, 37: 35–7.

Campbell, A., Converse, P.E. and Rogers, W.L. (1976) *The Quality of American Life*. New York: Russell Sage Foundation.

Campbell, D.T. (1969) Reforms as experiments, *American Psychologist*, 24: 409–29.

Campbell, D.T. and Fiske, D.W. (1959) Convergent and discriminant validation by the multitrait-multimethod marix, *Psychological Bulletin*, 56: 81–105.

Campbell, M., Snowdon, C., Francis, D. *et al.* (2007) Recruitment to randomised trials: strategies for trial enrolment and participation study (STEPS), report for Health Technology Assessment (Methodology Panel), *Health Technology Assessment*, 11(48).

Campbell, M.K. and Grimshaw, J.M. (1998) Cluster randomisation trials: time for improvement, *British Medical Journal*, 317: 1171–2.

Campbell, R. and Garcia, J. (eds) (1997) *The Organisation of Maternity Care: A Guide to Evaluation*. Hale: Hochland & Hochland.

Campbell, R., Pound, P., Morgan, M. *et al.* (2011) Evaluating meta-ethnography: systematic analysis and synthesis of qualitative research, *Health Technology Assessment*, 15: 43.

Campbell, R., Pound, P., Morgan, M. *et al.* (in press) Evaluating meta-ethnography: systematic analysis and synthesis of qualitative research, *Health Technology and Assessment*, 15(43): 1–164.

Campbell, R., Pound, P., Pope, C. *et al.* (2003) Evaluating meta-ethnography: a synthesis of qualitative research on lay experiences of diabetes and diabetes care, *Social Science and Medicine*, 56: 671–84.

Campbell, T. and Stanley, J.C. (1963) Experimental and quasi-experimental designs for research on teaching, in N.L. Gage (ed.) *Handbook of Research on Teaching*. Chicago: Rand McNally.

Campbell, T. and Stanley, J.C. (1966) *Experimental and Quasi-experimental Designs for Research*. Chicago: Rand McNally.

Cannell, C.C., Goves, R.M. and Miller, P.V. (1981) The effects of mode of data collection on health survey data, American Statistical Association, *Proceedings of the Social Statistics Section*, 1–6.

Cano, S.J., Lamping, D.L., Bamber, L. *et al.* (2012) The Anti-Clot Treatment Scale (ACTS) in clinical trials: cross-cultural validation in venous thromboembolism patients, *Health and QoL Outcomes*, 10: 120.

Carnevale, F.A., MacDonald, M.E., Bluebond-Langner, M. and McKeever, P. (2008) Using participant observation in pediatric health care settings: ethical challenges and solutions, *Journal of Child Health Care*, 12: 18–32.

Carneiro, I. and Howard, N. (2011) *Introduction to Epidemiology*. Maidenhead: Open University Press.

Carpiano, R.M. and Daley, D.M. (2006) A guide and glossary on post-positivist theory building for population health, *Journal of Epidemiology and Community Health*, 60: 564–70.

Carr-Hill, R. (1992) A second opinion: health-related quality of life measurement – Euro style, *Health Policy*, 20: 321–8.

Carter, S. and Henderson, L. (2005) Approaches to qualitative data collection in social science, in A. Bowling and S. Ebrahim (eds) *Handbook of Health Research Methods: Investigation, Measurement and Analysis*. Maidenhead: Open University Press.

Carter, Y., Shaw, S. and Thomas, C. (2000) *Randomised Controlled Trials and Multicentre Research: Master Classes in Primary Care Research*. London: Royal College of General Practitioners.

Cartwright, A. (1964) *Human Relations and Hospital Care*. London: Routledge & Kegan Paul.

Cartwright, A. (1978) Professionals as responders: variations in and effects of response rates to questionnaires 1961–77, *British Medical Journal*, 2: 1419–21.

Cartwright, A. (1983) *Health Surveys in Practice and in Potential*. London: King Edward's Hospital Fund for London.

Cartwright, A. (1988) Interviews or postal questionnaires? Comparisons of data about women's experiences with maternity services, *The Millbank Quarterly*, 66: 172–89.

Cartwright, A. (1992) Health services research, *Journal of Epidemiology and Community Health*, 46: 553–4.

Cartwright, A. and Anderson, R. (1980) *Patients and Their Doctors*. London: Tavistock.

Cartwright, A. and Anderson, R. (1981) *General Practice Revisited: A Second Study of Patients and Their Doctors*. London: Tavistock.

Cartwright, A. and Seale, C. (1990) *The Natural History of a Survey: An Account of the Methodological Issues Encountered in a Study of Life Before Death*. London: King Edward's Hospital Fund for London.

Cartwright, A. and Windsor, J. (1989) Who else responds to postal questionnaires? Are those involved in the subject of the study more likely to do so? *Community Medicine*, 11: 373–5.

Cattell, R.B. (ed.) (1966) *Handbook of Multivariate Experimental Psychology*. Chicago: Rand McNally.

Causley, M. (1967) *An Introduction to Benesh Movement Notation*. London: Max Parrish.

Cavanagh, S. and Chadwick, K. (2005) *Health Needs Assessment: A Practical Guide.* London: National Institute for Clinical Excellence. Available at: http://www.nice.org.uk/media/150/35/Health_Needs_Assessment_A_Practical_Guide.pdf

Chadwick, D.J., Gillatt, D.A. and Gingell, J.C. (1991) Medical or surgical orchidectomy: the patients' choice, *British Medical Journal*, 302: 572.

Chalmers, I. (1990) Under-reporting research is scientific misconduct, *Journal of the American Medical Association*, 263: 1405–8.

Chalmers, I. (1995) What do I want from health research and researchers when I am a patient? *British Medical Journal*, 310: 1315–18.

Chalmers, I. and Altman, D. (eds) (1995a) *Systematic Reviews*. London: British Medical Journal Publishing Group.

Chalmers, I. and Altman, D. (1995b) Foreword, in I. Chalmers and D. Altman (eds) *Systematic Reviews*. London: British Medical Journal Publishing Group.

Chambers, R. (1998) *Clinical Effectiveness Made Easy: First Thoughts on Clinical Governance.* Oxford: Radcliffe Medical Press.

Champion, V.L. (1984) Instrument development for health belief model constructs, *Advances in Nursing Science*, 6: 73–85.

Chandola, T. and Jenkinson, C. (2000) The new UK National Statistics socioeconomic classification (NS-SEC): investigating social class differences in self-reported health status, *Journal of Public Health Medicine*, 22: 182–90.

Chandra, A., Blanchard, J.C. and Ruder, T. (2013) *District of Columbia Health Needs Assessment.* Santa Monica, CA: Rand.

Chantler, C., Cochrane, G.M. and Wickings, I. (1989) Translating good ideas into appropriate action, in A. Hopkins (ed.) *Appropriate Investigation and Treatment in Clinical Practice*. London: Royal College of Physicians of London.

Chapple, E.D. (1949) The interaction chronograph: its evolution and present application, *Personnel*, 25: 295–307.

Charlton, J. and Murphy, M. (eds) (1997) *The Health of Adult Britain 1841–1994*, vols 1 and 2. London: The Stationery Office.

Charlton, J., Wallace, M. and White, I. (1994) Long-term illness: results from the 1991 census, *Population Trends*, 75, 18–25.

Charmaz, K. (1983) Loss of self: a fundamental form of suffering in the chronically ill, *Sociology of Health and Illness*, 5: 168–95.

Charmaz, K. (2000) Grounded theory: objectivist and constructivist methods, in N.K. Denzin and Y.S. Lincoln (eds) *Handbook of Qualitative Research*, 2nd edn. Thousand Oaks, CA: Sage, pp. 509–34.

Charmaz, K. (2003) Grounded theory, in J.A. Smith (ed.) *Qualitative Psychology: A Practical Guide to Research Methods*. London: Sage, pp. 81–110.

Chassin, M.R. (1989) How do we decide whether an investigation or procedure is appropriate?, in A. Hopkins (ed.) *Appropriate Investigation and Treatment in Clinical Practice*. London: Royal College of Physicians of London.

Chassin, M.R., Kosecoff, J., Park, R.E. *et al.* (1987) Does inappropriate use explain geographic variations in the use of health services? A study of three procedures, *Journal of the American Medical Association*, 258: 2533–7.

Chatellier, G., Zapletal, E., Lemaitre, D. *et al.* (1996) The number needed to treat: a clinically useful nomogram in its proper context, *British Medical Journal*, 312: 426–9.

Ciliska, D. (2005) Educating for evidence-based practice. *Journal of Professional Nursing*, 21(6): 345–50.

Clark, P. and Bowling, A. (1989) Observational study of quality of life in NHS nursing homes and a long stay ward for the elderly, *Ageing and Society*, 9: 123–48.

Clark, P. and Bowling, A. (1990) Quality of everyday life in long stay institutions for the elderly: an observational study of long stay hospital and nursing home care, *Social Science and Medicine*, 30: 1201–10.

Clarke, H.H. and Schober, M.F. (1992) Asking questions and influencing answers, in J.M. Tanur (ed.) *Questions about Questions: Inquiries into the Cognitive Bases of Surveys*. New York: Russell Sage Foundation.

Clarke, M. and Kurinczuk, J.J., for the Committee of Heads of Academic Departments of Public Health Medicine (1992) Health services research: a case of need or special pleading? *British Medical Journal*, 304: 1675–6.

Clausen, J.A. (1986) *The Life Course: A Sociological Perspective*. New York: Prentice-Hall.

Clinical Accountability, Service Planning and Evaluation (CAPSE) (1988) *CASPE's Patient Satisfaction Questionnaire*. London: King's Fund.

Clinical Resource and Audit Group (1994) *The Interface Between Clinical Audit and Management.* Edinburgh: Scottish Office.

Coast, J., Smith, R. and Lorgelly, P. (2008a) Should the capability approach be applied in health economics? *Health Economics*, 17: 667–70.

Coast, J., Smith, R. and Lorgelly, P. (2008b) Welfarism, extra-welfarism and capability: the spread of ideas in health economics, *Social Science and Medicine*, 67: 1190–8.

Cochrane Collaboration Handbook (1994) *Preparing and Maintaining Systematic Reviews*, vol. VI, ed. A. Oxman. Oxford: The Cochrane Centre.

Cochrane Database of Systematic Reviews (1995) *Disc Issue 1*. London: British Medical Journal Publishing Group/Update Software.

Cockerham, W.C. (1995) *Medical Sociology*, 6th edn. Englewood Cliffs, NJ: Prentice Hall.

Cockerham, W.C., Abel, T. and Lüeschen, G. *et al.* (1993) Max Weber, formal rationality, and health lifestyles, *Sociological Quarterly*, 34: 413–25.

Cockerham, W.C. and Scambler, G. (2010) Medical sociology and sociological theory, in W.C. Cockerham (ed.) *The New Blackwell Companion to Medical Sociology*. Chichester: Wiley-Blackwell, pp. 3–26.

Cohen, G., Forbes, J. and Garraway, M. (1996) Can different patient satisfaction survey methods yield consistent results? Comparison of three surveys, *British Medical Journal*, 313: 841–4.

Cohen, J. (1968) Weighted kappa: nominal scale agreement with provision for scaled disagreement or partial credit, *Psychological Bulletin*, 70: 213–20.

Cohen, J. (1977) *Statistical Power Analysis for the Behavioral Sciences*. New York: Academic Press.

Cohen, S., Kessler, R.C. and Underwood Gordon, L. (1998) *Measuring Stress: A Guide for Health and Social Scientists*. Oxford: Oxford University Press.

Colvez, A. (1996) Disability-free life expectancy, in S. Ebrahim and A. Kalache (eds) *Epidemiology in Old Age*. London: British Medical Journal Publishing Group.

Colvez, A. and Blanchet, M. (1983) Potential gains in life expectancy free of disability: a tool for health planning, *International Journal of Epidemiology*, 12: 86–91.

Conrad, P. and Bury, M. (1997) Anselm Strauss and the sociological study of chronic illness: a reflection and appreciation. *Sociology of Health and Illness*, 19: 373–6.

Conover, W.J. (1999) *Practical Nonparametric Statistics*, 3rd edn. New York: John Wiley and Sons Inc.

Cook, T.D. and Campbell, D.T. (1979) *Quasi-experimentation: Design and Analysis Issues for Field Settings*. Chicago: Rand McNally.

Cookson, R. (2003) Willingness to pay methods in health care: a sceptical view. *Health Economics*, 12: 891–4.

Cooley, C.H. (1964) *Human Nature and the Social Order*. New York: Schocken.

Coomarasamy, A., Latthe, P., Papaioannou, S., Publicover, M., Gee, H. and Khan, K.S. (2001) Critical appraisal in clinical practice: sometimes irrelevant, occasionally invalid, *Journal of the Royal Society of Medicine*, 94: 573–7.

Cornfield, J. (1978) Randomisation by group: a formal analysis, *American Journal of Epidemiology*, 108: 100–2.

Cornwell, J. (1984) *Hard Earned Lives: Accounts of Health and Illness from East London*. London: Tavistock Publications.

Cosper, R. (1972) Interviewer effect in a survey of drinking practices, *Sociological Quarterly*, 13: 228–36.

Coste, J., Guillemin, F., Pouchot, J. and Fermanian, J. (1997) Methodological approaches to shortening composite measurement scales, *Journal of Clinical Epidemiology*, 50: 247–52.

Coulter, A. (1987) Lifestyles and social class: implications for primary care, *Journal of the Royal College of General Practitioners*, 37: 533–6.

Coulter, A. (2006) Examining health expectations, *Health Expectations*, 9: 1–2.

Coulter, A., Klassen, A., Mackenzie, I.Z. and McPherson, K. (1993) Diagnosis dilation and curettage: is it used appropriately? *British Medical Journal*, 306: 236–9.

Cox, B.D., Blaxter, M., Buckle, A.L.J. *et al.* (1987) *The Health and Lifestyle Survey*. London: Health Promotion Research Trust.

Cox, B.D., Huppert, F.A. and Whichelow, M.J. (1993) *The Health and Lifestyle Survey: Seven Years On*. Aldershot: Dartmouth Publishing.

Cox, D.R. (1958) *Planning of Experiments*. New York: Wiley.

Craig, P., Dieppe, P., MacIntyre, S. *et al.* (2008) Developing and evaluating complex interventions, *British Medical Journal*, 337: a1655.

Craig, J.V. and Smyth, R.L. (eds) (2007) *The Evidence-Based Practice Manual for Nurses*, 2nd edn. Edinburgh: Churchill Livingstone Elsevier.

Crawley, S. and Pring, L. (2000) When did Mrs Thatcher resign? The effects of ageing on the dating of public events, *Memory*, 8: 111–21.

Cresswell, J.W. (2009) *Research Design: Qualitative, Quantitative, and Mixed Methods Approaches*, 3rd edn. Thousand Oaks, CA: Sage.

Creswell, J.W. and Plano Clark, V.L. (2007) *Designing and Conducting Mixed Methods Research.* Thousand Oaks, CA: Sage.

Creswell, J.W. and Plano Clark, V.L. (2011) *Designing and Conducting Mixed Methods Research,* 2nd edn. Thousand Oaks, CA: Sage.

Crichton, N.J. (1993) The importance of statistics in research design, in G.T. Lewith and D. Aldridge (eds) *Clinical Research Methodology for Complementary Therapies.* London: Hodder & Stoughton.

Crombie, I.K. (1996) *Pocket Guide to Critical Appraisal.* London: BMJ Books.

Cronbach, L.J. (1946) Response sets and test validity, *Educational Psychological Measurement,* 61: 475–94.

Cronbach, L.J. (1951) Coefficient alpha and the internal structure of tests, *Psychometrika,* 22: 293–6.

Cronbach, L.J. (1987) Social inquiry by and for earthlings, in W.R. Shadish and C.S. Reichardt (eds) *Evaluative Studies.* London: Sage.

Crow, R., Gage, H., Hampson, S. *et al.* (1999) The role of expectancies in the placebo effect and their use in the delivery of health care: a systematic review, *Health Technology Assessment,* 3(3).

Crow, R., Gage, H., Hampson, S. *et al.* (2002) The measurement of satisfaction with health care: implications for practice from a systematic review of the literature, *Health Technology Assessment,* 6(32).

Crowne, D.P. and Marlow, D. (1960) A new scale of social desirability independent of psychopathology, *Journal of Consulting Psychology,* 24: 349–54.

Cullinan, P. (2005) Evidence-based health care: systematic reviews, in A. Bowling and S. Ebrahim (eds) *Handbook of Health Research Methods: Investigation, Measurement and Analysis.* Maidenhead: Open University Press.

Culyer, A.J. (1995) Need: the idea won't do – but we still need it, *Social Science and Medicine,* 40: 727–30.

Culyer, A.J. and Wagstaff, A. (1991) *Need, Equality and Social Justice,* discussion paper 90. York: Centre for Health Economics, University of York.

Currer, C. and Stacey, M. (eds) (1986) *Concepts of Health, Illness and Disease: A Comparative Perspective.* Oxford: Berg.

Curtis, S. and Taket, A. (1996) *Health and Societies: Changing Perspectives.* London: Arnold.

Czaja, R. and Blair, J. (2005) *Designing Surveys.* Thousand Oaks, CA: Sage.

Dale, C.E., Bowling, A., Adamson, J., *et al.* (2013) Predictors of patterns of change in health-related quality of life in older women over 7 years: evidence from a prospective cohort study. *Age and Ageing,* 42: 312–18.

Datta, S., Foss, A.J.E., Grainge, M.J., Gregson, R.M. *et al.* (2008) The importance of acuity, stereopsis, and contrast sensitivity for health-related quality of life in elderly women with cataracts, *Investigative Ophthalmology and Visual Science,* 49: 1–6.

Davey, B. (1994) The nature of scientific research, in K. McConway (ed.) *Studying Health and Disease,* 2nd edn. Buckingham: Open University Press.

Davey Smith, G. and Phillips, A.N. (1992) Confounding in epidemiological studies: why 'independent effects may not be all they seem', *British Medical Journal,* 305: 757–9.

Davies, A.M. (1991) *The Evolving Science of Health Systems Research: From Research to Decision Making. Case Studies on the Use of Health Systems Research, Programme on Health Systems Research and Development.* Geneva: WHO.

Davies, A.R. and Ware, J.E. (1991) *GHAA's Consumer Satisfaction Survey and User's Manual.* Washington, DC: Group Health Association of America.

Davison, C., Davey Smith, G. and Frankel, S. (1991) Lay epidemiology and the prevention paradox: the implications of coronary candidacy for health education, *Sociology of Health and Illness,* 13: 131–9.

Dawes, M., Davies, P., Gray A., Mant, J. *et al.* (2004) *Evidence-Based Practice: A Primer for Health Care Professionals,* 2nd edn. London: Churchill Livingstone Elsevier.

Dawn, A.G. and Lee, P.P. (2004) Patient expectations for medical and surgical care: a review of the literature and applications to ophthalmology, *Survey of Ophthalmology,* 49: 513–24.

Dean, A.G., Dean, J.A., Coulombier, D. *et al.* (1995) *Epi Info Version 6: A Word-processing, Database and Statistics Program for Public Health on IBM-compatible Microcomputers.* Atlanta, GA: Centers for Disease Control and Prevention.

de Bruin, A., Picavet, H.S.J. and Nossikov, A. (1996) *Health Interview Surveys: Towards International Harmonization of Methods and Instruments.* Copenhagen: WHO.

Deeks, J. (1996) What is an odds ratio? *Bandolier, Evidence-Based Health Care,* 3: 6–7.

Deeks, J., Dinnes, J., D'Amico, R.D., Sowden, A.J., Sakarovitch, C., Song, F., Petticrew, M. and

Altman, D.G. (2003) Evaluating non-randomised studies, *Health Technology Assessment*, 7(27).

Deeks, J., Glanville, J. and Sheldon, T. (1996) *Undertaking Systematic Reviews of Research on Effectiveness*. York: NHS Centre for Reviews and Dissemination, University of York.

Dehue, T. (2000) From deception-trials to control-reagents: the introduction of the control group about a century ago, *American Psychologist*, 55: 264–9.

Dehue, T. (2001) Establishing the experimenting society: the historical origin of social experimentation according to the randomised controlled design, *American Journal of Psychology*, 114: 283–302.

Delgado-Rodríguez, M. and Llorca, J. (2004) Bias, *Journal of Epidemiology and Community Health*, 58: 635–41.

Denzin, N.K. (1970) *The Research Act in Sociology*. London: Butterworth.

Denzin, N.K. (1971) The logic of naturalistic inquiry, *Social Forces*, 50: 166–82.

Denzin, N.K. (1978) *Sociological Methods: A Sourcebook*, 2nd edn. New York: McGraw-Hill.

Denzin, N.K. (1989) *The Research Act: A Theoretical Introduction to Sociological Methods*, 3rd edn. Englewood Cliffs, NJ: Prentice Hall.

Department of Health (1993a) *Research for Health*. London: Department of Health.

Department of Health (1993b) *Clinical Audit: Meeting and Improving Standards in Healthcare*. London: NHS Management Executive.

Department of Transport (1994) *Value of Time Savings and Accident Prevention*. London: Department of Transport.

d'Houtard, A. and Field, M.G. (1984) The image of health: variations in perception by social class in a French population, *Sociology of Health and Illness*, 6: 30–60.

d'Houtard, A., Field, M.G., Tax, B. and Gueguen, R. (1990) Representations of health in two Western European populations, *International Journal of Health Sciences*, 1–4: 243–55.

DiCenso, A., Guyatt, G. and Ciliska, D. (eds) (2005) *Evidence-Based Nursing: A Guide to Clinical Practice*. St. Louis, MO: Elsevier Mosby.

Dickens, C. ([1861] 1958) *The Uncommercial Traveller*. Oxford: Oxford University Press.

Diener, E. (1994) Assessing subjective well-being: progress and opportunities, *Social Indicators Research*, 3: 2.

Diener, E., Sandvik, E., Pavot, W., et al. (1991) Response artefacts in the measurement of subjective well-being. *Social Indicators Research*, 24: 35–56.

Dingwall, R., Eekelaar, J. and Murray, T. (1983) *The Protection of Children: State Intervention and Family Life*. Padstow: T.J. Press.

Dobbs, J. and Breeze, E. (1993) Effect on response of including a reply card with advance letters: an enforced experiment, *Survey Methods Bulletin*, 32: 18–19.

Dolan, P. (1997) Modelling valuations for EuroQoL health states, *Medical Care*, 35: 1095–8.

Dolan, P., Gudex, C., Kind, P. and Williams, A. (1993) The valuation of health states: a comparison of methods, paper presented at the Fifth European Health Services Research Conference, Maastricht, December.

Doll, H., McPherson, K., Davies, J., Flood, A. et al. (1991) Reliability of questionnaire responses as compared with interview in the elderly: views on the outcome of transurethral resection of the prostate, *Social Science and Medicine*, 33: 1303–8.

Donabedian, A. (1980) *Explorations in Quality Assessment and Monitoring*, Vol. 1, *The Definition of Quality and Approaches to its Assessment*. Ann Arbor, MI: Health Administration Press.

Donaldson, C. (1993) *Theory and Practice of Willingness to Pay for Health Care*, Discussion Paper 01/93. Aberdeen: Health Economics Research Unit, University of Aberdeen.

Donaldson, C., Atkinson, A., Bond, J. and Wright, K. (1988) QALYs and the long term care for elderly people in the UK: scales for assessment of quality of life, *Age and Ageing*, 17: 379–87.

Donner, A. (1992) Sample size requirements for stratified cluster randomisation designs, *Statistics in Medicine*, 11: 743–50.

Donner, A. and Klar, N. (1994) Cluster randomisation trials in epidemiology: theory and application, *Journal of Statistics, Planning and Inference*, 42: 37–56.

Donner, A. and Klar, N. (2000) *Design and Analysis of Cluster Randomisation Trials in Health Research*. London: Arnold.

Donovan, J. and Sanders, C. (2005) Key issues in the analysis of qualitative data in health services research, in A. Bowling and S. Ebrahim (eds) *Handbook of Health Research Methods: Investigation, Measurement and Analysis*. Maidenhead: Open University Press.

Dooley, D. (1995) *Social Research Methods*. Englewood Cliffs, NJ: Prentice Hall.

Doyal, L.A. (1979) A matter of life and death: medicine, health and statistics, in I. Miles and

J. Evans (eds) *Demystifying Social Statistics*. London: Pluto Press.

Doyal, L.A. and Gough, I. (1991) *A Theory of Social Need*. London: Macmillan.

Drummond, M. (1994) *Economic Analysis Alongside Controlled Trials*. Leeds: NHS Executive, Department of Health.

Drummond, M.F., O'Brien, B., Stoddart, G.L. and Torrance, G.W. (1997) *Methods for the Economic Evaluation of Health Care Programmes*, 2nd edn. Oxford: Oxford University Press.

Drummond, M.F., Sculpher, M.J. and Torrance, G.W. (2005) *Methods for the Economic Evaluation of Health Care*, 3rd edn. Oxford: Oxford University Press.

Dunne, M.P., Martin, N.G. and Bailey, J.M. (1997) Participation bias in a sexuality survey: psychological and behavioural characteristics of responders and non-responders, *International Journal of Epidemiology*, 26: 844–54.

Dunnell, K. and Cartwight, A. (1972) *Medicine Takers, Prescribers and Hoarders*. London: Routledge & Kegan Paul.

Durkheim, E. (1951) *Suicide* (ed. G. Simpson, trans. J.A. Spaulding and G. Simpson). New York: Free Press. First published in 1897 as *Le Suicide*.

Durkin, K. (1985) *Television, Sex Roles and Children*. Milton Keynes: Open University Press.

Durkin, K. (1986) Sex roles and the mass media, in D.J. Hargreaves and A.M. Colley (eds) *The Psychology of Sex Roles*. London: Harper & Row.

Eagly, A.H. and Chaiken, S. (1993) *The Psychology of Attitudes*. Fort Worth, TX: Harcourt Brace Jovanovich.

Earl-Slater, A. (2004) *Lay Involvement in Health and Other Research*. Oxford: Radcliffe Medical Press.

Ebrahim, S. (1990) Case-control studies in rehabilitation, *Clinical Rehabilitation*, 4: 95–101.

Ebrahim, S. (2000) Do not resuscitate decisions: flogging dead horses or a dignified death? *British Medical Journal*, 320: 1155–6.

Edelmann, R.J. (1996) Attitude measurement, in D.F.S. Cormack (ed.) *The Research Process in Nursing*, 3rd edn. Oxford: Blackwell Scientific Publications.

Edelmann, R.J. (2000) *Psychosocial Aspects of the Health Care Process*. Harlow: Prentice Hall.

Edgar, A., Salek, S., Shickle, D. and Cohen, D. (1998) *The Ethical QALY: Ethical Issues in Healthcare Resource Allocations*. Haselmere: Euromed Communications.

Edwards, A.G.K. and Elwyn, G. (1999) How should effectiveness of risk communication to aid patients' decisions be judged? A review of the literature, *Medical Decision Making*, 19: 428–34.

Edwards, A.G.K., Elwyn, G.J., Covey, J. *et al.* (2001) Presenting risk information: a review of the effects of 'framing' and other manipulations on patient outcomes. *Journal of Health and Community*, 6: 61–82.

Edwards, A.L. (1957) *The Social Desirability Variable in Personality Assessment*. New York: Dryden Press.

Edwards, S.J.L., Braunholtz, D.A., Lilford, R.J. and Stevens, A.J. (1999) Ethical issues in the design and conduct of cluster randomised controlled trials, *British Medical Journal*, 318: 1407–9.

Eckenrode, J. and Hamilton, S. (2000) One-to-one support interventions, in S. Cohen, L.G. Underwood and B.H. Gottlieb (eds) *Social Support Measurement and Interventions: A Guide for Health and Social Scientists*. Oxford: Oxford University Press.

Egger, M., Davey Smith, G. and Phillips, A.N. (1997) Meta-analysis: principles and procedures, *British Medical Journal*, 315: 1533–7.

Egger, M., Jüni, P., Bartlett, C., Holenstein, F. and Sterne, J. (2003) How important are comprehensive literature searches and the assessment of trial quality in systematic reviews? Empirical study, *Health Technology Assessment*, 7(1).

Egger, M., Schneider, M. and Davey Smith, G. (1998) Spurious precision? Meta-analysis of observational studies, *British Medical Journal*, 316: 140–5.

Eklund, K. and Wilhelmson, K. (2009) Outcomes of coordinated and integrated interventions targeting frail elderly people: a systematic review of randomised controlled trials, *Health and Social Care in the Community*, 17: 447–58.

Ekman, P. and Friesen, W. (1978) *FACS Investigator's Guide*. Palo Alto, CA: Consulting Psychologists Press.

Elder, J.P., Ayala, G.X. and Harris, S. (1999) Theories and intervention approaches to health-behavior change in primary care, *American Journal of Preventive Medicine*, 17: 275–84.

Elliot, D. (1991) *Weighting for Non-response: A Survey Researcher's Guide*. London: Office of Population Censuses and Surveys.

Elliot, D. (1994) A note on confidence intervals for differences in proportions, *Survey Methods Bulletin*, 34: 1–2.

Emerson, E. and Hatton, C. (1994) *Moving Out: Relocation from Hospital to Community*. London: HMSO.

Emslie, C., Hunt, K. and Watt, G. (2000) 'It's a family affair': lay understandings of a 'family history' of heart disease, in *ESRC Findings from the Health Variations Programme*, no. 6. Lancaster: Department of Social Science, Lancaster University.

Ende, J., Kazis, L., Ash, A. and Moskowitze, M.A. (1989) Measuring patients' desire for autonomy: decision-making and information-seeking preferences among medical patients, *Journal of General Internal Medicine*, 4: 23–30.

Erikson, E.H. and Erikson, J.M. (1997) *The Life Cycle Completed*. New York: W.W. Norton & Company, Inc.

Eriksson, I., Undén, A.L. and Elofsson, S. (2001) Self-rated health: comparisons between three different measures. Results from a population study, *International Journal of Epidemiology*, 30: 326–33.

Erlandson, D.A., Harris, E.L., Skipper, B.L. and Allen, S.D. (1993) *Doing Naturalistic Inquiry: A Guide to Methods*. Newbury Park, CA: Sage.

Etzioni, A. (1993) *The Spirit of Community*. London: Fontana.

European Concerted Action on Harmonization of Health Expectancy Calculation in Europe (1996) *Practical Guide on Health Expectancy Calculation: Sullivan Method. Subcommittee on Research Design and Calculation Methods*. Paris: Institut National d'Etudes Démographiques.

European Union Agency for Fundamental Rights (2009) *EU-MIDIS Technical Report Methodology, Sampling and Fieldwork*. Vienna: European Union Agency for Fundamental Rights.

EuroQoL Group (1990) EuroQol: a new facility for the measurement of health-related quality of life, *Health Policy*, 16: 199–208.

Evans, R.G. (1990) The dog in the night time: medical practice variations and health policy, in T.F. Anderson and G. Mooney (eds) *The Challenges of Medical Practice Variations*. Basingstoke: Macmillan.

Evidence-Based Medicine (1995) Purpose and procedure (abbreviated), *Evidence-Based Medicine*, 1: 2.

Evidence-based Medicine Working Group (1992) Evidence-based medicine: a new approach to teaching the practice of medicine, *Journal of the American Medical Association*, 268: 2420–5.

Farquhar, M. (1995) Elderly people's definitions of quality of life, *Social Science and Medicine*, special issue on 'Quality of Life', 10: 1439–46.

Farrar, S. and Donaldson, C. (1996) Health economics, in S. Ebrahim and A. Kalache (eds)

Epidemiology in Old Age, London: British Medical Journal Publishing Group.

Fazio, R.H. (1990) Multiple processes by which attitudes guide behavior: the MODE model as an integrative framework, in M.P. Zanna (ed.) *Advances in Experimental Social Psychology*, vol. 23. San Diego, CA: Academic Press.

Featherstone, K. and Donovan, J.L. (1998) Random allocation or allocation at random? Patients' perspectives of participation in a randomised controlled trial, *British Medical Journal*, 317: 1177–80.

Feeny, D. (2005) The health utilities index: a tool for assessing health benefits, *Patient Reported Outcomes*, 34: 2–6.

Feeny, D., Furlong, W., Boyle, M. *et al.* (1995) Multi-attribute health status classification systems, *Health Utilities Index, Pharmacoeconomics*, 7: 490–502.

Feeny, D.H., Torrance, G.W. and Furlong, W.J. (1996) Health Utilities Index, in B. Spiker (ed.) *Quality of Life and Pharmacoeconomics in Clinical Trials*, 2nd edn. Philadelphia, PA: Lippincott-Raven.

Feldman, M.S. (1995) *Strategies for Interpreting Qualitative Data*, Qualitative Research Methods, Series 33. Thousand Oaks, CA: Sage.

Fennell, G., Phillipson, C. and Evers, H. (1994) *The Sociology of Old Age*. Maidenhead: Open University Press.

Fielding, J. (1993) Coding and managing data, in N. Gilbert (ed.) *Researching Social Life*. London: Sage.

Fielding, N. (1993) Ethnography, in N. Gilbert (ed.) *Researching Social Life*. London: Sage.

Filmer, P., Philipson, M., Silverman, D. and Walsh, D. (1972) *New Directions in Sociological Theory*. London: Collier-Macmillan.

Fink, A., Kosecoff, J., Chassin, M. and Brook, R. (1984) Consensus methods: characteristics and guidelines for use, *American Journal of Public Health*, 74: 979–83.

Fishbein, M. (1967) Attitude and the prediction of behavior, in M. Fishbein (ed.) *Readings in Attitude Theory and Measurement*. New York: Wiley.

Fisher, R.A. (1935) *The Design of Experiments*. Edinburgh: Oliver & Boyd.

Fisk, J., Brown, M., Sketris, I. *et al.* (2005) A comparison of health utility measures for the evaluation of multiple sclerosis treatments, *Journal of Neurology, Neurosurgery and Psychiatry*, 76: 58–63.

Fitzpatrick, R. (1990) Measurement of patient satisfaction, in A. Hopkins and D. Costain (eds)

Measuring the Outcomes of Medical Care. London: Royal College of Physicians of London.

Fitzpatrick, R. (1994) Health needs assessment, chronic illness and the social sciences, in J. Popay and G. Williams (eds) *Researching the People's Health*. London: Routledge.

Fitzpatrick, R., Bowling, A., Gibbons, E. *et al*. (2006) *A Structured Review of Patient-reported Measures in Relation to Selected Chronic Conditions, Perceptions of Quality of Care and Carer Impact*. Oxford: Patient-reported Health Instruments Group, National Centre for Health Outcomes Development (Oxford site), Unit of Health-Care Epidemiology, Department of Public Health, University of Oxford.

Fitzpatrick, R., Davey, C., Buxton, M. and Jones, D.R. (1998) Evaluating patient-based outcome measures for use in clinical trials, *Health Technology Assessment*, 2: 1–74.

Fitzpatrick, R. and Hopkins, A. (1983) Problems in the conceptual framework of patient satisfaction research: an empirical exploration, *Sociology of Health and Illness*, 5: 297–311.

Fitzpatrick, R., Norquist, J.M., Jenkinson, C., Reeves, B.C., Morris, R.W. and Murray, D.W. (2004) A comparison of Rasch with Likert scoring to discriminate between patients' evaluations of total hip surgery, *Quality of Life Research*, 13: 331–8.

Fleisher, M.L. (1989) *Warehousing Violence*. Newbury Park, CA: Sage.

Fleiss, J.L. (1981) The measurement of inter-rater agreement, in J.L. Fleiss (ed.) *Statistical Methods for Rates and Proportions*. New York: Wiley.

Flesch, R. (1948) A new readability yardstick, *Journal of Applied Psychology*, 32: 221–33.

Floyd, C.B. and Livesey, A. (1975) Self-observation in general practice – the bleep method, *Journal of the Royal College of General Practitioners*, 25: 425–31.

Flynn, T.N. (2010) Using conjoint analysis and choice experiments to estimate QALY values: issues to consider. *Pharmacoeconomics*, 28: 711–22.

Folkman, S. and Lazarus, R.S. (1980) An analysis of coping in a middle-aged community sample, *Journal of Health and Social Behavior*, 21: 219–39.

Folkman, S. and Lazarus, R.S. (1988) *Manual of the Ways of Coping Questionnaire*. Palo Alto, CA: Consulting Psychologists Press.

Folkman, S., Lazarus, R.S., Gruen, R.J. and DeLongis, A. (1986) Appraisal, coping, health status

and psychological symptoms, *Journal of Personality and Social Psychology*, 50: 571–9.

Foster, G.M. and Anderson, B.G. (1978) *Medical Anthropology*. New York: Wiley.

Foster, K., Jackson, B., Thomas, M. *et al*. (1995) *General Household Survey 1993*. Norwich: HMSO.

Fowler, F.J. (2009) *Survey Research Methods*. Thousand Oaks, CA: Sage.

Fowler, F. and Mangione, T. (1986) *Reducing Interviewer Effects on Health Survey Data*. Rockville, MD: National Center for Health Services Research and Health Care Technology Assessment.

Fox, A.J., Goldblatt, P.O. and Adelstein, A.M. (1982) Selection and mortality differentials, *Journal of Epidemiology and Community Health*, 36: 69–79.

Fox-Rushby, J. and Cairns, J. (2005) *Economic Evaluation*. Maidenhead: Open University Press.

Francis, J., Fisher, M. and Rutter, D. (2011) *Reablement: A Cost-Effective Route to Better Outcomes*. Research briefing 36. London: Social Care Institute of Excellence.

Francis, J.J., Eccles, M.P., Johnston, M. *et al*. (2004) *Constructing Questionnaires Based on the Theory of Planned Behaviour*. Newcastle: Centre for Health Services Research, University of Newcastle upon Tyne.

Franke, R.H. and Kaul, J.D. (1978) The Hawthorne experiments: first statistical interpretation, *American Sociological Review*, 43: 623–43.

Frankel, S. (1991) Health needs, health care requirements and the myth of infinite demand, *Lancet*, 337: 1588–9.

Frankfort-Nachmias, C. and Nachmias, D. (1992) *Research Methods in the Social Sciences*, 4th edn. London: Edward Arnold.

Freedman, L. (1996) Bayesian statistical methods: a natural way to assess clinical evidence, *British Medical Journal*, 313: 569–70.

Frewer, L.J., Howard, C., Hedderley, D. and Shepherd, R. (1998a) Methodological approaches to assessing risk perceptions associated with food-related hazards, *Risk Analysis*, 18: 95–102.

Frewer, J.L., Howard, C. and Shepherd, R. (1998b) The influence of initial attitudes on reponse to communication about genetic engineering in food production, *Agriculture and Human Values*, 15: 15–30.

Friedson, E. (1970) *Profession of Medicine: A Study in the Sociology of Applied Knowledge*. New York: Dodd Mead.

Fries, J.F., Spitz, P.W. and Young, D.Y. (1982) The dimensions of health outcomes: the Health

Assessment Questionnaire, disability and pain scales, *Journal of Rheumatology*, 9: 789–93.

Frogberg, D. and Kane, R. (1989) Methodology for measuring health-state preferences, III: population and context effects, *Journal of Clinical Epidemiology*, 42: 585–92.

Fuller, R., Dudley, N. and Blacktop, J. (2001) Risk communication and older people – understanding of probability and risk information by medical in-patients aged 75 and older, *Age and Ageing*, 30: 473–6.

Furlong, W., Feeny, D., Torrance, G.W. *et al.* (1998) *Multiplicative Multi-Attribute Utility Function for the Health Utilities Index Mark 3 (HU13) System: A Technical Report*. Hamilton, Ontario: McMaster University Centre for Health Economics and Policy Analysis.

Gardner, M.J. and Altman, D.G. (1986) Confidence intervals rather than *P* values: estimation rather than hypothesis testing, *British Medical Journal*, 292: 746–50.

Garfinkel, H. (1967) *Studies in Ethnomethodology*. Cambridge: Polity Press.

Garratt, A.M., Bjaertnes, Ø.A., Krogstad, U. and Gulbrandsen, P. (2005) The outpatient experiences questionnaire (OPEQ): data quality, reliability and validity in patients attending 52 Norwegian hospitals, *Quality and Safety in Health Care*, 14: 433–7.

Gecas, V. (1989) The social psychology of self-efficacy, *Annual Review of Sociology*, 15: 291–316.

Gelber, R.D. and Goldhirsh, A. (1986) A new endpoint for the assessment of adjuvant therapy in postmenopausal women with operable breast cancer, *Journal of Clinical Oncology*, 4: 1772–9.

Gelber, R.D., Richard, D. and Goldhirsh, A. (1989) Comparison of adjuvant therapies using quality of life considerations, *International Journal of Technology Assessment in Health Care*, 5: 401–13.

George, L.K., Blazer, D.G., Hughes, D.C. and Fowler, N. (1989) Social support and the outcome of major depression, *British Journal of Psychiatry*, 154: 478–85.

Gerard, K., Ryan, M. and Amaya-Amaya, M. (2008) Introduction, in M. Ryan, K. Gerard and M. Amaya-Amaya (eds) *Using Discrete Choice Experiments to Value Health and Health Care*. Dordrecht: Springer.

Gerhardt, U. (1987) Parsons, role theory, and health interaction, in G. Scambler (ed.) *Sociological Theory and Medical Sociology*. London: Tavistock.

Gerhardt, U. (1996) Narratives of normality: end-stage renal-failure patients' experience of their transplant options, in S.J. Williams and M. Calnan (eds) *Modern Medicine: Lay Perspectives and Experiences*. London: University College London Press.

Gerrard, M. and Warner, T.D. (1991) Antecedents of pregnancy among women Marines, *Journal of the American Academy of Sciences*, 80: 1015.

Giddens, A. (ed.) (1974) *Positivism and Sociology*. London: Heinemann.

Gigerenzer, G. and Edwards, A. (2003) Simple tools for understanding risks: from innumeracy to insight, *British Medical Journal*, 327: 741–4.

Glaser, B. and Strauss, A. (1965) *Time for Dying*. Chicago: Aldine.

Glaser, B. and Strauss, A.L. (1967) *The Discovery of Grounded Theory: Strategies for Qualitative Research*. New York: Aldine Publishing.

Glaser, B. and Strauss, A. (1968) *Awareness of Dying*. Chicago: Aldine.

Glynn, J.R. (1993) A question of attribution, *Lancet*, 342: 530–2.

Goffman, E. (1959) *The Presentation of Self in Everyday Life*. New York: Anchor.

Goffman, E. (1961) *Asylums*. New York: Doubleday.

Goffman, E. (1968) *Stigma: Notes on the Management of Spoiled Identity*. Harmondsworth: Penguin.

Goldberg, D. and Williams, P. (1988) *A User's Guide to the General Health Questionnaire*. Windsor: NFER-Nelson.

Goldberg, P., Guëguen, A., Schmaus, A. *et al.* (2001) Longitudinal study of associations between perceived health status and self-reported diseases in the French Gazel Cohort, *Journal of Epidemiology and Community Health*, 55: 233–8.

Goldstein, H. (1995) *Multilevel Statistical Models*. London: Edward Arnold.

Gonzalez Morganti, K., Bauhoff, S., Blanchard, J.C. *et al.* (2013) *The Evolving Role of Emergency Departments in the United States*. Santa Monica, CA: RAND Corporation.

Gore, S.M. (1981) Assessing clinical trials – trial size, *British Medical Journal*, 282: 1687–9.

Gosden, T.B., Black, M.E., Mead, N.J. and Leese, B.M. (1997) The efficiency of specialist outreach clinics in general practice: is further evaluation needed? *Journal of Health Services Research and Policy*, 3: 174–9.

Government Statisticians' Collective (1979) How official statistics are produced: views from the inside, in I. Miles and J. Evans (eds) *Demystifying Social Statistics*. London: Pluto Press.

Gowers, E.A. (1954) *The Complete Plain Words*. Harmondsworth: Penguin.

Gracely, R.H., Dubner, R., Deeter, W.R. and Wolskee, P.J. (1985) Clinical expectations influence placebo analgesia, *Lancet*, i: 43.

Graham, H. (1976) Smoking in pregnancy: the attitudes of expectant mothers, *Social Science and Medicine*, 10: 399–405.

Graham, H. (1984) Surveying through stories, in C. Bell and H. Roberts (eds) *Social Researching: Politics, Problems, Practices*. London: Routledge & Kegan Paul.

Graham, H. (ed.) (2000) *Understanding Health Inequalities*. Buckingham: Open University Press.

Grammatik 5 (1992) Reference Software Inc 330 Townsend Street Suite 123 San Francisco, CA.

Granger, C.V., Deutsch, A. and Linn, R. (1998) Rasch analysis of the functional independence measure (FIM) mastery test, *Archives of Physical Medicine and Rehabilitation*, 79: 52–7.

Grant, A. (1989) Reporting controlled trials, *British Journal of Obstetrics and Gynaecology*, 96: 397–400.

Green, J. (2005) Analysing qualitative data, in J. Green and J. Browne (eds) *Principles of Social Research*. Maidenhead: McGraw-Hill.

Green, J. and Brown, J. (2005) *Principles of Social Research*. Maidenhead: Open University Press.

Greenfield, S. (1989) The state of outcome research: are we on target? *New England Journal of Medicine*, 320: 1142–3.

Greenglass, E. (2002) Proactive coping, in E. Frydenberg (ed.) *Beyond Coping: Meeting Goals, Vision, and Challenges*. Oxford: Oxford University Press.

Greenland, S. (2000) Principles of multilevel modelling, *International Journal of Epidemiology*, 29: 158–67.

Griffiths, J.M., Black, N.A., Pope, C. *et al.* (1998) What determines the choice of procedure in stress incontinence surgery? The use of multilevel modelling, *International Journal of Health Technology Assessment*, 14: 431–45.

Griffiths, R. (1983) *NHS Management Inquiry* (Griffiths Report). London: Department of Health and Social Security.

Griffiths, R. (1988) Does the public service serve? The consumer dimension, *Public Administration*, 66: 195–204.

Grootendorst, P., Feeny, D. and Furlong, W. (2000) Health Utilities Index Mark 3: evidence of construct validity for stroke and arthritis in a population health survey, *Medical Care*, 38: 290–9.

Groves, R.M. (1979) Actors and questions in telephone and personal interview surveys, *Public Opinion Quarterly*, 43: 190–205.

Groves, R.M. and Couper, M.P. (1998) *Non-Response in Household Interview Surveys*. New York: Wiley.

Groves, R.M., Fowler, F.J., Couper, M.P. *et al.* (2009) *Survey Methodology*. Chichester: John Wiley & Sons Ltd.

Grundy, E. (1996) Populations and population dynamics, in R. Detels, W. Holland, J. McEwan and G.S. Omenn (eds) *Oxford Textbook of Public Health*. Oxford: Oxford University Press.

Grundy, E. and Bowling, A. (1991) The sociology of ageing, in R. Jacoby and C. Oppenheimer (eds) *Psychiatry in the Elderly*. Oxford: Oxford University Press.

Grundy, E. and Holt, G. (2001) The socio-economic status of older adults: how should one measure it in studies of inequalities? *Journal of Epidemiology and Community Health*, 55: 895–904.

Grundy, E. *et al.* (1999) *Disability in Great Britain*, Department of Social Security Research Report No. 94. Leeds: Corporate Document Services.

Guariano, P., Lamping, D.L., Elbourne, D. *et al.* (2005) A brief measure of perceived understanding of informed consent in a clinical trial was validated, *Journal of Clinical Epidemiology*, 59: 608–14.

Gudagnol, E. and Ward, P. (1998) Patient participation in decision-making, *Social Science and Medicine*, 47(3): 329–39.

Gudex, C., Dolan, P.H., Kind, P. *et al.* (1997) Valuing health states: interviews with the general public, *European Journal of Public Health*, 7: 441–8.

Gunnell, D., Berney, L., Holland, P. *et al.* (2000) How accurately are height, weight and leg length reported by the elderly, and how closely are they related to measurements recorded in childhood? *International Journal of Epidemiology*, 29: 456–64.

Gunnell, D., Fernando, R., Hewagama, M. *et al.* (2007) The impact of pesticide regulations on suicide in Sri Lanka, *International Journal of Epidemiology*, 36: 1235–42.

Guttman, L. (1944) A basis for scaling quantitative data, *American Sociological Review*, 9: 139–50.

Guttman, L. (1950) The third component of scalable attitudes, *International Journal of Opinion and Attitude Research*, 4: 285–7.

Guyatt, G.H. (1993) The philosophy of health-related quality of life translation, *Quality of Life Research*, 2: 461–5.

Guyatt, G.H., Berman, L.B., Townsend, M. *et al.* (1987a) A measure of quality of life for clinical trials in chronic lung disease, *Thorax*, 42: 773–8.

Guyatt, G., Cairns, J., Churchill, D., Cook, D. *et al.* (1992) Evidence-based medicine: a new approach to teaching the practice of medicine, *Journal of the American Medical Association*, 268: 2420–5.

Guyatt, G.H., Mitchell, A., Irvine, E.J. *et al.* (1989a) A new measure of health status for clinical trials in inflammatory bowel disease, *Gastroenterology*, 96: 804–10.

Guyatt, G.H., Nogradi, S., Halcrow, S. *et al.* (1989b) Development and testing of a new measure of health status for clinical trials in heart failure, *Journal of General Internal Medicine*, 4: 101–7.

Guyatt, G.H., Sackett, D.L., Cook, D.J. and The Evidence-Based Medicine Working Group (1993) Users' guides to the medical literature: II. How to use an article about therapy or prevention: A. Are the results of the study valid? *Journal of the American Medical Association*, 270: 2598–601.

Guyatt, G.H., Walter, S. and Norman, T.G. (1987b) Measuring change over time: assessing the usefulness of evaluative instruments, *Journal of Chronic Diseases*, 40: 171–8.

Hall, E.T. (1965) A system for the notation of proxemic behaviour, *American Anthropologist*, 65: 1003–26.

Hall, G.M. (ed.) (1994) *How to Write a Paper*. London: British Medical Journal Publishing Group.

Hall, J.A. and Dornan, M.C. (1988) What patients like about their medical care and how often they are asked: a meta-analysis of the satisfaction literature, *Social Science and Medicine*, 27: 935–9.

Hallal, J. (1982) The relationship of health beliefs, health locus of control and self concept to the practice of breast self-examination in adult women, *Nursing Research*, 31: 137–49.

Hammersley, M. (1995) *The Politics of Social Research*. London: Sage.

Hammersley, M. and Atkinson, P. (1983) *Ethnography: Principles in Practice*. London: Tavistock Publications.

Handley, M.A., Schillinger, D. and Shiboski, S. (2011) Quasi-experimental designs in practice-based research settings: design and implementation considerations, *Journal of the American Board of Family Medicine*, 24: 589–96.

Hanley, J.A. and McNeil, B.J. (1982) The meaning and use of the area under a Receiver Operating Characteristic (ROC) curve, *Radiology*, 143: 29–36.

Hanley, N., Ryan, M., and Wright, R. (2003) Estimating the monetary value of health care: lessons from environmental economics, *Health Economics*, 2: 3–16.

Harlow, S.D. and Linet, M.S. (1989) Agreement between questionnaire data and medical records, *American Journal of Epidemiology*, 129: 233–48.

Harries, A. and Stiggelbout, A. (2005) Approaches to measuring patients' decision-making, in A. Bowling and S. Ebrahim (eds) *Handbook of Health Research Methods: Investigation, Measurement and Analysis*. Maidenhead: Open University Press.

Harries, C. and Kostopoulou, O. (2005) Psychological approaches to measuring and modelling clinical decision-making, in A. Bowling and S. Ebrahim (eds) *Handbook of Health Research Methods: Investigation, Measurement and Analysis*. Maidenhead: Open University Press.

Harris, D. and Guten, S. (1979) Health protective behaviour: an explanatory study, *Journal of Health and Social Behavior*, 20: 17–29.

Hart, E. and Bond, M. (1995) *Action Research for Health and Social Care: A Guide to Practice*. Buckingham: Open University Press.

Hart, J.T. (1971) The inverse care law, *Lancet*, ii: 405–12.

Hayden, C., Boaz, A. and Taylor, F. (1999) *Attitudes and Aspirations of Older People: A Qualitative Study*. Warwick: Warwick Business School on behalf of the Department of Social Security.

Hays, R.D. and Hadhorn, D. (1992) Responsiveness to change: an aspect of validity, not a separate dimension, *Quality of Life Research*, 1: 73–5.

Hays, R.D., Morales, L. and Reise, S. (2000) Item response theory and health outcomes measurement in the 21st century, *Medical Care*, 38: S28–42.

Hays, R.J. and Bennett, S. (1999) Sample size calculations for cluster-randomised trials, *International Journal of Epidemiology*, 28: 319–26.

Hayward, J. (1975) *Information: A Prescription against Pain*. London: Royal College of Nursing.

Health, A. (1995) Non-response in panel surveys, *Survey Methods Briefing*, 37: 34–5.

Hedley, A., Wong, C., Thach, T. *et al.* (2002) Cardiorespiratory and all-cause mortality after restrictions on sulphur content in fuel in Hong Kong: an intervention study. *The Lancet*, 360: 1646–52.

Heimel, C. (1995) *If You Leave Me Can I Come Too?* London: Picador.

Heistaro, S., Jousilahti, P., Vartiainen, E. *et al.* (2001) Self-rated health and mortality: a long term prospective study in east Finland, *Journal of Epidemiology and Community Health*, 55: 227–32.

Helman, C.G. (1978) 'Feed a cold, starve a fever': folk models of infection in an English suburban community, and their relation to medical treatment, *Culture, Medicine and Psychiatry*, 2: 107–37.

Helman, C.G. (1990) *Culture, Health and Illness*, 2nd edn. London: Wright.

Helmstater, G.C. (1964) *Principles of Psychological Measurement*. New York: Appleton-Century-Crofts.

Hemingway, H., Stafford, M., Stansfeld, S., Shipley, M. and Marmot, M. (1997) Is the SF-36 a valid measure of change in population health? Results from the Whitehall II study, *British Medical Journal*, 315: 1273–9.

Henle, M. and Hubble, M.B. (1938) 'Egocentricity' in adult conversation, *Journal of Social Psychology*, 9: 227–34.

Hennekens, C.H. and Buring, J.E. (1987) *Epidemiology in Medicine*. Boston, MA: Little, Brown.

Hennekens, C.H., Buring, J.E., Manson, J.E. *et al.* (1996) Lack of effect of long-term supplementation with beta-carotene on the incidence of malignant neoplasms and cardiovascular disease, *New England Journal of Medicine*, 334: 1145–9.

Herbert, R.D. and Bø, K. (2005) Analysis of quality of interventions in systematic reviews, *British Medical Journal*, 331: 507–9.

Herzlich, C. (1973) *Health and Illness: A Social Psychological Analysis*. New York: Academic Press.

Hicks, N.R. (1994) Some observations on attempts to measure appropriateness of care, *British Medical Journal*, 309: 731–3.

Higginson, I. (1994) Quality of care and evaluating services, *International Review of Psychiatry*, 6: 5–14.

Higginson, I. (2000) The quality of expectation: healing, palliation or disappointment, *Journal of the Royal Society of Medicine*, 93: 609–10.

Hill, A.B. (1965) The environment and disease: association or causation? *Proceedings of the Royal Society of Medicine*, 58: 295–300.

Hill, S., Harries, U. and Popay, J. (1995) Is the SF-36 suitable for routine health outcomes assessment in health care for older people? Evidence from preliminary work in community-based health services in England, *Journal of Epidemiology and Community Health*, 50: 94–8.

Hobart, J.C., Riazi, A., Lamping, D.L. *et al.* (2004) Improving the evaluation of therapeutic interventions in multiple sclerosis: development of a patient-based measure of outcome, *Health Technology Assessment*, 8(9).

Hoffman, S.C., Burke, A.E., Heizlsouer, K.J. and Comstock, G. (1998) Controlled trial of the effect of length, incentives, and follow-up techniques on response to a mailed questionnaire, *American Journal of Epidemiology*, 148: 1007–11.

Holm, L. and Smidt, S. (1997) Uncovering social structures and status differences in health systems, *European Journal of Public Health*, 7: 373–8.

Holmes, T.H. and Rahe, R.H. (1967) The Social Readjustment Rating Scale, *Journal of Psychosomatic Research*, 11: 213–18.

Holsti, O.R. (1968) Content analysis, in G. Lindzey and E. Aronson (eds) *The Handbook of Social Psychology*. Reading, MA: Addison-Wesley.

Holt-Lunstad, J., Smith, T.B. and Layton, J.B. (2010) Social relationships and mortality risk: a meta-analytic review. *PLoS Medicine*, 27(7):e1000316.

Holtgraves, T. (2004) Social desirability and self-reports: testing models of socially desirable responding, *Personality and Social Psychology Bulletin*, 30: 161–72.

Homans, G. (1964) Contemporary theory in sociology, in R.E.L. Faris (ed.) *Handbook of Modern Sociology*. Chicago: Rand McNally.

Hopewell, S., Clarke, M., Moher, D. *et al.* (2008) CONSORT for reporting randomized controlled trials in journal and conference abstracts: explanation and elaboration. *PLoS Medicine*, 5: e20.

Hopkins, A. (1990) *Measuring the Quality of Medical Care*. London: Royal College of Physicians of London.

Hopkins, A. (on behalf of the Working Group of the NHS Management Executive) (1993) What do we mean by appropriate health care? *Quality in Health Care*, 2: 117–23.

Hopkins, A., Menken, M., DeFriese, G.H. and Feldman, A.G. (1989) Differences in strategies for the diagnosis and treatment of neurological disease among British and American neurologists, *Archives of Neurology*, 46: 1142–8.

Hornsby-Smith, M. (1993) Gaining access, in N. Gilbert (ed.) *Researching Social Life*. London: Sage.

Horswill, M.S. and McKenna, F.P. (1998) *Risk Taking: The Participant's Perspective. Full Report of*

Research Activities and Results. Reading: Department of Psychology, University of Reading.

Hosmer, D.W. and Lemeshow, S. (1999) *Applied Survival Analysis: Regression Modelling of Time to Event Data*. New York: Wiley.

Houghton, A., Bowling, A., Clarke, K., Hopkins, A. and Jones, I. (1996) Does a dedicated discharge coordinator improve the quality of hospital discharge? *Quality in Health Care*, 5: 89–95.

Houghton, A., Bowling, A., Jones, I. and Clarke, K. (1997) Appropriateness of admission and the last 24 hours of hospital care in medical wards in an East London teaching group hospital, *International Journal for Quality in Health Care*, 8: 543–53.

Houle, C. and Berthelot, J.M. (2000) A head-to-head comparison of the Health Utilities Index Mark 3 and the EQ-5D for the population living in private households in Canada, *Quality of Life Newsletter*, 24: 5–6.

Howard, K.I. and Forehand, G.G. (1962) A method of correcting item–total correlations for the effect of relevant item inclusion, *Education Psychology Measures*, 22: 731–5.

Hröbjartsson, A. and Gøtzsche, P.C. (2001) Is the placebo powerless? An analysis of clinical trials comparing placebo with no treatment, *New England Journal of Medicine*, 344: 1594–602.

Hughes, J. (1990) *The Philosophy of Social Research*. London: Longman.

Hughes, J.A. (1976) *Sociological Analysis: Methods of Discovery*. London: Nelson.

Humphrey, R. (1993) Life stories and social careers: ageing and social life in an ex-mining town. *Sociology*, 27: 166–78.

Humphreys, L. (1970) *Tearoom Trade: Impersonal Sex in Public Places*. Chicago: Aldine.

Humphriss, R.L., Baguley, D.M., Anderson, G. and Wagstaff, S. (2004) Hyperventilation in the vestibular clinic: use of the Nijmegen questionnaire, *Clinical Otolaryngology*, 29, 232.

Hunninghake, D.B., Darby, C.A. and Probstfield, J.L. (1987) Recruitment experience in clinical trials: literature survey and annotated bibliography, *Controlled Clinical Trials*, 8: 6S–30S.

Hunt, S. (1976) The food habits of Asian immigrants, in *Getting the Most Out of Food*. Burgess Hill: Van den Berghs & Jurgens.

Hunt, S.M., McEwan, J. and McKenna, S.P. (1986) *Measuring Health Status*. Beckenham: Croom Helm.

Hunter, D.J. and Long, A.F. (1993) Health research, in W. Sykes, M. Bulmer and M. Schwerzel (eds) *Directory of Social Research Organizations in the UK*. London: Mansell.

Hunter, D.J.W., McKee, C.M., Sanderson, C.F.B. and Black, N.A. (1994) Appropriateness of prostatectomy: a consensus panel approach, *Journal of Epidemiology and Community Health*, 48: 58–64.

Hutchings, A., Raine, R., Sanderson, C. and Black, N. (2005) An experimental study of determinants of the extent of disagreement within clinical guideline development groups, *Quality and Safety in Health Care*, 14: 240–5.

Hutton Commission (2000) ICM poll on the NHS, cited in *The Guardian*, 18 April: 19.

Hyde, M., Wiggins, R.D., Higgs, P. *et al.* (2003) A measure of quality of life in early old age: the theory, development and properties of a needs satisfaction model (CASP-19), *Ageing and Mental Health*, 7: 186–94.

Hyland, M.E. (1996) Diary assessments of quality of life, *Quality of Life Newsletter*, 16: 8–9.

Hyland, M.E. and Crocker, G.R. (1995) Validation of an asthma quality of life diary in a clinical trial, *Thorax*, 50: 724–30.

Hyman, H.H., Cobb, W.J., Feldman, J.J. *et al.* (1954) *Interviewing in Social Research*. Chicago: University of Chicago Press.

Idler, E.L. and Angel, R.J. (1990) Self-rated health and mortality in the NHANES-1 epidemiologic follow-up study, *American Journal of Public Health*, 80: 446–52.

Illich, I. (1976) *Medical Nemesis: Limits to Medicine*. Harmondsworth: Penguin.

International Journal of Health Science (1996) Recommendations of the conference 'Measuring Social Inequalities in Health', sponsored by the National Institutes of Health, 28–30 September 1994, *International Journal of Health Science*, 26: 521–7.

Interstudy (1994) Randomised clinical trials, in *Compendium of the Interstudy Quality Edge: General Health Status Measures, Data for Health Decisions, the Presentation of Health Status Data*. St Paul, MN: Decisions Resources.

Jacobson, B. and Amos, A. (1985) *When Smoke Gets in Your Eyes: Cigarette Advertising Policy and Coverage of Smoking and Health in Women's Magazines*. London: British Medical Association Professional Division.

Jaesche, R., Singer, J. and Guyatt, G.H. (1990) A comparison of seven-point and visual analogue scales: data from a randomised trial, *Controlled Clinical Trials*, 11: 43–51.

James, M. (1994) Historical research methods, in K. McConway (ed.) *Studying Health and Disease*. Buckingham: Open University Press.

Janzen, J.A., Silvius, J., Jacobs, S. *et al.* (2006) What is a health expectation? Development of a pragmatic conceptual model from psychological theory, *Health Expectations*, 9: 37–48.

Jefferys, M. (1996) The development of medical sociology in theory and practice in Western Europe, 1950–1990, *European Journal of Public Health*, 6: 94–8.

Jenkins, V.A., Fallowfeld, L.J., Souhami, A. and Sawtell, M. (1999) How do doctors explain randomised clinical trials to their patients? *European Journal of Cancer*, 35: 1187–93.

Jenkinson, C. (1991) Why are we weighting? A critical examination of the use of item weights in a health status measure, *Social Science and Medicine*, 32: 1413–16.

Jenkinson, C., Coulter, A., Reeves, R., Bruster, S. and Richards, N. (2003) Properties of the Picker Patient Experience questionnaire in a randomised controlled trial of long versus short form survey instruments, *Journal of Public Health Medicine*, 25: 197–201.

Jenkinson, C., Gray, A., Doll, H. *et al.* (1997) Evaluation of index and profile measures of health status in a randomised controlled trial: comparison of the SF-36, the EuroQoL and disease-specific measures, *Medical Care*, 35: 1109–18.

Jenkinson, C. and McGee, H. (1998) *Health Status Measurement: A Brief but Critical Introduction*. Oxford: Radcliffe Medical Press.

Jenkinson, C., Ziebland, S., Fitzpatrick, R. *et al.* (1991) Sensitivity to change of weighted and unweighted versions of two health status measures, *International Journal of Health Sciences*, 2: 189–94.

Jerusalem, M. and Schwarzer, R. (1992) Self-efficacy as a resource factor in stress appraisal process, in R. Schwarzer (ed.) *Self-efficacy: Thought Control of Action*. Washington, DC: Hemisphere.

Jitapunkel, S., Kunanusont, C., Phoolcharoen, W., Suriyawongpaisal, S. and Ebrahim, S. (2003) Disability-free life expectancy of elderly people in a population undergoing demographic and epidemiologic transition, *Age and Ageing*, 32: 401–5.

Johnson, A.G. (ed.) (1995) *The Blackwell Dictionary of Sociology*. Oxford: Blackwell Publishers.

Johnson, M., Wright, S. and Weinman, J. (1995) *Measures in Health Psychology: A User's Portfolio*. Windsor: NFER-Nelson.

Jones, I.R. (1995) Health care need and contracts for health services, *Health Care Analysis*, 3: 91–8.

Jones, J. and Hunter, D. (1996) Consensus methods for medical and health services research, in N. Mays and C. Pope (eds) *Qualitative Research in Health Care*. London: British Medical Journal Publishing Group.

Jones, L.J. (1994) *The Social Context of Health and Health Work*. Basingstoke: Macmillan.

Jorm, A.F. and Henderson, A.S. (1992) Memory bias in depression: implications for risk factor studies relying on self-reports of exposure, *International Journal of Methods in Psychiatric Research*, 2: 31–8.

Jung, T. and Wickrama, K.A.S. (2008) An introduction to latent class growth analysis and growth mixture modeling, *Social and Personality Psychology Compass*, 2(1): 302–17.

Juniper, E.F., Guyatt, G.H., Willan, A. and Griffith, L.E. (1994) Determining a minimal important change in a disease-specific quality of life questionnaire, *Journal of Clinical Epidemiology*, 47: 81–7.

Kahn, K.L., Kosecoff, J., Chassin, M.R. *et al.* (1988) Measuring the appropriateness of the use of a procedure: can we do it? *Medical Care*, 26: 415–22.

Kahn, S.R., Lamping, D.L., Ducruet, T. *et al.* (2006) VEINES-QOL/sym questionnaire was a reliable and valid disease-specific quality of life measure for deep venous thrombosis, *Journal of Clinical Epidemiology*, 59: 1049–56.

Kahneman, D. and Tversky, A. (1983) Choices, values and frames, *American Psychologist*, 39: 341–50.

Kaiser, H. (1970) A second generation Little Jiffy, *Psychometrika*, 35: 401–15.

Kaiser, H. (1974) An index of factorial simplicity, *Psychometrika*, 39: 31–6.

Kalton, G. (1983) *Compensating for Missing Survey Data*. Ann Arbor, MI: Institute for Social Research, University of Michigan.

Kaplan, R.M. and Anderson, J.P. (2004) The general health policy model: an integrated approach, in B. Spilker (ed.) *Quality of Life and Pharmacoeconomics in Clinical Trials*, 2nd edn. Philadelphia, PA: Lippincott-Raven.

Kaplan, R.M., Atkins, C.J., Times, R. *et al.* (1984) Validity of Quality of Wellbeing Scale as an outcome measure in chronic obstructive pulmonary disease, *Journal of Chronic Diseases*, 37: 85–95.

Kaplan, R.M. and Bush, J.W. (1982) Health-related quality of life measurement for evaluation research and policy analysis, *Health Psychology*, 1: 61–80.

Kaplan, R.M., Bush, J.W. and Berry, C.C. (1976) Health status: types of validity and the Index of Well-being, *Health Services Research*, 11: 478–507.

Kaplan, R.M., Bush, J.W. and Berry, C.C. (1978) The reliability, stability and generalisability of a health status index, *Proceedings of the American Statistical Association, Social Statistics Section*, 704–9.

Karnofsky, D.A., Abelmann, W.H., Craver, L.F. *et al.* (1948) The use of nitrogen mustards in the palliative treatment of carcinoma, *Cancer*, 1: 634–56.

Kasl, S. and Cobb, S. (1966) Health behavior, illness behavior and sick role behavior, *Archives of Environmental Health*, 12: 246–66.

Katz, M.H. (1999) *Multivariable Analysis: A Practical Guide for Clinicians*. Cambridge: Cambridge University Press.

Katz, S., Ford, A.B., Moskowitz, R.W. *et al.* (1963) Studies of illness in the aged: the index of ADL – a standardized measure of biological and psychosocial function, *Journal of the American Medical Association*, 185: 914–19.

Kazis, L.E., Anderson, J.J. and Meenan, R.F. (1989) Effect sizes for interpreting changes in health status, *Medical Care*, 27: S178–89.

Keat, R. (1979) Positivism and statistics in social science, in J. Irvine, I. Miles and J. Evans (eds) *Demystifying Social Statistics*. London: Pluto Press.

Kelle, U. (ed.) (1995) *Computer-aided Qualitative Data Analysis*. London: Sage.

Kelle, U. and Laurie, H. (1995) Computer use in qualitative research and issues of validity, in U. Kelle (ed.) *Computer-aided Qualitative Data Analysis*. London: Sage.

Keller, S.D. and Ware, J.E. (1996) Questions and answers about SF-36 and SF-12, *Medical Outcomes Trust Bulletin*, 4: 3.

Kelley, H.H. (1972) Attribution in social interaction, in E.E. Jones *et al.* (eds) *Attribution: Perceiving the Causes of Behavior*. Morristown, NJ: General Learning Press.

Kelly, A. and Bebbington, A. (1993) Proceed with caution: the use of official sources of cost information in social services departments, in A. Netten and J. Beecham (eds) *Costing Community Care: Theory and Practice*. Aldershot: Ashgate Publishing.

Kelly, G.A. (1955) *The Psychology of Personal Constructs: A Theory of Personality*. New York: Norton.

Kemm, J.R. and Booth, D. (1992) *Promotion of Healthier Eating: How to Collect and Use Information for Planning, Monitoring and Evaluation*. London: HMSO.

Kennedy, G.J., Kelman, H.R. and Thomas, C. (1991a) Persistence and older persons, *The Gerontologist*, 31: 735–45.

Kennedy, G.J., Kelman, H.R. and Thomas, C. (1991b) Persistence and remission of depressive symptoms in late life, *American Journal of Psychiatry*, 148: 174–8.

Kennelly, C. and Bowling, A. (2001) Suffering in deference: a focus group study of older cardiac patients' preferences for treatment and perceptions of risk, *Quality and Safety in Health Care*, 10: i23–8.

Kerry, S.M. and Bland, J.M. (1998a) Trials which randomise practices 1: how should they be analysed? *Family Practice*, 15: 80–3.

Kerry, S.M. and Bland, J.M. (1998b) Statistics notes: sample size in cluster randomisation, *British Medical Journal*, 316: 549.

Kessler, R. and Mroczek, D. (1995) Measuring the effects of medical interventions, *Medical Care*, 33: AS109–19.

Kind, P. (1996) The EuroQol instrument: an index of health-related quality of life, in B. Spilker (ed.) *Quality of Life and Pharmacoeconomics in Clinical Trials*, 2nd edn. Philadelphia, PA: Lippincott-Raven.

Kind, P., Dolan, P., Gudex, C. and Williams, A. (1998) Variations in population health status: results from a United Kingdom national questionnaire survey, *British Medical Journal*, 316: 736–41.

Kind, P., Rosser, R.M. and Williams, A. (1982) Valuation of quality of life: some psychometric evidence, in M.W. Jones-Lee (ed.) *The Value of Life and Safety*. Amsterdam: Elsevier.

King, M., Nazareth, I., Lampe, F. *et al.* (2005a) Conceptual framework and systematic review of the effects of participants' and professionals' preferences in randomised controlled trials, *Health Technology Assessment*, 9: 1–186.

King, M., Nazareth, I., Lampe, F. *et al.* (2005b) Impact of participant and physician intervention preferences on randomized trials, *Journal of the American Medical Association*, 293: 1089–99.

Kingery, D.W. (1989) Sampling strategies for surveys of older adults, in F.J. Fowler (ed.) *Health*

Survey Research Methods. Rockville, MD: National Center for Health Services Research and Health Care Technology Assessment.

Kinsella, K. (1996) Demographic aspects, in S. Ebrahim and A. Kalache (eds) *Epidemiology in Old Age*. London: British Medical Journal Publishing Group.

Kippax, S. and Crawford, J. (1993) Flaws in the theory of reasoned action, in D.J. Terry, C. Gallois and M.M. Mccamish (eds) *The Theory of Reasoned Action: Its Application to AIDS Preventive Behaviour*. New York: Pergamon.

Kirk, J. and Miller, M. (1986) *Reliability and Validity in Qualitative Research*, Qualitative Research Methods Series, 1. London: Sage.

Kirkup, B. and Forster, D. (1990) How will health needs be measured in districts? Implications for variations in hospital use, *Journal of Public Health Medicine*, 12: 45–50.

Kitsuse, J. and Cicourel, A. (1963) A note on the official use of statistics, *Social Problems*, 11: 131–9.

Kitzinger, J. (1994) The methodology of focus group interviews: the importance of interaction between research participants. *Sociology of Health and Illness*, 16: 103–21.

Kitzinger, J. (1995) Introducing focus groups, *British Medical Journal*, 311: 299–302.

Kitzinger, J. (1996) Introducing focus groups, in N. Mays and C. Pope (eds) *Qualitative Research in Health Care*. London: British Medical Journal Publishing Group.

Kitzinger, J. and Barbour, R.S. (1999) Introduction: the challenge and promise of focus groups, in R.S. Barbour and J. Kitzinger (eds) *Developing Focus Group Research: Politics, Theory, Practice*. London: Sage.

Klepacz, A. (1991) Activity and health survey: possible effects on response of different versions of the advance letter, *Survey Methods Bulletin*, 29: 29–32.

Kline, P. (1986) *A Handbook of Test Construction*. London: Methuen.

Kline, P. (1993) *The Handbook of Psychological Testing*. London: Routledge.

Knapp, M. (1993) Background theory, in A. Netten and J. Beecham (eds) *Costing Community Care: Theory and Practice*. Aldershot: Ashgate Publishing.

Koch, T. (2000) The illusion of paradox: commentary on 'Albrecht, G.L. and Devlieger, P.L. (1998) The disability paradox: high quality of life against all odds, *Social Science and Medicine*, 48: 977–88', *Social Science and Medicine*, 50: 757–9.

Koch, T., Jenkin, P. and Kralik, D. (2004) Chronic illness self-management: locating the 'self', *Journal of Advanced Nursing*, 48: 484–92.

Koller, M., Lorenz, W., Wagner, K. *et al.* (2000) Expectations and quality of life of cancer patients, *Journal of the Royal Society of Medicine*, 93: 621–8.

Koos, E. (1954) *The Health of Regionville: What People Thought and Did About It*. New York: Columbia University Press.

Korman, N. and Glennerster, H. (1990) *Hospital Closure: A Political and Economic Study*. Buckingham: Open University Press.

Körmendi, E. and Noordhoek, J. (1989) *Data Quality and Telephone Interviews: A Comparative Study of Face-to-face and Telephone Data Collecting Methods*. Copenhagen: Danmarks Statistik.

Kravitz, R.L., Callahan, E.J., Paterniti, D. *et al.* (1996) Prevalence and sources of patients' unmet expectations for care, *Annals of Internal Medicine*, 125: 730–7.

Krieger, N., Williams, D.R. and Moss, N.E. (1997) Measuring social class in US public health research: concepts, methodologies, and guidelines. *Annual Review of Public Health*, 18: 341–78.

Kuh, D., Ben-Schlomo, B., Lynch, J., *et al.* (2003) Life course epidemiology. *Journal of Epidemiology and Community Health*, 57: 778–83.

Kühberger, A. (1998) The influence of framing on risky decisions: a meta-analysis, *Organizational Behaviour and Human Decision Processes*, 75: 23–55.

Kuhn, T.S. (1970) *The Structure of Scientific Revolutions*, 2nd expanded edn. Chicago: University of Chicago Press.

Kuhn, T.S. (1972) Scientific paradigms, in B. Barnes (ed.) *Sociology of Science: Selected Readings*. Harmondsworth: Penguin.

Kwok, O-M., Underhill, A.T., Berry, J.W. *et al.* (2008) Analyzing longitudinal data with multilevel models: an example with individuals living with lower extremity intra-articular fractures, *Rehabilitation Psychology*, 53: 370–86.

Lahelma, E., Karisto, A. and Rahkonen, O. (1996) Analysing inequalities: the tradition of socioeconomic public health research in Finland, *European Journal of Public Health*, 6: 87–93.

Lakey, B. and Cohen, S. (2000) Social support theory and measurement, in S. Cohen, L.G. Underwood and B.H. Gottlieb (eds) *Social Support Measurement and Interventions: A Guide for Health and Social Scientists*. Oxford: Oxford University Press.

Lambert, N., Rowe, G., Bowling, A., Ebrahim, S., Thomson, R., Laurence, M. and Dalrymple, J. (2004) Reasons underpinning patients' preferences for various angina treatments, *Health Expectations*, 6: 246–56.

Lancaster, T., Sheppherd, S. and Silagy, C. (1997) Systematic reviews and meta-analyses, in C. Jenkinson (ed.) *Assessment and Evaluation of Health and Medical Care: A Methods Text*. Buckingham: Open University Press.

Lancet (1863) The *Lancet* investigation into the administration of the outpatient department of the London hospitals, No. II: St. Bartholomew's Hospital. *Lancet*, 23 October: 578–9.

Langlie, J.K. (1977) Social networks, health beliefs and preventive health behavior, *Journal of Health and Social Behavior*, 18: 244–60.

Last, J.M. (1963) The iceberg: completing the clinical picture in general practice, *Lancet*, ii: 28–31.

Last, J.M. (1988) *A Dictionary of Epidemiology*. Oxford: Oxford University Press.

Lau, R. and Ware, J. (1981) Refinements in a measure of health specific locus of control beliefs, *Medical Care*, 19: 1147–57.

Laurence, J. (2013) What's wrong with you? It depends where you live. *The Independent*, Thursday 12 September 2013 (online) at: www.independent.co.uk (accessed 12 September 2013).

Lawlor, D.A., Bedford, C., Taylor, M. and Ebrahim, S. (2002) Agreement between measured and self-reported weight in older women: results for the British Women's Heart and Health Study, *Age and Ageing*, 31: 169–74.

Lawton, M.P. (1972) The dimensions of morale, in D. Kent, R. Kastenbaum and S. Sherwood (eds) *Research, Planning and Action for the Elderly*. New York: Behavioral Publications.

Lawton, M.P. (1983) The dimensions of well-being. *Experimental Aging Research*, 9: 65–72.

Lawton, M.P. (1991) A multidimensional view of quality of life in frail elders, in J.E. Birren, J.E. Lubben, J.C. Rowe and G.E. Deutchman (eds) *The Concept and Measurement of Quality of Life in the Frail Elderly*, New York: Academic Press, pp. 4–27.

Lawton, M.P. (1994) Quality of life in Alzheimer's disease, *Alzheimer's Disease and Associated Disorders*, 8(Suppl. 3): 138–50.

Lawton, M.P. (1997) Assessing quality of life in Alzheimer's disease research. *Alzheimer's Disease and Associated Disorders*, 1: 91–9.

Lazarus, R.S. and Folkman, S. (1984) *Stress, Appraisal and Coping*. New York: Springer.

Le Grand, J. (1982) *The Strategy of Equality*. London: Allen & Unwin.

Le Grand, J. (2003) From pawn to queen: an economics perspective, in A. Oliver (ed.) *Equity in Health and Health Care: Views from Ethics, Economics and Political Science*. Proceedings from a meeting of the Health Equity Network. London: The Nuffield Trust for Research and Policy Studies in Health Services.

Lee, R.M. (2000) *Unobtrusive Methods in Social Research*. Buckingham: Open University Press.

Lefcourt, H.M. (1982) *Locus of Control: Current Trends in Theory and Research*. Hillsdale, NJ: Lawrence Erlbaum Associates.

Leff, J. (1991) The relevance of psychosocial risk factors for treatment and prevention, in P.E. Bebbington (ed.) *Social Psychiatry: Theory, Methodology and Practice*. London: Transaction Publishers.

Leidberg, G.M., Eddy, L. and Burckhardt, C.S. (2012) Validity testing of the quality of life scale, Swedish version: focus group interviews of women with fibromyalgia, *Occupational Therapy International*, 19: 167–75.

Lemert, E. (1967) *Human Deviance, Social Problems and Social Control*. Englewood Cliffs, NJ: Prentice Hall.

Lessler, J.T. and Kalsbeek, W.D. (1992) *Nonsampling Errors in Surveys*. New York: Wiley.

Leufer, T. and Cleary-Holdforth, J. (2009) Evidence-based practice: improving patient outcomes, *Nursing Standard*, 23(32): 35–9.

Levi, P. (1990) The interview, in P. Levi (ed.) *The Mirror Maker: Stories and Essays by Primo Levi*. London: Methuen.

Lewin, K. (1946) Action research and minority problems, in G.W. Lewin (ed.) *Resolving Social Conflicts: Selected Papers on Group Dynamics by Kurt Lewin*. New York: Harper & Brothers.

Lewis, S.J., Davey Smith, G. and Ebrahim, S. (2005) Genetics, health and population genetics research, in A. Bowling and S. Ebrahim (eds) *Handbook of Health Research Methods: Investigation, Measurement and Analysis*. Maidenhead: Open University Press.

Ley, P. (1988) *Communicating with Patients*. London: Croom Helm.

Leydon, G.M., Boulton, M., Moynihan, C. *et al.* (2000) Cancer patients' information needs and information seeking behaviour: in-depth interview study, *British Medical Journal*, 320: 909–13.

Liang, M., Fossel, A.H. and Larson, M.G. (1990) Comparison of five health status instruments for orthopaedic evaluation, *Medical Care*, 28: 632–42.

Liberatos, P., Link, B.G. and Kelsey, J.L. (1988) The measurement of social class in epidemiology, *Epidemiologic Reviews*, 10: 87–121.

Light, R.J. and Pillemar, D.B. (1984) *Summing Up: The Science of Reviewing Research*. Cambridge, MA: Harvard University Press.

Likert, R. (1932) A technique for the measurement of attitudes, *Archives of Psychology*, 22: 1–55.

Lilford, R.J. and Braunholtz, D. (1996) The statistical basis of public policy: a paradigm shift is overdue, *British Medical Journal*, 313: 603–7.

Lilienfeld, D.E. (2000) John Snow: the first hired gun, *American Journal of Epidemiology*, 152: 4–9.

Lim, S.S., Dandona, L., Hoisington, J.A. *et al.* (2010) India's Janani Suraksha: a conditional cash transfer scheme to increase births in health facilities: an impact evaluation, *Lancet*, 375: 2009–23.

Lindelow, M., Hardy, R. and Rogers, B. (1997) Development of a scale to measure symptoms of anxiety and depression in the general population: the Psychiatric Symptom Frequency (PSF) Scale, *Journal of Epidemiology and Community Health*, 51: 549–57.

Linder-Pelz, S. (1982) Towards a theory of patient satisfaction, *Social Science and Medicine*, 16: 577–82.

Lipman, A. (1967) Chairs as territory. *New Society*, 20 April: 564–6.

Little, R.J.A. and Rubin, D.B. (1987) *Statistical Analysis with Missing Data*. New York: Wiley.

Liu, S., Lee, I.-M., Linson, P. *et al.* (2000) A prospective study of physical activity and risk of prostate cancer in US physicians, *International Journal of Epidemiology*, 29: 29–35.

Lloyd, A. (2003) Threats to the estimation of benefit: are preference elicitation methods accurate? *Health Economics*, 12: 393–402.

Lloyd, A.J., Hayes, P.D., London, N.J.M., Bell, P.R.F. and Naylor, A.R. (1999) Patients' ability to recall risk associated with treatment options, *Lancet*, 353: 645.

Locker, D. and Dunt, D. (1978) Theoretical and methodological issues in sociological studies of consumer satisfaction with medical care, *Social Science and Medicine*, 12: 283–92.

Locket, T. (1996) *Health Economics for the Uninitiated*. Oxford: Radcliffe Medical Press.

Lockwood, M. (1988) Quality of life and resource allocation, in J.M. Bell and S. Mendus (eds) *Philosophy and Medical Welfare*. Cambridge: Cambridge University Press.

Lofland, J. and Lofland, L.H. (1995) *Analyzing Social Settings*, 3rd edn. Belmont, CA: Wadsworth Publishing Company.

Logan, R.L. and Scott, P.J. (1996) Uncertainty in clinical practice: implications for quality and costs of health care, *Lancet*, 347: 595–8.

Lohr, K.N. (1988) Outcomes measurement: concepts and questions, *Inquiry*, 25: 37–50.

Lohr, K.N., Brook, R.H., Kamberg, C.J. *et al.* (1986) *Use of Medical Care in the Rand Health Insurance Experiment: Diagnosis- and Service-specific Analyses in a Randomised Controlled Trial*, Report No. R-3469-HHS. Santa Monica, CA: Rand.

Lonkila, M. (1995) Grounded theory as an emerging paradigm for computer assisted qualitative data analysis, in U. Kelle (ed.) *Computer-aided Qualitative Data Analysis*. London: Sage.

Lorig, K.R. and Holman, H. (2003) Self-management education: history, definition, outcomes, and mechanisms, *Annals of Behavioral Medicine*, 26: 1–7.

Ludlow, L.H. and Haley, S.M. (1995) Rasch model logits: interpretation, use, and transformation, *Educational Psychological Measures*, 55: 967–75.

Lugon, M. and Secker-Walker, J. (1999) *Clinical Governance: Making It Happen*. London: Royal Society of Medicine Press.

Lynch, J., Due, P., Muntaner, C. and Dowey Smith, G. (2000) Social capital – is it a good investment strategy for public health? *Journal of Epidemiology and Community Health*, 54: 404–8.

Lyons, R.A., Wareham, K., Lucas, M. *et al.* (1999) SF-36 scores vary by method of administration: implications for study design, *Journal of Public Health Medicine*, 21: 41–5.

Macaulay, A.C., Commanda, L.E., Freeman, W.L. *et al.* (1999) Participatory research maximises community and lay involvement, *British Medical Journal*, 319: 774–8.

Macdonald, K. and Tipton, C. (1993) Using documents, in N. Gilbert (ed.) *Researching Social Life*. London: Sage.

Mackenzie, E.J., Shapiro, S. and Yaffe, R. (1985) The utility of synthetic and regression estimation: techniques for local planning, *Medical Care*, 23: 1–13.

Mahoney, F.I. and Barthel, D.W. (1965) Functional evaluation: the Barthel Index, *Maryland State Medical Journal*, 14: 61–5.

Mailbach, E., Flora, J.A. and Nass, C. (1991) Changes in self-efficacy and health behavior in response to minimal contact community health campaign, *Health Communication*, 3: 1–15.

Malley, J.N., Towers, A-M., Netten, A.P. *et al.* (2012) An assessment of the construct validity of the ASCOT measure of social care-related QoL with older people. *Health and QoL Outcomes*, 10: 21.

Mallinson, S. (1998) The Short-Form 36 and older people: some problems encountered when using postal administration, *Journal of Epidemiology and Community Health*, 52: 324–8.

Manderbacka, K. (1998) How do respondents understand survey questions on ill-health? *European Journal of Public Health*, 8: 319–24.

Mann, A. (1991) Epidemiology, in R. Jacoby and C. Oppenheimer (eds) *Psychiatry in the Elderly*. Oxford: Oxford Medical Publications.

Manstead, A.S.R. and McCulloch, C. (1981) Sex-role stereotyping in British television advertisements, *British Journal of Social Psychology*, 20: 171–80.

Manton, K.G. (1992) Mortality and life expectancy changes among the oldest old, in R.M. Suzman, D.P. Willis and K.G. Manton (eds) *The Oldest Old*. New York: Oxford University Press.

Marks, D. (2002) Perspectives on evidence-based practice, paper presented at Health Development Agency, Public Health Evidence Steering Group, London, 17 October. Available at: www.nice.org.uk/niceMedia/pdf/persp_evid_dmarks.pdf.

Marks, R., Allegrante, J.P. and Lorig, K. (2005) A review and synthesis of research evidence for self-efficacy-enhancing interventions for reducing chronic disability: implications for health education practice (part I), *Health Promotion and Practice*, 6: 37–43.

Martin, D.C., Dierh, E., Perin, E.V. and Koepsell, T.D. (1993) The effect of matching on the power of randomised community intervention studies, *Statistics in Medicine*, 12: 329–38.

Martin, R.A. (2005) Epidemiological study designs for health research and evaluation, in A. Bowling and S. Ebrahim (eds) *Handbook of Health Research Methods: Investigation, Measurement and Analysis*. Maidenhead: Open University Press.

Marx, K. ([1933] 1967) *Capital: A Critique of Political Economy*, Vol. 1. London: Dent.

Maxwell, M., Heaney, D., Howie, J.G.R. and Noble, S. (1993) General practice fundholding: observations on prescribing patterns and costs using the defined daily dose method, *British Medical Journal*, 307: 1190–4.

Maxwell, R. (1989) Towards appropriate clinical practice: some reflections, in A. Hopkins (ed.) *Appropriate Investigation and Treatment in Clinical Practice*. London: Royal College of Physicians of London.

Maxwell, R.J. (1984) Quality assessment in health, *British Medical Journal*, 288: 1471.

May, T. (1993) *Social Research: Issues, Methods and Process*. Buckingham: Open University Press.

Mays, N. and Pope, C. (1996) Rigour and qualitative research, in N. Mays and C. Pope (eds) *Qualitative Research in Health Care*. London: BMJ Publishing Group.

Mays, N. and Pope, C. (2000) Quality in qualitative health research, in N. Mays and C. Pope (eds) *Qualitative Research in Health Care*, 2nd edn. London: BMJ Publishing Group.

McColl, E., Steen, I.N., Meadows, K.A. *et al.* (1995) Developing outcome measures for ambulatory care: an application to asthma and diabetes, *Social Science and Medicine*, special issue on 'Quality of Life', 10: 1339–48.

McConway, K. (1994a) Some basic ideas of demography and epidemiology, in K. McConway (ed.) *Studying Health and Disease*. Buckingham: Open University Press.

McConway, K. (1994b) Analysing numerical data, in K. McConway (ed.) *Studying Health and Disease*. Buckingham: Open University Press.

McGettigan, P., Sly, K., O'Connell, D., Hill, S. and Henry, D. (1999) The effects of information framing on the practices of physicians, *Journal of General Internal Medicine*, 14: 633–42.

McHorney, C.A., Kosinski, M. and Ware, J.E. (1994) Comparisons of the costs and quality of norms for the SF-36 Health Survey collected by mail versus telephone interview: results from a national survey, *Medical Care*, 32: 551–67.

McKee, M., Britton, A., Black, N. *et al.* (1999) Interpreting the evidence: choosing between randomised and non-randomised studies, *British Medical Journal*, 319: 312–15.

McKenna, F.P. (1993) 'It won't happen to me': unrealistic optimism or illusion of control? *British Journal of Psychology*, 84: 39–50.

McKinlay, J.B. and McKinlay, S.M. (1972) Some social characteristics of lower working class utilisers and under-utilisers of maternity care services, *Journal of Health and Social Behavior*, 13: 369–81.

McKinley, R.K., Stevenson, K., Adams, S. and Manku-Scott, T.K. (2002) Meeting patient expectations of care: the major determinant of satisfaction with out-of-hours primary medical care, *Family Practice*, 19: 333–8.

McKinney, P.A., Alexander, F.E., Nicholson, C. *et al.* (1991) Mothers' reports of childhood vaccinations and infections and their concordance with general practitioner records, *Journal of Public Health Medicine*, 13: 13–22.

McNeil, B.J., Pauker, S.G., Sox, H.C. and Tversky, A. (1982) On the elicitation of preferences for alternative therapies, *New England Journal of Medicine*, 306: 1259–62.

McShine, R., Lesser, G.T. and Likourezos, A. (2000) Older Americans hold on to life dearly, *British Medical Journal*, 320: 1206–7 (letter).

Mead, G.H. (1934) *Mind, Self and Society*. Chicago: University of Chicago Press.

Meadows, K., Bentzen, N. and Touw-Otten, F. (1997) Cross-cultural issues: an outline of the important principles in establishing cross-cultural validity in health outcome assessment, in A. Hutchinson, N. Bentzen and C. König-Zahn (eds) *Cross Cultural Health Outcome Assessment: A User's Guide*. Hull: Department of Public Health, University of Hull.

Mechanic, D. (1959) Illness and social disability: some problems of analysis, *Pacific Sociological Review*, 2: 37–41.

Mechanic, D. (1978) *Medical Sociology: A Selective View*. New York: Free Press.

Mechanic, D. (1979) The stability of health and illness behavior: results from a 16-year follow up, *American Journal of Public Health*, 69: 832–92.

Medical Research Council (1995) *Principles in the Assessment and Conduct of Medical Research and Publicising Results*. London: Medical Research Council.

Medical Research Council (1998) *MRC Guidelines for Good Clinical Practice in Clinical Trials*. London: Medical Research Council.

Medical Research Council (2000) *A Framework for Development and Evaluation of RCTs for Complex Interventions to Improve Health*. London: Medical Research Council.

Medical Research Council (2008) *Developing and Evaluating Complex Interventions: New Guidance*. Prepared by P. Craig, P. Dieppe, S. Macintyre, *et al.* London: Medical Research Council.

Medical Research Council (2011) *Using Natural Experiments to Evaluate Population Health Interventions: Guidance for Producers and Users of Evidence*. London: MRC. Available at: www.mrc.ac.uk/naturalexperimentsguidance (accessed 27 September 2013).

Meenan, R.F., Gertman, P.M. and Mason, J.H. (1980) Measuring health status in arthritis: the arthritis impact measurement scales, *Arthritis and Rheumatism*, 23: 146–52.

Mehrez, A. and Gafni, A. (1989) Quality-adjusted life-years, utility theory and healthy years equivalents, *Medical Decision Making*, 9: 142–9.

Meijer, R.R. and Sijtsma, K. (1990) Theoretical and empirical comparisons of the Mokken and Rasch approaches to IRT, *Applied Psychological Measurement*, 14: 282–98.

Melnyk, B.M., Fineout-Overholt, E., Stillwell, S. and Williamson, K. (2010) Evidence-based practice: step by step: the seven steps of evidence-based practice, *American Journal of Nursing*, 110: 51–3.

Merriam, S.B. (1988) *Case Study Research in Education: A Qualitative Approach*. San Francisco, CA: Jossey-Bass.

Merton, R.K. (1968) *Social Theory and Social Structure*, revised edn. New York: Free Press.

Michels, K.B., Welch, A.A., Luben, R. *et al.* (2005) Measurement of fruit and vegetable consumption with diet questionnaires and implications for analysis and interpretation, *American Journal of Epidemiology*, 161: 987–94.

Midthjell, K., Holmen, J., Bjórndal, A. and Lund-Larsen, G. (1992) Is questionnaire information valid in the study of a chronic disease such as diabetes? The Nord-Tróndelag Diabetes Study, *Journal of Epidemiology and Community Health*, 46: 537–42.

Miles, I. and Irvine, J. (1979) The critique of official statistics, in I. Miles and J. Evans (eds) *Demystifying Social Statistics*. London: Pluto Press.

Milgram, S. (1963) Behavioural study of obedience, *Journal of Abnormal and Social Psychology*, 67: 371–8.

Miller, B. and McFall, S. (1991) Stability and change in the informal task support network of frail older persons, *The Gerontologist*, 31: 735–45.

Minichiello, V., Aroni, R. and Hays, T.N. (2008) *In-depth Interviewing*. Melbourne, VIC: Pearson Education Australia.

Mirowsky, J. and Ross, C.E. (1991) Eliminating defence and agreement bias from measures of the Sense of Control Index: a 2 × 2 index, *Social Psychology Quarterly*, 54: 127–45.

Mishra, S.I., Dooley, D., Catalano, R. and Serxner, S. (1993) Telephone health surveys: potential bias from noncompletion, *American Journal of Public Health*, 83: 94–9.

Mitchie, S., van Stralen, M.M. and West, R. (2011) The behaviour change wheel: a new method for characterising and designing behaviour change interventions. *Implementation Science*, 6: 42. doi: 10.1186/1748-5908-6-42.

Mock, C., Acheampong, F., Adjei, S. and Koepsell, T. (1999) The effect of recall on estimation of incidence rates for injury in Ghana, *International Journal of Epidemiology*, 28: 750–5.

Moher, D., Hopewell, S. and Schulz, K.F. (2010) CONSORT 2010 explanation and elaboration: updated guidelines for reporting parallel group randomised trials. *British Medical Journal*, 340: c869.

Moher, D., Pham, B., Lawson, M.L. and Klassen, T.P. (2003) The inclusion of reports of randomised trials published in languages other than English in systematic reviews, *Health Technology Assessment*, 7(41).

Moher, D., Schulz, K.F., Altman, D. for the CONSORT Group (2001) The CONSORT Statement: revised recommendations for improving the quality of reports of parallel-group randomised trials, *Journal of the American Medical Association*, 285: 37–41.

Mok, M. (1995) Sample size requirements for 2-level designs in educational research, Institute of Education, University of London, *Multilevel Modelling Newsletter*, 7: 11–15.

Mokken, R.J. (1971) *A Theory and Procedure of Scale Analysis*. Berlin: De Gruyter,

Montgomery, A.A., Fahey, T., Peters, T.J., Mackintosh, C. *et al.* (1998) Evaluation of cardiovascular risk in hypertensive patients in primary care, paper presented at Society for Social Medicine, annual conference, Cardiff, September.

Moon, G. *et al.* (2000) *Epidemiology: An Introduction*. Buckingham: Open University Press.

Moon, G., Subramanian, S.V., Jones, K. *et al.* (2005) Area-based studies and the evaluation of multilevel influences on health outcomes, in A. Bowling and S. Ebrahim (eds) *Handbook of Health Research Methods: Investigation, Measurement and Analysis*. Maidenhead: Open University Press.

Mooney, G. (1992) *Economics, Medicine and Health Care*. London: Harvester Wheatsheaf.

Moore, T.H. (1922) Further data concerning sex differences, *Journal of Abnormal and Social Psychology*, 17: 210–14.

Moos, R.H. and Schaefer, J.A. (1984) The crisis of physical illness: an overview and conceptual approach, in R.H. Moos (ed.) *Coping with Physical Illness: New Perspectives*, vol. 2. New York: Plenum Press.

Morgan, M. (1996) Perceptions of anti-hypertensive drugs among cultural groups, in S.J. Williams and M. Calnan (eds) *Modern Medicine: Lay Perspectives and Experiences*. London: University College London Press.

Morgan, D.L. (2007) Paradigms lost and pragmatisms regained: methodological implications of combining qualitative and quantitative methods. *Journal of Mixed Methods Research*, 1: 48–76.

Moriarty, J. (2010) *Qualitative Methods Overview*. London: National Institute for Health Research: School for Social care Research, Methods Review 1. eprints.lse.ac.uk/41199/1/SSCR_Methods_Review_1-1.pdf.

Mortimer, L. and White, A. (1996) *Ethnic Group Question: Findings from Focus Group Discussions*. London: Office for National Statistics.

Moscovice, I., Armstrong, P. and Shortell, S. (1988) Health services research for decision-makers: the use of the Delphi technique to determine health priorities, *Journal of Health Politics, Policy and Law*, 2: 388–410.

Moser, C.A. and Kalton, G. (1971) *Survey Methods in Social Investigation*, 2nd edn. London: Heinemann.

Mossad, S.B., Mackin, M.L., Medendorp, S.V. *et al.* (1996) Zinc gluconate lozenges for treating the common cold, *Annals of Internal Medicine*, 125: 81–8.

Muggah, H., Hunter, A.G., Ivey, B. and Cox, D.M. (1987) Difficulties encountered in a randomisation trial of CVS versus amniocentesis for prenatal diagnosis, *Clinical Genetics*, 32: 235–9.

Muir Gray, J.A. (1997) *Evidence-Based Health Care: How to Make Health Policy and Management Decisions*. London: Churchill Livingstone.

Mulholland, H. (1985) Surreal and symbolic elements in advertising: probing consumer response, in *Proceedings of the 28th Annual Conference of the Market Research Society*, Brighton, 19–22 March. London: The Market Research Society.

Murphy, E., Dingwall, R., Greatbatch, D. *et al.* (1998) Qualitative research methods in health technology assessment: a review of the literature, *Health Technology Assessment*, 2: 1–276.

Murray, S.A. and Graham, L.J. (1995) Practice based data health needs assessment: use of four methods in a small neighbourhood, *British Medical Journal*, 310: 1443–8.

Naji, S. (1994) Integrated care for diabetes: clinical, psychosocial, and economic evaluation (Diabetes Integrated Care Evaluation Team), *British Medical Journal*, 308: 1208–12.

Nancarrow, C. and Brace, I. (2000) Saying the 'right thing': coping with social desirability bias in marketing research, *Bristol Business School Teaching and Research Review*, 3: 1–11.

Nathanson, C.A. (1975) Illness and the feminine role, *Social Science and Medicine*, 9: 57–62.

Nathanson, C.A. (1977) Sex, illness and medical care, *Social Science and Medicine*, 11: 13–25.

National Organization on Disability (1994) *NOD/Harris Survey of Disabled Americans*. New York: National Organization on Disability.

Navarro, V. (1976) *Medicine under Capitalism*. New York: Prodist.

Navarro, V. (1986) *Crisis, Health and Medicine: A Social Critique*. New York: Tavistock Publications.

Nease, R.F., Kneeland, T., O'Connor, G.T. *et al.* (1995) Variation in patient utilities for outcomes of the management of chronic stable angina, *Journal of the American Medical Association*, 273: 1185–90.

Nederhof, A.J. (1985) Methods of coping with social desirability bias: a review. *European Journal of Social Psychology*, 15: 263–80.

Netten, A. and Beecham, J. (eds) (1993) *Costing Community Care: Theory and Practice*. Aldershot: Ashgate Publishing Ltd.

Netten, A., Burge, P., Malley, J. *et al.* (2012) Outcomes of social care for adults: developing a preference-weighted measure. *Health Technology Assessment*, 16(16).

Netten, A., Smith, P., Healey, A. *et al.* (2002) *OPUS: A Measure of Social Care Outcome for Older People*, PSSRU Research Summary No. 23. Canterbury: Personal Social Services Research Unit, University of Kent.

Newman, M.A. (1995) *Report into the Cardiac Rehabilitation and Secondary Prevention Needs for Coronary Bypass Patients*. York: North Yorkshire Health Authority Research Report.

Newman, S.C. (1988) A Markov process interpretation of Sullivan's index of morbidity and mortality, *Statistics in Medicine*, 7: 787–94.

NHS Executive (1999) *National Surveys of NHS Patients, General Practice 1998*. London: Department of Health.

NHS Health Survey Advice Centre (1996) Progress on the postal survey, *Briefing*, 4: 4–5.

NHS Management Executive (1991) *Moving Forwards: Needs, Services and Contracts*. London: NHSME.

NICE (National Institute for Health and Clinical Excellence) (2004) *Guide to the Methods of Technology Appraisal*. London: NICE.

Nolan, M. and Grant, G. (1993) Service evaluation, *Journal of Advanced Nursing*, 18: 9.

Nolte, E., McKee, M. and Wait, S. (2005) Describing and evaluating health systems, in A. Bowling and S. Ebrahim (eds) *Handbook of Health Research Methods: Investigation, Measurement and Analysis*. Maidenhead: Open University Press.

Nord, E. (1992) An alternative to QALYs: the saved young life equivalent (SAVE), *British Medical Journal*, 305: 875–7.

Norman, G.R., Neufeld, V.R., Walsh, A. *et al.* (1985) Measuring physicians' performances by using simulated patients, *Journal of Medical Education*, 60: 925–34.

Norusis, M.J. (1993) *SPSS for Windows: Base System User's Guide*. Chicago: Statistical Package for the Social Sciences Inc.

Nunnally, J. (1994) *Psychometric Theory*, 3rd edn. New York: McGraw-Hill.

Oakley, A. (1974) *The Sociology of Housework*. Oxford: Martin Robertson.

Oakley, A. (2006) Process evaluation in randomised controlled trials of complex interventions. *British Medical Journal*, 332: 413.

O'Boyle, C.A., McGee, H., Hickey, A. *et al.* (1992) Individual quality of life in patients undergoing hip replacement, *Lancet*, 339: 1088–91.

O'Conner, A., Rostom, A., Fiset, V. *et al.* (1999) Decision aids for patients facing health treatment or screening decisions: systematic review, *British Medical Journal*, 319: 731–4.

Office for National Statistics (2004) *Focus on Older People*. London: ONS.

Office of Population Censuses and Surveys (1980) *Classification of Occupations*. London: HMSO.

Office of Population Censuses and Surveys (1990) *Standard Occupational Classification*, vols 1–2. London: HMSO.

Office of Population Censuses and Surveys (1991) *Standard Occupational Classification*, vol. 3. London: HMSO.

Office of Technology Assessment, US Congress (1983) *The Impact of Randomised Clinical Trials on Health Policy and Medical Practice*, OTA-BP-H22. Washington, DC: US Government Printing Office.

Ogden, J. (1995) Psychosocial theory and the creation of the risky self, *Social Science and Medicine*, 40: 409–15.

Ogden, J. (1996) *Health Psychology: A Textbook*. Buckingham: Open University Press.

Oliver, A. (ed.) (2003) Introduction, in A. Oliver (ed.) *Equity in Health and Health Care: Views from*

Ethics, Economics and Political Science. Proceedings from a meeting of the Health Equity Network. London: The Nuffield Trust for Research and Policy Studies in Health Services.

Oliver, S., Clarke-Jones, L., Rees, R. *et al.* (2004) Involving consumers in research and agenda development-setting for the NHS: developing an evidence-based approach, *Health Technology Assessment*, 8(15).

Olsen, J. on behalf of the IEA European Questionnaire Group (1998) Epidemiology deserves better questionnaires, *International Journal of Epidemiology*, 27: 935.

Omran, A.R. (1971) The epidemiological transition: a theory of the epidemiology of population change, *The Milbank Memorial Fund Quarterly*, 49: 509–38.

Ong, B.N. and Humphris, G. (1994) Prioritising needs with communities: rapid appraisal methodologies in health, in J. Popay and G. Williams (eds) *Researching the People's Health*. London: Routledge.

Ong, B.N., Humphris, G., Annet, H. and Rifkin, S. (1991) Rapid appraisal in an urban setting: an example from the developed world, *Social Science and Medicine*, 32: 909–15.

Oppenheim, A.N. (1992) *Questionnaire Design, Interviewing and Attitude Measurement*. London: Pinter Publishers.

Oppenheimer, G.M. (1988) In the eye of the storm: the epidemiological construction of AIDS, in E. Fee and D.M. Fox (eds) *AIDS: The Burdens of History*. Berkeley, CA: University of California Press.

O'Rourke, A. (2005) Critical appraisal, in A. Bowling and S. Ebrahim (eds) *Handbook of Health Research Methods: Investigation, Measurement and Analysis*. Maidenhead: Open University Press.

Orrell, M., Hancock, G., Woods, B. *et al.* (2007) A cluster randomised trial to reduce the unmet needs of people with dementia living in residential care, *International Journal of Geriatric Psychiatry*, 22: 1–8.

Osgood, C.E. (1953) *Method and Theory in Experimental Psychology*. New York: Oxford University Press.

Osgood, C.E., Suci, G.J. and Tannenbaum, P.H. (1957) *The Measurement of Meaning*. Urbana, IL: University of Illinois Press.

Oxman, A.D. (1995) Checklists for review articles, in I. Chalmers and D.G. Altman (eds) *Systematic Reviews*. London: British Medical Journal Publishing Group.

Oxman, A.D. (ed.) (1996) Section VI: preparing and maintaining systematic reviews, in *Cochrane Collaboration Handbook*. Oxford: Cochrane Collaboration and Health Information Research Unit, University of Oxford.

Oxman, T.E., Berkman, L.F., Kasl, S. *et al.* (1992) Social support and depressive symptoms in the elderly, *American Journal of Epidemiology*, 135: 356–68.

Packwood, T. (1995) Clinical audit in four therapy professions: results of an evaluation, in K. Walshe (ed.) *Evaluating Clinical Audit: Past Lessons, Future Directions*, International Congress and Symposium Series 212. London: The Royal Society of Medicine Press.

Pallant, J. (2007) *SPSS Survival Manual: A Step by Step Guide to Data Analysis Using SPSS*, 3rd edn. Maidenhead: Open University Press.

Park, P. (1999) People, knowledge, and change in participatory research, *Management Learning*, 30: 141–57.

Parker, M. (2001) The ethics of evidence-based patient choice, *Health Expectations*, 4: 87–91.

Parkin, F. (1979) *Marxism and Class Theory: A Bourgeois Critique*. London: Tavistock Publications.

Parry, O., Thomson, C. and Fowkes, G. (1999) Life course data collection: qualitative interviewing using the life grid. *Sociological Research Online*, 4; www.socresonline.ork.uk/4/4parry.html.

Parsons, T. (1951) *The Social System*. Glencoe, IL: Free Press.

Patel, R.P. and Taylor, S.D. (2002) Factors affecting medication adherence in hypertensive patients, *Annals of Pharmacotherapy*, 36: 40–5.

Patsopoulos, N. (2011) A pragmatic view on pragmatic trials. *Dialogues in Clinical Neuroscience*, 13(2): 217–224.

Patrick, D.L. (2003) Patient-reported outcomes (PROs): an organizing tool for concepts, measures, and applications, *Quality of Life Newsletter*, 31: 1–5.

Patton, M.Q. (1990) *Qualitative Evaluation and Research Methods*. Newbury Park, CA: Sage.

Paulhus, D.L. and Moore, R.J. (1991) Enhancement and denial in socially desirable responding, *Journal of Personality and Social Psychology*, 60: 307–17.

Pawson, R. and Tilley, N. (1997) *Realistic Evaluation*. London: Sage.

Payer, L. (1988) *Medicine and Culture: Varieties of Treatment in the United States, England, West Germany, and France*. New York: Henry Holt.

Pearlin, L.I. (1999) Stress and mental health: a conceptual overview, in A.V. Horwitz and T.L. Scheid (eds) *Handbook for the Study of Mental Health: Social Contexts, Theories and Systems.* Cambridge: Cambridge University Press.

Pearlin, L.I., Menaghan, E., Leiberman, M. and Mullan, J. (1981) The stress process. *Journal of Health and Social Behavior*, 22: 337–56.

Pearlin, L.I. and Pioli, M.F. (2003) Personal control: some conceptual turf and future directions, in S.H. Zarit, L.I. Pearlin and K.W. Schaie (eds) *Personal Control in Social and Life Course Context*. New York: Springer.

Peckham, M. (1991) Research and development for the NHS, *Lancet*, 338: 367–71.

Péron, Y. (1992) A stage in the promotion of disability-free life expectancy as a health indicator, in J.M. Robine, M. Blanchet and J.E. Dowd (eds) *Health Expectancy* (first workshop of the International Healthy Life Expectancy Network (REVES)), Studies on Medical and Population Subjects No. 54. London: HMSO.

Perry, L., Kendrick, D., Morris S. *et al.* (2011) Completion and return of fall diaries varies with participants' level of education, first language, and baseline fall risk. *Journals of Gerontology A: Biological Science and Medical Sciences*, 67: 210–14.

Perry, S. and Kalberer, J.T. (1980) The NIH consensus development program and the assessment of health care technologies: the first two years, *New England Journal of Medicine*, 303: 169–72.

Petty, R.E. and Cacioppo, J.T. (1981) *Attitudes and Persuasion: Classic and Contemporary Approaches*. Dubuque, IA: WC Brown.

Pfaffenberger, B. (1988) *Microcomputer Applications in Qualitative Research*, Qualitative Research Methods, Series 14. Newbury Park, CA: Sage.

Phillips, C. (1996) So what is a QALY? *Bandolier, Evidence-based Health Care*, 24: 7.

Phillips, D. (1986) Assessing dependency in old people's homes, *Social Services Research*, 6: 23–47.

Pickin, C. and St Leger, S. (1993) *Assessing Health Need Using the Life Cycle Framework*. Buckingham: Open University Press.

Pilkonis, P.A., Imler, S.D. and Rubinsky, P. (1985) Dimensions of life stress in psychiatric patients, *Journal of Human Stress*, 11: 5–10.

Pill, R. and Stott, N.C.H. (1985) Choice or chance: further evidence on ideas of illness and responsibility for health, *Social Science and Medicine*, 20: 981–91.

Pill, R. and Stott, N.C.H. (1988) Invitation to attend a health screening in a general practice setting: the views of a cohort of non-attenders, *Journal of the Royal College of General Practitioners*, 38: 57–60.

Plato (1987) *The Republic*, trans. with an introduction by D. Lee. London: Penguin.

Pocock, S.J. (1983) *Clinical Trials: A Practical Approach*. Chichester: Wiley.

Pocock, S.J. (1985) Current issues in the design and interpretation of clinical trials, *British Medical Journal*, 290: 39–42.

Pocock, S.J., Hughes, M.J. and Lee, R.J. (1987) Statistical problems in the reporting of clinical trials: a survey of three medical journals, *New England Journal of Medicine*, 317: 426–32.

Pommier, J., Guével, M-R. and Jourdan, D. (2010) Evaluation of health promotion in schools: a realistic evaluation approach using mixed methods. *BMC Public Health*, 10: 43.

Popay, J. and Williams, G. (1993) Methodology in health services research (letter), *British Medical Journal*, 306: 1069.

Popay, J. and Williams, G. (1994) Introduction, in J. Popay and G. Williams (eds) *Researching the People's Health*. London: Routledge.

Pope, C. (1992) What use is medical sociology to health services research? *Medical Sociology News*, 18: 25–7.

Pope, C. (2005) Conducting ethnography in medical settings, *Medical Education*, 39: 1180–7.

Pope, C. and Mays, N. (1993) Opening the black box: an encounter in the corridors of health services research, *British Medical Journal*, 306: 315–18.

Pope, C., Mays, N. and Popay, J. (2007) *Synthesising Qualitative and Quantitative Health Evidence: A Guide to Methods*. Maidenhead: Open University Press.

Popper, K.R. (1959) *The Logic of Scientific Discovery*. London: Hutchinson.

Porter, T.M. (1986) *The Rise of Statistical Thinking, 1820–1900*. Princeton, NJ: Princeton University Press.

Potter, J. and Wetherell, M. (1987) *Discourse and Social Psychology*. London: Sage.

Pound, P., Ebrahim, S., Sandercock, P., Bracken, M.B. *et al.* (2004) Where is the evidence that animal research benefits humans? *British Medical Journal*, 328: 514–17.

Powell-Tuck, J., MacRae, K.D., Healy, M.J.R. *et al.* (1986) A defence of the small clinical trial: evaluation of three gastroenterological studies, *British Medical Journal*, 292: 599–602.

Power, M., Harper, A., Bullinger, M. and the WHO Quality of Life Group (1999) The World Health

Organization WHOQOL-100: tests of the universality of quality of life in 15 different cultural groups worldwide, *Health Psychology*, 18: 495–505.

Power, M., Quinn, K., Schmidt, S. and WHOQOL-OLD Group. (2005) Development of WHOQOL-OLD module, *Quality of Life Research*, 14: 2197–214.

Pravikoff, D.S., Tanner, A.B. and Pierce, S.T. (2005) Readiness of U.S. nurses for evidence-based practice, *American Journal of Nursing*, 105(9): 40–51.

Prein, G. and Kelle, U. (1995) Introduction: using linkages and networks for theory building, in U. Kelle (ed.) *Computer-aided Qualitative Data Analysis*. London: Sage.

Pringle, M. and Rothera, I. (1996) Practicality of recording patient ethnicity in general practice: descriptive intervention study and attitude survey, *British Medical Journal*, 312: 1080–2.

Prior, L. (1987) Policing the dead: a sociology of the mortuary, *Sociology*, 21: 355–76.

Prochasksa, J.O. and DiClemente, C.C. (1992) Stages of change in the modification of problem behaviors, *Progress in Behavior Modification*, 28: 183–218.

Prochaska, J.O. and Velicer, W.F. (1997) The transtheoretical model of health behaviour change, *American Journal of Health Promotion*, 12: 38–48.

Propp, V.I. (1968) *The Morphology of the Folktale*, 2nd revised edn (ed. L.A. Wagner). Austin, TX: University of Texas Press.

Puddephatt, A.J. (2006) Special: an interview with Kathy Charmaz: on constructing grounded theory, *Qualitative Sociology Review*, 2: 5–20.

Puffer, S., Torgerson, D. and Watson, J. (2003) Evidence of risk of bias in cluster randomised trials: review of recent trials published in three general medical journals, *British Medical Journal*, 327: 785–9.

Puhan, M., Schünemann, H., Wong, E. *et al.* (2007) The standard gamble showed better construct validity than the time trade-off, *Journal of Clinical Epidemiology*, 60: 1029–33.

Punch, M. (1986) *Politics and Ethics of Fieldwork*. London: Sage.

Purcell, N.J. and Kish, L. (1979) Estimation for small domains, *Biometrics*, 35: 365–84.

Qureshi, H., Nocon, A. and Thompson, C. (1994) *Measuring Outcomes of Community Care for Users and Carers: A Review*. York: Social Policy Research Unit, University of York.

Rabbitt, P., Donlan, C., Bent, N. *et al.* (1993) The University of Manchester Age and Cognitive Performance Research Centre and North East Age Research Longitudinal Programmes, 1982–1997, *Zeitschrift für Gerontologie*, 26: 176–83.

Radley, A. (1989) Style, discourse and constraint in adjustment to chronic illness, *Sociology of Health and Illness*, 11: 231–52.

Radley, A. (1996) The critical moment: time, information and medical expertise in the experience of patients receiving coronary bypass surgery, in S.J. Williams and M. Calnan (eds) *Modern Medicine: Lay Perspectives and Experiences*. London: University College London Press.

Raine, R., Sanderson, C., Hutchings, A. *et al.* (2004) An experimental study of determinants of group judgments in clinical guideline development, *Lancet*, 364: 429–37.

Randall, C. (2010) e-Society, *Social Trends* 41. Newport, Wales: Office for National Statistics.

Rao, J.K., Weinberger, M. and Kroenke, K. (2000) Visit-specific expectations and patient-centred outcomes, *Archives of Family Medicine*, 9: 1148–55.

Rasbash, J. and Woodhouse, G. (1995) *MLn Command Reference*. London: Institute of Education, University of London.

Rasch, G. ([1960] 1980) *Probabilistic Models for Some Intelligence and Attainment Tests*. Expanded edition (1980) with foreword and afterword by B.D. Wright. Chicago: The University of Chicago Press.

Reed, J. and McCormack, B. (2012) Independence and autonomy: the foundation of care, in J. Reed, C.L. Clarke, and A. MacFarlane (eds) *Nursing Older Adults*. Maidenhead: Open University Press.

Reese, P.R. and Joseph, A. (1995) Quality translations – no substitution for psychometric evaluation, *Quality of Life Research*, 4: 573–4.

Rehm, J. (1998) Measuring quantity, frequency and volume of drinking, *Alcoholism: Clinical and Experimental Research*, 22: 45–145.

Rehm, J., Greenfield, T.K., Walshe, G. *et al.* (1999) Assessment methods for alcohol consumption, prevalence of high risk drinking and harm: a sensitivity analysis, *International Journal of Epidemiology*, 28: 219–24.

Rembold, C.M. (1998) Number needed to screen: development of a statistic for disease screening, *British Medical Journal*, 317: 307–12.

Resch, K.I., Ernst, E. and Garrow, J. (2000) A randomised controlled study of reviewer bias against an unconventional therapy, *Journal of the Royal Society of Medicine*, 93: 164–7 (and see editorial p. 163).

Rethans, J.J. (1994) To what extent do clinical notes by general practitioners reflect actual medical performance? A study using simulated patients, *British Journal of General Practice*, 44: 153–6.

Reynolds, P.D. (1979) *Ethical Dilemmas and Social Science*. San Francisco: Jossey-Bass.

Richards, T.I. and Richards, L. (1990) *Manual for Mainframe NUD.IST Software Version 2.1*. Melbourne: Replee.

Riordan, J. and Mockler, D. (1996) Audit of care programming in an acute psychiatric admission ward for the elderly, *International Journal of Geriatric Psychiatry*, 11: 109–18.

Rippetoe, P.A. and Rogers, R.W. (1987) Effects of components of protection motivation theory on adaptive and maladaptive coping with a health threat, *Journal of Personality and Social Psychology*, 52: 596–604.

Ritchie, J. and Spencer, L. (1994) Qualitative data analysis for applied policy research, in A. Bryman and R.G. Burgess (eds) *Analysing Qualitative Data*. London: Routledge.

Roberts, H. and Pearson, J. (1993) Impact of a postcard versus a questionnaire as a first reminder in a postal lifestyle survey, *Journal of Epidemiology and Community Health*, 47: 334–5.

Robine, J.M. (1992) Disability-free life expectancy, in J.M. Robine, M. Blanchet and J.E. Dowd (eds) *Health Expectancy*. First workshop of the International Healthy Life Expectancy Network (REVES), Studies on Medical and Population Subjects, no. 54. London: HMSO.

Robinson, D. (1971) *The Process of Becoming Ill*. London: Routledge & Kegan Paul.

Robinson, E.J., Kerr, C.E.P., Stevens, A.J. *et al.* (2005) Lay public's understanding of equipoise and randomisation in randomised controlled trials, *Health Technology Assessment*, 9(8).

Robinson, K.A. and Dickersin, K. (2002) Development of a highly sensitive search strategy for the retrieval of reports of controlled trials using PubMed, *International Journal of Epidemiology*, 31: 150–3.

Rockwood, K., Stolee, P., Robertson, D. and Shillington, E.R. (1989) Response bias in a health status survey of elderly people, *Age and Ageing*, 18: 177–82.

Roderick, P., Nicholson, T., Armitage, A. *et al.* (2005) An evaluation of the costs, effectiveness and quality of renal replacement therapy provision in rural satellite units in England and Wales, *Health Technology Assessment*, 9(24).

Roe, B. (1993) Undertaking a critical review of the literature, *Nurse Researcher*, 1: 31–42.

Roethlisberger, F.J. and Dickson, W.J. (1939) *Management and the Worker*. Cambridge, MA: Harvard University Press.

Rogers, R.W. (1983) Cognitive and physiological processes in fear appeals and attitude change: a revised theory of protection motivation, in J.T. Cacioppo and R.E. Petty (eds) *Social Psychophysiology: A Source Book*. New York: Guilford Press.

Rogers, R.W. and Mewborn, C.R. (1976) Fear appeals and attitude change: effects of noxiousness, probability of occurrence, and the efficacy of coping responses, *Journal of Personality and Social Psychology*, 34: 54–61.

Rohde, P. (2000) Age-related distortion, *Journal of the Royal Society of Medicine*, 93: 35–6.

Rose, D. and Pevalin, D.J. (eds) (2002) *A Researcher's Guide to the National Statistics Socio-economic Classification*. London: Sage.

Rosenberg, M. (1969) The conditions and consequences of evaluation research, in R. Rosenthal and R.L. Rosnow (eds) *Artifact in Behavioral Research*. New York: Academic Press.

Rosenhan, D.L. (1973) On being sane in insane places, *Science*, 179: 250–8.

Rosenstock, I.M. (1966) Why people use health services, *The Milbank Memorial Fund Quarterly*, 44: 94–124.

Rosenstock, I.M. (1974) The health belief model and preventive health behaviour, *Health Education Monographs*, 2: 354–86.

Rosenthal, R. (1976) *Experimenter Effects in Behavioral Research*. New York: Irvington.

Rosenthal, R., Percinger, G.W., Vikan-Kline, L. and Fode, K.L. (1963) The effects of early data returns on data subsequently obtained by outcome-biased experimenters, *Sociometry*, 26: 487–93.

Roscoe, J.A., Bushunow, P., Morrow, G.R. *et al.* (2004) Patient expectation is a strong predictor of severe nausea after chemotherapy, *Cancer*, 11: 2701–8.

Ross, M. and Olson, J.M. (1981) An expectancy attribution model of the effects of placebos, *Psychological Review*, 88: 408–37.

Rosser, R.M. and Watts, V.C. (1972) The measurement of illness, *Journal of the Operational Research Society*, 29: 529–40.

Rothman, K.J. (1986) *Modern Epidemiology*. Boston, MA: Little, Brown.

Rotter, J.B. (1954) *Social Learning and Clinical Psychology*. Englewood Cliffs, NJ: Prentice Hall.

Rotter, J.B. (1966) Generalised expectancies for internal vs. external control of reinforcement. *Psychological Monographs*, 80: 1–21.

Rowe, A., McClelland, A. and Billingham, K. (2001) *Community Health Needs Assessment. An Introductory Guide for the Family Health Nurse in Europe*. Copenhagen: WHO.

Rowe, G., Lambert, N., Bowling, A. *et al.* (2005) Ascertaining patients' preferences for treatment for angina using a modified repertory grid method, *Social Science and Medicine*, 60: 2585–95.

Rowntree, B.S. (1902) *Poverty: A Study of Town Life*. London: Longman.

Rozensky, R.H. and Honor, L.F. (1982) Notation systems for coding nonverbal behavior: a review, *Journal of Behavioral Assessment*, 4: 119–32.

Rubin, D.B. (1987) *Multiple Imputation for Nonresponse in Surveys*. New York: Wiley & Sons.

Rubin, H.J. and Rubin, I.S. (1995) *Qualitative Interviewing: The Art of Hearing Data*. Thousand Oaks, CA: Sage.

Rubin, H.R., Gandek, B., Rogers, W.H. *et al.* (1993) Patients' ratings of outpatient visits in different practice settings: results from the Medical Outcomes Study, *Journal of the American Medical Association*, 270: 835–40.

Rundall, I.G. and Wheeler, J.R. (1979) The effect of income on use of preventive care: an evaluation of alternative explanations, *Journal of Health and Social Behavior*, 20: 397–406.

Russell, I.T. and Wilson, B.J. (1992) Audit: the third clinical science, *Quality in Health Care*, 1: 51–5.

Ruta, D.A., Garratt, A.M., Leng, M. *et al.* (1994) A new approach to the measurement of quality of life: the Patient-Generated Index, *Medical Care*, 32: 1109–26.

Ryan, M. (1996) *Using Consumer Preferences in Health Care Decision Making*. London: Office of Health Economics.

Ryan, M. and Farrar, S. (2000) Using conjoint analysis to elicit preferences for health care, *British Medical Journal*, 320: 1530–3.

Ryan, M. and Hughes, J. (1997) Using conjoint analysis to assess women's preferences for miscarriage management, *Health Economics*, 6: 261–73.

Ryan, M., Netten, A., Skatun, D. and Smith, P. (2006) Using discrete choice experiments to estimate a preference-based measure of outcome: an application to social care for older people, *Journal of Health Economics*, 25: 927–44.

Rycroft-Malone, J., Fontenla, M., Bick, D. and Seers, K. (2010) A realistic evaluation: the case of

protocol-based care, *Implementation Science*, 5: 38.

Sackett, D.L. (1979) Bias in analytic research, *Journal of Chronic Diseases*, 32: 51–63.

Sackett, D.L. and Naylor, C.D. (1993) Should there be early publication of ancillary studies prior to the first primary report of an unblinded randomised clinical trial? *Journal of Clinical Epidemiology*, 46: 395–402.

Sackett, D.L., Rosenberg, W.M.C., Gray, J.A.M. and Richardson, W.S. (1996) Evidence based medicine: what it is and what it isn't, *British Medical Journal*, 312: 71–2.

Sackett, D.L., Strauss, S.E., Richardson, W.S., Rosenberg, W. and Haynes, R.B. (2000) *Evidence Based Medicine: How to Practice and Teach EBM*, 2nd edn. Edinburgh: Churchill Livingstone.

Sadler, G.R., Lee, H-C., Lim, R., S-H. and Fullerton, J. (2010) Recruiting hard-to-reach United States population sub-groups via adaptations of snowball sampling strategy, *Nursing and Health Science*, 12: 369–74.

Sallis, J.F., Fortmann, S.P., Soloman, D.S. *et al.* (1984) Increasing returns of physician surveys, *American Journal of Public Health*, 74: 1043 (letter).

Sanderson, C., Haglund, B.J.A., Tillgren, P. *et al.* (1996) Effect and stage models in community intervention programmes and the development of the model for management of intervention programme preparation (MMIPP), *Health Promotion International*, 11: 143–56.

Sandler, D.P. (2000) John Snow and modern day environmental epidemiology, *American Journal of Epidemiology*, 152: 1–3.

Sandvik, H. (1995) *Female Urinary Incontinence: Studies of Epidemiology and Management in General Practice*. Bergen: Department of Public Health and Primary Health Care, University of Bergen.

Sarason, I.G., Levine, H.M., Basham, R.B. *et al.* (1983) Assessing social support: the Social Support Questionnaire, *Journal of Personality and Social Psychology*, 44: 127–39.

Sartre, J.P. (1969) Itinerary of thought, *New Left Review*, 58.

SAS (1990) *SAS Language: Reference, Version 6*. Cary, NC: SAS Institute Inc.

Saunders, L. (1954) *Cultural Differences and Medical Care*. New York: Russell Sage Foundation.

Say, R.E. and Thomson, R. (2003) The importance of patient preferences in treatment decisions –

challenges for doctors, *British Medical Journal*, 327: 542–5.

Scambler, G. (1984) Perceiving and coping with stigmatising illness, in R. Fitzpatrick, J. Hinton, S. Newman et al. (eds) *The Experience of Illness*. London: Tavistock.

Scambler, G. (2009) Health-related stigma, *Sociology of Health and Illness*, 31: 441–5.

Scambler, G. and Hopkins, A. (1986) Being epileptic: coming to terms with stigma, *Sociology of Health and Illness*, 8: 26–43.

Scambler, G. and Hopkins, A. (1988) Accommodating epilepsy in families, in R. Anderson and M. Bury (eds) *Living with Chronic Illness: The Experience of Patients and Their Families*. London: Unwin Hyman.

Schegloff, E.A. and Sacks, H. (1974) Opening up closings, in R. Turner (ed.) *Ethnomethodology*. Harmondsworth: Penguin.

Scheirer, M.F. and Carver, C.S. (1985) Optimism, coping and health: assessment and implications of generalised outcome expectancies, *Health Psychology*, 4: 219–47.

Scheirer, M.F. and Carver, C.S. (1987) Dispositional optimism and physical wellbeing: the influence of generalised outcome expectancies on health, *Journal of Personality*, 55: 169–210.

Scherer, K. and Ekman, P. (eds) (1982) *Handbook of Methods in Nonverbal Behavior Research*. Cambridge: Cambridge University Press.

Schneider, J. and Conrad, P. (1981) Medical and sociological typologies: the case of epilepsy, *Social Science and Medicine*, 15A: 211–19.

Schulman, B.A. (1979) Active patient orientation and outcomes in hypertensive treatment, *Medical Care*, 17: 267–80.

Schultz, K.F., Chalmers, I., Hayes, R.J. and Altman, D.G. (1995) Empirical evidence of bias: dimensions of methodologic quality associated with estimates of treatment effects in controlled trials, *Journal of the American Medical Association*, 273: 408–12.

Schwartz, L.M., Woloshin, S. and Birkmeyer, J.D. (2005) How do elderly patients decide where to go for major surgery? Telephone interview survey, *British Medical Journal*, 331: 821.

Schwarzer, R. (1992) Self-efficacy in the adoption and maintenance of health behaviors: theoretical approaches and a new model, in R. Schwarzer (ed.) *Self-efficacy: Thought Control of Action*. Washington, DC: Hemisphere.

Schwarzer, R. (1993) *Measurement of Perceived Self-efficacy: Psychometric Scales for Cross-cultural Research*. Berlin: Freie Universität, Institut für Psychologie.

Schwarzer, R. and Fuchs, R. (1995) Self-efficacy and health behaviours, in M. Connor and P. Norman (eds) *Predicting Health Behaviour*. Buckingham: Open University Press.

Scientific Software Development (1997) *Atlas of Visual Qualitative Data Analysis Management Theory Building: User's Guide and Reference*. Berlin: Scientific Software Development.

Scott, E.A. and Black, N. (1991) When does a consensus exist in expert panels? *Journal of Public Health Medicine*, 13: 35–9.

Scourfield, J. and Pithouse, A. (2006) Lay and professional knowledge in social work: reflections from ethnographic research on child protection, *European Journal of Social Work*, 9: 323–37.

Sculpher, M. (2004) Economic evaluation, in N. Fulop, P. Allen, A. Clarke and N. Black (eds) *Studying the Organisation and Delivery of Health Services*. London: Routledge.

Seale, C., Charteris-Black, J., MacFarlane, A. and McPherson, A. (2010) Interviews and Internet forums: a comparison of two sources of qualitative data, *Qualitative Health Research*, 20: 595–606.

Secretaries of State for Health, Wales, Northern Ireland and Scotland (1989a) *Working for Patients*. London: HMSO.

Secretaries of State for Health, Wales, Northern Ireland and Scotland (1989b) *Contracts for Services and Role of District Health Authorities*. London: HMSO.

Seedhouse, D. (1985) *Health: The Foundations for Achievement*. Chichester: Wiley.

Seedhouse, D. (1994) *Fortress NHS: A Philosophical Review of the National Health Service*. Chichester: Wiley.

Seeman, M. (1983) Alienation motifs in contemporary theorizing: the hidden continuity of classic themes, *Social Psychology Quarterly*, 46: 171–84.

Seidel, J. and Clarke, J.A. (1984) The ETHNOGRAPH: a computer program for the analysis of qualitative data, *Qualitative Sociology*, 7: 110–25.

Seligman, M.E.P. (1975) *Helplessness: On Depression, Development and Death*. San Francisco, CA: Freeman.

Senn, S. (1993) *Cross-over Trials in Clinical Research*. Chichester: Wiley.

Senn, S. (1995) Crossover at the crossroads, *Applied Clinical Trials*, 4: 25–9.

Senn, S. (1997) *Statistical Issues in Drug Development*. Chichester: Wiley.

Senn, S. (1998) Cross-over trials, in *Wiley Encylopedia of Biostatistics*. Chichester: Wiley.

Shavers, V.L. (2007) Measurement of socioeconomic status in health disparities research, *Journal of the National Medical Association*, 99: 1013–23.

Shaw, C. (1980) Aspects of audit 1: the background, *British Medical Journal*, 280: 1256–8.

Shaw, C. (1989) *Medical Audit: A Hospital Handbook*, 2nd edn. London: King's Fund Centre.

Shaw, M. (2005) Finding and using secondary data on the health and health care of populations, in A. Bowling and S. Ebrahim (eds) *Handbook of Health Research Methods: Investigation, Measurement and Analysis.* Maidenhead: Open University Press.

Shea, B.J., Grimshaw, J.M., Wells, G.A. *et al.* (2007) Development of AMSTAR: a measurement tool to assess the methodological quality of systematic reviews, *BMC Medical Research Methodology*, 7: 10.

Sheeran, P. and Abraham, C. (1995) The health belief model, in M. Conner and P. Norman (eds) *Predicting Health Behaviour*. Buckingham: Open University Press.

Shontz, F.C. (1975) *The Psychological Aspects of Physical Illness and Disability*. New York: Macmillan.

Schulz, K.F., Altman, D.G., Moher, D. and CONSORT Group (2010) CONSORT 2010 statement: updated guidelines for reporting parallel group randomised trials, *British Medical Journal*, 340: c332.

Sidell, M. (1995) *Health in Old Age*. Buckingham: Open University Press.

Siegel, S. (1956) *Nonparametric Statistics for the Behavioural Sciences*. London: McGraw-Hill.

Siegman, A.W. and Feldstein, S. (1987) *Nonverbal Behavior and Communication*. Hillsdale, NJ: Lawrence Erlbaum.

Sijtsma, K. (2005) Nonparametric item response theory models, *Encyclopedia of Social Measurement*, 2: 875–81.

Sijtsma, K. and Molenaar, I.W. (2002) *Introduction to Nonparametric Item Response Theory*. New York: Sage Publications.

Silverman, D. (1993) *Interpreting Qualitative Data: Methods for Analysing Talk, Text and Interaction*. London: Sage.

Silverstein, F.E., Graham, D.Y., Senior, J.R. *et al.* (1995) Misoprostol reduces serious gastrointestinal complications in patients with rheumatoid arthritis receiving nonsteroidal anti-inflammatory drugs, *Annals of Internal Medicine*, 123: 241–9.

Singer, P.A., Tasch, E.S., Stocking, C. *et al.* (1991) Sex or life: tradeoffs between quality and quantity of life, *Journal of Clinical Oncology*, 9: 328–34.

Skinner, H. (1992) Life-style assessment and change: theory, what theory?, in F. Indiver (ed.) *Assessing Interventions, Traditional and Innovative Methods*. London: Sage.

Slagsvold, B. and Sørensen, A. (2008) Age, education, and the gender gap in the sense of control, *International Journal of Aging and Human Development*, 67: 25–42.

Slevin, M., Mossman, J., Bowling, A. *et al.* (1995) Volunteers or victims: patients' views of randomised cancer clinical trials, *British Journal of Cancer*, 71: 1270–4.

Slovic, P., Fischoff, B. and Lichenstein, S. (1977) Behavioral decision theory, *Annual Review of Psychology*, 28: 1–39.

Slymen, D.J. and Hovell, M.F. (1997) Cluster versus individual randomisation in adolescent tobacco and alcohol studies: illustrations for design decisions, *International Journal of Epidemiology*, 26: 765–71.

Smart, B. (1976) *Sociology, Phenomenology, and Marxian Analysis: A Critical Discussion of the Theory and Practice of a Science of Society*. London: Routledge & Kegan Paul.

Smidth, M., Christensen, M.B., Olesen, F. and Vedsted P. (2013) Developing an active implementation model for a chronic disease management program, *International Journal of Integrated Care*, 13: e020.

Smith, G.R., Rost, K. and Kashner, T.M. (1995) A trial of the effect of a standardized psychiatric consultation on health outcomes and costs in somatizing patients, *Archives of General Psychiatry*, 52: 238–43.

Smith, R. (1990) Crisis in American health care, *British Medical Journal*, 300: 765.

Smith, S., Sinclair, D., Raine, R. and Reeves, B. (2005) *Health Care Evaluation.* Maidenhead: Open University Press.

Smith, S.C., Lamping, D.L., Banerjee, S. *et al.* (2005) Measurement of health-related quality of life for people with dementia: development of a new instrument (DEMQOL) and an evaluation of current methodology, *Health Technology Assessment*, 9(10).

Smithells, R.W., Sheppard, S., Schorah, C.J. *et al.* (1980) Possible prevention of neural-tube defects by periconceptional vitamin supplementation, *Lancet*, i: 339–40.

Snape, D. and Spencer, L. (2003) *Case Study Research in Practice*. London: Sage.

Snow, J. (1860) *On the Mode of Communication of Cholera*, 2nd edn. London: John Churchill (facsimile of 1936 reprinted edition published in 1965 by Hafner, New York).

Snowdon, C., Garcia, J. and Elbourne, D. (1998) Reactions of participants to the results of a randomised controlled trial: exploratory study, *British Medical Journal*, 317: 21–6.

Soper, K. (1981) *On Human Needs*. Brighton: Harvester.

Soper, K. (1993) A theory of human need, *New Left Review*, 197: 113–28.

Spiegelhalter, D.J., Myles, J.P., Jones, D.R. and Abrams, K.R. (2000) Bayesian methods in health technology assessment: a review, *Health Technology Assessment*, 4(38).

Sprangers, M.A.G. and Schwartz, C.E. (1999) Integrating response shift into health-related quality of life research: a theoretical model, *Social Science and Medicine*, 48: 1507–15.

Stacey, M. (1976) The health service consumer: a sociological misconception, *Sociological Review Monograph*, 22: 194–200.

Stacey, M. (1986) Concepts of health and illness and the division of labour in health care, in C. Currer and M. Stacey (eds) *Concepts of Health, Illness and Disease: A Comparative Perspective*. Oxford: Berg.

Stake, R.E. (1995) *The Art of Case Study Research*. London: Sage.

Standing Committee on Postgraduate Medical Education (1989) *Medical Audit: The Educational Implications*. London: SCOPME.

Stanford, J.L. *et al.* (2000) Urinary and sexual function after radical prostatectomy for clinically localized prostate cancer: the prostate cancer outcomes study, *Journal of the American Medical Association*, 283: 354–60.

Stanton, A.L. (1987) Determinants of adherence to medical regimens by hypertensive patients, *Journal of Behavioral Medicine*, 10: 377–94.

Statistics Watch (1998) Prospects, *Statistics Watch*, 35: 4.

Steen, N. and McColl, E. (1996) Developing and testing symptom based outcome measures, in A. Hutchinson, E. McColl, A. Christie, and C. Riccalton (eds) *Health Outcome Measures in Primary and Out-Patient Care*. Amsterdam: Harwood Academic Publishers, pp. 23–44.

Stevens, A. (1991) *Assessing Health Care Needs*, a DHA Project discussion paper. London: NHS Management Executive.

Stevenson, R.C., Pharoah, P.O.D., Cooke, R.W.I. and Sandhu, B. (1991) Predicting costs and outcomes of neonatal intensive care for very low birth-weight infants, *Public Health*, 105: 121–6.

St Leger, A.S., Schnieden, H. and Wadsworth-Bell, J.P. (1992) *Evaluating Health Services' Effectiveness*. Buckingham: Open University Press.

Stocking, B. (1992) Promoting change in clinical care, *Quality in Health Care*, 1: 56–60.

Stocking, B., Jennet, B. and Spiby, J. (1991) Criteria for change, in *The History and Impact of Consensus Development Conferences in the UK*. London: King's Fund Centre.

Stott, N.C.H. and Pill, R. (1983) *A Study of Health Beliefs, Attitudes and Behaviour among Working Class Mothers*. Cardiff: Department of General Practice, Welsh National School of Medicine.

Strauss, A. and Corbin, J. (1990) *Basics of Qualitative Research: Grounded Theory Procedures and Techniques*. Thousand Oaks, CA: Sage.

Strauss, A. and Glaser, B.G. (1975) *Chronic Illness and the Quality of Life*. St Louis, MO: Mosby.

Strauss, R. (1957) The nature and status of medical sociology, *American Sociological Review*, 22: 200–4.

Streiner, G.L. and Norman, D.R. (2003) *Health Measurement Scales: A Practical Guide to Their Development and Use*, 3rd edn. Oxford: Oxford University Press.

Streiner, G.L. and Norman, D.R. (2008) *Health Measurement Scales: A Practical Guide to Their Development and Use*, 4th edn. Oxford: Oxford University Press.

Stringer, E.T. (1996) *Action Research: A Handbook for Practitioners*. London: Sage.

Stroebe, W. (2000) *Social Psychology and Health*, 2nd edn. Buckingham: Open University Press.

Stroebe, W. and Stroebe, M.S. (1995) *Social Psychology and Health*. Buckingham: Open University Press.

Suchman, L. and Jordan, B. (1992) Validity and the collaborative construction of meaning in face-to-face surveys, in J.M. Tanur (ed.) *Questions about Questions: Inquiries into the Cognitive Bases of Surveys*. New York: Russell Sage Foundation.

Sudman, S. and Bradburn, N.M. (1983) *Asking Questions*. New York: Jossey-Bass.

Sudnow, D. (1968) Normal crimes, in E. Rubington and M. Weinberg (eds) *Deviance: The Interactionist Perspective*. New York: Macmillan.

Sullivan, D.F. (1971) A single index of mortality and morbidity, *Health Service Management Association Health Reports*, 86: 347–54.

Sung, L., Greenberg, M.L., Doyle, J.J. et al. (2003) Construct validation of the Health Utilities Index and the Child Health Questionnaire in children undergoing cancer chemotherapy, *British Journal of Cancer*, 88: 1185–90.

Survey Research Center (1976) *Interviewer's Manual*, revised edn. Ann Arbor, MI: University of Michigan, Survey Research Center, Institute for Social Research.

Sutton, S.R. (1998) How ordinary people in Great Britain perceive the health risks of smoking, *Journal of Epidemiology and Community Health*, 52: 338–9.

Sutton, S.R. (1999) How accurate are smokers' perceptions of risk? *Health, Risk and Society*, 1: 223–30.

Svanborg, A. (1996) Conduct of long term cohort sequential studies, in S. Ebrahim and A. Kalache (eds) *Epidemiology in Old Age*. London: British Medical Journal Publishing Group.

Swinscow, T.D.V. and Campbell, M.J. (2001) *Statistics at Square One*. Oxford: Blackwell BMJ Books.

Tabachnick, B.G. and Fidell, L.S. (1996) *Using Multivariate Statistics*, 3rd edn. New York: HarperCollins.

Tansey, J. and O'Riordan, T. (1999) Cultural theory and risk: a review, *Health, Risk and Society*, 1: 71–90.

Tanur, J.M. (ed.) (1992) *Questions About Questions: Inquiries into the Cognitive Bases of Surveys*. New York: Russell Sage Foundation.

Taylor, D., Bury, M., Campling, N. et al. (2006) *A Review of the Use of the Health Belief Model (HBM), the Theory of Reasoned Action (TRA), the Theory of Planned Behaviour (TPB) and the Trans-theoretical Model (TTM) to Study and Predict Health Related Behaviour Change*. London: School of Pharmacy.

Taylor, S. and Ashworth, C. (1987) Durkheim and social realism: an approach to health and illness, in G. Scambler (ed.) *Sociological Theory and Medical Sociology*. London: Tavistock Publications.

Taylor, S.E. (1983) Adjustment to threatening events: a theory of cognitive adaptation, *American Psychologist*, 38: 1161–73.

Terwee, C.B., Mokkink, L.B., Knol, D.L. et al. (2012) Rating the methodological quality in systematic reviews of studies on measurement properties: a scoring system for the COSMIN checklist, *Quality of Life Research*, 21: 651–7.

Thomas, A.J. (2010) *The Lambeth Cholera Outbreak of 1848–1849*. Jefferson, NC: McFarlane and Company, Inc., Publishers.

Thompson, P. (1988) *The Voice of the Past: Oral History*. Oxford: Oxford University Press.

Thompson, S.G. (1995) Why sources of heterogeneity in meta-analyses should be investigated, in I. Chalmers and D.G. Altman (eds) *Systematic Reviews*. London: British Medical Journal Publishing Group.

Thunedborg, K., Allerup, P., Bech, P. and Joyce, C.R.B. (1993) Development of the repertory grid for measurement of individual quality of life in clinical trials, *International Journal of Methods in Psychiatric Research*, 3: 45–56.

Thurstone, L.L. (1927) Law of comparative judgement, *Psychology Review*, 34: 93–7.

Thurstone, L.L. (1928) Attitudes can be measured, *American Journal of Sociology*, 33: 529–54.

Thurstone, L.L. (1952) Autobiography, in E.G. Boring, H.S. Langfeld, H. Werner and R.M. Yerkes (eds) *A History of Psychology in Autobiography*, vol. 4. Englewood Cliffs, NJ: Prentice Hall.

Tilling, K., Peters, T. and Sterne, J. (2005) Key issues in the statistical analysis of quantitative data in research on health and health services, in A. Bowling and S. Ebrahim (eds) *Handbook of Health Research Methods: Investigation, Measurement and Analysis*. Maidenhead: Open University Press.

Titler, M.G. (2008) The evidence for evidence-based practice implementation, in R.G. Hughes (ed.) *Patient Safety and Quality: An Evidence-Based Handbook for Nurses*. Rockville, MD: Agency for Healthcare Research and Quality.

Titler, M.G., Kleiber, C., Steelman, V.J. et al. (2001) The Iowa model of evidence-based practice to promote quality care, *Critical Care Nursing Clinics of North America*, 13(4): 497–509.

Titmuss, R.M. (1968) *Commitment to Welfare*. London: Allen & Unwin.

Torgerson, D.J., Donaldson, C. and Reid, D.M. (1994) Private versus social opportunity cost of time: valuing time in the demand for health care, *Health Economics*, 3: 149–55.

Torgerson, D.J., Klaber-Moffett, J. and Russell, I.T. (1996) Patient preferences in randomised trials: threat or opportunity? *Journal of Health Services Research and Policy*, 1: 194–7.

Torgerson, D.J. and Roland, M. (1998) What is Zelen's design? *British Medical Journal*, 316: 606.

Torgerson, D.J. and Sibbald, B. (1998) What is a patient preference trial? *British Medical Journal*, 316: 360.

Torrance, G.W. (1976) Social preferences for health states, and empirical evaluation of three measurement techniques, *Socio-Economic Planning Science*, 10: 129.

Torrance, G.W. (1986) Measurement of health state utilities for economic appraisal: a review, *Journal of Health Economics*, 3: 1–30.

Torrance, G.W., Boyle, M.H. and Horwood, S.P. (1982) Application of multiattribute utility theory to measure social preferences for health states, *Operations Research*, 30: 1043–69.

Townsend, P. (1979) *Poverty in the United Kingdom*. Harmondsworth: Penguin.

Townsend, P. and Davidson, N. (1982) *Inequalities in Health: The Black Report*. Harmondsworth: Penguin.

Townsend, P., Phillimore, P. and Beattie, A. (1988) *Health and Deprivation: Inequality and the North*. London: Routledge.

Trauer, T. and Mackinnon, A. (2001) Why are we weighting? The role of importance ratings in quality of life measurement, *Quality of Life Research*, 10: 579–85.

Tugwell, P., Bombardier, C., Buchanan, W.W. *et al.* (1987) The MACTAR Patient Preference Disability Questionnaire, *Journal of Rheumatology*, 14: 446–51.

Turner, E.H., Matthews, A.M., Linardatos, E. *et al.* (2008) Selective publication of antidepressant trials and its influence on apparent efficacy, *New England Journal of Medicine*, 358: 252–60.

Vandenbroucke, J.P. (1999) Case reports in an evidence-based world, *Journal of the Royal Society of Medicine*, 92: 159–63.

Vandenbroucke, J.P. (2000) The testimony of Doctor Snow, *American Journal of Epidemiology*, 152: 10–12.

Van Schuur, W.H. and Kiers, H.A.L. (1994) Why factor analysis often is the incorrect model for analysing bipolar concepts, and what model to use instead, *Applied Psychological Measurement*, 18: 97–110.

Varkevisser, C.M., Pathmanathan, I. and Brownlee, A. (1991) *Designing and Conducting Health Systems Research Projects: Health Systems Research Training Services*. Geneva: WHO, International Development Research Centre.

Victora, C.G., Habicht, J.P. and Bryce, J. (2004) Evidence-based public health: moving beyond randomized trials, *American Journal of Public Health*, 94: 400–5.

Volkart, E.H. (1951) *Social Behavior and Personality*. New York: Social Science Research Council.

von Elm, E., Altman, D.G., Egger, M., Pocock, S.J., Götzsche, P.C., Vandenbroucke, J.P., for the STROBE Initiative (2007) Strengthening the reporting of observational studies in epidemiology (STROBE) statement: guidelines for reporting observational studies. *British Medical Journal*, 335: 806–8.

Wade, D.T. and Halligan, P.W. (2004) Do biomedical models of illness make for good healthcare systems? *British Medical Journal*, 329: 1398–401.

Wadsworth, M. (1986) Serious illness in childhood and its association with later life achievements, in R. Wilkinson (ed.) *Class and Health*. London: Tavistock, pp. 50–74.

Wadsworth, M.E.J., Butterfield, W.J.H. and Blaney, R. (1971) *Health and Sickness: The Choice of Treatment. Perception of Illness and Use of Services in an Urban Community*. London: Tavistock Publications.

Waitzkin, H. (1983) *The Second Sickness: Contradictions of Capitalist Health Care*. New York: The Free Press.

Wales, E. and Brewer, B. (1976) Graffiti in the 1970s. *Journal of Social Psychology*, 99: 115–23.

Walker, A. (1987) The poor relation: poverty among older women, in C. Glendenning and J. Millar (eds) *Women and Poverty in Britain*. Hemel Hempstead: Harvester Wheatsheaf.

Wallston, B.S., Alagna, S.W., De Vellis, B.M. and De Vellis, R.F. (1983) Social support and physical illness, *Health Psychology*, 2: 2367–91.

Wallston, B.S. and Wallston, K.A. (1981) Social psychological models of health and behaviour: an examination and integration, in G. Sanders and J. Suls (eds) *The Social Psychology of Health and Illness*. Hillsdale, NJ: Lawrence Erlbaum.

Wallston, B.S., Wallston, K.A., Kaplan, G.D. and Maides, S.A. (1976) Development and validation of the Health Locus of Control (HLC) Scale, *Journal of Consulting and Clinical Psychology*, 44: 580–5.

Wallston, K., Wallston, B.S. and De Vellis, R. (1978) Development of the multidimensional health locus of control (MHLC) scales, *Health Education Monographs*, 6: 160–71.

Walshe, K. (1995) The traits of success in clinical audit, in K. Walshe (ed.) *Evaluating Clinical Audit: Past Lessons, Future Directions*, International Congress and Symposium Series 212. London: The Royal Society of Medicine Press.

Walter, F.S., James, T. and Matanowski, M.D. (1987) The validity of questionnaire-reported work history in live respondents, *Journal of Occupational Medicine*, 29: 795–800.

Ware, J.E., Brook, R.H., Rogers, W.H. *et al.* (1987) *Health Outcomes for Adults in Prepaid and*

Fee-for-Service Systems of Care: Results from the Health Insurance Experiment, Report no. R-3459-HHSt. Santa Monica, CA: Rand.

Ware, J.E., Harris, W.J., Gandek, B. *et al.* (1997b) *MAP-R for Windows: Multitrait/multi-item Analysis Programme – Revised Users' Guide*. Boston, MA: Health Assessment Laboratory.

Ware, J.E. and Hays, R.D. (1988) Methods for measuring patient satisfaction with specific medical encounters, *Medical Care*, 26: 393–402.

Ware, J.E., Kosinski, M. and Keller, S.D. (1995) *SF-12: How to Score the SF-12. Physical and Mental Health Summary Scales*. Boston, MA: The Health Institute, New England Medical Center.

Ware, J.E., Snow, K.K., Kosinski, M. and Gandek, B. (1997a) *SF-36 Health Survey: Manual and Interpretation Guide*. Boston, MA: The Health Institute, New England Medical Center.

Ware, J.E., Snow, K.K., Kosinski, M. and Gandek, B. (1993) *SF-36 Health Survey: Manual and Interpretation Guide*. Boston, MA: The Health Institute, New England Medical Center.

Ware, J.E. and Snyder, M.K. (1975) Dimensions of patient attitudes regarding doctors and medical care services, *Medical Care*, 13: 669–82.

Wasson, J.H., Reda, D.J., Bruskewitz, R.C. *et al.*, for the Veterans Affairs Cooperative Study Group on Transurethral Resection of the Prostate (1995) A comparison of transurethral surgery with watchful waiting for moderate symptoms of benign prostatic hyperplasia, *New England Journal of Medicine*, 332: 75–9.

Weaver, A. and Atkinson, P. (1994) *Microcomputing and Qualitative Data Analysis*. Aldershot: Avebury.

Web, S.A. (2001) Some considerations on the validity of evidence-based practice in social work. *British Journal of Social Work*, 31: 57–79.

Webb, E.J., Campbell, D.T., Schwartz, R.D. and Sechrest, L. (1966) *Unobtrusive Measures: Nonreactive Research in the Social Sciences*. Chicago: Rand McNally College Publishing Company.

Webb, E.J., Campbell, D.T., Schwartz, R.D. and Sechrest, L. (2000) *Unobtrusive Measures*, revised edn. Thousand Oaks, CA: Sage.

Webb, C. and Kevern, J. (2001) Focus groups as a research method: a critique of some aspects of their use in nursing research, *Journal of Advanced Nursing*, 33: 798–805.

Webber, G.C. (1990) Patient education: a review of the issues, *Medical Care*, 28: 1089–103.

Weber, M. (1946) *From Max Weber: Essays in Sociology* (ed. and trans. H.H. Gerth and C. Wright Mills). New York: Oxford University Press.

Weber, M. (1964) *The Theory of Social and Economic Organization* (trans. A.M. Henderson and T. Parsons). New York: Free Press.

Weber, M. (1978) *Economy and Society*, vols 1 and 2 (ed. G. Roth and C. Wittich). Berkeley, CA: University of California Press.

Weber, M. (1979) *Max Weber on Capitalism, Bureaucracy and Religion: A Selection of Texts* (ed. S. Andreski). London: Allen & Unwin.

Week, J. (2001) If you must drill a hole in someone's head, make sure it's worthwhile, *Guardian 2*, 19 April.

Weinstein, M.C. and Fineberg, H.V. (1980) *Clinical Decision Analysis*. Philadelphia, PA: WB Saunders.

Weinstein, N.D. (1984) Why it won't happen to me: perception of risk factors and illness susceptibility, *Health Psychology*, 3: 431–57.

Weinstein, N.D., Rothman, A. and Sutton, S.R. (1998) Stage theories of human behavior: conceptual and methodological issues, *Health Psychology*, 17: 290–9.

Weitzman, E.A. and Miles, M.B. (1995) *Computer Programs for Qualitative Data Analysis*. Thousand Oaks, CA: Sage.

Wells, E. and Marwell, G. (1976) *Self Esteem*. Beverly Hills, CA: Sage.

Wells, K.B., Burnam, M.A., Leake, B. and Robins, L.N. (1988) Agreement between face-to-face and telephone-administered versions of the depression section of the NIMH diagnostic interview schedule, *Journal of Psychiatric Research*, 22: 207–20.

Wennberg, J.E., Mulley, A.G., Hanley, D. *et al.* (1988) An assessment of prostatectomy for benign urinary tract obstruction: geographic variations and the evaluation of medical care outcomes, *Journal of the American Medical Association*, 259: 3027–30.

Westermeyer, J.F. (2013) Predictors and characteristics of successful aging among men: a 48-year longitudinal study, *International Journal of Aging and Human Development*, 76: 323–45.

White, M. and Elander, G. (1992) Translation of an instrument: the US-Nordic Family Dynamics Nursing Research Project, *Scandinavian Journal of Caring Science*, 6: 161–4.

Whitehead, M. (1987) *The Health Divide*. London: Health Education Council.

Whitehead, M. (1994) Who cares about equity in the NHS? *British Medical Journal*, 308: 1284–7.

WHOQOL Group (1993) *Measuring Quality of Life: The Development of the World Health Organi-*

zation Quality of Life Instrument (WHOQOL). Geneva: WHO.

WHOQOL Group (1998a) The World Health Organization Quality of Life Assessment (WHOQOL): development and general psychometric properties, *Social Science and Medicine*, 46: 1569–85.

WHOQOL Group (1998b) Development of the World Health Organization WHOQOL-BREF Quality of Life Assessment, *Psychological Medicine*, 28: 551–8.

Whyte, W.F. (1943) *Street Corner Society*. Chicago: University of Chicago Press.

Wicker, A.W. (1969) Attitudes versus actions: the relationship of verbal and overt behavioural responses to attitude objects, *Journal of Social Issues*, 25: 41–78.

Wiggins, D. and Dermen, S. (1987) Needs, need, needing, *Journal of Medical Ethics*, 13: 62–8.

Wilcock, G.K. (1979) The prevalence of osteoarthritis of the hip requiring total hip replacement in the elderly, *International Journal of Epidemiology*, 8: 247–50.

Wilkinson, R. (1992) Income distribution and life expectancy, *British Medical Journal*, 304: 165–8.

Wilkinson, R. (2000) Inequality and the social environment: a reply to Lynch *et al.*, *Journal of Epidemiology and Community Health*, 54: 411–13.

Williams, A. (1992) Priorities – not needs, in A. Corden, G. Robertson and K. Tolley (eds) *Meeting Needs*. Aldershot: Avebury Gower.

Williams, A. and Kind, P. (1992) The present state of play about QALYs, in A. Hopkins (ed.) *Measures of the Quality of Life and Uses to Which Such Measures May Be Put*. London: Royal College of Physicians.

Williams, R. (1990) *A Protestant Legacy*. Oxford: Clarendon Press.

Williams, S. (1987) Goffman, interactionism, and the management of stigma in everyday life, in G. Scambler (ed.) *Sociological Theory and Medical Sociology*. London: Tavistock Publications.

Willis, G.B. (2005) *Cognitive Interviewing: A Tool for Improving Questionnaire Design*. Thousand Oaks, CA: Sage Publications, Inc.

Wills, T.A. (1985) Supportive functions of interpersonal relationships, in S. Cohen and S.L. Syme (eds) *Social Support and Health*. Orlando, FL: Academic Press.

Wilson, D.K., Purdon, S.E. and Wallston, K.A. (1988) Compliance to health recommendations: a theoretical overview of message framing. *Health Education Research*, 3: 161–71.

Winslow, C.M., Solomon, D.H., Chassin, M.R. *et al.* (1988) The appropriateness of carotid endarterectomy, *New England Journal of Medicine*, 318: 721–7.

Wolfe, F. and Hawley, D.J. (1997) Measurement of the quality of life in rheumatic disorders using the EuroQol, *British Journal of Rheumatology*, 36: 786–93.

Wolff, B.B. and Langley, S. (1977) Cultural factors and the responses to pain, in D. Landy (ed.) *Culture, Disease and Healing: Studies in Medical Anthropology*. New York: Macmillan.

Wolf-Maier, K., Cooper, R.S., Kramer, H.K. *et al.* (2004) Hypertension treatment and control in five European countries, Canada, and the United States, *Hypertension*, 43: 10–17.

Wood, J. and Freemantle, N. (1999) Choosing an appropriate unit of analysis in trials of interventions that attempt to influence practice, *Journal of Health Services Research and Policy*, 4: 44–8.

World Bank (1993) *World Development Report 1993: Investing in Health*. Oxford: Oxford University Press.

World Health Organization (1947) *Constitution of the World Health Organization*. Geneva: WHO.

World Health Organization (1948) *Official Records of the World Health Organization, No. 2*. Geneva: WHO.

World Health Organization (1992) *International Classification of Diseases*, vols I–III, 10th edn. Geneva: WHO.

World Health Organization (1996) *Health Interview Surveys: Towards International Harmonisation of Methods and Instruments*, WHO regional publications, European series No. 58. Copenhagen: WHO.

Wragg, J.A., Robinson, E.J. and Lilford, R.J. (2000) Information presentation and decision to enter clinical trials: a hypothetical trial of hormone replacement therapy, *Social Science and Medicine*, 51: 453–62.

Wright, B.D. and Linacre, J.M. (1989) Observations are always ordinal, measurements, however, must be interval, *Archives of Physical Medicine and Rehabilitation*, 70: 857–60.

Wright, B.D. and Masters, G.N. (1982) *Rating Scale Analysis*. Chicago: MESA Press.

Wright, K. (1993) The dangers of inappropriate or poor quality information, in J. Beecham and A. Netten (eds) *Community Care in Action: The Role of Costs*. Canterbury: Personal Social Services Research Unit, University of Kent at Canterbury.

Wright, S.J. (1990) Conceptions and dimensions of health, in R. Shute and G. Penny (eds)

Psychology and Health Promotion. Proceedings of the Welsh Branch of the British Psychological Society Conference on 'Psychology and Health Promotion'. Cardiff: British Psychological Society (Welsh Branch).

Wrigley, E.A. and Schofield, R.S. (1981) *Population History of England 1541–1871: A Reconstruction*. Cambridge: Cambridge University Press.

Yates, J.F. (1992) *Risk-taking Behaviour*. Chichester: Wiley.

Yin, R.K. (2003) *Case Study Research: Design and Methods*, 3rd edn. Thousand Oaks, CA: Sage.

Young, A. (1983) The relevance of traditional medical cultures to modern primary health care, *Social Science and Medicine*, 17: 1205–11.

Yudkin, P. and Stratton, I.M. (1996) How to deal with regression to the mean in intervention studies, *Lancet*, 347: 241–3.

Zborowski, M. (1952) Cultural components in response to pain, *Journal of Social Issues*, 8: 16–30.

Zelen, M. (1979) A new design for randomized clinical trials. *New England Journal of Medicine*, 300: 1242–45.

Zhu, K., McKnight, B., Stergachis, A. *et al.* (1999) Comparison of self-report data and medical records data: results from a case-control study on prostate cancer, *International Journal of Epidemiology*, 28: 409–17.

Zola, I.K. (1966) Culture and symptoms – an analysis of patients' presenting complaints, *American Sociological Review*, 31: 615–30.

Index

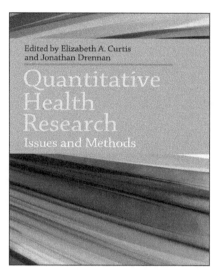

QUANTITATIVE HEALTH RESEARCH
Issues and Methods

Elizabeth A. Curtis and Jonathan Drennan

9780335245734 (Paperback)
August 2013

eBook also available

This book is a detailed and comprehensive guide to undertaking quantitative health research at postgraduate and professional level. It takes you through the entire research process, from designing the project to presenting the results and will help you execute high quality quantitative research that improves and informs clinical practice.

Key features:

- Ethical considerations of research
- Designing and planning quantitative research projects
- Data measurement and collection

www.openup.co.uk

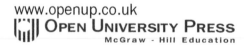

OPEN UNIVERSITY PRESS
McGraw - Hill Education

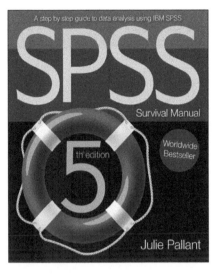

SPSS SURVIVAL MANUAL
Fifth Edition

Julie Pallant

9780335262588 (Paperback)
August 2013

eBook also available

In her bestselling guide, now covering up to version 21 of the SPSS software,
Julie Pallant guides you through the entire research process, helping you choose the
right data analysis technique for your project. From the formulation of research
questions, to the design of the study and analysis of data, to reporting the results,
Julie discusses basic and advanced statistical techniques. She outlines each
technique clearly, with step by step procedures for performing the analysis, a
detailed guide to interpreting data output and an example of how to present the
results in a report.

Key features:

- Fully revised and updated to accommodate changes to IBM SPSS version
  21 procedures, screens and output
- Additional recommended readings and websites have been added
- Supported by a website with sample data and guidelines on report writing

www.openup.co.uk
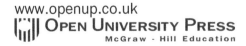 OPEN UNIVERSITY PRESS
McGraw - Hill Education

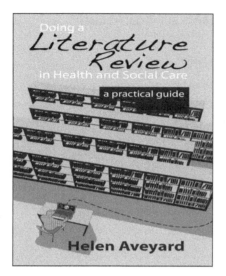

Doing a Literature Review in Health and Social Care
A Practical Guide
Third Edition

Helen Aveyard

9780335263073 (Paperback)
January 2014

eBook also available

This bestselling book is a step-by-step guide to doing a literature review in health and social care. It is vital reading for all those undertaking their undergraduate or postgraduate dissertation or any research module which involves a literature review. The book provides a practical guide to doing a literature review from start to finish.

Key features:

- Even more examples of real life research scenarios
- More emphasis on how to ask the right question
- New and updated advice on following a clear search strategy

www.openup.co.uk
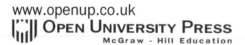 OPEN UNIVERSITY PRESS
McGraw - Hill Education